Classification and Clustering in Biomedical Signal Processing

Nilanjan Dey
Techno India College of Technology, India

Amira Ashour
Tanta University, Egypt

A volume in the Advances in Medical Technologies and Clinical Practice (AMTCP) Book Series

Medical Information Science Reference
An Imprint of IGI Global

Published in the United States of America by
Medical Information Science Reference (an imprint of IGI Global)
701 E. Chocolate Avenue
Hershey PA, USA 17033
Tel: 717-533-8845
Fax: 717-533-8661
E-mail: cust@igi-global.com
Web site: http://www.igi-global.com

Library of Congress Cataloging-in-Publication Data

Library of Congress Cataloging-in-Publication Data

Names: Dey, Nilanjan, 1984- editor. | Ashour, Amira, 1975- editor.
Title: Classification and clustering in biomedical signal processing / Nilanjan Dey and Amira Ashour, editors.
Description: Hershey, PA : Medical Information Science Reference, 2016. | Includes bibliographical references and index.
Identifiers: LCCN 2016000045| ISBN 9781522501404 (hardcover) | ISBN 9781522501411 (ebook)
Subjects: LCSH: Diagnostic imaging. | Signal processing. | Biomedical engineering.
Classification: LCC RC78.7.D53 C536 2016 | DDC 616.07/54--dc23 LC record available at http://lccn.loc.gov/2016000045

This book is published in the IGI Global book series Advances in Medical Technologies and Clinical Practice (AMTCP) (ISSN: 2327-9354; eISSN: 2327-9370)

British Cataloguing in Publication Data
A Cataloguing in Publication record for this book is available from the British Library.

All work contributed to this book is new, previously-unpublished material. The views expressed in this book are those of the authors, but not necessarily of the publisher.

For electronic access to this publication, please contact: eresources@igi-global.com.

Advances in Medical Technologies and Clinical Practice (AMTCP) Book Series

Srikanta Patnaik
SOA University, India
Priti Das
S.C.B. Medical College, India

ISSN: 2327-9354
EISSN: 2327-9370

Mission

Medical technological innovation continues to provide avenues of research for faster and safer diagnosis and treatments for patients. Practitioners must stay up to date with these latest advancements to provide the best care for nursing and clinical practices.

The **Advances in Medical Technologies and Clinical Practice (AMTCP) Book Series** brings together the most recent research on the latest technology used in areas of nursing informatics, clinical technology, biomedicine, diagnostic technologies, and more. Researchers, students, and practitioners in this field will benefit from this fundamental coverage on the use of technology in clinical practices.

Coverage

- Neural Engineering
- Telemedicine
- Medical Imaging
- Medical Informatics
- Clinical Data Mining
- E-Health
- Patient-Centered Care
- Biomedical Applications
- Diagnostic Technologies
- Biomechanics

IGI Global is currently accepting manuscripts for publication within this series. To submit a proposal for a volume in this series, please contact our Acquisition Editors at Acquisitions@igi-global.com or visit: http://www.igi-global.com/publish/.

The Advances in Medical Technologies and Clinical Practice (AMTCP) Book Series (ISSN 2327-9354) is published by IGI Global, 701 E. Chocolate Avenue, Hershey, PA 17033-1240, USA, www.igi-global.com. This series is composed of titles available for purchase individually; each title is edited to be contextually exclusive from any other title within the series. For pricing and ordering information please visit http://www.igi-global.com/book-series/advances-medical-technologies-clinical-practice/73682. Postmaster: Send all address changes to above address.

Titles in this Series

For a list of additional titles in this series, please visit: www.igi-global.com

Virtual Reality Enhanced Robotic Systems for Disability Rehabilitation
Fei Hu (University of Alabama, USA) Jiang Lu (University of Houston -Clear Lake, USA) and Ting Zhang (University of Alabama, USA)
Medical Information Science Reference • copyright 2016 • 383pp • H/C (ISBN: 9781466697409) • US $210.00 (our price)

Software Innovations in Clinical Drug Development and Safety
Partha Chakraborty (Cognizant Technology Solutions, India) and Amit Nagal (GVK Bioscience, India)
Medical Information Science Reference • copyright 2016 • 305pp • H/C (ISBN: 9781466687264) • US $225.00 (our price)

Handbook of Research on Holistic Perspectives in Gamification for Clinical Practice
Daniel Novák (Czech Technical University in Prague, Czech Republic) Bengisu Tulu (Worcester Polytechnic Institute, USA) and Håvar Brendryen (Norwegian Center for Addiction Research, University of Oslo, Norway)
Medical Information Science Reference • copyright 2016 • 636pp • H/C (ISBN: 9781466695221) • US $340.00 (our price)

Optimizing Assistive Technologies for Aging Populations
Yosry S. Morsi (Swinburne University of Technology, Australia) Anupam Shukla (ABV - Indian Institute of Information Technology and Management Gwalior, India) and Chandra Prakash Rathore (Oracle India Private Limited, India)
Medical Information Science Reference • copyright 2016 • 494pp • H/C (ISBN: 9781466695306) • US $220.00 (our price)

Modern Concepts and Practices in Cardiothoracic Critical Care
Adam S. Evans (Icahn School of Medicine at Mount Sinai, USA) Gregory E. Kerr (Weill Cornell Medical College, USA) Insung Chung (Icahn School of Medicine at Mount Sinai, USA) and Robin Varghese (Icahn School of Medicine at Mount Sinai, USA)
Medical Information Science Reference • copyright 2015 • 1110pp • H/C (ISBN: 9781466686038) • US $415.00 (our price)

Recent Advances in Assistive Technologies to Support Children with Developmental Disorders
Nava R. Silton (Marymount Manhattan College, USA)
Medical Information Science Reference • copyright 2015 • 424pp • H/C (ISBN: 9781466683952) • US $210.00 (our price)

Table of Contents

Section 5
Assortment of Medical Imaging Applications-Based Classification

Section 6
Wireless Systems for Healthcare

Detailed Table of Contents

Microscopic image analysis plays a foremost role for understanding biological processes, diagnosis of diseases and cells/ tissues identification. Microscopic image classification is one of the challenging tasks that have a leading role in the medical domain. In this chapter, an overview on different classification techniques elaborated with microscopic images is presented to guide the reader through the advanced knowledge of major quantitative image classification approaches. Applied examples are conducted to classify different Albino rats' samples captured using light microscope for three different organs, namely hippocampus, renal and pancreas. The Bag-of-Features (BoF) technique was employed for features extraction and selection. The BoF selected features were used as input to the multiclass linear support vector machine classifier. The proposed classifier achieved 94.33% average classification accuracy for the three classes. Additionally, for binary classification the achieved average accuracy was 100% for hippocampus and pancreas sets classification.

Medical image analysis is an area which has witnessed an increased use of machine learning in recent times. In this chapter, the authors attempt to provide an overview of applications of machine learning techniques to medical imaging problems, focusing on some of the recent work. The target audience comprises of practitioners, engineers, students and researchers working on medical image analysis, no prior knowledge of machine learning is assumed. Although the stress is mostly on medical imaging problems, applications of machine learning to other proximal areas will also be elucidated briefly. Health informatics is a relatively new area which deals with mining large amounts of data to gain useful insights. Some of the common challenges in health informatics will be briefly touched upon and some of the efforts in related directions will be outlined.

Most of medical images not only have noise but also have blur. This problem reduces the quality of images and influences diagnostic process of medical specialists because a small detail in a medical image is very useful for treatment process. This chapter explores the new generation wavelets, which provides the basic framework for the development of adaptive techniques to improve the quality of medical images. The process of the method for improving medical images includes: decompose of medical images in nonsubsampled contourlet domain and calculate the coefficients of Bayesian thresholding combined with Lucy Richard to reconstruct the medical images. For demonstrating the superiority of the method, the results of the proposed method are compared with the results of the other methods in new generation wavelet domain.

Section 2
Filtering and Thresholding for Medical Image Quality Improvement

Today, medical image processing and analysis are highly active research fields boosted by rapid technical developments in medical imaging field. This chapter describes common procedures such as thresholding methods and clustering algorithms (both non-hierarchical and hierarchical approaches) used for digital image processing, with specific reference to brain magnetic resonance images. These techniques represent starting points for other sophisticated methods such as segmentation and classification. The results, which are an outcome of these methods, are used for classification of neurodegenerative diseases such as Alzheimer, Pick's, Huntington's or cerebral calcinosis. A number of applications together with the code listing are provided with the aim to make the subject accessible and practical. The MATLAB software will help the readers to identify and choose the best solution for a particular problem.

The level set method (LSM) has been widely used in image segmentation due to its intrinsic nature which allows handling complex shapes and topological changes easily. We propose a new level set algorithm, which is based on probabilistic c mean objective function which incorporates intensity inhomogeneity in image and robust to noise. The computational complexity of the proposed LSM is greatly reduced by using highly parallelizable lattice Boltzmann method (LBM). So the proposed algorithm is effective and highly parallelizable. The proposed LSM is implemented using Experimental results demonstrate the performance of the proposed method.

Advancing techniques in image processing has led to many inventions and provides valuable support especially in medical fields to identify and analyze the diseases. MRI images are chosen for detection of brain tumor as they are used in soft tissue determinations. Brain tumor is one of the severe diseases in the field of medicine. Early identification of disease increases the chances for successful treatment. Classification and Segmentation plays a vital role in identifying the disease. First, image Pre-processing is used to enhance the image quality. Subsequently, Decomposition is performed using Dual-Tree Complex Wavelet Transform to analysis texture of an image and features are extracted using Gray-Level Co-Occurrence Matrix. Then, Neuro-Fuzzy and Neural Network can be used to categorize the types of Brain Tumor such as normal, benign and malignant. Finally, tumor region is detected using Kernel weighted clustering method by segmenting the brain tissues and also to find the size of the tumor.

There is certain to be a significant increase in the use of registration, retrieval and registration based retrieval of medical images in healthcare. But there is a related major concern that these initiatives are narrowly policy or technology led rather than evidence based or case based reasoning. Or else, either they will be based on old paradigm structures without considering the new paradigms that they create. It is planned to look at the image registration and retrieval from a unified perspective based on their performance for clinical diagnosis and treatment. It is concluded with an experiment carried out on

In this study, the effect of slow and fast music on the heart rate variability and conduction pathway of the heart was studied. The results indicated an increase in the parasympathetic dominance as the volunteers were made to listen to music. The magnitude of the parasympathetic activity was higher when the volunteers were made to listen to fast music. This indicates that slow and fast music affected the sympatho-vagal balance in different proportions. The analysis of the ECG signal and wavelet transformed ECG signal suggested an alteration in the conduction pathway of the heart.

Non-invasive diagnostic imaging methods for diagnosis of pathological conditions is increasingly gaining popularity resulting from speedy and effective recovery during follow up in several clinical trials. The accuracy of the diagnosis depends on the experience and knowledge of physicians conducting the trial. In such scenario, the need for quantitative measures for details such as shape and size of tissue can assist physicians for better intuitive understanding of tissue and its pathologies. Computer aided diagnosis (CAD) tool incorporating methods for segmentation, texture analysis and area computation can increase the accuracy of diagnosis by providing quantitative analysis of the image. This chapter briefly describes issues and challenges for building the CAD tool followed by brief description about the methods involved. The methods are validation are also discussed briefly. To summarize the work, brief discussion about a new software or CAD tool for diagnosis of pathologies supraspinatus tendon with the help of ultrasound images is provided. The new software has an intuitive user interface which is easy, quick and suitable for medical work.

Surface EMG (sEMG) signals from the palmaris longus, flexor carpi radialis and flexor carpi ulnaris muscles were recorded using an in-house developed EMG signal acquisition system. The bandwidth of the acquisition system was 1500 Hz. The extracted sEMG signal was processed using Discrete Wavelet Transform (DWT). The features of the extracted and the wavelet processed signals were determined and were used for probable classification using Artificial Neural Network (ANN). A classification efficiency of more than 90% was achieved using ANN classifiers. The results suggested that the sEMG may be successfully used for designing efficient control system.

The current study discusses about the development of an EMG based wireless control system for the patients suffering from high-level motor disability. Surface EMG (sEMG) signals were processed in the time domain and using discrete wavelet transforms (DWT). The statistical features of the signals (sEMG, envelope of the squared sEMG and wavelet processed sEMG) were determined and analyzed. The analysis of the features suggested that the features of the envelope of the squared sEMG signals were sufficient to be used for high-efficiency classification and control signal generation. A hall-effect sensor based switching mechanism was introduced for controlling the duration of the activation of the device. The control signals were wirelessly transmitted to the assistive device (robotic vehicle). The training and the subsequent use of the developed control system were easy.

Preface

Advanced techniques in image processing have led to many inventions and provide valuable support especially in medical fields to identify and analyze the diseases. Biomedical imaging is an essential part of early diagnosis, detection and treatment for assorted diseases, as it is considered as the first step for proper management of medical pathological conditions. Therefore, the role of medical signal/ image processing augments the ability to improve the visibility of significant features in a medical image which facilitate the diagnosis process and remove/ reduce unwanted information. Thus, the need for powerful instruments for detecting, sorting, transmitting, analyzing, and displaying images becomes a must. Miscellaneous modalities such has Echo Cardiograph, Magnetic Resonance Imaging (MRI), Computed Tomography (CT) and X-ray are encompassed various paradigms dedicated to diagnosing the diseases. These instruments greatly support biologists, medical scientists, biochemists, and physicians as they produce the required signals and images ambulated to extract the required features. Non-invasive diagnostic imaging schemes for patients' pathological condition diagnosis is increasingly developed due to the promising results and follows up in several clinical trials for treatment. The accuracy of the diagnosis depends on the experience and knowledge of physicians. In such scenario, the need for quantitative measures for details such as shape and size of tissue can assist physicians for better intuitive understanding of tissue and its pathologies. Computer aided diagnosis (CAD) tool incorporating methods for segmentation, texture analysis and area computation can increase the accuracy of the diagnosis by providing quantitative analysis of the image.

The basic processes such as filtering, enhancement, clustering, classification, and combining images different modalities, can assist scanning, diagnosis, research, and treatment. Thus, pattern recognition techniques play a crucial role. Automated image processing facilities accurate detection with less computational time. Often this involves identifying structures such as a tumor or lesions.

Clustering and classification are the foremost subdivisions of pattern recognition techniques. Using these techniques, samples can be classified according to a precise property by measurements indirectly related to the property of interest. Numerous computational and cognitive applications, especially medical imaging requires objects to be grouped into disjoint sets and classification for further processing. Clustering is a statistical technique by which objects of similar nature are grouped together. Similarity means that the objects have similar shape, dimensions, magnitude, direction (vectors) and color. Clustering achieved its importance as it is the preprocessing step in numerous procedures. Thus, there is an increasing necessity to simplify the process and its mathematical interpretations. Afterward, the classification rule can be used to predict the property in samples that are not part of the original training set. Moreover, there is a significant increase in the use of registration, retrieval and registration based retrieval of medical images in healthcare.

Consequently, there is an urgent need for edited wide collection of the major techniques of clustering and classification in the biomedical field. It compacts with methods and approaches that involve clustering, classification and pattern recognition. Additionally, these methods are use to support computer-aided diagnosis systems. Also, it will specify the principals of pattern recognition and medical image applications.

OBJECTIVE OF THE BOOK

This book elaborates the foremost techniques of classification and clustering. It deals, principally, with methods and approaches that involve medical signals/image and signal analysis, image retrieval, biomedical images feature extraction, etc. and their algorithms. As well as, it includes miscellaneous techniques of various modalities in medical imaging techniques and the computer-aided diagnosis (CAD) systems. This book endeavors to endow with significant frameworks and the most recent empirical research findings in the area. It is written for professionals who desire to improve their understanding and developing automated systems for medical imaging classification and clustering. Progressions of this field will assist to intensify interdisciplinary discovery in medical image processing, CAD systems, medical device improvements, aid doctors and physicians in diagnosis, early detection of diseases.

ORGANIZATION OF THE BOOK

The book consists of and introductory chapter followed by sixteen chapters that are organized in six sections as shown below. The first two chapters focus on the concept and applications for the medical image processing with more focus on the classification and clustering. The second section, consists of Chapters 3 and 4, relates to the filtering and thresholding for medical image quality improvement. The third section of the book encloses two chapters that introduced the classification and clustering of Magnetic Resonance Imaging. The fourth section contains two chapters concerning medical image database retrieval. From Chapter 9 till Chapter 13, the fifth section introduces several medical imaging applications based classification. The last three chapters are included in section 6, which focuses on wireless systems for healthcare.

Introduction Chapter: Includes the main concept of image analysis and processing in the medical domain is introduced, with referring to the different non-invasive automated medical image modalities. The authors elaborated the classification and clustering various applications in the biomedical area. The intention is to state the biomedical image classification and clustering in its context.

Section 1: Introduction to Classification and Clustering

This section elaborates the fundamental concepts of the image processing in the biomedical domain with various applications. The intention is to state the biomedical image classification and clustering in its context. Since, the classification process has several techniques that support various. Thus, the aim is to emphasize the role of the classifier selection on the classification accuracy and performance.

Table 1. Organization of the book

<table>
<tr><th colspan="30">Section 1: Introduction to Classification and Clustering</th></tr>
<tr><td colspan="15">Chapter 1
Bag-of-Features in Microscopic Images Classification</td><td colspan="15">Chapter 2
An overview of Machine Learning in Medical Image Analysis: Trends in health informatics</td></tr>
<tr><th colspan="30">Section 2: Filtering and Thresholding for Medical Image Quality Improvement</th></tr>
<tr><td colspan="15">Chapter 3
The Combination of Adaptive Filters to Improve the Quality of Medical Images in New Wavelet Domain</td><td colspan="15">Chapter 4
Intensity – based classification and related methods in brain MR images</td></tr>
<tr><th colspan="30">Section 3: Classification and Clustering of Magnetic Resonance Imaging</th></tr>
<tr><td colspan="15">Chapter 5
GPU based Level Set Method for MRI Brain Tumor Segmentation Using Modified Probabilistic Clustering</td><td colspan="15">Chapter 6
Classification of Magnetic Resonance image and segmentation of brain tissues for tumor detection</td></tr>
<tr><th colspan="30">Section 4: Medical Image Retrieval</th></tr>
<tr><td colspan="15">Chapter 7
Analysais and Comparaison of Developed 2D Medical Image Database Design Using Registration Scheme, Retrieval Scheme and Bag-of-Visual-Words</td><td colspan="15">Chapter 8
Multimodal indexing and information retrieval system based on mammographic image analysis: Gabor model in digital Learning</td></tr>
<tr><th colspan="30">Section 5: Assortment of Medical Imaging Applications Based Classification</th></tr>
<tr><td colspan="6">Chapter 9
Effect of Slow and Fast Music on the Autonomic Nervous System and Cardiac Health: A Preliminary Investigation</td><td colspan="6">Chapter 10
Development of Ultrasound Imaging CAD Tool for Assessment of Pathologies in Supraspinatus Tendon</td><td colspan="6">Chapter 11
New Imaging and Computational Technology as a guide for CatheterAblation of Incessant Tachyarrhythmias</td><td colspan="6">Chapter 12
An Optimized Graph Based Metagenomic Gene Classification Approach: Metagenomic Gene Analysis</td><td colspan="6">Chapter 13
Classification of Surface Electromyogram Signals Acquired from the Forearm of a Healthy Volunteer</td></tr>
<tr><th colspan="30">Section 6: Wireless Systems for Healthcare</th></tr>
<tr><td colspan="10">Chapter 14
Development of a Surface EMG Based Control System for Controlling Assistive Devices: A Study on Robotic Vehicle</td><td colspan="10">Chapter 15
Development of Bluetooth, Xbee and Wi-Fi Based Wireless Control Systems for Controlling Electric-Powered Robotic Vehicle Wheelchair Prototype</td><td colspan="10">Chapter 16
Wireless Body Area Networks Combined with Mobile Cloud Computing in Healthcare: A Survey</td></tr>
</table>

Chapter 1: This chapter included an overview on several classification techniques employed in microscopic image classification to guide the reader to advanced aspects concerning image classification approaches. Additionally, an applied examplewasintroduced to classify different Albino rats' samples captured using light microscope taken from three different organs, namely hippocampus, renal and pancreas. The Bag-of-Features (BoF) technique was used for features extraction and selection, which then classified using the multiclass linear support vector machine classifier. The proposed classifier realized 94.33% average classification accuracy for the three classes. For binary classification of the hippocampus and pancreas sets, the attained average accuracy was 100%.

Chapter 2: Health informatics is a relatively new area which deals to mining large amounts of data to gain useful insights. The authors provided an overview of machine learning applications. Medical imaging problems using machine learning are the main concern of this chapter. Some of the common challenges in health informatics were briefly discussed.

Section 2: Filtering and Thresholding for Medical Image Quality Improvement

Improving the quality of the medical images is an essential issue for accurate further image analysis and processing such as classification and clustering. The incorporated noise during medical images acquisition using various modalities degrades the human interpretation and the automated analysis of the images. This section presented filtering and thresholding approaches that considered starting points for other sophisticated methods such as segmentation, classification and clustering.

Chapter 3: The chapter discussed the effect of noise and blur which reduces the image quality and influences the medical diagnosis process. The authors explored new wavelets generation to provide the basic framework for the adaptive techniques development to improve the medical imagesquality. Medical images decomposition in non-sub-sampled contourlet domain and the calculation of Bayesian thresholding coefficients combined with Lucy Richard to reconstruct the medical images were proposed. The dataset was collected from several hospitals to test different cases: motion blur combined with Gaussian noise and Gaussian blur combined with Gaussian noise. The experimental results compared the proposed method to other approaches in the wavelet domain and new generation wavelet transform such as ridgelet, curvelet and contourlet domain. The results of the proposed method were superior to those of the other methods. The authors recommended in the medical image domain to carefully select the threshold value to preserve the image information.

Chapter 4: This chapter depicted widespread procedures such as thresholding schemes and clustering algorithms for digital image processing. These schemes represent the initial step for other sophisticated methods such as segmentation and classification. A specific reference was directed to brain magnetic resonance images. The authors proposed a method to classify neurodegenerative diseases such as Alzheimer, Pick's, Huntington's or cerebral calcinosis. The MATLAB code used to solve such problem was listed to assist the reader to identify and choose the best solution for a particular problem.

Section 3: Classification and Clustering of Magnetic Resonance Imaging

Accurate and efficient diagnosis in diminutive time period is a significant issue of brain magnetic resonance imaging (MRI) classification and cluttering. This section outlines the MRI Brain Tumor Segmentation based on various approaches such as Modified Probabilistic Clustering and Kernel weighted clustering.

Chapter 5: The authors proposed a new level set algorithm (LMS) based on probabilistic C- mean objective function which included intensity in-homogeneity in the image and robust to noise. The proposed LSM computational complexity is greatly reduced by using highly parallelizable lattice Boltzmann method (LBM). The LSM is then implemented using a graphics processing units (NVIDIA) to fully take the advantage of the LBM local nature. After carrying out exhaustive results, comparison to Li method in terms of the consumed time proved the superiority of the proposed method.

Chapter 6: Brain tumor is one of the severe diseases that require early diagnosis for successful treatment. Classification and segmentation play a vital role in identifying the disease. In the present chapter, image Pre-processing is elaborated for image quality enhancement the image quality, followed by decomposition using Dual-Tree Complex Wavelet Transform to analysis the image texture. Features are extracted using Gray-level co-occurrence matrix, which used in the classification process. Neuro-Fuzzy and Neural Network are employed to categorize the types of the brain tumor into normal, benign and malignant. Finally, tumor regions are detected using Kernel weighted clustering method by segmenting the brain tissues with determining the tumor size.

Section 4: Medical Image Retrieval

With the extensive dissemination of medical images archiving and communication systems in hospitals, the amount of medical imaging data is hastily increased. Effective image retrieval methods are required to manage these complex and huge image databases. This section is concerned with medical image database retrieval.

Chapter 7: This chapter is extensively discussed the registration and retrieval for monomodal images. Retrieval techniques, Bag-of-Visual-Words and registration techniques are considered in an interoperable manner to design a successful computer assisted diagnostic system. The authors aim to disseminate the knowledge of creating the patient database and a basis healthcare setup for the clinical diagnosis. Thus, the goal of this chapter is to provide an overview of various strategies to design a system based on a proposed model. The experiment results are carried out on five types of anatomical (radiology) images. Bag-of-visual-words approach is employed in the retrieval technique for modality images than content based retrieval techniques. The results proved that Affine with B-Spine and Bag-of-visual-words are more appropriate for modality images in registration based retrieval.

Chapter 8: The main objective of this chapter is to design an intelligent application to assist medical professionals in the decision-making on tumor diagnosis based on mammography scanner. A suggested new indexing approach on medical image scanner databases, which joined the texture characteristics analysis process with the descriptive information, is proposed. A characteristics vector is used in the proposed model to represent the morphological processing result on the image texture. The used application context is based on mammographic image analysis (MIAS) in databases. The texture analysis of the image is based on the Gabor wavelets filter. The proposed system included both offline and online processes for each image in MIAS databases. The similarities are built between the image-query and images in MIAS databases using the same Gabors' algorithms implementation. A database of 320 mammographies is conducted in the evaluation step. The results provided a set of criteria in image representations based on the Gabor's Wavelets, semantic attributes and significant ratios in the system recall and precision.

Section 5: Assortment of Medical Imaging Applications Based Classification

Medical images are considered the main component in the patient's health record. They are associated with manipulation, processing and handling by computers. Medical imaging is involved in both diagnosis and therapy. One of the major processes is the automated classification, which plays an implicative role in several applications. This section focuses on a variety of applications based medical image classification using different modalities. Besides, an example for Ultrasound Imaging computer-aided detection development is introduced.

Chapter 9: This chapter studies the effect of slow and fast music on the heart rate variability. The authors calculated the statistical features of the time domain and wavelet transform of the electrocardiogram (ECG) signals. Additionally, the artificial neural network (ANN) was employed for classification, which achieved classification efficiency of more than 80%.The experimental results indicated that slow and fast music affected the sympatho-vagal balance in different proportions. Additionally, the authors concluded that listening to music affects the conduction pathway of the heart.

Chapter 10: This chapter is briefly described the issues and challenges for building the Computer aided diagnosis (CAD) tool. A new CAD tool for supraspinatus tendon diagnosis using ultrasound images is provided. The results proved the intuitive user interface of the new software which is easy, quick and suitable for medical applications.

Chapter 11: This chapter reported the results of the 3D electroanatomical mapping (EAM) system of the atrial tachyarrhythmias (AT) for more than 500 consecutive patients. Patients underwent electroanatomical-mapping systems, which combined electrophysiological and spatial information to provide accurate reconstruction of the whole atria with real-time activation sequence guiding RFA for continuous transmural linear lesions. The mapping discriminated obviously and rapidly between micro-macro-reentrant (>80%) and focal mechanisms. The EAM technology allowed the determination of both mechanism and location of arrhythmia with successful elimination of complex arrhythmogenic substrates.

Chapter 12: This chapter supported the Gene analysis and assembly problem in the field of bioinformatics. Assembly is a computationally very exhaustive process that consumes long time to produce the sequence of a more complex organism. A variety of techniques are used to address the problem. Thus, the authors used graph reduction rule to build a de Bruijn graph. The results found accurate solution of large scale sequencing trims space complexity and generates optimal gene assembly.

Chapter 13: The current chapter introduced the electromyography signal (sEMG) classification recorded from the skin surface above the palmaris longus, flexor carpi radialis and flexor carpi ulnaris muscles by flexing fingers in different combinations and durations. The authors used an in-house developed EMG signal acquisition system. The extracted sEMG signal was processed using Discrete Wavelet Transform (DWT). The extracted features and the wavelet processed signals are used for probable classification using Artificial Neural Network (ANN). The results established 90% classification efficiency using the ANN classifier. The results suggested that the sEMG can be used efficiently for designing efficient control system.

Section 6: Wireless Systems for Healthcare

Recently, wireless control devices design and development become essential to support healthcare applications. This section provides a study on Wireless Control Systems for Controlling Electric-Powered Robotic Vehicle Wheelchair Prototype as well as wireless body area networks combined with mobile cloud computing as applications in the healthcare domain.

Chapter 14: The current study proposed a simple surface EMG based control system for wireless control of the wheelchair movement as well as other rehabilitative devices. The Surface EMG (sEMG) signals are processed in the time domain and using discrete wavelet transforms (DWT). The statistical features of the signals are determined and analyzed, where the features of the squared sEMG signals envelope are sufficient for high-efficiency classification and control signal generation. A hall-effect sensor based switching mechanism is introduced for controlling the duration of the activation of the device. The control signals are wirelessly transmitted to the robotic vehicle.

Chapter 15: In this chapter, multiple control systems are developed using wireless communication protocols, such as the Bluetooth, Xbee and Wi-Fi. The Xbee and Bluetooth protocols are used to design mechanical switch based control systems. Additionally, an android application based control systems is developed using Bluetooth and Wi-Fi protocols. A robotic vehicle is used as an electric-powered wheelchair prototype. For obstacle and pothole detection, the ultrasonic sensors and infrared sensors are integrated with the robotic vehicle, respectively. L-shaped corridor is used to test the control systems for identifying the suitable wireless communication protocol to powerfully guide the robotic vehicle through a scheduled navigational pathway. Both Xbee and Wi-Fi technology based control systems have the ability to guide the robotic vehicle through the corridor.

Chapter 16: In this chapter, a theoretical study on the combination of wireless body area network (WBAN) and mobile cloud computing (MCC) in healthcare was presented. Cloud computing is used to achieve much more user friendly device that manage the information. The combination of WBAN and the MCC promised better performance to the users immediately. The authors wired the sensor which executed the necessary medical tests and provided the information through devices, such as mobile phones and tablets.

This book is expected to assist researchers, academicians and engineering in healthcare informatics, medical imaging, biology and medical devices design. It addressed innovative conceptual framework for various applications. The book is expected to serve as a reference for the post-graduated students as it offers the requisite knowledge for understanding the classification and clustering along with their applications. This book is based on a research studies carried out by experienced academicians and is expected to shed new insights for researchers; academicians, students and improves understanding of biomedical image classification and clustering concept.

The editors,

Nilanjan Dey
Techno India College of Technology, India

Amira Ashour
Tanta University, Egypt

Acknowledgment

A clear purpose will unite you as you move forward, values will guide your behavior, and goals will focus your energy. – Kenneth H. Blanchard

The Editors,

We would like to say 'THANK YOU' to our parents for endless support, guidance and love through all our life stages. We are heartiest thankful to our beloved family members for standing beside us throughout our career, move our career forward through editing this book. Our great thanks to our students, who have put in their time and effort to support and contribute in some manner. We dedicate this book to all of them.

We would like to express our gratitude to the all people support, share, talked things over, read, wrote, offered comments, allowed us to quote their remarks and assisted in editing, proofreading and design; through the book journey.

We believe that the team of authors provides the perfect blend of knowledge and skills that went into authoring this book. We thank each of the authors for devoting their time, patience, perseverance and effort towards this book; we think that it will be a great asset to the all researchers in this field!

We are grateful to the IGI-publisher team, who showed us the ropes to start and continue. Without that knowledge we wouldn't have ventured into starting this book, which ultimately led to this! Their trusting for us, their guide and providing the necessary time and resource, gave us the freedom to manage this book and.

Last, but definitely not least, we'd like to thank our readers, who gave us their thrust and hope our work inspired and guide them.

Acknowledgment

A clear purpose will unite you as you move forward, values will guide your behavior, and goals will focus your energy. – Kenneth H. Blanchard

The Editors,

Nilanjan Dey
Techno India College of Technology, India

Amira Ashour
Tanta University, Egypt

Introduction

INTRODUCTION

Digital image processing becomes progressively more essential in the medical domain and health care (Semmlow and Griffel, 2014). For disease diagnosis or pathological study, medical imaging is involved to create images and obtain significant information about the biological structures or body functions using specialized modalities and techniques. Biomedical signal/ image analysis and processing are one of the most imperative visualization and interpretation processes in biology and medicine.

Recently, various powerful algorithms and instruments for acquiring, detecting, transmitting, storing, analyzing, processing and displaying images have been developed (Rangayyan, 2004). Consequently, scientists and physicians can attain quantitative measurements that support medical diagnoses and scientific hypotheses. In addition to the original medical imaging modalities such as Computed Tomography (CT), Magnetic Resonance Imaging (MRI), MR angiography (MRA), Ultrasound, Positron Emission Tomography (PET) and X-ray (Pan, 2010), nowadays other imaging modalities such as endoscopy or radiography are equipped with digital sensors. Moreover, microscopic images are commonly used in medicine and biology for cells/ tissues structure representation.

Medical images are extremely cooperative for accurate diseases diagnosis, pathological lesion detection, supports the human body anatomy and to deduce different problems in the medical domain. Typically, digital images are composed of individual pixels which have discrete color/ brightness values. These images are then efficiently processed and objectively evaluated after their acquisition and transmission if required. To transmit these images to many places at the same time, communication networks and protocols are to be used. Such systems and protocols are the Picture Archiving and Communication Systems (PACS) and the Digital Imaging and Communications in Medicine (DICOM) protocol; respectively (Erberich *et al.*, 2007).

To acquire and extract accurate information from the medical images, analysis and processing biomedical image data is to be executed. Therefore, complex processing procedures are to be performed concerning several phases, such as data acquisition, preprocessing, segmentation, feature extraction, classification, clustering and registration. New technologies for medical data acquisition and storage provided large datasets for statistical analysis, which requires efficient pattern recognition methods. Image classification systems have received a recent boost and become one of the most interesting research areas. Medical image classification has an important role for diagnosis, treatment and medical teaching (Sonka *et al.*, 2014). Additionally, medical images' clustering involves finding a structure in a cluster with data having no label, which is important for example to recognize damaged areas in tissues. Various procedures have been developed for clustering in different fields such as medicine, engineering, data mining (Liu *et al.*, 2011). Nevertheless, there is no standard technique of clustering for ideal results for all of the medical imaging applications.

The main concern of the current chapter is to introduce the different modalities used for medical images acquisition and the concept of the medical image analysis/ processing. Besides presenting the concept of medical image processing and analysis, classification and clustering with various applications in the medical domain are also explained.

BACKGROUND

Medical Image Modalities

Medical imaging is concerning with numerous technologies to view the human body for diagnoses and monitor medical conditions. Consequently, wide variety of modalities in medical imaging techniques can be employed. Each modality provided different information about the organ/ area of the body under study or treatment, which related to possible disease/ injury. The imaging modality selection for a targeted

Table 1. Comparison between common medical imaging modalities

Instrument/Concept	Limitations that Affect Its Image Quality
Magnetic Resonance Imaging (MRI) • Uses radio waves and magnetic field to create detailed images of organs and tissues. • MRI highly efficient in diagnosing a number of conditions by showing the difference between normal and diseased soft tissues of the body. • MRI uses strong magnetic fields to cause water molecules to resonate. It is very good at imaging soft tissues, such as the heart, lungs, liver and other organs.	• Implanted medical devices that contain metal may malfunction or cause problems during an MRI exam. • MRI cannot image classifications and bone and cannot always distinguish between cancerous and non-cancerous anomalies.
Computed Tomography (CT) • Combines multiple X-ray projections taken from different angles to produce detailed cross-sectional images of areas inside the body. • CT images allow physicians to get precise, 3-D views of certain parts of the body, such as soft tissues, the pelvis, blood vessels, the lungs, the brain, the heart, abdomen and bones. • CT is often the preferred method of diagnosing many cancers, such as liver, lung and pancreatic cancers.	• Enable to view very fine details in soft tissues such as muscles or ligaments (MRI might be more appropriate in such situations). • Patient motion during a CT scan can cause the images to be "blurry". • Metal artifacts in the body can cause 'streaks' in the image. Flat tumors may also be harder to image with a CT scan.
X-RAY • Uses ionizing radiation to produce images of a person's internal structure by sending X-ray beams through the body, which are absorbed in different amounts depending on the density of the material. • Radiation Therapy is a type of device which also utilizes X-rays, gamma rays, electron beams or protons.	• The two dimensional nature of the images can lead to false positives. • Technicians often take two images, one from the front and one from the side. • Not good for distinguishing anomalies in dense tissue. • The resolution of an x-ray is not very high.
Ultrasound (Medical Sonography or Ultrasonography) • Uses high frequency sound waves to create images inside the body. • The ultrasound machine sends sound waves into the body and is able to convert the returning sound echoes into a picture. • Ultrasound technology produces audible sounds of blood flow, allowing medical professionals to use both sound and visuals to assess a patient's health.	• Ultrasound can be blocked by bone, and so is not useful in imaging past the ribs of the chest. • Ultrasound imaging will not be useful for evaluating the digestive. • The clarity of an ultrasound attenuates as it passes through tissue (not useful for imaging deep within the body). • The resolution of an ultrasound is fairly limited. • The accuracy of an ultrasound depends to a large degree on the skill of the technician and radiologist.

Figure 1. Medical images classification structure

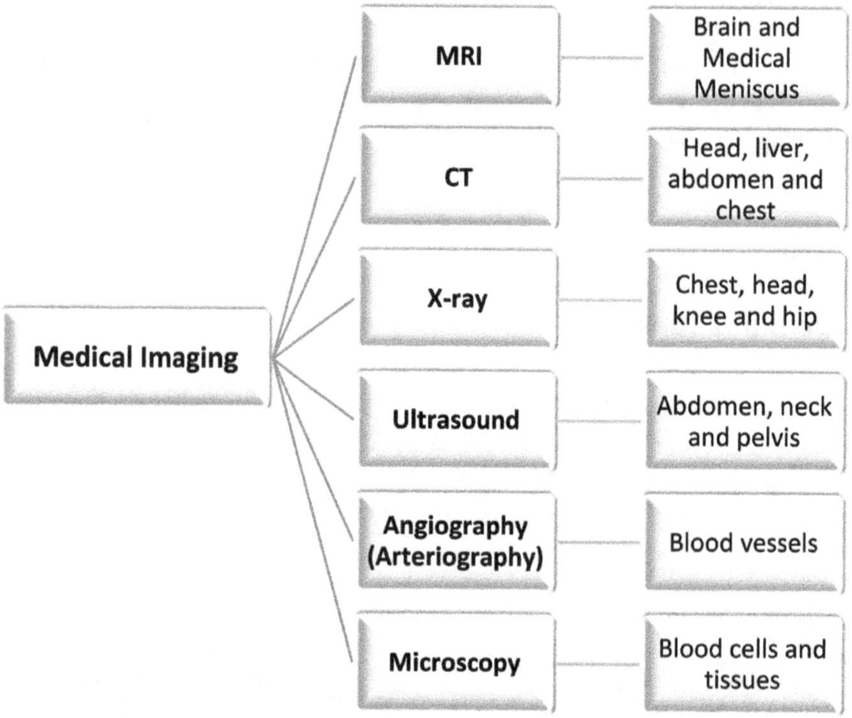

clinical study requires medical insights specific to organs under study (Giedd *et al.*, 1999; Gohagan *et al.*, 2005; Linton *et al.*, 2014; Turkington *et al.*, 2014; Nørgaard *et al.*, 2014; Dey *et al.*, 2015; Hore *el al.*, 2015). Figure 1 illustrates the different modalities that can be used for medical imaging with referring to the body part under test by each device.

A comparison between some of these modalities and their limitations that affects the image is demonstrated in Table 1.

For more reliable and accurate assessment, the images from different multiple modalities can be considered using medical images fusion (Singh and Khare, 2014; James and Dasarathy, 2014).

Medical Image Analysis and Processing

Biomedical image processing refers to the provision of digital image processing for biomedical sciences. Image analysis considered high-level image processing, while, low-level processing refers to techniques which can be realized without prior knowledge on the specific images content (Deserno, 2011). Image processing can be considered as the transformation of an image into another modified (enhanced) image. On the other hand, image analysis is the transformation of an image to produce information representing a description for the original image. Thus, the main purpose of the image processing is to produce images which are more reliable and simple for subsequent analysis.

Medical images are used to derive coherent visualizations and models. Image analysis sequence starts from the acquisition, proceeds to restoration and segmentation to conclude with analysis. The steps of biomedical image processing are addressed as follows: i) image formation: start from medical image

Figure 2. Image processing modules

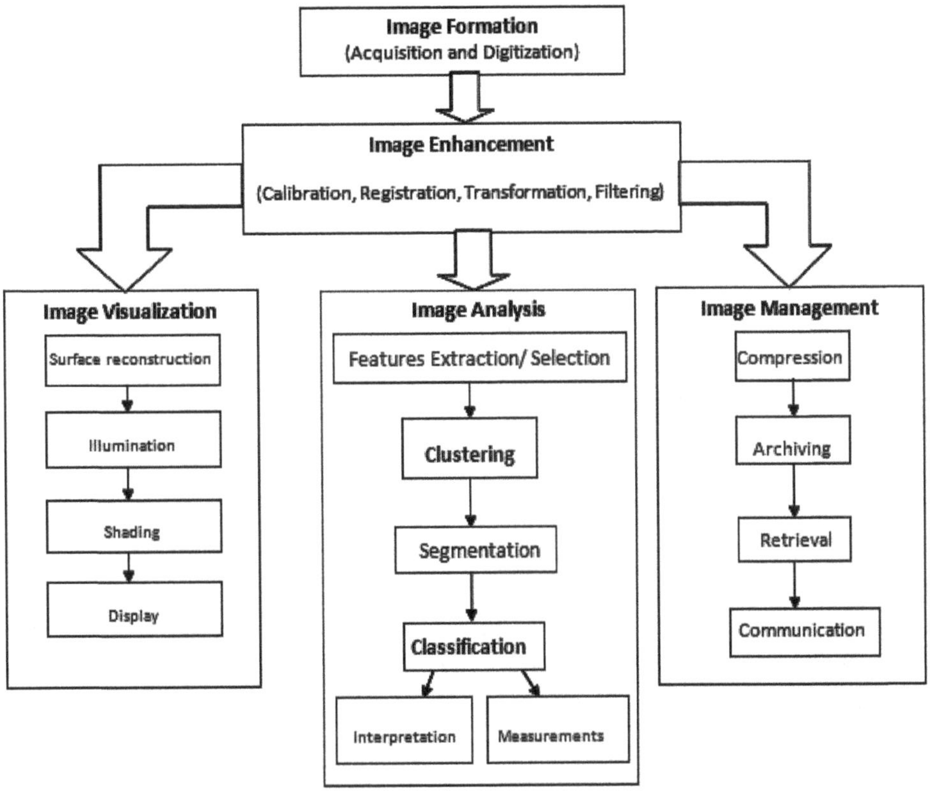

capturing to digital image matrix formation, ii) image visualization (image enhancement): manipulates the image matrix to obtain optimized output of the image, iii) image analysis: includes all the steps of processing, which are used for quantitative measurements as well as abstract interpretations of biomedical images and iv) image management: includes techniques that provide the efficient storage, communication, transmission, archiving, and access (retrieval) of image data as well as including telemedicine methods. These modules of the image processing are demonstrated in Figure 2.

From Figure 2, it is clear that image analysis requires a priori knowledge of the nature and content of the images. This knowledge about the image is further integrated into algorithms at a higher level of abstraction. Thus, image analysis process of is very precise. High-level image processing consists of schemes at the texture, region, object, and scene levels (Xu *et al.*, 2002).

It is obvious that image analysis techniques entail features extraction to aid in the object's identification and to emphasize the image information at particular level. Afterwards, description (feature selection) can be performed to extract the attributes that result in some quantitative information of interest. Features selection is also important for data size reduction. Subsequently, the extracted features are aggregated into a list which acts as the input to a clustering algorithm. Clustering algorithms then presents a depiction of the grouping structures which discovered within the objects. This description consists of a list containing labeled clusters to which it has been assigned. Thus, after features extraction, the features are organized into groups (clusters) of approximately shared features.

Segmentation methods are used to isolate the desired object from the scene. Thus, measurements can be performed on it subsequently. Segmentation partitions the image into its constituent connected regions or objects. The segmentation level to which the subdivision is carried depends on the problem being solved (Tsechpenakis *et al.*, 2007; Dey *et al.*, 2012; Samanta *et al.*, 2012; Roy *et al.*, 2014). In medical image processing, the segmentation is performed for example to discriminate between healthy anatomical structures and pathological tissues. Depending on the level of feature extraction required after segmentation, the segmentation procedure can be categorized into pixel, edge, and texture or region-oriented or hybrid (combination of single procedures).

According to the image analysis steps in Figure 2, the classification/detection task is to be executed after the segmentation step. Classification is to assign particularly specified classes of objects to all connected regions obtained from the segmentation process.

Image analysis mainly engages feature extraction and selection, clustering, segmentation, representation and description, classification or recognition (Lotufo *et al.*, 2011).

MAIN FOCUS OF THE CHAPTER

Based on the pervious detailed description of the image analysis steps, it is clear that both image clustering and classification play significant role in the image analysis/ processing module. Therefore, this chapter focuses on an extensive representation for the clustering/ classification of the medical images supported with related literatures.

Clustering

Clustering involves finding a structure in a cluster with data having no label. It is the process of assigning a cluster label for every object. Therefore, it is required to search on a specific label to find out which objects belong to it. However, based on the used clustering paradigm, there are other ways of describing the discovered structure. These paradigms become an open research domain to suggest different assumptions and approaches. Such clustering paradigms are:

1. Hierarchical clustering (HCA), which produces a tree-like description of the clustering structure. Cutting the tree at any level produces a partition of the objects (Thies *et al.*, 2003; TamijeSelvy *et al.*, 2011),
2. Graph-theoretic clustering, which views the objects as nodes in a weighted network, or graph (Cordella *et al.*, 2005; Peng *et al.*, 2013),
3. Mixture Models clustering, which assumes the objects as generated by a mixture of probability distributions (Penny and Friston, 2003; Greenspan *et al.*, 2006),
4. Partitional cluistering, wherer Clusters are disjoint partition of objects. An object belongs to only one cluster (Gath and Iskoz, 1995), and
5. Fuzzy clustering, where an object possesses varying degrees of membership with more than one cluster (Tabakov, 2006; Mahmoud *et al.*, 2013).

Extensive studies were conducted concerning medical images clustering applications. Dey's team has extensive work on segmentation based clustering. In 2012, they employed Fuzzy C-Means (FCM) for blood vessels segmentation in retinal images to provide early glaucoma detection/ diagnosis. The authors compared the results of an expert ophthalmologist hand-drawn ground-truths and segmented image using the proposed method. The experimental results established that the segmented blood vessels have with sensitivity, specificity, PPV, PLR and accuracy of 99.62%, 54.66%, 95.08%, 219.72 and 95.03%, respectively (Dey *et al.*, 2012). Additionally, Dey *et al.*, (2013) proposed appropriate selection of the Region of Non-Interest based on Fuzzy C-Means (FCM) clustering for segmentation and Harris corner detection, to improve retention of diagnostic value lost in watermarking to embed ownership information. Afterwards, the present watermark is embedded in the selected area of RONI based on alpha blending technique. The results prove that the generated watermarked image achieved acceptable level of imperceptibility, where the distortion was compared to the original image. The Peak signal-to-noise ratio (PSNR) of the original image versus the watermarked image was calculated to prove the efficacy of the proposed method. Bose *et al.*, (2013) proposed to images segmentation using multi-threaded programming and k-means clustering. Parts of images were considered as a thread and k-means clustering was used to segment them on every thread. The proposed method results were compared to segmentation results without multithreading. The obtained results were very much promising. Azween *et al.*, (2014) proposed an ensemble clustering algorithm with supervised classification of clinical data for untimely coronary artery disease diagnosis.

Zhou *et al.* (2014) introduced medium mathematics system to process fuzzy information for image segmentation. The authors established the medium similarity measure based on the measure of medium truth degree (MMTD) and used the pixel correlation and its neighbors to identify the medium membership function. An improved FCM medical image segmentation algorithm based on the MMTD which considered some spatial features was employed. The experimental results proved that the proposed algorithm was robust to noise than the standard FCM, with more certainty and less fuzziness. Thus, the authors suggested employing the proposed method to segment the medical images efficiently in various applications.

Classification

Image classification research aspires to find images representations to be automatically used for images categorization into a finite set of classes. Generally, algorithms for image classification requires preprocessing, which involve relevant features extraction and images segmentation into sub-components based on some prior knowledge about their context. Medical image classification plays an important role in diagnosis and treatment. An extensive explanation of the different classifiers with applied example is introduced in Chapter 2. Thus, in the current chapter the most common classifiers for the medical applications are mentioned, such as:

1. Neural network (NN) classifier, which neural networks are data driven self-adaptive methods in which they can adjust themselves to the data, without any explicit specification of functional or distributional form with the underlying model (Tech and Korrapati, 2010),
2. Support Vector Machines (SVM), which is a binary classifier (classify two classes) by finding the maximum separating hyper plane between the two classes (Vanitha and Venmathi, 2011) and

3. Neuro Fuzzy classifier, where Neuro fuzzy systems are fuzzy systems that uses artificial NNs theory in to determine their properties (fuzzy sets and fuzzy rules) by processing data samples (Bhardwaj and Siddhu, 2013).

Previous studies were very useful to conduct several classifiers in medical image classification applications as follows. Zacharaki *et al.* (2009) investigates pattern classification methods to distinguish between different types of brain tumors, namely primary gliomas from metastases, and also for grading of gliomas. A computer-assisted classification method combining conventional MRI and perfusion MRI was developed and used for differential diagnosis using Support Vector Machines (SVMs) with recursive feature elimination. The proposed method consisted of several steps: region of interest (ROI) definition, feature extraction, feature selection and classification. Tumor shape and intensity characteristics as well as rotation invariant texture features, were the extracted features. 102 brain tumors histologically images were involved in this study. The binary SVM classification accuracy, sensitivity, and specificity, assessed by leave-one-out cross-validation, were respectively 85%, 87%, and 79%. Multi-class classification was also performed via one-versus-all voting scheme.

Othman *et al.* (2011) used discrete wavelet transformation to obtain the feature related to MRI images. An advanced kernel based schemes such as SVM for the classification of volume of MRI data as normal and abnormal was deployed. In the same year, Vanitha and Venmathi (2011) developd an automatic tool to identify microbiological types without human supervision. The Bacteriophage typing and the fluorescent imaging methods were used to extract representative feature profiles. The bacterial types were identified by human experts by reading the feature profiles. These methods were time consuming and prone to errors. The bacterial image features were extracted, and then the SVM was used for classifying the Bacterial types. Results proved that the SVM have high approximation capability and much faster convergence.

Hosseini and Zekri (2012) conducted an extensive review for the adaptive neuro-fuzzy inference system (ANFIS) classifier for medical image classification during the past 16 years. The authors revealed that the ANFIS is a fuzzy inference system (FIS) implemented in the framework of an adaptive fuzzy neural network. It joins the FIS explicit knowledge representation with the artificial neural networks learning power. Thus, the ANFIS integrates best features of fuzzy systems and neural networks. A brief comparison with other classifiers, main advantages and drawbacks of this classifier are investigated.

FUTURE RESEARCH DIRECTIONS

Image processing have many purposes such as i) image enhancement to reduce the noise or sharpening images, ii) pattern recognition for automatic detection of a certain shape/ texture in the images and identify objects, iii) data reduction to easily handled and interpreted information, e.g., the reduction of an image to a set of objects, features, or a set of measurements, iv) image synthesis, which refers to reconstructing a three-dimensional scene from two-dimensional images, v) combination of images (fusion), refers to combining images of two different modalities (types) from the same scene involves registration, and vi) Data compression to reduce the images size and speed up image transmission across a network.

There are major challenges in biomedical image processing that can be addressed and to be considered as future points and recommendations to be covered by researches as follows.

- **Semantic Gap:** Refers to the inconsistency between the cognitive interpretation of a diagnostic image by the physician (high level) and the simple structure of discrete pixels, which is used in computer programs to represent an image (low level). Thus, it is difficult to formulate a priori knowledge, using medical images that can be integrated directly and easily into automatic algorithms of image processing. In the medical domain, there are three main aspects hindering bridging this gap, namely (Lotufo *et al.*, 2011): i) Heterogeneity of images: it can be largely eliminated using correction algorithms, but this runs the risk of destroying the subtle features of the real image (Lee, 1983), ii) Unknown delineation of objects: where the biological structures cannot be separated from the background due to the diagnostically or therapeutically relevant object is represented by the entire image. This leads to segmentation problem even if the objects were definable in the biomedical images. This problem is due to the shape or borderline itself is represented fuzzily or only partly. In addition to these medical images inherent properties, which complicate their high-level processing, special requirements related to the process has its limitations, where iii) Robustness and reliability of algorithms (medical process): it is required that images which cannot be processed correctly, must be automatically, rejected and withdrawn from further processing. Consequently, all images that have not been rejected must be evaluated correctly.
- Texture analysis plays a supportive rather than a comprehensive role in the future of medical image interpretation. The robustness of texture analysis makes it particularly attractive for monitoring disease progression or treatment response with time.
- Features selection is a recommended step for size and consuming time reduction.
- Fuzzy c-means (FCM) is one of the trendy clustering algorithms for medical image segmentation. However, FCM is highly vulnerable to noise due to not considering the spatial information in image segmentation, which needs to be resolved for efficient segmentation.
- Automatic medical image classification is a progressive field in image classification, and it is expected to be more developed in the future with further new algorithms.
- Automatic diagnosis is a promising can assist pathologists by providing second opinions and reducing their workload. These automated system need to cover all medical imaging aspects and to replace all manual or semi-automated existing systems (where, currently, segmentation is often carried out manually by experienced clinicians or radiologists).
- Image fusion is a promising process.
- More focus should direct to processing images (data) in four dimensional (4D) domains.
- On-line medical images atlases can be found for many medical domains including dermatology, ophthalmology, radiology, cytopathology and gastroenterology. The complete volume of medical image data is valuable for numerous challenges and opportunities.

CONCLUSION

Medical imaging domain gains its importance with the increasing need to automated and efficient diagnosis in a short period of time. It is a promising plays a significant role in medical diagnosis, treatment, executing, and evaluating surgical and radiotherapeutical procedures. The extracted information from the medical images captured by various modalities may include geometric models of anatomical structures, functional descriptions of anatomical structures, or diagnostic assessment. Most medical imaging modalities provided data in two spatial dimensions (2D) as well as in time. In addition, data in three spatial dimensions (3D) as well as in time (called 4D) are becoming common and promising trend. The large amount of data involved necessitates the identification or segmentation of the objects of interest before further analysis can be made. The result of this segmentation process is the grouping or labeling of pixels into meaningful regions or objects.

Additionally, medical image retrieval system is to provide a tool for radiologists to retrieve the images similar to query image in content. Classification is an essential part in retrieval system that utilizes image processing, pattern recognition and classification methods in order to distinguish between normal and abnormalities due to tumor. Support Vector Machines using the correlation kernel, Polinomial kernel, Gaussian kernel and Radial basis function (RBF) kernel all pay important role in each application and provide satisfactory results. SVM proved its efficiency over neural networks and RBF classifiers. Unlike neural networks, SVM model does not need hypothesizing number of neurons in the middle layer or defining the centre of Gaussian functions in RBF. SVM uses an optimum linear separating hyperplane to separate two set of data in a feature space. This optimum hyperplane is produced by maximizing minimum margin between the two sets. Conversely, Neural network techniques are more useful in automatically analyzing the images by training the networks. Data mining techniques are also playing equal role in keeping the image databases and making analysis on the set of images.

Nilanjan Dey
Techno India College of Technology, India

Amira Ashour
Tanta University, Egypt

REFERENCES

Azween, A., Kausar, N., & Dey, N. (2014). Ensemble clustering algorithm with supervised classification of clinical data for early diagnosis of coronary artery disease. *J. Med. Imaging Health Inf*, 226-239.

Bhardwaj, A., & Siddhu, K. K. (2013). An Approach to Medical Image Classification Using Neuro Fuzzy Logic and ANFIS Classifier. *International Journal of Computer Trends and Technology*, *4*(3).

Bose, S., Mukherjee, A., Chakraborty, S., Samanta, S., & Dey, N. (2013, December). Parallel image segmentation using multi-threading and k-means algorithm. In *Computational Intelligence and Computing Research (ICCIC), 2013 IEEE International Conference on* (pp. 1-5). IEEE.

Cordella, L. P., Percannella, G., Sansone, C., & Vento, M. (2005, June). A graph-theoretical clustering method for detecting clusters of micro-calcifications in mammographic images. In *Computer-Based Medical Systems, 2005. Proceedings. 18th IEEE Symposium on* (pp. 15-20). IEEE.

Deserno, T. M. (2011). Fundamentals of biomedical image processing. In *Biomedical Image Processing* (pp. 1–51). Springer Berlin Heidelberg.

Dey, N., Ashour, A. S., Ashour, A. S., & Singh, A. (2015). Digital Analysis of Microscopic Images in Medicine. *Journal of Advanced Microscopy Research*, *10*, 1–13.

Dey, N., Das, P., Biswas, D., Maji, P., Das, A., & Chaudhuri, S. S. (2013). Visible Watermarking within the Region of Non-Interest of Medical Images Based on Fuzzy C-Means and Harris Corner Detection. In *The Fourth International Workshop Communications Security & Information Assurance* (CSIA-2013) (pp. 161-168). Springer.

Dey, N., Roy, A. B., Pal, M., & Das, A. (2012). FCM Based Blood Vessel Segmentation Method For Retinal Images. *International Journal of Computer Science and Network*, *1*(3).

Erberich, S. G., Silverstein, J. C., Chervenak, A., Schuler, R., Nelson, M. D., & Kesselman, C. (2007). Globus MEDICUS-federation of DICOM medical imaging devices into healthcare Grids. *Studies in Health Technology and Informatics*, *126*, 269.

Gath, I., & Iskoz, A. S. (1995, March). Clustering of non-convex patterns for medical imaging. In *Electrical and Electronics Engineers in Israel, 1995., Eighteenth Convention of* (pp. 1-2). IEEE.

Giedd, J. N., Blumenthal, J., Jeffries, N. O., Castellanos, F. X., Liu, H., Zijdenbos, A., & Rapoport, J. L. (1999). Brain development during childhood and adolescence: A longitudinal MRI study. *Nature Neuroscience*, *2*(10), 861–863.

Gohagan, J. K., Marcus, P. M., Fagerstrom, R. M., Pinsky, P. F., Kramer, B. S., & Prorok, P. C.Lung Screening Study Research Group. (2005). Final results of the Lung Screening Study, a randomized feasibility study of spiral CT versus chest X-ray screening for lung cancer. *Lung Cancer (Amsterdam, Netherlands)*, *47*(1), 9–15.

Greenspan, H., Ruf, A., & Goldberger, J. (2006). Constrained Gaussian mixture model framework for automatic segmentation of MR brain images. *IEEE Transactions on Medical Imaging*, *25*(9), 1233–1245.

Hore, S., Chakroborty, S., Ashour, A. S., Dey, N., Ashour, A. S., Sifaki-Pistolla, D., & Chaudhuri, S. R. B. et al. (2015). Finding contours of Hippocampus Brain Cell using Microscopic Image Analysis. *Journal of Advanced Microscopy Research*, *10*(2).

Hosseini, M. S., & Zekri, M. (2012). Review of medical image classification using the adaptive neuro-fuzzy inference system. *Journal of Medical Signals and Sensors*, *2*(1), 49.

James, A. P., & Dasarathy, B. V. (2014). Medical image fusion: A survey of the state of the art. *Information Fusion*, *19*, 4–19.

Lee, J. S. (1983). Digital image smoothing and the sigma filter. *Computer Vision Graphics and Image Processing*.

Linton, K. M., Taylor, M. B., & Radford, J. A. (2014). Response evaluation in gastrointestinal stromal tumours treated with imatinib: Misdiagnosis of disease progression on CT due to cystic change in liver metastases. *The British Journal of Radiology*.

Liu, Y., Wu, X., & Shen, Y. (2011). Automatic clustering using genetic algorithms. *Applied Mathematics and Computation*, *218*(4), 1267–1279.

Lotufo, R. A., Rittner, L. R., Audigier, R. M., Saúde, A. V., & Machado, R. C. (2011). Morphological Image processing applied in biomedicine. In T. M. Deserno (Ed.), *Biomedical Image Processing* (pp. 107–128). Springer.

Mahmoud, H., Masulli, F., & Rovetta, S. (2013). Feature-based medical image registration using a fuzzy clustering segmentation approach. In *Computational Intelligence Methods for Bioinformatics and Biostatistics* (pp. 37–47). Springer Berlin Heidelberg.

Nørgaard, B. L., Leipsic, J., Gaur, S., Seneviratne, S., Ko, B. S., Ito, H., & Achenbach, S. et al. (2014). Diagnostic performance of noninvasive fractional flow reserve derived from coronary computed tomography angiography in suspected coronary artery disease: the NXT trial (Analysis of Coronary Blood Flow Using CT Angiography: Next Steps). *Journal of the American College of Cardiology*, *63*(12), 1145–1155.

Othman, M. F. B., Abdullah, N. B., & Kamal, N. F. B. (2011, April). MRI brain classification using support vector machine. In *Modeling, Simulation and Applied Optimization (ICMSAO), 2011 4th International Conference on* (pp. 1-4). IEEE.

Pan, T. (2010). Fundamentals of Medical Imaging. *Journal of Nuclear Medicine*, *51*(11), 1821–1821.

Peng, B., Zhang, L., & Zhang, D. (2013). A survey of graph theoretical approaches to image segmentation. *Pattern Recognition*, *46*(3), 1020–1038.

Penny, W., & Friston, K. (2003). Mixtures of general linear models for functional neuroimaging. *IEEE Transactions on Medical Imaging*, *22*(4), 504–514.

Rangayyan, R. M. (2004). *Biomedical image analysis*. CRC Press.

Roy, P., Goswami, S., Chakraborty, S., Azar, A. T., & Dey, N. (2014). Image Segmentation using Rough Set theory: A Review. *International Journal of Rough Sets and Data Analysis*, *1*(2), 62–74.

Samanta, S., Dey, N., Das, P., Acharjee, S., & Chaudhuri, S. S. (2012). Multilevel Threshold Based Gray Scale Image Segmentation using Cuckoo Search. *International Conference on Emerging Trends in Electrical, Communication and Information Technologies*.

Semmlow, J. L., & Griffel, B. (2014). *Biosignal and medical image processing*. CRC Press.

Singh, R., & Khare, A. (2014). Fusion of multimodal medical images using Daubechies complex wavelet transform–A multiresolution approach. *Information Fusion*, *19*, 49–60.

Sonka, M., Hlavac, V., & Boyle, R. (2014). *Image processing, analysis, and machine vision*. Cengage Learning.

Tabakov, M. (2006, September). A fuzzy clustering technique for medical image segmentation. In *Evolving Fuzzy Systems, 2006 International Symposium on* (pp. 118-122). IEEE.

TamijeSelvy, P., Palanisamy, V., & Purusothaman, T. (2011). Performance Analysis of Clustering Algorithms in Brain Tumor Detection of MR Images. *European Journal of Scientific Research*, *63*(3).

Tech, K. R. M., & Korrapati, R. B. (2010). Neural Network Based Classification and Diagnosis of Brain Hemorrhages. *International Journal of Artificial Intelligent and Expert Systems, 7*.

Thies, C., Malik, A., Keysers, D., Kohnen, M., Fischer, B., & Lehmann, T. M. (2003, May). Hierarchical feature clustering for content-based retrieval in medical image databases. In *Medical Imaging 2003* (pp. 598–608). International Society for Optics and Photonics.

Tsechpenakis, G., Wang, J., Mayer, B., & Metaxas, D. (2007). Coupling CRFs and Deformable Models for 3D Medical Image Segmentation. *IEEE Mathematical Methods in Biomedical Image Analysis*, 1-8.

Turkington, J. R. A., Paterson, A., Sweeney, L. E., & Thornbury, G. D. (2014). Neck masses in children. *The British Journal of Radiology*.

Vanitha, L., & Venmathi, A. R. (2011). Classification of medical images using support vector machine. In *International Conference on Information and Network Technology* (Vol. 4, pp. 63-67). Academic Press.

Xu, R., Luo, L., & Ohya, J. (2002). *Segmentation of brain MRI, A Text Book of Advances in brain Imaging*. In Tech Publishers.

Zacharaki, E. I., Wang, S., Chawla, S., Soo Yoo, D., Wolf, R., Melhem, E. R., & Davatzikos, C. (2009). Classification of brain tumor type and grade using MRI texture and shape in a machine learning scheme. *Magnetic Resonance in Medicine*, *62*(6), 1609–1618.

Zhou, N., Yang, T., & Zhang, S. (2014). An improved FCM medical image segmentation algorithm based on MMTD. *Computational and Mathematical Methods in Medicine*.

Section 1

Introduction to Classification and Clustering

Chapter 1
Bag-of-Features in Microscopic Images Classification

Samsad Beagum
Taif University, Saudi Arabia & Karpagam University, India

Amira S. Ashour
Tanta University, Egypt & Taif University, Saudi Arabia

Nilanjan Dey
Techno India College of Technology, India

ABSTRACT

Microscopic image analysis plays a foremost role for understanding biological processes, diagnosis of diseases and cells/ tissues identification. Microscopic image classification is one of the challenging tasks that have a leading role in the medical domain. In this chapter, an overview on different classification techniques elaborated with microscopic images is presented to guide the reader through the advanced knowledge of major quantitative image classification approaches. Applied examples are conducted to classify different Albino rats' samples captured using light microscope for three different organs, namely hippocampus, renal and pancreas. The Bag-of-Features (BoF) technique was employed for features extraction and selection. The BoF selected features were used as input to the multiclass linear support vector machine classifier. The proposed classifier achieved 94.33% average classification accuracy for the three classes. Additionally, for binary classification the achieved average accuracy was 100% for hippocampus and pancreas sets classification.

INTRODUCTION

Medical and biological image analysis/ processing provide a forum for the dissemination of extensive research results. Medical imaging advances so promptly to develop more techniques and algorithms that facilities accurate analysis. Image enhancement, restoration, registration, segmentation and classification are considered the main digital image processing requirements for medical applications. Various medical imaging modalities and acquisition systems are used to capture medical images. Such modalities are the X-ray, Magnetic resonance imaging (MRI), Computed tomography (CT), Endoscopy, Ultrasound and Positron emission tomography (PET).

DOI: 10.4018/978-1-5225-0140-4.ch001

Recently, microscopic imaging technology becomes one of the utmost extensively used research tools to assist physicians in diagnosis/ prognoses of the patient conditions as well as the biologists in understanding the complex processes of cells (Mohapatra *et al.*, 2010). Histology is concerned with the study of microscopic structure of cells and tissues. Cells and tissues analysis assists the diagnosis of a vast number of diseases. Manual analysis has numerous evaluation drawbacks such as time consuming, less accuracy and dependency on the operator skills. Otherwise, the automated analysis performed quickly and provided precise results.

Image analysis elaborates complex algorithms to count, identify and characterize cellular shape, color, and tissue samples' quantity using image pattern recognition schemes. Tissue image analysis can be employed to ensure/ measure the presence of cancer cells in a biopsy of a malignant tumor and determine the recurrence prediction rate of cancer. Conventional image analysis and processing tools are involved in histology image analysis. It includes preprocessing, image segmentation, feature extraction and classification. Since, texture characterizes any geometric structure of the image gray levels. Thus, texture is imperative in many application of computer image analysis for the classification of segmented images based on local spatial variations of intensity of color (Smitha *et al.*, 2011). Texture analysis provides significant information on the spatial character of the gray levels and the relationship with their neighborhood.

Classification is the most imperative aspect of texture analysis that interests with the search for a specific texture among different predefined texture categories. It is performed using statistical methods and algorithms that describe the texture descriptors and then perform the classification process. Medical and microscopic image databases contain images of different modalities taken under varied conditions with variable accuracy of annotation that can be used for image classification. There is an exponential increase in medical images classification using different classifiers and algorithms. Several classifiers are engaged for the classification process such as: Support Vector Machine (SVM), artificial neural network (ANN), Probabilistic Neural Network, nearest neighbor classifier, and K-means.

Generally, image classification techniques can be categorized into two main groups, namely supervised classification and unsupervised classification. Supervised classifier (parametric method), which requires an exhaustive training phase of the classifier parameters. It involves the act of obtaining the information class of data sets, and classifying the test data by identifying training data's best possible match (Supardi *et al.*, 2012). In contrast, unsupervised classifier does not require training and relies directly on the data to execute the classification process (Oren *et al.*, 2008). Figure 1 illustrates these two main classification categories.

Figure 1. Various medical image classification techniques

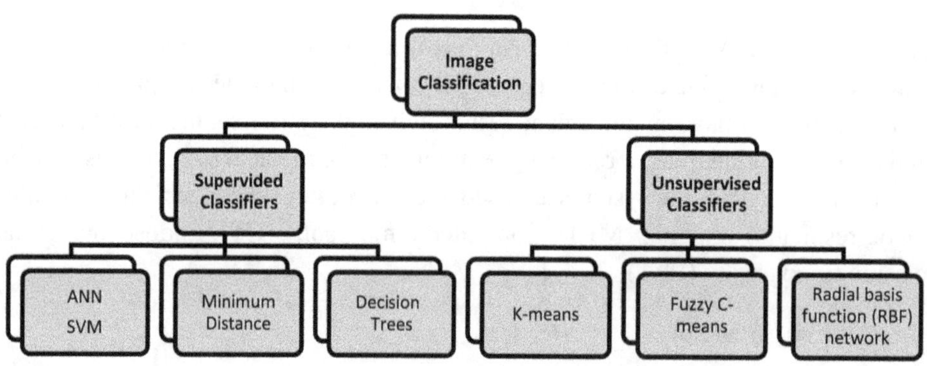

Neural Network is one of the most essential classification tools for medical images. Recently, numerous advanced techniques based on neural network are considered for classification such as Fuzzy logic, Artificial Neural Network, Radial Basis function neural network (RBFNN), Multi layer Neural Network (MLNN), Polynomial Neural Network (PNN). Additionally, hybrid classification techniques are such as Neuro-Fuzzy technique, Neuro-Genetic Technique and Adaptive Neuro- Fuzzy Inference system (ANFIS) (Hota *et al.*, 2013). SVM is a binary classifier that classifies two classes by finding the maximum separating hyper plane between them. Bag-of-Features (BoF) is also called bag of words, which represents an order-less distribution of local image features sampled from an image.

The main contribution of the current chapter is to highlight various works that has been performed on microscopic images classification using various techniques. Then, an applied example has been included using the BOF classifier. A database of albino rats' hippocampus, renal and pancreas images are used to test the classification process. The images were captured using light microscope in the Anatomy and Embryology Department of Medicine Faculty, Tanta University, Egypt.

The structure of the remaining sections is as follows. Background to provide extensive clarification for the classification process with literature review related to the microscopic images classification. Afterwards, the main focus of the chapter, included the proposed applied example using the BOF classifier is presented. Then, solutions and recommendations section containing the obtained results and their discussion is conducted. Finally, the future research directions and the conclusion sections are introduced.

BACKGROUND

Numerous fields of medicine, technology and physics elaborate microscopic image analysis. Typically, the input image may have 1024x1024 pixels resolution, although objects of interest have 50x50 pixels resolution. Consequently, detection and classification become complex due to the objects of interest strong variability, poor resolution and noisy background. These drawbacks required development in the recognition systems to be able to deal with the variability within each class as well as the variability between the classes.

Classification is one of the imperative machine learning areas which collect unprocessed data and categorizes it into definite classes based on set of parameters (Islam *et al.*, 2007). Classification structure usually applies either statistical or syntactic approach according to the pattern's statistical characteristics. The classification process generally entails training and testing datasets which contains different features or traits such that pattern can be recognized. Generally, classification techniques are significant to partition a feature space of an image using data with known labels. Feature extraction is considered the main step to enhance the image presentation to achieve image classification process. Several studies were concerned with microscopic image analysis and features extraction (Dey *et al.*, 2015a; 2015b; Kotyk *et al.*, 2015a; Hore *et al.*, 2015; Nandi *et al.*, 2015; Kotyk *et al.*, 2015b, Kotyk *et al.*, 2015c).

Recently, with the rapid machine learning algorithms improvement, some medical/ microscopic image processing applications have adopted further techniques to improve the detection and classification performance. Several intelligent techniques were elaborated by the researchers to classify microscopic images to detect abnormalities and diagnose several critical diseases. Such techniques are as follows.

Artificial Neural Networks (ANNs)

Neural networks have several advantages over the conventional techniques lie in their ability to solve problems that do not have an algorithmic solution or if the available solution is too complex to be found. Neural networks are well suited for prediction, pattern recognition and classification. ANNs have been applied in the medical area for clinical diagnosis, image analysis/ interpretation and drug development. Extensive studies were conducted on the microscopic images classification for different applications as follows.

Schnorrenberg *et al.* (1997) introduced a new system for computer–aided biopsy analysis, which interested with the system's nuclear classification module based on a feed-forward neural network. A set of six local and global features were used as input to the classifier. These features were the two chromaticity indices, optical density, a variance based texture measure, global nuclei density mean, and the variance. The nuclei classification module output was a membership label in a zero to four grading method for each detected nucleus. The training phase was performed in a supervised fashion to classify the nuclear feature vectors. The sample data were contained 3015 nuclei from 28 images that were classified by human expert. The neural network achieved 72% classification accuracy. Pascual-Montano *et al.* (2001) suggested a self-organizing neural network for electron microscopy (EM) images classification of biological macromolecules. Two different data sets have been used, namely 2458 rotational power spectra of individual negative stain images of the G40P helicase of Bacillus subtilis bacteriophage SPP1, and the other contained 2822 cryoelectron images of SV40 large T-antigen. The results proved that the proposed technique was successful and allowed the exploring of complex patterns in a succinct, informative, and objective manner.

Phukpattaranont and Boonyaphiphat (2006) performed cancer cells segmentation from breast cancer microscopic tissue images. Back propagation neural network was employed to classify pixels based on their color contents. To separate cancer cells and eliminate spike noise, cell size as well as morphological operations was considered. The experimental results proved that the proposed method achieved outstanding segmentation with microscopic images under both low and high histological noise conditions. Kruk *et al.* (2007) extracted individual cells from colon tissue by applying morphological operations and watershed algorithm. These extracted cells were then fed into the neural network classifiers for succeeding recognition of colon cell types. The results proved 6% mean discrepancy rate. Gallegos-Funes *et al.* (2009) introduced the potential of the Rank M-Type Radial Basis Function (RMRBF) neural network in the Pap smear microscopic images classification. Simulation results proved that the RMRBF neural network has improved the classification capabilities compared to other RBF based algorithms. The proposed classifier had about 20% error in the detection of the Cervical intra-epithelial neoplasia (CIN) 2 or 3. Furthermore, it provided high classification efficiency into 3 groups, namely normal, CINs and CIS (carcinoma-in-situ) cells. Jurrus *et al.* (2010) proposed a novel scheme for neuron membrane detection. A serial ANN classifier was conducted to close gaps in the weak membranes and suppress intracellular structures using increasingly non-local information with every ANN in the series. To increase the classifier flexibility, raw image intensities sampled through a stencil were used as inputs to the series ANN. These inputs were then trained to detect neuron membranes in the datasets with extensively different characteristics. The experimental results established that stencil utilization achieved significantly better results, where for the same features number, a stencil provided context information for a larger neighborhood. Due to the proposed scheme capability to close gaps in weak areas of elongated structures, Jurrus *et al.* suggested similar classifier approach can be used for segmenting long tubular structures such as vasculature in MRI.

Chen (2012) proposed two methods for microscopic image segmenting and classification. These methods were the radial basis function neural network (RBF) with fuzzy initialization and the graph-based discrete approach. The experimental results illustrated that RBF neural network was easy to implement, and the training procedure was very fast. Additionally, to accelerate the procedure of parameters and structure selection, the RBF neural network employed the fuzzy mean algorithm. Meanwhile, the graphed-based discrete method was used to perform the cellular extraction segmentation problem. Mohamad *et al.* (2014) suggested an automatic bacteria identification framework to classify bacteria into three classes, namely Cocci, Vibrio and Bacilli from microscopic morphology using the Naïve Bayes classifier. First, the system was trained using a set of microscopic images containing Cocci, Bacilli, and Vibrio that normalized to emphasize the diameter and shape features. Edge-based descriptors were extracted from the input images. Afterward, the Naïve Bayes classifier was conducted to perform probabilistic inference based on the input descriptors. The authors used 64 images for each class of bacteria in the training set and 222 images as test set, where no images overlapped between the training set and the test set. The system proved its ability to accurately discriminate the three classes of bacteria and rejecting images that did not belong to any of the three classes. The results established the efficiency of this two-step automatic bacteria identification approach that can be extended to identify a variety of other types of bacteria.

Support Vector Machine (SVM)

Support Vector Machines (SVMs) are widely known and have achieved high classification performance in various applications, including blood/ tissue cells sorting, cell yeast cells on suspension in bioreactors, cells in culture using fluorescent microscopy and on sections of brain tumors (Wang *et al.*, 2003; Glotsos *et al.*, 2004; Wang *et al.*, 2008).

Ronneberger *et al.* (2000) extracted 3D invariant features for pollen grains captured images using fluorescence microscope. The dataset of 350 pollen samples were taken from trees. A SVM was employed to classify the acquired pollen images after feature extraction. The results indicated 8% error rate. Additionally, the authors concluded that the 3D analysis is not suitable for a real-time application. By the same year, El-Naqa *et al.* (2002) employed SVMs to detect microcalcifications in mammogram images. The proposed classifier achieved sensitivity as high as 94% at an error rate of one false-positive cluster per image. The SVM outperformed all the other methods considered within the study. Luo *et al.* (2004) extracted features by considering granulometric measurements, invariant moments, and domain specific features for recognizing plankton images. The particles did not have clear contours and there were many unidentifiable objects that must be removed. After feature extraction, the authors applied a feature selection procedure to reduce the number of features. The SVM was then employed to classify the images dataset. The SVM achieved 76% overall average accuracy, but with a high error rate of 42% the unidentifiable particles.

Rahman *et al.* (2006) proposed a multi-class classification system based on pairwise coupling of some binary SVM to predict the categories of test images, which used later for annotation. Thus, the SVMs were used for medical image annotation and retrieval achieving an automatic image annotation of 56.7% accuracy and 72.96% retrieval accuracy. Wei *et al.* (2007) developed in situ probe on-line monitoring for parameters describing cell growth such as cell density and viability during fermentation processes. The authors separated cells from background by applying two support vector machine based classifiers. The proposed method was also distinguished living cells from dead ones. The suggested classifiers achieved high accuracy and stability. In situ experiments proved strong correlation between results attained by the probe and those by other standard methods. Tabesh *et al.* (2007) introduced a study of image features for cancer diagnosis and Gleason grading of the histological images of prostate. In diagnosis, the tissue image was classified into the tumor and non-tumor classes. The used image sets consisted of 367 and 268 color images for the diagnosis and Gleason grading problems; respectively. The images were captured from representative areas of hematoxylin and eosin-stained tissue retrieved from tissue microarray cores or whole sections. The authors aggregated texture, color and morphometric cues at the global and histological object levels for classification. The comparative results of the performance of Gaussian, K-nearest neighbor, Linear and support vector machine classifiers together with the sequential forward feature selection algorithm proved that the Linear classifier outperformed the other mentioned classifiers when used to classify Gleason grading in terms of the accuracy. On diagnosis, five-fold cross-validation estimated an accuracy of 96.7%. On Gleason grading, the achieved accuracy of classification into low- and high-grade classes was 81.0%.

Li *et al.* (2013) introduced an automatic classification technique for the Environmental Microorganisms (EMs) for content-based image analysis. Edge Histograms, Internal Structure Histograms, Fourier Descriptors, extended Geometrical Features were employed to describe the shapes of the EMs observed in the microscopic images. Multi-class SVM was applied to EMs represented by the mentioned features for classification. A comprehensive experiment with a ground truth of manually segmented microscopic EM images was conducted. The results established best classification result of 89.7% with high robustness.

K-Nearest Neighborhood Classifier

K-nearest neighbor (KNN) is broadly used as an effective classification model. Jafari-Khouzani and Soltanian-Zadeh (2003) extracted features based on wavelet packets, multi-wavelets, and co-occurrence matrices combined with a KNN classifier. The authors classified pathological images of prostate into grades 2 through 5. The classification distance metric was optimized using simulated annealing algorithm. The results reported 97% accuracy using the leave-one-out (LOO) procedure for error estimation. Shen *et al.* (2008) proposed a machine-aided classification technique for microscope images of cataractous lens. Color information of cataractous lens with different hardness degrees was investigated. The KNN classifiers were used to classify different cataractous lens' hardness degrees. Real microscope images of phacoemulsifieation were used for testing the proposed method. The results proved 92.5% recognition rate. Yu *et al.* (2011) designed an automated classification algorithm for microscopic images of yeast cells in a microfluidic channel environment. The k-nearest-neighbor algorithm, linear support vector machine and the distance-based classification were the classifiers used. To reduce background noise, the images were enhanced. Then, robust segmentation algorithm was used to extract geometrical features including compactness, axis ratio and the bud size. These features were applied for classification. The system performance under different illumination and focusing conditions were examined.

Kumar *et al.* (2015) proposed a framework for automated detection and classification of cancer from microscopic biopsy images. The KNN method was employed for images classification into normal and cancerous categories. The proposed framework performance was evaluated using well-known parameters for four fundamental tissues (muscular, connective, epithelial and nervous) of randomly selected 1000 microscopic biopsy images. Various classification approaches have been tested, namely the KNN, fuzzy KNN, support vector machine (SVM), and random forest based classifiers. The comparative study established that the SVM provided average results for all the tissues types but not better than the KNN. The

Fuzzy KNN was comparatively a less good classifier, while the KNN classifier was performing better for all categories of the test data cases. Among all categories of test cases, further it was found that the proposed method was performing better for connective tissues type samples. Based on the performance metrics measures for connective tissues dataset, the proposed method was achieved 0.92, 0.94, 0.82, 0.88, 0.76 and 0.72 in terms of the average accuracy, specificity, sensitivity, F-measure, and Matthews's Correlation Coefficient (MCC); respectively.

Fuzzy Logic

Fuzzy classification is the process of grouping elements into a fuzzy set. It can be involved in various applications as follows. Begelrnan *et al.* (2004) presented a semi-supervised training of fuzzy logic engine technique to connect a set of parameters for nucleus segmentation. Each parameter for itself was detected using a set of fuzzy logic rules. Hildebrand and Ploch (2011) described the steps for steel production starting from image capturing using microscopic images classification using fuzzy logic based classifiers. Haralick feature analysis and fuzzy logic based classification were able to automate the quality control process. The microstructure was analyzed to assess the processed steel products quality. Results showed classification rate of 82% correct classifications. In the same year, Hiremath and Iranna (2011) suggested a new technique based on active contours for segmentation and fuzzy rule based classification of microscopic images of esophagus tissues. The images were acquired from the human esophagus abnormal regions detected using endoscopy. The proposed approach was used for classification of Squamous Cell Carcinoma (SCC) of esophagus, namely well-, moderately- and poorly- differentiated SCC. For cell nuclei segmentation, multi-grid active contour method was employed. Additionally, three geometric features were used feature extraction and a fuzzy rule based classifier for the SCC classification. The results established the proposed method efficacy.

Lijiya *et al.* (2013) proposed new classification method to automate the karyotyping based on Fuzzy c-means (FCM) algorithm combined with a labeling chart. The Karyotyping has a significant role to identify genetic disorders due to structural changes in chromosomes. Multiplex fluorescence in-situ hybridization (M-FISH) method provided more accurate karyotyping. The classification results indicated that the proposed method improved the running time and accuracy.

Classification Techniques Based Meta-Heuristic Algorithms

Optimization is a generally encountered mathematical problem in all engineering disciplines. Meta-heuristics optimization algorithms are based on the iterative improvement of either a population of solutions (as in Evolutionary algorithms (EA), Swarm based algorithms) or a single solution (as Tabu Search). Mostly, meta-heuristics employs randomization and local search to solve a given optimization problem (Binitha and Sathya, 2012). Several meta-heuristic approaches have been used in image classification and analysis such as the Genetic algorithm (GA), Particle swarm optimization (PSO), Ant Colony Optimization (ACO), Fish Swarm Algorithm and Firefly algorithm (FA).

Marinakis *et al.* (2008) proposed a scheme to classify the pap-smear cells based meta-heuristic algorithm, namely the particle swarm optimization (PSO). The pap-smear cells are samples of human cells stained using Papanicolaou method to diagnose pre-cancerous cell changes before they progress to invasive carcinoma. The authors used two databases consisting of 917 and 500 images of pap-smear cells. Each cell was represented by 20 features, where the cells fall into seven classes. The achieved goal was to distinguish normal from abnormal cells. The PSO algorithm was used to find the best possible performing feature subset. This algorithm was combined with a number of nearest neighbor based classifiers. The experimental results demonstrated that the proposed classification accuracy generally outperformed other applied intelligent methods. Dhasal *et al.* (2012) proposed a feature sampling technique to reduce the unclassified region of multi-class classification during image classification. Ant colony optimization (ACO) algorithm for proper feature sub set selection was conducted. The authors designed ACO-SVM to alleviate the SVM drawbacks.

Singh (2013) presented a method for nano-particles microscopic image analyzes by edge detection using Ant Colony Optimization (ACO) algorithm. The optimization algorithm was employed to obtain a well-connected image edge map. This method was applied on the atomic force microscope (AFM) images of Cerium Oxide (CeO2) nano-particles and SEM image of ZnO nanoparticles. The results illustrated that the edges obtained in the images can be used to classify the particles, to determine the particles' sizes/ shapes and to distinguish particles in agglomerates more precisely. Sweidan *et al.* (2015) proposed a bio-inspired optimization classification model by using the fish gills microscopic images to evaluate the water pollution and to determine the water quality. Wavelet transforms and edge detection algorithms have been used for feature extraction. For optimizing feature selection, the Case-based reasoning (CBR) was employed along with the Gray Wolf Optimization (GWO) algorithm. The datasets employed for the experiment contained real sample microscopic images for fish gills exposed to copper and water pH in different histopathlogical stages. The experimental results proved that 97.2% average accuracy was achieved by the proposed GWO-CBR classification model.

Hybrid Techniques

As an example for hybrid system for microscopic images classification, Gan (2011) designed, implemented and evaluated a hybrid classifier that discriminates between three classes of colonic histopathological images namely, normal, adenomatous polyp, and cancerous lesions. The proposed hybrid classifier system was realized by combining the fuzzy logic, artificial neural networks and genetic algorithms to tackle the classification problem. Textural features represented by Haralick were used as input to the classifier system. The system implementation included two parts: feature selection and classification. Variance ratios derived from scatter matrices and GA were used and compared to select the candidate feature sets. The Kohonen self-organizing map was used in the fitness function of the GA. In the classification part, a hybrid neuro-fuzzy adaptive network (ANFIS) was used. For performance evaluation, the test dataset should be different from the used training dataset. The results demonstrated the robustness of the proposed hybrid algorithms.

Bag-of-Features Model

Recently, Bag-of-features (BoF) approach become popular for content based image classification. It is developed from the Texton methods in texture analysis. It has the advantages of simplicity and good performance. BoF methods have been applied to image classification, image retrieval, object detection, and even visual localization for robots. BoF characterized by the use of an orderless collection of image features. Lazebnik *et al.* (2003) employed a sparser bag-of-features approach, using Scale-Invariant Feature Transform (SIFT) descriptors over Harris-affine key-points. The authors avoided the global quantization by comparing histograms using Earth Movers Distance. Fergus *et al.* (2005) demonstrated the ability of the geometry-free bag-of-features approaches to localize the images. Nowak *et al.* (2006) treated images as loose collections of independent patches. The authors sampled a representative set of patches from the image, evaluated a visual descriptor vector for each patch independently, and used the resulting distribution of samples in descriptor space as a characterization of the image. Bag-of-Features was used to demonstrate the representative selection of commonly used test databases with large numbers of samples, random sampling provided equal/better classifiers than the sophisticated multi-scale interest operators.

Researches involved BoF for classification are as follows. Zhang *et al.* (2005) performed a large-scale quantitative evaluation of BoF representations for both texture recognition and image classification using SVM classifier kernels. The authors suggested a mix of detectors and features with corresponding types of information. Jiang *et al.* (2007) evaluated several factors that impact BoF image classification using SVMs. The experimental results indicated that most notable factors affected the BoF performance, namely the feature detector selection, the vector weighting scheme, and the SVM kernel.

The preceding extensive literature review established that various classifiers can be involved for microscopic images classification for broad range of applications. Additionally, no prior studies elaborated the BoF technique for microscopic images classification.

MAIN FOCUS OF THE CHAPTER

The first contribution of the current chapter is the previous broad background that focused on the different types of classifiers employed for microscopic images classification. Afterward, the second contribution is to provide an applied example for microscopic images classification. For this goal, a dataset of 180 Albino rats' samples from hippocampus, renal and pancreas with 60 images from each class are used for classification. The samples were acquired using light microscope in the Anatomy department, Tanta University, Egypt.

Proposed System

The proposed microscopic images classification system applied the Bag-of-Features (bag-of-words model (BoW)) technique under Matlab R2015b. Generally, the BoF technique handles the image features as words.

The pre-defined three input data sets are passed through the Bag-of-Features technique for features extraction. BoF can be considered as a histogram representation method based on independent features. For features detection, good descriptor which has the ability to handle rotation, intensity, scale and affine variations is to be used. The Speeded up Robust Features (SURF) are extracted to represent each image category. Then, the k-means clustering is used to reduce the number of features for proper classification and to reduce the classification time. The encode approach is then applied to produce a histogram that of the image. Thus, each image is encoded into a feature vector using the BoF. The feature vector of an image represents the histogram of visual word occurrences contained in the image. This histogram considered a basis for training the classifier, as it encoded the image into a feature vector.

The encoded training images from each set are fed into a classifier training process. BoF is supported by the multi-class linear SVM classifier from the Statistics and Machine Learning Toolbox in Matlab. Figure 2 demonstrates the proposed classifier block diagram using BoF.

Figure 2. Proposed microscopic images classification using BoF technique

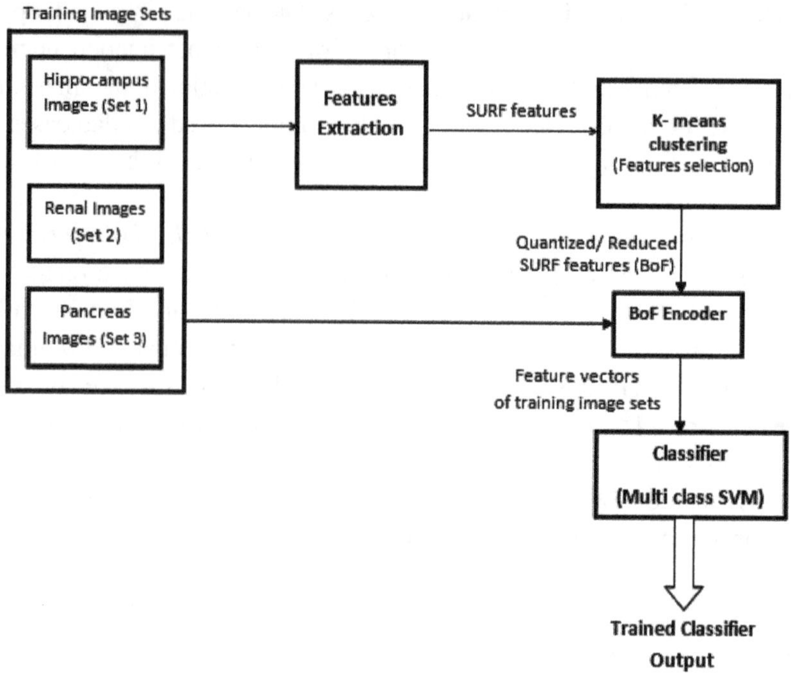

The following algorithm illustrated the steps of the proposed approach for microscopic images classification.

SOLUTIONS AND RECOMMENDATIONS (RESULTS AND DISCUSSION)

The main objective of the present study was the classification of different rats' cell structures from different organs. This study concerned with the classification of the Albino rats' microscopic images from hippocampus, renal and pancreas into three categories using the BoF technique that based on the multiclass linear SVM. Matlab R2015a (Version 8.6) software was employed. The algorithm was ex-

Table 1. Algorithm: microscopic images classification based BoF technique

Start
Input the image sets (180 images of the three hippocampus, renal and pancreas images (60 images from each class))
Separate the images into training, validation and testing data
Create the Bag-of-Features from the three image sets
• Extract the SURF features from all images using the Grid selection method
• Reduce the number of features using K-means clustering
Start Training Phase
Encode the images to produce a histogram
Feed the encoded images from each category into the multiclass linear SVM classifier
End of training phase
Evaluate Classifier Performance
End

Figure 3. Samples of the dataset images from the three classes: left images are hippocampus samples (set 1), middle images are renal samples (set 2) and the right images are pancreas samples (set 3).

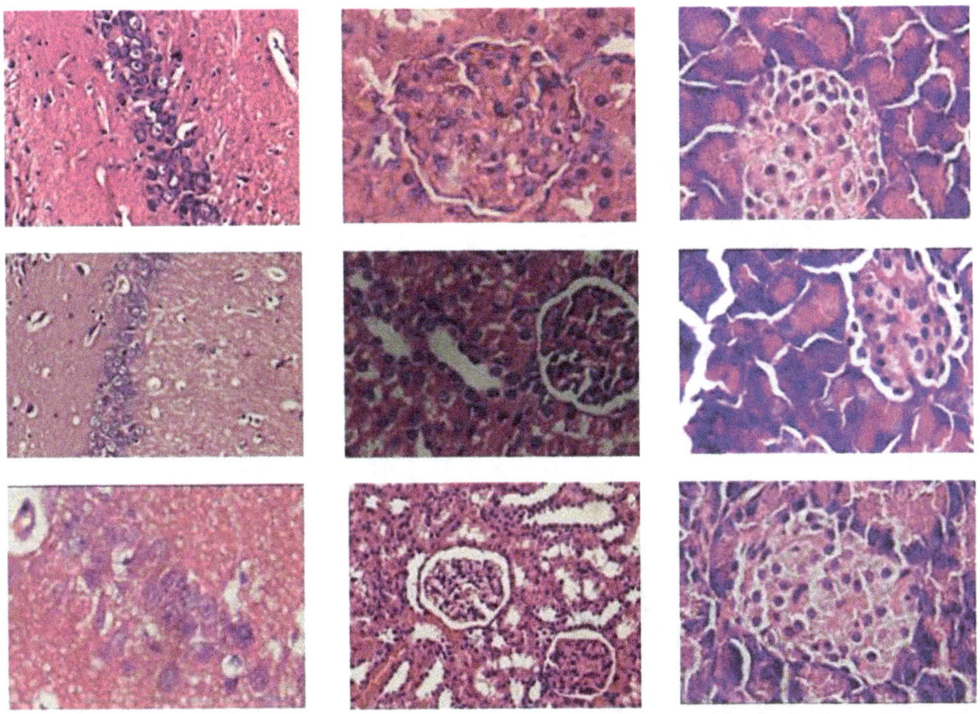

ecuted using Windows 7 platform having 6 GB RAM, Intel Core i5-2410M CPU 2.30GHz processor. The conducted dataset were composed of colored rats' specimens obtained using light microscope. The data set consists of 60 rat microscopic images pool form each class. The images were captured in the Anatomy and Embryology department, faculty of medicine, Tanta University, Egypt.

Samples from the Three Categories

Figure 3 illustrates examples from the dataset used for the classification process. The Left column in Figure 3 represents samples of set 1 which contains hippocampus images. The middle column represented renal images from set 2. While, samples for the pancreas (set 3) are represented in the right column of Figure 3.

Histogram of Visual Word Occurrences

Figure 4 illustrates the output of the encoding step when plotting 1x500 feature vector of each. Figure 4 a), c), e) are the image samples from each class and Figure 4 b), d), f) are the histogram of visual word rate contained in each corresponding image.

Figure 4. a), c), e) are the image samples from each class: hippocampus image, renal image and pancreas image; respectively; b), d), f) are the histogram of visual word occurrence (rate) contained in each correspondence images; respectively.

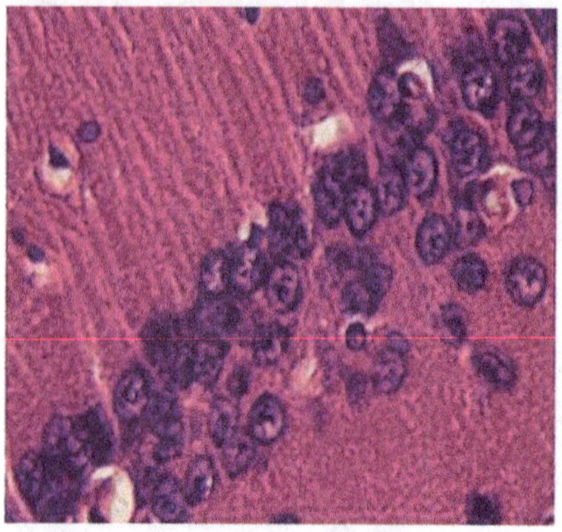

a)

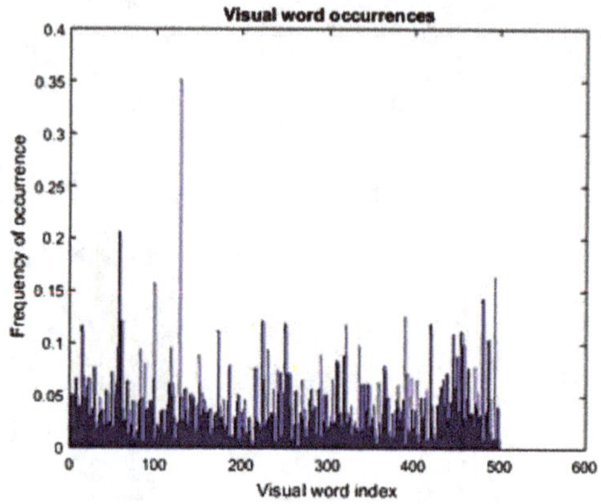

b)

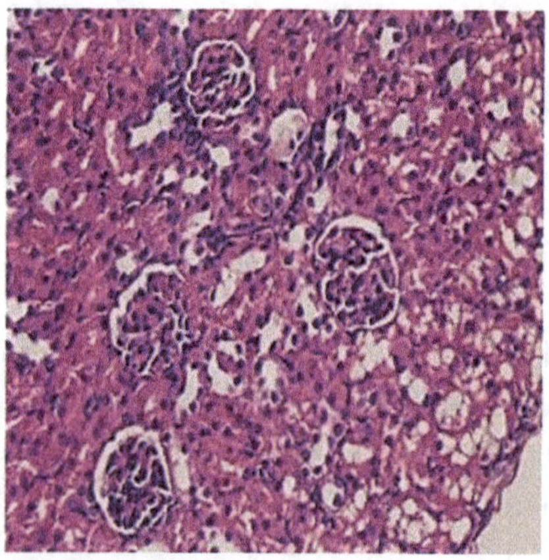

c)

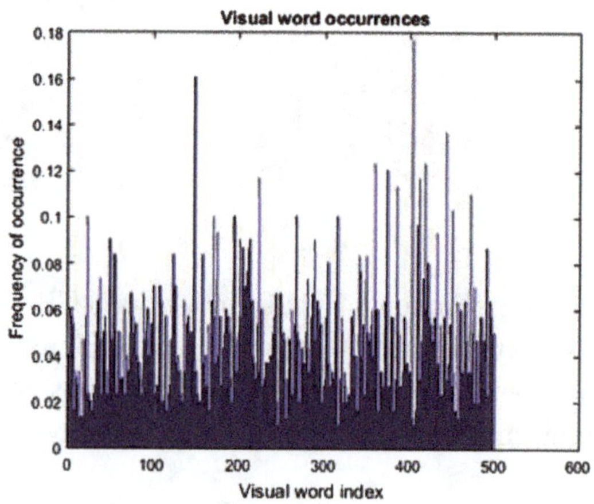

d)

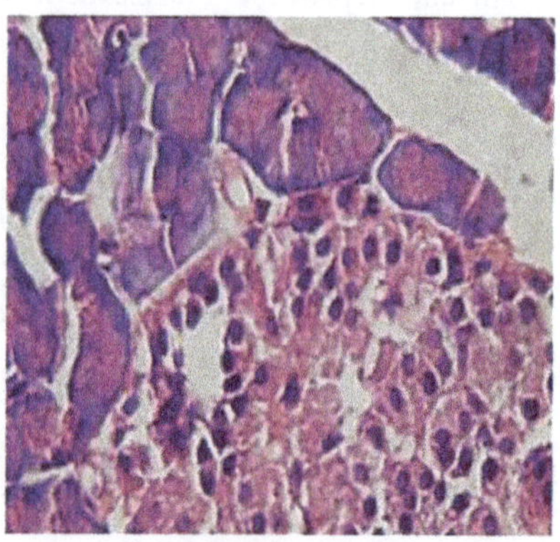

e)

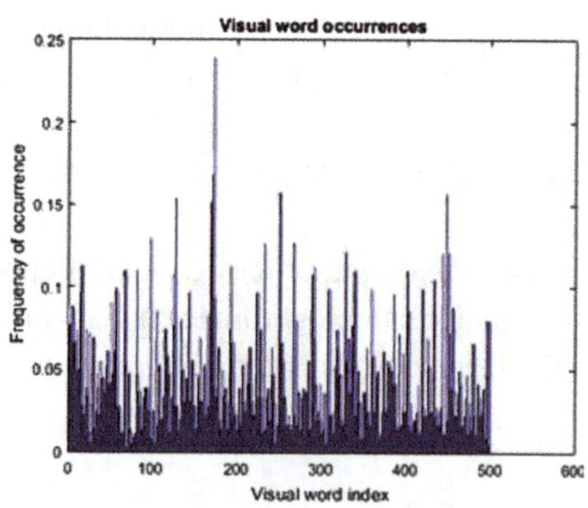

f)

Classification using BoF Technique and Performance Evaluation

For classification purpose each image set is divided into 70% of the images (42 images) are used for feature extraction and training, 30% for validation and test (18 images) in each image set.

Performance evaluation is compulsory in all automated classification systems. It is conducted to evaluate the ability of the used classifier to classify the dataset into proper categories. In fact, performance metrics such as the accuracy, specificity, and sensitivity are calculated from a confusion matrix as shown in Table 2. The confusion matrix contains information about actual and predicted classifications performed by the classification system for performance evaluation. Generally, the confusion matrix entries can be defined as follows:

- True positive (T_p) is the number of positive instances categorized as positive (Correctly identified 'positive').
- False positive (F_p) is the number of negative instances categorized as positive (Incorrectly identified 'positive').
- False negative (F_n) is the number of positive instances categorized as negative (Incorrectly rejected 'negative').
- True negative (T_n) is the number of negative instances categorized as negative (Correctly rejected 'negative').

Thus, for each class the confusion matrix entries are calculated. Then, the other performance metrics can be calculated as follows:

- The accuracy is defined as a ratio of sum of the instances classified correctly to the total number of instances. It is expressed as:

$$Accuracy = \frac{T_P + T_N}{T_P + F_P + F_N + T_N} \times 100\% \tag{1}$$

- Precision is defined as the ratio of correctly classified data in positive class to the total number of data classified as to be in positive class. It is expressed as:

$$Precision = \frac{T_P}{T_P + F_P} \tag{2}$$

where, the Positive prediction value (PPV) is equal to the precision.

Table 2. Typical example of confusion matrix of a binary classification problem

		Predicted Class	
		Positive	**Negative**
Actual Class	**Positive**	T_P	F_P
	Negative	F_N	T_N

- Recall (TP rate) is defined as the ratio of T_p to the total number of instances classified under positive class. It is calculated by:

$$Recall = \frac{T_P}{T_P + F_N} \tag{3}$$

where, the sensitivity is measures the proportion of positives that are correctly identified, which is the same as the recall.

- F-measure is defined as a combined representation of Precision and Recall. It is given by:

$$F - measure = 2 * \frac{Precision * Recall}{Precision + Recall} \tag{4}$$

- Specificity is the true negative rate, which measures the proportion of negatives that are correctly identified.

$$Specificity = \frac{T_N}{T_N + F_P} \tag{5}$$

- Negative prediction value (NPV) is given by:

$$NPV = \frac{T_N}{T_N + F_N} \tag{6}$$

Different scenarios are depicted as follows to study and evaluate the classifier performance.

Experiment 1: Binary Classification between Hippocampus and Renal Sets.

The classifier is used to classify between the hippocampus and renal images. The confusion matrix obtained is illustrated in Table 3.

Table 3. Confusion matrix classifying hippocampus and renal sets

	Renal	**Hippocampus**
Renal	**0.94**	0.06
Hippocampus	0.11	**0.89**

Table 4. Confusion matrix classifying hippocampus and pancreas sets

	Pancreas	Hippocampus
Pancreas	1	0
Hippocampus	0	1

It is reported that the effective classification accuracy is 92% for classifying set 1 and set2. Using the previous formulas for the other metrics, it is found that the achieved sensitivity (recall) of 0.90, specificity of 0.94, precision (PPV) 0.94, NPV of 0.89, and the F-measure has the value of 0.91.

Experiment 2: Binary Classification between Pancreas and Hippocampus.

The classifier is used to classify between the hippocampus and pancreas images. The confusion matrix obtained is illustrated in Table 4.

It is reported that the effective classification accuracy is 100% for classifying set 1 and set3. Using the previous formulas for the other metrics, it is found that the achieved sensitively, specificity, precision (PPV), recall, F-measure and the NPV all have value of 1.

Experiment 3: Binary Classification between Renal and Pancreas.

The classifier is used to classify between the renal and pancreas images. The confusion matrix obtained is illustrated in Table 5.

It is reported that the effective classification accuracy is 100% for classifying set 2 and set3. Using the previous formulas for the other metrics, it is found that the achieved sensitively, specificity, precision (PPV), recall, F-measure and the NPV all have value of 1.

Experiment 4: Classify the Three Datasets.

To classify the three sets, namely hippocampus, renal and pancreas, the confusion matrix will have the form represented in Table 6.

To evaluate the classifier performance in the training, the confusion matrix is calculated. Table 7 contains the calculated confusion matrix in the training phase.

The achieved average accuracy in the training phase is 98.66%.

The performance evaluation during the validation phase of the trained classifier using the confusion matrix in Table 8.

The achieved average accuracy in the validation phase is 94.33%.

Table 5. Confusion matrix classifying renal and pancreas sets

	Renal	Pancreas
Renal	1	0
Pancreas	0	1

Table 6. Confusion matrix of the three categories classification problem

		Predicted Class		
		Hippocampus	**Renal**	**Pancreas**
Actual Class	**Hippocampus**	T_{hippo}	F_{hippo}	F_{hippo}
	Renal	F_{renal}	T_{renal}	F_{renal}
	Pancreas	F_{panc}	F_{panc}	T_{panc}

Table 7. Confusion matrix of the three categories classification problem in the training phase

		Predicted Class		
		Hippocampus	**Renal**	**Pancreas**
Actual Class	**Hippocampus**	**0.98**	0.02	0.00
	Renal	0.02	**0.98**	0.00
	Pancreas	0.00	0.00	**1.00**

Table 8. Confusion matrix of the three categories classification problem in the validation phase

		Predicted Class		
		Hippocampus	**Renal**	**Pancreas**
Actual Class	**Hippocampus**	**0.94**	0.06	0.00
	Renal	0.00	**0.89**	0.11
	Pancreas	0.00	0.00	**1.00**

From the preceding results it is established that using the BoF technique achieved classification accuracy of 94.33% when classifying the three classes. The accuracy achieved was 100% for the binary classification of the hippocampus and pancreas or to classify renal and pancreas, while 92% accuracy to classify the hippocampus and the renal sets.

FUTURE RESEARCH DIRECTIONS

Microscopic analysis of biological particles, cells and tissues aims to identify/ classify these objects based on their variable shape and texture, and very low contrast and resolution. Furthermore, the images background can be highly variable. Thus, the recognition and classification of these images are challenging task. Additionally, from the previous literatures it is reported that the traditional techniques of bacterial classification depends on phenotypic identification using gram staining, culture methods as well as biochemical process. Nevertheless, these bacterial identification techniques can be used only for organisms which are cultivated in vitro and illustrate unique biochemical attributes, which are not appropriate for patterns that have been used as a characteristic of any known groups of microorganism.

Development of fully automatic detection and classification of abnormal cells and tissues in the pathological microscopic image samples is a demanding process. Several future directions can be reported as follows:

1. Elaborate meta-heuristic optimization algorithms to increase the efficiency of the classifiers parameters selection,
2. Design and implement more efficient feature extraction and selection algorithms,
3. Employing hybrid classification techniques to take the advantages of the various approaches, and
4. More focus should be given to the misclassification conditions and how to measure and overcome.

It is recommended to use large classification dataset for more accurate classification. Additionally, since the classification accuracy is not a reliable metric for assessing the performance of a classifier as it may produce misleading results when the numbers of samples in different classes vary greatly. Thus, it is suggested to use several metrics to evaluate the performance of the classification method.

Moreover, the current applied classification example proved the efficiency of the BoF technique, which applied with any microscopic images classification. As well the classification of different cells structures can be used further to specify certain rules that concern each class during de-noising for example.

CONCLUSION

Due to progression in treatment modalities, the use of advanced microscopy for automated detection and classification for precise pathologies has been established in recent years to facilitate medical accurate diagnosis. Typically, all computer-aided diagnosis (CAD) systems rely on image processing and machine learning techniques to classify the acquired images into normal and abnormal classes or any other required classes. For these objectives, considerable features are extracted from the segmented tissue/ cell images. Then, these features are fed to the classifiers. Image classification based automated techniques are more accurate, reliable and less time consuming compared to the manual investigation of the microscopic samples. This chapter carried out an extensive literature review for several studies on different classifier methods that classify the microscopic histopathological images or any microscopic images in various applications.

An applied example concerning the use of BoF technique for albino rats' image samples was conducted. The SURF features of each image category were extracted and then the K-means clustering was employed for features reduction and selection. The multi-class linear SVM classifier was used as a part from the BoF technique. The experimental results established the efficiency of the used method, which achieved 94.33% average accuracy for three sets classification, while 100% for the binary classification of the hippocampus and pancreas or to classify renal and pancreas and 92% to classify the hippocampus and the renal sets.

ACKNOWLEDGMENT

We acknowledge Dr. Ahmed Salah Ashour, Anatomy and Embryology Department of Medicine Faculty, Tanta University, Egypt for providing us with the database of albino rats' hippocampus, renal and pancreas images.

REFERENCES

Azar, J. C., Simonsson, M., Bengtsson, E., & Hast, A. (2015). Automated Classification of Glandular Tissue by Statistical Proximity Sampling. *International Journal of Biomedical Imaging*, *2015*, 1–11. doi:10.1155/2015/943104

Begelrnan, G., Gur, E., Rivli, E., Rudzsky, M., & Zalevsky, Z. (2004, October). Cell nuclei segmentation using fuzzy logic engine. *2004 International Conference on Image Processing, ICIP'04*, *5*, 2937-2940. doi:10.1109/ICIP.2004.1421728

Binitha, S., & Sathya, S. S. (2012). A survey of bio inspired optimization algorithms. *International Journal of Soft Computing and Engineering*, *2*(2), 137–151.

Chen, Y. (2012). Microscopic Image Segmenting and Classification with RBF Neural Network. *2012 International Symposium on Information Science and Engineering (ISISE)*. doi:10.1109/ISISE.2012.78

Dey, N., Ashour, A. S., Ashour, A. S., & Singh, A. (2015a). Digital Analysis of Microscopic Images in Medicine. *Journal of Advanced Microscopy Research*, *10*(1), 1–13. doi:10.1166/jamr.2015.1229

Dey, N., Ashour, A. S., & Hassanien, A. E. (2015b). *Generation of Feature Detectors and their Numerous Applications: A Recap. Image Feature Detectors Foundations, Innovations, and Applications. Springer.*

Dhasal, P., Shrivastava, S. S., Gupta, H., & Kumar, P. (2012). An Optimized Feature Selection for Image Classification Based on SVM-ACO. *International Journal of Advanced Computer Research*, *2*(3), 123–128.

El-Naqa, I., Yang, Y. Y., Wernick, M. N., Galatsanos, N. P., & Nishikawa, R. (2002). Support vector machine learning for detection of microcalcifications in mammograms. *IEEE Transactions on Medical Imaging*, *21*, 1552–1563. doi:10.1109/TMI.2002.806569 PMID:12588039

Fergus, R., Fei-Fei, L., Perona, P., & Zisserman, A. (2005). *Learning object categories from Google's image search*. Academic Press.

Gallegos-Funes, F. J., Gómez-Mayorga, M. E., Lopez-Bonilla, J. L., & Cruz-Santiago, R. (2009). Rank M-type radial basis function (RMRBF) neural network for Pap smear microscopic image classification. *Apeiron (Montreal, Quebec)*, *16*(4), 542–554.

Gan Lim, L. (2011). *Automatic Classification Of Colonic Histophathological Images Using Adaptive Neuro-Fuzzy Networks And Genetic Algorithms*. (PhD Thesis). Coventry University.

Glotsos, D., Spyridonos, P., Petalas, P., Cavouras, D., Ravazoula, P., Dadioti, P., & Nikiforidis, G. et al. (2004). Computer-based malignancy grading of astrocytomas employing a support vector machine classifier, the who grading system and the regular hematoxylineosin diagnostic staining procedure. *Analytical and Quantitative Cytology and Histology*, *26*(2), 77–83. PMID:15131894

Hildebrand, L., & Ploch, T. (2011). Image Based Analysis of Microstructures Using Texture Detection and Fuzzy Classifiers. In Integrated Systems, Design and Technology 2010, (pp. 313-319). doi:10.1007/978-3-642-17384-4_25

Hiremath, P. S., & Iranna, Y. H. (2011). Fuzzy rule based classification of microscopic images of squamous cell carcinoma of esophagus. *International Journal of Computers and Applications*, *25*(11), 30–33. doi:10.5120/3156-4366

Hore, S., Chakroborty, S., Ashour, A. S., Dey, N., Ashour, A., Sifaki-Pistolla, D., & Chaudhuri, S. R. B. et al. (2015). Finding contours of Hippocampus Brain Cell using Microscopic Image Analysis. *Journal of Advanced Microscopy Research*, *10*(2), 93–103. doi:10.1166/jamr.2015.1245

Hota, H.S., Shukla S.P., & Kiran, G. K. (2013). Review of Intelligent Techniques Applied for classification and preprocessing of Medical Image Data. *International Journal of Computer Science Issues, 10*(3).

Islam, M. J., Wu, Q. M. J., Ahmadi, M., & Sid-Ahmed, M. A. (2007). Investigating the Performance of Naive- Bayes Classifiers and K- Nearest Neighbor Classifiers. *International Conference on Convergence Information Technology*, 1541-1546. doi:10.1109/ICCIT.2007.148

Jafari-Khouzani, K., & Soltanian-Zadeh, H. (2003). Multiwavelet grading of pathological images of prostate. *IEEE Transactions on Bio-Medical Engineering*, *50*(6), 697–704. doi:10.1109/TBME.2003.812194 PMID:12814236

Jiang, Y. G., Ngo, C. W., & Yang, J. (2007). Towards optimal bag-of-features for object categorization and semantic video retrieval. *6th ACM international conference on Image and video retrieval*, 494-501.

Jurrus, E., Paiva, A. R., Watanabe, S., Anderson, J. R., Jones, B. W., Whitaker, R. T., & Tasdizen, T. et al. (2010). Detection of neuron membranes in electron microscopy images using a serial neural network architecture. *Medical Image Analysis*, *14*(6), 770–783. doi:10.1016/j.media.2010.06.002 PMID:20598935

Kotyk, T., Ashour, A. S., Chakraborty, S., Dey, N., & Balas, V. E. (2015c). *Apoptosis Analysis in Classification Paradigm: A Neural Network based Approach.* Healthy World Conference 2015 - A Healthy World for a Happy Life, Kakinada, India.

Kotyk, T., Dey, N., Ashour, A. S., Balas-Timar, D., Chakraborty, S., Ashour, A. S., & Tavares, J. M. (2015a). Measurement of the Glomerulus Diameter and Bowman's Space Width of Renal Albino Rats. [In-press]. *Computer Methods and Programs in Biomedicine*. doi:10.1016/j.cmpb.2015.10.023 PMID:26796351

Kotyk, T., Dey, N., Ashour, A. S., Victoria, A. D. C., Hassanien, A. E., Gaber, T., & Snasel, V. (2015b) Detection of Dead stained microscopic cells based on Color Intensity and Contrast. *International Conference on Advanced Intelligent Systems and Informatics*. Beni Suef University.

Kruk, M., Osowski, S., & Koktysz, R. (2007) Recognition of colon cells using ensemble of classifiers. *Proceedings of International Joint Conference on Neural Networks*, 288–293. doi:10.1109/IJCNN.2007.4370970

Kumar, R., Srivastava, R., & Srivastava, S. (2015). Detection and Classification of Cancer from Microscopic Biopsy Images Using Clinically Significant and Biologically Interpretable Features. *Journal of Medical Engineering*, *2015*, 1–14. doi:10.1155/2015/457906

Lazebnik, S., Schmid, C., & Ponce, J. (2003). Affine-invariant local descriptors and neighborhood statistics for texture recognition. *Computer Vision*, 649–655.

Li, C., Shirahama, K., Grzegorzek, M., Ma, F. J., & Zhou, B. (2013, September). Classification of environmental microorganisms in microscopic images using shape features and support vector machines. *2013 20th IEEE International Conference on Image Processing* (ICIP), (pp. 2435-2439).

Lijiya, A., Sreejithlal, G. S., & Govindan, V. K. (2013). M-FISH Image Segmentation and Classification using Fuzzy Logic. *International Journal of Computers and Applications*, *70*(25).

Luo, T., Kramer, K., Goldgof, D. B., Hall, L. O., Samson, S., Remsen, A., & Hopkins, T. (2004). Recognizing plankton images from the shadow image particle profiling evaluation recorder. *IEEE Transactions on Systems, Man, and Cybernetics*, *34*(4), 1753–1762. doi:10.1109/TSMCB.2004.830340 PMID:15462442

Marinakis, Y., Marinaki, M., & Dounias, G. (2008). Particle swarm optimization for pap-smear diagnosis. *Expert Systems with Applications*, *35*(4), 1645–1656. doi:10.1016/j.eswa.2007.08.089

Mohamad, A., Jusoh Awang, N., Zaw, Z., & Shoon, L. W. (2014). Bayesian prokaryote classification from microscopic images. *Computer Applications: An International Journal*, *1*(1), 1–9.

Mohapatra, S., Patra, D., & Satpathi, S. (2010). Image analysis of blood microscopic images for acute leukemia detection. *2010 International Conference on Industrial Electronics, Control & Robotics (IECR)*, (pp. 215-219). doi:10.1109/IECR.2010.5720171

Nandi, D., Ashour, A. S., Samanta, S., Chakraborty, S., Salem, M., & Dey, N. (2015). Principal Component Analysis in Medical Image Processing: A Study. *International Journal of Image Mining*, *1*(1), 65. doi:10.1504/IJIM.2015.070024

Nowak, E., Jurie, F., & Triggs, B. (2006). Sampling strategies for bag-of-features image classification. In Computer Vision–ECCV 2006, (pp. 490-503). Springer Berlin Heidelberg. doi:10.1007/11744085_38

Oren, B. (2008). *Defense of Nearest-Neighbor Based Image Classification*. Weizmann Institute of Science.

Pascual-Montano, A., Donate, L. E., Valle, M., Barcena, M., Pascual-Marqui, R. D., & Carazo, J. M. (2001). A novel neural network technique for analysis and classification of EM single-particle images. *Journal of Structural Biology*, *133*(2), 233–245. doi:10.1006/jsbi.2001.4369 PMID:11472094

Phukpattaranont, P., & Boonyaphiphat, P. (2006, October). Segmentation of cancer cells in microscopic images using neural network and mathematical morphology. *International Joint Conference SICE-ICASE*, (pp. 2312-2315). doi:10.1109/SICE.2006.315360

Rahman, M. M., Desai, B.C., & Bhattacharya, P. (2006). Supervised machine learning based medical image annotation and retrieval. In Accessing Multilingual Information Repositories (LNCS) (pp. 692–701). Berlin: Springer.

Ronneberger, O., Heimann, U., Schultz, E., Dietze, V., Burkhardt, H., & Gehrig, R. (2000). Automated pollen recognition using gray scale invariants on 3D volume image data. *Second European Symposium on Aerobiology*.

Schnorrenberg, F., Pattichis, C., Kyriacou, K., & Schizas, C. (1997). Computer-aided detection of breast cancer nuclei. *IEEE Transactions on Information Technology in Biomedicine*, *1*(2), 128–140. doi:10.1109/4233.640655 PMID:11020815

Shen, H., Hao, H., Wei, L., & Wang, Z. (2008, December). An image based classification method for cataract. *International Symposium on Computer Science and Computational Technology* (vol. 1, pp. 583-586). doi:10.1109/ISCSCT.2008.78

Singh, S. (2013). Microscopic Image Analysis of Nanoparticles by Edge Detection Using Ant Colony Optimization. *IOSR Journal of Computer Engineering*, *11*(3), 84–89. doi:10.9790/0661-1138489

Smitha, P., Shaji, L., & Mini, M. G. (2011). A review of medical image classification technique. In *International conference on VLSI, Communication & Intrumrnataiom*, (pp. 34-38).

Supardi, N. Z., Mashor, M. Y., Harun, N. H., Bakri, F. A., & Hassan, R. (2012). Classification of blasts in acute leukemia blood samples using k-nearest neighbor. *2012 IEEE 8th International Colloquium on Signal Processing and its Applications* (CSPA), (pp. 461-465). IEEE.

Sweidan, A. H., El-Bendary, N., Hassanien, A. E., Hegazy, O. M., & Mohamed, A. E.-K. (2015). Grey Wolf Optimizer and Case-Based Reasoning Model for Water Quality Assessment. *1st International Conference on Advanced Intelligent System and Informatics (AISI2015)*.

Tabesh, A., Teverovskiy, M., Pang, H. Y., Kumar, V. P., Verbel, D., Kotsianti, A., & Saidi, O. (2007). Multifeature prostate cancer diagnosis and Gleason grading of histological images. Medical Imaging. *IEEE Transactions on*, *26*(10), 1366–1378.

Wang, H., Zheng, C., Li, Y., Zhu, H., & Yan, X. (2003). Application of support vector machines to classification of blood cells. *Sheng Wu Yi Xue Gong Cheng Xue Za Zhi*, *20*(3), 484–487. PMID:14565019

Wang, M., Zhou, X., Li, F., Huckins, J., King, R. W., & Wong, S. T. C. (2008). Novel cell segmentation and online SVM for cell cycle phase identification in automated microscopy. *Bioinformatics (Oxford, England)*, *24*(1), 94–101. doi:10.1093/bioinformatics/btm530 PMID:17989093

Wei, N., You, J., Friehs, K., Flaschel, E., & Nattkemper, T. W. (2007). An in situ probe for on-line monitoring of cell density and viability on the basis of dark field micfroscopy in conjunction with image processing and supervised machine learning. *Biotechnology and Bioengineering*, *97*(6), 1489–1500. doi:10.1002/bit.21368 PMID:17274069

Yu, B. Y., Elbuken, C., Ren, C. L., & Huissoon, J. P. (2011). Image processing and classification algorithm for yeast cell morphology in a microfluidic chip. *Journal of Biomedical Optics*, *16*(6), 066008–066008. doi:10.1117/1.3589100 PMID:21721809

Zhang, J., Marszalek, M., Lazebnik, S., & Schmid, C. (2005). *Local features and kernels for classification of texture and object categories: A comprehensive study.* Technical Report RR-5737. Inria.

KEY TERMS AND DEFINITIONS

Classification: A topic of pattern recognition in computer vision. It is the analysis of the numerical properties of various image features and organizes data into categories.

Feature Extraction: The transforming the existing features into a lower dimensional space.

Feature Selection: The selection of a subset of the existing features without a transformation in order to decrease the dimensions and reduce the processing time.

Features: Inherent properties of data, independent of coordinate frames.

Image Analysis: The extraction of meaningful information from images; mainly from digital images by means of digital image processing techniques.

Image Processing: The analysis and manipulation of a digitized image, especially in order to improve its quality.

Supervised Classification: A parametric method requires an exhaustive training phase of the classifier parameters. It involves the act of obtaining the information class of data sets, and classifying the test data by identifying the training data which achieve best possible match.

Support Vector Machine (SVM): A binary classifier that classifies two classes by finding the maximum separating hyper plane between them.

Unsupervised Classification: The classification process which does not require training. It relies directly on the data to execute the classification process.

Chapter 2
An Overview of Machine Learning in Medical Image Analysis:
Trends in Health Informatics

Anand Narasimhamurthy
BITS Pilani – Hyderabad, India

ABSTRACT

Medical image analysis is an area which has witnessed an increased use of machine learning in recent times. In this chapter, the authors attempt to provide an overview of applications of machine learning techniques to medical imaging problems, focusing on some of the recent work. The target audience comprises of practitioners, engineers, students and researchers working on medical image analysis, no prior knowledge of machine learning is assumed. Although the stress is mostly on medical imaging problems, applications of machine learning to other proximal areas will also be elucidated briefly. Health informatics is a relatively new area which deals with mining large amounts of data to gain useful insights. Some of the common challenges in health informatics will be briefly touched upon and some of the efforts in related directions will be outlined.

INTRODUCTION

Machine Learning (ML) aspires to provide computational methods for accumulating, updating and changing knowledge in the intelligent systems and particular learning mechanisms that assist to induce knowledge from the data. It is useful in cases where direct algorithmic solutions are unavailable, there is lack of formal models, or the knowledge about the application domain is inadequately defined. Although the term machine learning is widely used, a precise definition is elusive. Wernick et al. (2010) define machine learning as a unified concept subsuming various important problems in statistical methods of automated decision making and modeling and being concerned with

DOI: 10.4018/978-1-5225-0140-4.ch002

1. The development of algorithms that quantify relationships within existing data, and
2. The use of these identified patterns to make predictions based on new data.

Machine learning is closely allied with disciplines such as pattern recognition and data mining; it utilizes techniques from areas such as numerical optimization and computational statistics. It is thus convenient to think of machine learning as an "umbrella" encompassing various methods and techniques. Figure 1 illustrates the overlap between the various disciplines taken from a data mining primer course SAS Institute offered in 1998. While this illustrates the considerable overlap between the various disciplines, considering that machine learning as well as the other allied disciplines are evolving continuously, we must expect the diagram to change almost year to year or even become irrelevant. Machine learning and data mining overlap significantly, many of the sub tasks and techniques are common; some authors prefer to make a distinction in that data mining is considered to focus more on exploratory analysis. Machine learning and pattern recognition can be considered as two facets of the same field (Bishop, 2006). In its initial phases at least, pattern recognition was considered as a spin-off of Artificial Intelligence (the diagram in Figure 1 also suggests this); however they have evolved along different directions, and it is fair to say that pattern recognition and artificial intelligence techniques in use at present are significantly different. Artificial Intelligence (AI) is predominantly rule based while pattern recognition tends to favor statistical methods. The techniques in these disciplines are not mutually exclusive though. Neural networks which were initially developed within the AI community are an integral part of pattern recognition. Deep Learning (Hinton, Osindero & Teh, 2006) can be considered as a modern update to Artificial Neural Networks, although the foundations date back to 1950s and 60s, there have been significant developments since 2006 and as a result Deep Learning methods are being used extensively in many applications.

A practical way to think of machine learning is in terms the tasks involved in an actual application. Almost all machine learning tasks include the steps of pre-processing and feature extraction. Pre-processing may include cleaning up noisy data, dealing with missing fields and other steps required to convert the raw data to a more suitable form. The feature extraction step consists of extracting and/or computing the required attributes relevant for the specific problem. Note that there may be additional computations applied to the data. These may include applying transformations, dimensionality reduction and feature selection to name

Figure 1. A diagram illustrating overlap between various disciplines

Source: Looking backwards, looking forwards: SAS, data mining, and machine learning, Polly Mitchell-Guthrie, August 22, 2014.

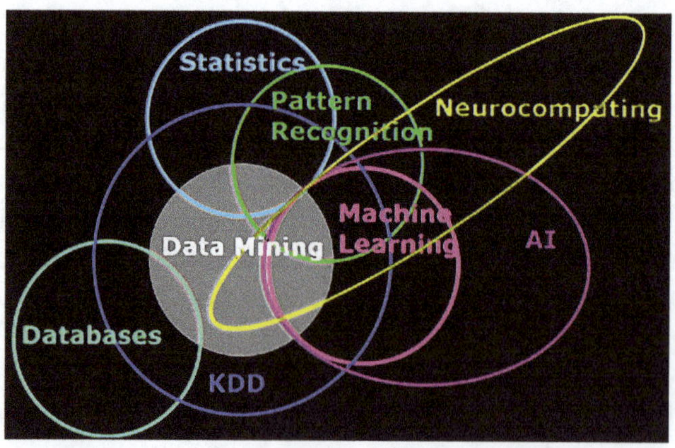

Figure 2. A schematic block diagram illustrating typical steps in classification, namely training/learning and test/classification steps

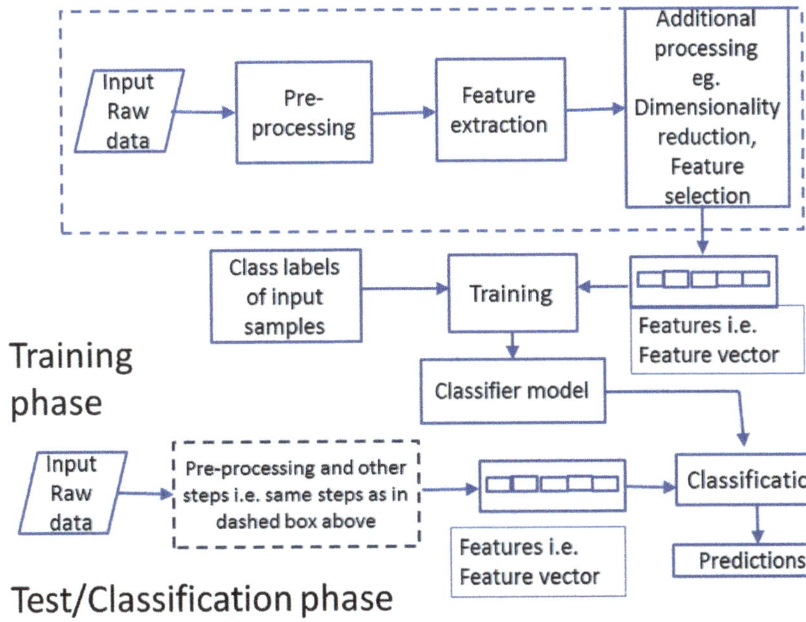

a few. Classification and clustering account for a large number of machine learning sub tasks. These fall under supervised and unsupervised learning methods respectively. In classification, there is a predefined set of class labels and the goal is to accurately assign the correct class label to a previously unseen instance. Figure 2 is a generic block diagram illustrating the typical steps in classification. The modules shown in the dash box are common steps in most machine learning applications. In addition to pre-processing and feature extraction, classification tasks additionally involve training and prediction. For training, the inputs are the feature vectors (obtained from the raw input data) and the class labels. The "trained" classifier model is then used to make predictions on new previously unseen data samples. Note that the same pre- processing and other steps need to be applied to the new unseen data also.

As a realistic example of classification, consider the problem of automatically identifying whether a lesion which has been imaged is benign or malignant, thus there are two predefined classes. Assume that images of lesions which have been annotated by an expert are available (note that the expert may have labelled them as benign or malignant, based on possibly other information and not necessarily just the image itself). In this case we say that training data (samples along with class labels) is available. Suppose an image of a lesion from a new patient is available, the goal is then to automatically predict correctly whether the lesion is benign or malignant. The machine learning task in this case is classification and the classifier "trained" using the available training data is used to make predictions on new test samples. Presumably attributes of the lesion such as shape characteristics, size etc. may be relevant for classifying a lesion, these are referred to as features and the process of computing these is referred to as "feature extraction". The output of the feature extraction step is a "feature vector", the order in which the attributes are stored matters. For example, assume that lesion is represented as <sh1,size1> where sh1 and size1 represent a shape and size attribute respectively for that lesion, another lesion2 should also be represented as <sh2,size2> and not say <size2,sh2> .

Figure 3. A toy example with simulated data illustrating classification; illustration of data which is (a) linearly separable (b) separable but not linearly separable

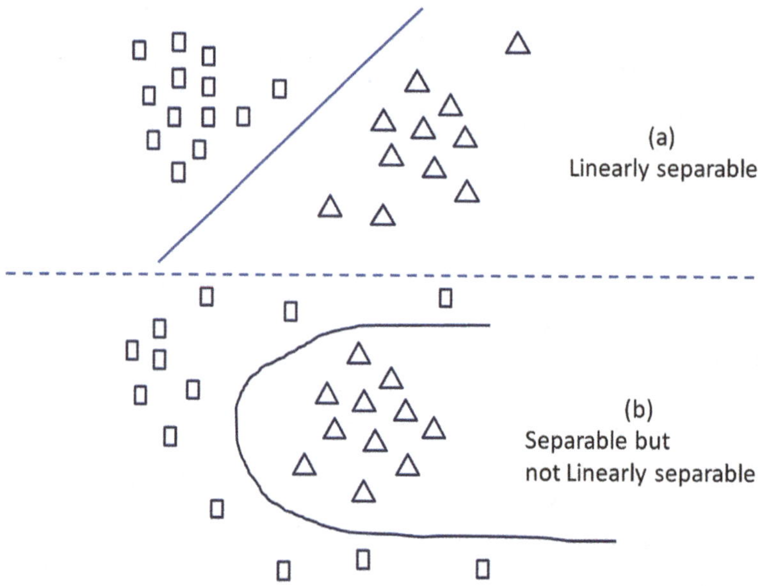

The feature vectors thus obtained can be thought of as either points or vectors in a high dimensional space (if there are more than three features, we cannot visualize this space however the relevant mathematical tools and techniques generalize to these high dimensional spaces). One can then simplistically think of the training procedure as figuring out where one draws the line (more generally a decision boundary) that "optimally" separates different classes. This is illustrated with a toy example with two classes in Figure 3. In general, the decision boundary could be non-linear as illustrated in Figure 3b. Also, note that unlike the toy examples shown in Figure 3, data may not be separable; in general the aim is to obtain a classifier model that provides a good trade-off between accuracy on training set and good generalization i.e. the ability to classify unseen test data well. The practical issues in this regard are highlighted in subsequent sections.

Unsupervised learning covers those tasks where there are no class labels, most often because there may not be a pre-defined set of classes. In fact often the goal is an exploratory analysis with the aim of finding out if there are any "natural" groups or clusters exhibited in the data. For instance, in the lesion image example above, one may want to group lesions based on how similar they are. The groups may indicate different broad classes of lesions for example. In the area of bioinformatics, in many experiments involving gene expression data, the first step is to group genes based on similarity of expression patterns. It can then be a basis for further investigation as to whether genes showing similar expression patterns are involved in similar functions. Clustering methods are widely used in these types of analyses. A wide variety of clustering approaches are available in the literature, two well-known methods are the k-means and hierarchical clustering. A large number of implementations of clustering methods are available; some require specifying the number of clusters as input, while others do not.

Medical image analysis is an area which has witnessed an increased use of machine learning in recent times. In the most recent edition of Medical Image Computing and Computer-Assisted Intervention (MICCAI), a premier conference in medical imaging, machine learning (8.3%) was one of the top five keywords among all submissions (others included segmentation (7.1%), MRI (6.6%) and CAD (4.9%)). This trend may be expected to continue at least into the near future as evidenced by special tracks in conferences (e.g. Machine Learning in Medical Imaging has been a track in MICCAI for six successive years), special topics courses offered in universities (e.g. Machine Learning in Medical Image and Signal Analysis offered in University of British Columbia) and research groups whose significant work focuses on machine learning for medical image analysis (examples include the Kenji Suzuki lab in University of Chicago and the Illinois Institute of Technology, Chicago).

Machine learning has been successfully applied to many medical image analysis applications such as Computer Aided Detection/Diagnosis (CADx/CADe) (e.g. (Roth et al., 2015); (Suzuki, Li, Sone & Doi, 2005); (Suzuki, Abe, MacMahon & Doi, 2006)), brain segmentation (Zhang, Brady & Smith,2001), localization (Criminisi et al., 2013) and various other tasks. Image registration and segmentation continue to be two major research areas in medical image analysis. Image registration is concerned with finding spatial/temporal correspondences between image data and/or models. ML has not been employed in a significant way for registration. There have, however, been studies in which manifold learning techniques have been used to pre-process image data, either prior to or alongside a more conventional registration method (Aljabar, Wolz & Rueckert, 2012). Image segmentation is concerned with identifying the boundaries of objects such as organs or abnormal regions (e.g. tumors) in images. While machine learning algorithms have been used either as the main component or as supportive tools to help to automate segmentation methods, recent applications of machine learning techniques to similar, related problems illustrate their potential. A few recent examples include localization of multiple anatomical structures within three-dimensional computed tomography (CT) scans using regression forests (Criminisi et al., 2013), cortical parcellation using spectral forests (Lombaert et al., 2015), automated pancreas segmentation using multi-level deep convolution networks (Roth et al., 2015) and carotid artery bifurcation detection on a head-neck CT dataset using a deep learning method (Zheng et al., 2015). It is fair to say that for people working on medical image analysis, machine learning methods would be a useful addition to their computational toolkit.

This chapter is organized as follows. In the Background section a broad overview of machine learning algorithms is provided. The main focus of this chapter is reviewing existing applications of machine learning to medical image analysis. It is difficult to cover in a single chapter, the breadth of machine learning applications even to well-known medical image analysis problems. Hence other related problems such as Content Based Image Retrieval, time series techniques and various other aspects related to the overall health care chain are not addressed here. The interested reader may consult a recent survey (Karaa & Dey, 2015) which covers various topics regarding image processing as a tool for disease identification and diagnosis. Another suggested reference is a recent survey which covers data mining techniques applied to processing of clinical data to detect cardiovascular diseases (Kausar et al., 2015).

While it is expected that machine learning will continue to play a useful role in medical imaging, it is to be noted that image data is only one type of information amongst a vast amount of possibly heterogeneous data. Mining useful and actionable information from heterogeneous data is a huge challenge; machine learning is expected to play a major role in this aspect. Accordingly, possible future directions are also outlined. Finally conclusions are presented.

BACKGROUND: MACHINE LEARNING TECHNIQUES

The aim of this section is to provide a bird's eye view of machine learning techniques and algorithms. Some of the general issues related to classification and clustering are discussed in the appendix. Categorization of machine learning algorithms is a difficult task, given the plethora of machine learning methods and also the many sub fields. Two useful ways of grouping are by the learning style or alternately by similarity in form or function (Brownlee, 2013). Figure 4 illustrates grouping by type of input data and learning style. A number of machine learning tasks can be subsumed under supervised and unsupervised learning. Supervised learning pertains to the situation where both the data and class labels are available i.e. annotated data is present. It encompasses tasks such as classification and regression. Classification is mainly concerned with discrete outputs; regression on the other hand is concerned with prediction of continuous valued outputs. Unsupervised learning is relevant to scenarios where no class labels are present, clustering is one of the main unsupervised learning tasks. Semi-supervised learning (Chapelle et al., 2006) can be regarded as "midway" between supervised and unsupervised learning. It refers to the scenario where there are a large number of data samples but only a small number of them have annotations or class labels. Other classes of learning techniques include reinforcement learning (this has strong connections with Artificial Intelligence), active learning, online learning, incremental learning and instance based learning.

Figure 4. A categorization of a few common machine learning tasks according to input data and "method of learning"

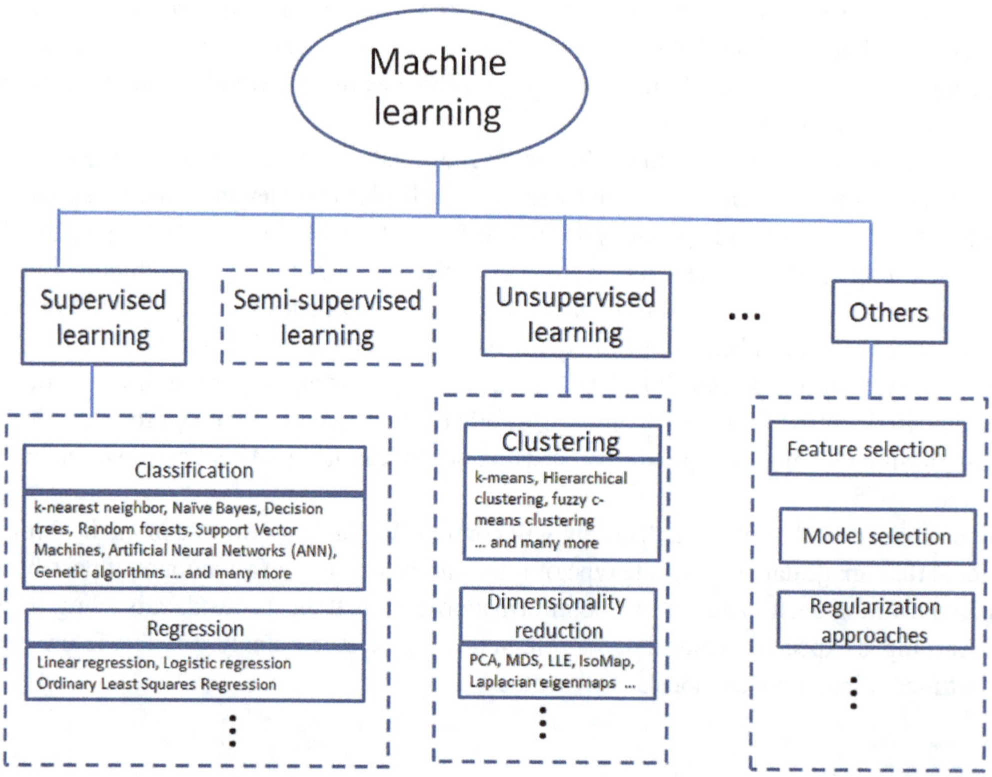

Table 1 illustrates grouping of some of the commonly used machine learning algorithms by similarity.

This is only intended to be representative but by no means exhaustive. Also the groupings are not mutually exclusive. For example, logistic regression can be used for both classification and regression. Similarly, the CART algorithm can be used to generate a decision tree for either classification or regression. In ensemble learning, the aim is to build an ensemble of predictors and combine the outputs in some way. Thus random forests can be categorized under ensemble algorithms, however they could also be grouped with decision trees since a random forest is an ensemble of decision trees. Algorithms related to time series analysis and other specialized applications such as text mining, natural language processing, recommender systems and so on have not been included; these areas have evolved into sub fields in their own right.

Table 1. A categorization of a few machine learning algorithms according to similarity in form

Category	Algorithms
Bayesian algorithms	• Naïve Bayes, Multinomial Naïve Bayes • Bayesian Network (BN) and Bayesian Belief Network (BBN)
Decision tree algorithms	• Classification and Regression Tree (CART) • Iterative Dichotomiser 3 (ID3) • C4.5 and C5.0 • Decision stump
Artificial Neural Network algorithms	• Perceptron • Back-propagation • Hopfield network
Deep learning algorithms	• Deep Boltzmann Machine (DBM) • Deep Belief Networks (DBN) • Convolutional Neural Network (CNN) • Stacked Auto-Encoders
Ensemble algorithms	• Boosting (e.g. AdaBoost) • Bagging • Gradient boosted Regression Trees (GBRT) • Random Forest
Instance based algorithms	• k-nearest neighbor (kNN) • Learning Vector Quantization (LVQ)
Regression algorithms	• Logistic regression • Multivariate Adaptive Regression Splines (MARS) • Ordinary Least Squares Regression (OLSR)
Clustering algorithms	• k-means • k-median • Hierarchical clustering • Expectation Maximization (EM)
Dimensionality reduction	• Principal Component Analysis (PCA) • Multidimensional scaling (MDS) • Local Linear Embedding (LLE)
Randomized search algorithms	• Simulated Annealing • Evolutionary algorithms e.g. Genetic Algorithms • Swarm Algorithms e.g. Particle Swarm Optimization, Ant Colony Optimization

MAIN FOCUS OF THE CHAPTER: MACHINE LEARNING APPLICATIONS IN MEDICAL IMAGE ANALYSIS

In this section a brief overview of the types of medical image analysis tasks where machine learning has been employed is provided. A few representative applications are summarized in Table 2, to provide an idea of the breadth of applications. This is by no means exhaustive and is a growing list since researchers continue to report results obtained using machine learning to their specific problems. In this context, an image refers to either a single 2D image or a 3D image volume depending on the context. Similarly the term pixel could either refer to a pixel or a voxel depending on the particular case.

CAD which encompasses CADe (Computer -Aided Detection) and CADx (Computer-Aided Diagnosis) has been a successful testbed as far as application of machine learning to medical image analysis is concerned. A suggested reference is (Suzuki, 2012a), it includes twenty contributed chapters mostly dealing with CAD and covering applications in breast, lung, brain, abdomen, and whole-body imaging.

Table 2. A small listing of applications of machine learning to medical image analysis problems

Reference	Broad Class of Problem/Modality	Details of Approach Used
(Roth et al., 2015)	Segmentation, abdominal computed tomography (CT) scans	A probabilistic bottom-up approach for pancreas segmentation using Multi-level deep convolutional networks (ConvNets).
(Wolterink et al., 2015)	Automatic coronary calcium scoring in non-contrast-enhanced ECG-triggered cardiac CT	• Features: Location features derived from estimated coronary artery positions, as well as size, shape and intensity features. • Both two class and multi class classifiers used. • Candidates that could not be labeled with high certainty were identified by entropy-based ambiguity detection and presented to an expert for review and possible relabeling. • System was evaluated with 530 test images.
(Zheng et al., 2015)	Method evaluated on head-neck CT data (3D). Approach is general and could potentially be applied anywhere.	• An efficient and robust deep learning algorithm capable of full 3D detection in volumetric data. • Deep learning based method. A shallow network (with one hidden layer) is used for the initial testing of all voxels to obtain a small number of promising candidates, followed by more accurate classification with a deep network. In addition, two approaches are proposed to speed up the evaluation of a network.
(Luo et al.,2014)	Liver segmentation, CT	A survey of various liver segmentation techniques in CT.
(Criminisi et al., 2013)	Localization, 3D CT	• Automatic detection and localization of multiple anatomical structures within three-dimensional computed tomography (CT) scans • Regression forests, an extension of random forest classifier used
(Xie & Tao, 2011)	White matter lesion segmentation from MR images. Inputs are T1, T2 and FLAIR images.	A fast, learning-based algorithm that only requires the user to provide a few regions of interest (ROI's) containing lesions.
(Xu et al.,2011)	CAD, CT colonography	False positive reduction in a CAD scheme for polyp detection
(Rubinov & Sporns, 2011)	rs-fMRI data	Characterization of complex functional brain networks using graph theoretic methods and complex network measures.
(Carneiro et al., 2008)	Ultrasound (fetal)	Automated segmentation & measurement of fetal anatomies
(Park et al.,2008)	Ultrasound (cardiac)	Automatic detection of view from cardiac ultrasound images
(Suzuki et al.,2006)	CAD, X ray	Automatic separation of ribs from soft tissue in chest X-rays (CXRs)
(Suzuki et al.,2005)	CAD, CT	Detection of lung nodules from CT images using Massive-Training Artificial Neural Networks (MTANN)

Localization and segmentation are common requirements in many medical image analysis scenarios. Image segmentation is concerned with identifying the boundaries of objects such as organs or abnormal regions (e.g. tumors) in images. Having the segmentation result enables shape analysis, detecting volume change, and making a precise radiation therapy treatment plan. The precision requirements vary depending on the actual application; in some applications only a gross localization of organs may be sufficient whereas in others a precise segmentation to within millimeter accuracy of anatomical structures may be required. Among some of the dominant mathematical models for segmentation are low level image feature based methods (thresholding, region growing, edge detection), Markov Random Fields (MRF) (Zhang et al., 2001) and deformable models (McInerney & Terzopoulos, 2008). There has been a significant amount of work related to liver segmentation from CT scans, many approaches including machine learning based ones have been used. A suggested reference on this topic is the survey by Luo et al. (Luo, 2014). Image registration may be atlas based or may involve matching two given image volumes. Applications of machine learning to registration are relatively few. A recent work uses a learning based approach for multi-modal US image registration (Oktay et al., 2015). A probabilistic edge map (PEM) image representation is generated from a structured decision forest (SDF). Learning the image representation from training data increases the robustness in US images and allows the registration to focus on the organs of interest. Other applications of machine learning to ultrasound data include automated view detection from cardiac images (Park, Zhou, Simopoulos & Comaniciu, 2008) and automated segmentation & measurement of fetal anatomies (Carneiro, Georgescu & Good, 2008).

Two crucial aspects in classification applications are the set of features and the choice of classifiers. The feature set is arguably more critical since a set of features without enough discriminative capability cannot yield good results even with sophisticated classifiers. Often times it may not be straightforward to articulate the feature set, even when there is good reason to believe that all the necessary information for classification is present in the image. In such situations when it is hard to articulate clear rules to classify, machine learning methods are a good choice, i.e. it is convenient to "throw data at the machine and let it figure it out". Such methods have been successfully used in many image processing tasks, for instance Moghaddam and Yang (2002) addressed the task of automatic gender classification from frontal face images using the Support Vector Machine (SVM) classifier. The images were preprocessed and reduced to a standard size, the pixel intensities in a pre-defined order formed the feature vector.

Pixel/voxel-based ML (PML) approaches have been used for various classification tasks in medical image analysis. These use as input information the pixel/voxel values in images directly instead of features calculated from segmented objects. It is claimed that pixel/voxel-based machine learning have advantages over the feature based machine learning, namely i) it can avoid errors caused by feature calculation and imprecise segmentation, ii) its performance can be better than common feature-based machine learning. In this class the advanced machine-learning techniques comprise neural edge enhancers, neural filters, convolution neural networks, massive training artificial neural networks, and shift-invariant neural networks. A suggested reference is a review article by Suzuki (Suzuki, 2012b) in which PMLs were surveyed and compared with each other as well as with other non-PML algorithms (i.e., ordinary feature-based classifiers) to make the similarities, differences, advantages and limitations clear.

The InnerEye research project spearheaded by Microsoft Research, Cambridge is one example of an enterprise level effort that employs machine learning for biomedical applications in a major way. It focuses on the automatic analysis of patients' medical scans. According to the description provided on their webpage *it uses state of the art machine learning techniques for the automatic delineation and measurement of healthy anatomy and anomalies, robust registration for monitoring disease progression, semantic navigation and visualization for improved clinical workflow and development of natural user interfaces for medical practitioners.*

An example of the work within this group is automatic detection and localization of multiple anatomical structures within three-dimensional computed tomography (CT) scans using regression forests (Criminisi et al., 2013). They use regression forests which are similar to the more popular classification forests, but trained to predict continuous, multi-variate outputs, where the training focuses on maximizing the confidence of output predictions. An extension of Random Decision Forests algorithm via improving its spatial representation with spectral features was used for cortical parcellation (Lombaert et al.,2015). Lombaert et al. report accuracy equivalent to the state of the art tool FreeSurfer in a fraction of its time (23 seconds versus 3 to 4 hours) for their data.

Graph based analysis is quickly becoming part of mainstream machine learning. A graph is a simple, yet powerful data structure; typically the nodes represent individual entities and edges between a pair of nodes represent strength of relationship between them. Although graph theory itself is not new and graphs have been extensively studied by mathematicians, computer scientists and others; graph based analysis is finding application in various tasks such as mining social network or mobile call subscriber data where a graph is a natural representation of the data. Complex network analysis has evolved as a research area in its own right. A small, non-exhaustive list of established topics in complex network analysis includes node centrality measures, identifying hubs and critical nodes, community detection, quantifying hierarchy and substructure within a graph analysis at different scales of a network and estimating the controllability of a system. Graph theoretic methods have been widely used in analysis of functional MRI (f-MRI) data. Graphs form a good abstraction and representation for brain connectivity where the nodes represent neural elements (neurons, brain regions etc.) and the edges represent some measure of structural or functional connectivity between nodes. Resting state functional connectivity MRI (rs-fcMRI), which measures spontaneous low-frequency fluctuations in blood oxygen level dependent (BOLD) signal in subjects at rest, has attracted particular attention for its ability to measure correlations in neural activity (via BOLD signal) between distant brain regions. Graph theoretic approaches are a natural and attractive choice for rs-fcMRI analysis since graph theoretic analyses can model properties at the level of the entire graph, subgraphs, or individual nodes, and because the brain itself is a complex network (Power et al., 2012). Although other approaches can be used, one of the most powerful and flexible approaches is the graph theoretic approach (Bullmore & Sporns, 2009; Rubinov & Sporns, 2011).

A significant body of literature has focused on understanding connectivity at a somewhat global level, often using established graph metrics. While a number of graph based metrics such as the clustering coefficient capture connectivity at a global level (integrated view), often it is necessary to examine changes at the local level (segregated view). One example of alteration in brain connectivity is the development of re-routings that restore functionality typically after a local injury. This may be especially important in the studies related to Traumatic Brain Injury (TBI). While graph theoretic concepts have been extensively used for understanding of brain connectivity, other models have also been applied.

Varoquaux et al. (2012) use Markov models in their fMRI study. Specifically, they examine the Markov structure of the fMRI signal to find realistic assumptions on the connectivity structure that are required to explain the observed functional connectivity. In particular they seek a decomposition of the Markov structure into segregated functional networks using decomposable graphs: a set of strongly-connected and partially overlapping cliques. They claim that their results highlight that Markov models are good tools to identify the structure of brain connectivity from fMRI signals, but for this purpose they must reflect the small-world properties of the underlying neural systems.

In addition to applications such as the above, graph based analysis is being applied in an increasing number of scenarios where there is a large amount of heterogeneous data. This is a common occurrence in hospitals where different types of patient data are stored; this may include scans, blood reports and patient examination data. While traditional database models are quite powerful, they are more suited for structured data. There have been a few efforts to deal with unstructured data by using graph based methods; in fact there are a few commercial graph databases. A couple of examples include the Neo4j by Neo Technology and the uRiKA graph database appliance by YarcData (established in 2012 as a division of Cray Inc.).

DISCUSSION

It is often difficult to choose the appropriate method for a particular task, given the vast and growing number of machine learning techniques available. While machine learning offers great potential it is important to understand the types of problems and scenarios tailor made for application of machine learning techniques and understand the suitability of these techniques for a given problem. Although it is nearly impossible to provide an exhaustive guide, a few suggestions are offered.

Among the broad medical imaging tasks, CADx/CADe tasks are most amenable for formulating as machine learning problems and thus ML has been applied extensively. In fact in the most recent MICCAI conference, there was one parallel track on Computer Aided Diagnosis focusing on Machine Learning.

Amongst other problems, registration is far less amenable for ML methods; thus ML may be used only in a supporting role. ML methods however may be useful in multi-modal registration (e.g. Oktay et al., 2015). For segmentation tasks, depending on precision required, a hybrid approach may be suitable i.e. a fast but less precise method such as graph cut or PML based method followed by a more precise but computationally expensive technique such as the Chan-Vese model (Chan & Vese, 2001) or a level set (Osher & Sethian, 1988) based method. Although a number of extensions have helped to significantly speed up these latter methods, they still require a good initialization which could be provided by the former. ML approaches could be useful for fast localization of gross structures in whole body or scout scans, these could serve as initialization for organ-specific processing. Criminisi et al. (2013) were able to achieve automatic detection and localization of multiple anatomical structures within three-dimensional computed tomography (CT) scans in typical run-times of only about 4 s on a conventional single-core machine.

Implications Related to Availability of Annotated Data

Supervised learning approaches typically require a large number of training samples, i.e. in terms of medical data a relatively large number of annotated samples which may not be available in many situations. In situations where the number of annotated samples is small but a large amount of unannotated data is available, semi-supervised learning is an option.

A relatively common situation in the medical scenario is the availability of a large amount of data but very few annotated samples (it is either too tedious or expensive to get expert annotation and hence it may be realistic to annotate only a small number of samples). A class of machine learning techniques known as semi-supervised learning as outlined in an earlier section is suitable for such a situation. While there have been successful applications of semi-supervised learning, generally more data is better; caution needs to be exercised. One example from the literature that takes a cautionary view of semi-supervised learning is the work of Cozman and Cohen (2006). They study the effect of modeling errors in semi-supervised learning, and show how modeling errors can lead to performance degradation. Among other researchers who have suggested a more measured approach, one suggestion is using unlabeled data only if the classifier obtained using labeled data is poor.

Suggestions for Classification Problems

A number of medical image analysis problems, especially CADx/CADe ones can be formulated as classification problems. A variety of classifiers are available, ranging from simple ones such as the k-nearest neighbor, Linear Discriminant Analysis (LDA), Naïve Bayes to more sophisticated ones such as Artificial Neural Networks, Genetic Algorithms (Holland,1975), Decision trees (Breiman & Friedman,1984), Support Vector Machines(SVM) (Vapnik,1995), AdaBoost (Freund & Schapire, 1999), Random forests (Breiman,2001) and Convolutional Neural Networks (CNN) (Krizhevsky, Sutskever & Hinton, 2013) . A detailed discussion is out of scope, accordingly the advantages/disadvantages of well-known classifiers are summarized in Table 3. Table 4 summarizes choices of classifiers according to criteria often dictated by the applications. For instance, many machine learning algorithms are "black boxes", while this may not be a concern in many applications, some "transparency" is desirable especially in biomedical applications i.e. it is not only important to arrive at the correct prediction but also be able to explain how or why that prediction was made. This influences the choice of features as well as classifier. If interpretability is a primary concern, decision tree or rule based classifiers are preferable; else powerful but "black-box" classifiers such as deep networks based ones or ensemble learning methods such as boosting or random forests can be used along with "weak" features. The "weak" features could either be easy to compute image features or pixel intensities as in PML methods.

FUTURE RESEARCH DIRECTIONS

It is to be expected that challenges in medical image analysis will persist and may require either extensions of existing techniques or novel approaches to address them. However, medical imaging is one part of the overall healthcare system. This may include anything from optimizing hospital schedules, post operative care, workflow improvements and so on. Health informatics is a relatively new area which deals with mining large amounts of data to gain useful insights. As defined by the U.S. National Library of Medicine, health informatics is the interdisciplinary study of the design, development, adoption, and application of IT-based innovations in healthcare services delivery, management, and planning. Invariably, large volumes of data need to be dealt with. This poses its own challenges, it may necessitate significant changes to existing approaches and sometimes redesigning ground up.

Table 3. Advantages/limitations of a few common classification techniques

Algorithm	Advantages	Limitations
Naïve Bayes	• Simple to implement and low computation overhead. • Can naturally deal with a mix of categorical and continuous features.	A simplistic classifier, may not capture complex decision surfaces, however often does well in practice.
k- nearest neighbour (kNN)	Training overhead is minimal.	• Not suitable where the data is high dimensional • Classification computation time is high.
Decision Trees	• Interpretability: Decision path taken for a particular sample is clearly interpretable. • Can naturally deal with a mix of categorical and continuous features.	• Tend to overfit. • If new training data is added and the algorithm is run, the decision tree could be completely different.
Random forests	• Much less prone to overfitting as compared to decision trees. • Can deal with uneven data sets that have missing variables. • Performs a feature selection as part of the algorithm itself, thus indicating which features provide good discrimination.	Classification result not as interpretable as in decision trees.
Support Vector Machine (SVM)	• Can deal with high dimensional data. • Provide good generalization capability. • Problem is convex. No local minima issues.	Limited interpretability. Although the support vectors may yield some insight, it is essentially a "black box" with regard to how a classification decision was made.
Artificial Neural Networks (ANN)	Can handle large amount of data; it has the ability to implicitly detect complex nonlinear relationships between dependent and independent variables.	• Prone to overfitting. • Mostly a "black box", very limited interpretability.
Deep learning	Capable of learning with large amounts of data. Are being increasingly used successfully in a wide variety of applications.	Mostly a "black box", very limited or no interpretability.
Genetic algorithms	Useful when the search space is very large and the function is non-convex.	• Convergence properties hard to prove. • No guarantees on goodness of solution with respect to the optimal solution.

Table 4. A listing of classifier choices depending on criteria (often dictated by the application)

Criteria	Classifier Choices
High dimensional data i.e. the number of features is large relative to number of samples.	• Instance based classifiers such as kNN methods may not work well. In general, density based methods are more severely affected by "curse of dimensionality" • Classifiers such as SVM are more suited for high dimensional data. Random forests and deep learning methods have been demonstrated on large data with many features.
Presence of categorical features	• Classifiers such as Naïve Bayes, Decision Tree and Random Forests can naturally deal with a mix of numerical and categorical features. • If other classifiers are preferred, one alternative is to combine the categorical features to form an additional numerical feature.
Interpretability vs black box	Many powerful classifiers such as Artificial Neural Networks and Deep Learning methods are "black boxes". If interpretability is a prime concern, following classifiers are good choices. • Decision trees • rule-based classifiers

While some of the health informatics problems may be suitable for application of machine learning, there are a number of challenges that need to be first surmounted. For instance, the exercise of meaningfully collating all the information related to a patient is still a big challenge. Although there are a few standardizations within PACS (Picture archiving and communication system) which allow for storing images from different modalities, in a typical hospital set up even seamlessly retrieving all relevant scans in say, a one year period along with patient history and displaying the information meaningfully is often a difficult proposition. Add to this, apart from imaging data, a significant amount of patient related data is often recorded to the extent of even genomic data becoming available. Aside from the large volume of data, the heterogeneity and other aspects pose significant challenges.

A significant amount of data is stored electronically as structured or unstructured text. Text mining now regarded as a specialty area in ML, focuses on extracting interesting and useful knowledge from textual data. The data could either be patient data recorded within a hospital system or more generally, archives of biomedical literature. Mining literature can be useful for medical researchers and doctors who want to identify whether cases similar to one they have encountered have been reported earlier. Another use is to identify information about particular genes and correlate them with results of an experiment. Thus there is a constant need for tools for automatic extraction of knowledge from large and growing volume of literature. An example of a recent work is an extension of genetic algorithm combined with a vector space model and an agglomorative algorithm for clustering abstracts in MEDLINE, the largest biomedical literature database (Karaa et al.,2015).

Correlating text data (e.g. patient reports) with image data (e.g. patient scans) is a challenging problem.

The Data Analytics for Medicine using Semi-Supervised Learning (DAMSEL) project (Beckerman, 2009) shown in Figure 5 is an example of an effort aimed at integrating multimodal data. It was created with the intention of addressing some of the existing gaps in technology for multi-modal data analytics. It involved the creation of a multi-modal architecture and tools for the analysis of biomedical data, including images and test reports. The target applications include mammography and abdominal aortic aneurysm (AAA). DAMSEL employs semi-supervised learning and incorporates both image analysis and text analysis methods along with a scalable architecture.

A possible route for addressing the various challenges is to adapt existing technologies to the particular scenario. One such example has been the adaptation of Kinect, Microsoft's touchless technology developed for gaming, to surgery. In many surgeries, a surgeon will need to consult medical images anywhere from once an hour to every few minutes. Surgeons have to either leave the operating room and scrub in again or rely on assistants to manipulate the computer for them. Thus a touchless technology such as Kinect would be of great advantage in sterile environments such as an operating theatre. Trials of Kinect were conducted by a surgeon at Guy's and St Thomas' hospital (Campbell, 2012). The initial trials were welcomed and assessments were optimistic. John Brennan, British Society for Endovascular Therapy opined that it is difficult to think of operating rooms in ten or 15 years' time where such advancements were just not the norm (Brimelow, 2012). It remains to be seen however how much and how soon such advancements will be adapted by the surgery community.

In this day and age no discussion is complete without at least a mention of Big Data. It is relatively common to have massive amounts of data running into peta and exa bytes. On the data analytics front, it appears at least at the moment that Big Data and Cloud computing technologies will continue to be a driving force for many application domains in the coming years. This is not surprising, given that most present day applications produce an enormous amount of data continuously. Big data is a broad term referring to a collection of information that is vast and complex and cannot be handled by traditional data processing tools. Apart from the enormous volume of data, the other challenges associated with Big Data are velocity and variety. Velocity refers to the speed at which data is continuously accumulated. Variety reflects the heterogeneous nature of the data; it could be a mix of structured and unstructured data and of different types/formats which are not easily integrated. Some people add a fourth V, namely veracity, namely that it is extremely difficult to perform quality control on such vast amounts of data.

Figure 5. A block diagram of the DAMSEL project
(Beckerman, 2009).

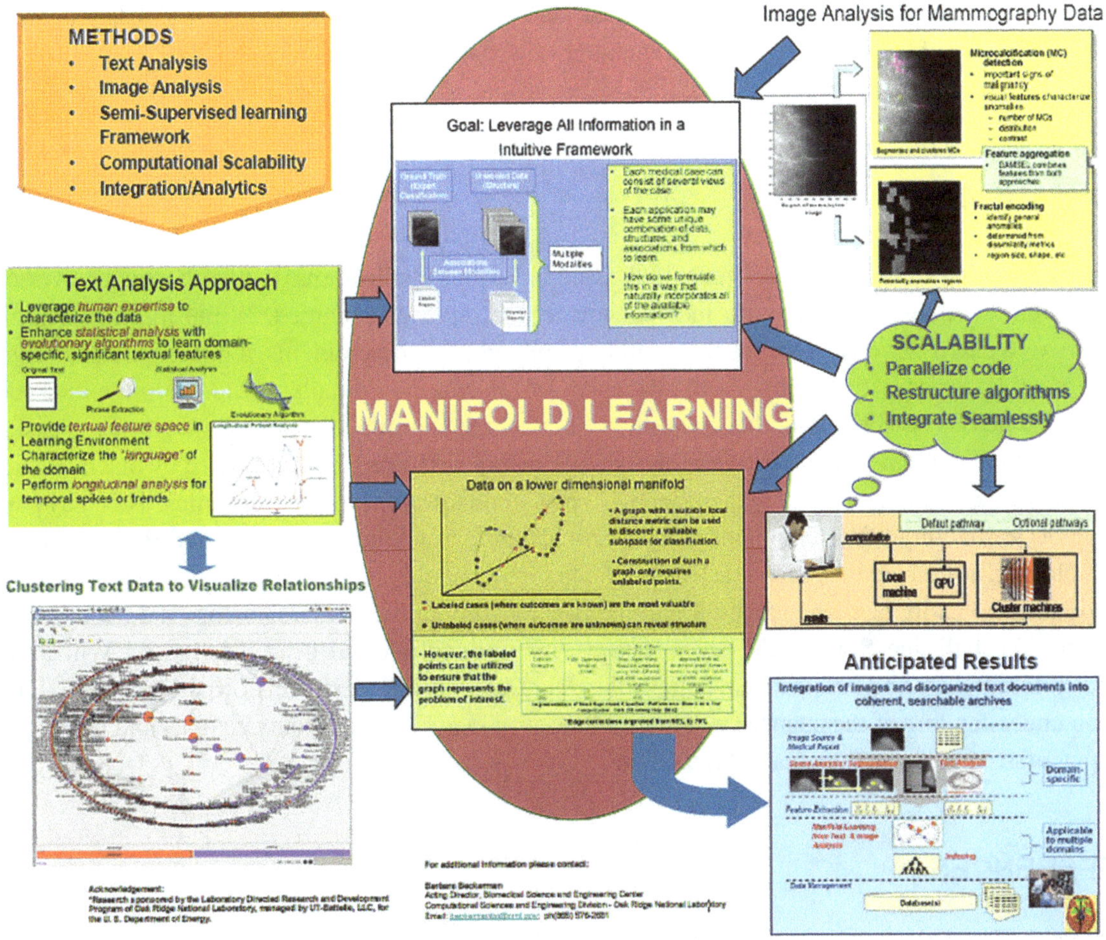

It is believed that Big Data has tremendous potential and there are a number of initiatives in leveraging Big Data for better health care. A major push in health care is the US is fueled by a $40 billion federal government effort to urge health care practitioners to have electronic records. Mayo Clinic, one of the largest private health systems in the USA, sees the emerging field of big data analytics as a crucial strategy to defend and reinforce its standing as an elite medical institution (Crosby,2014). Mayo Clinic has made a concerted effort to leverage Big Data; one prominent example is their Optum Labs project which is a partnership between Mayo and UnitedHealth, a $122 billion insurance corporation. Since the launch of the project, a growing number of partners have joined. The scale of the effort and the potential are immense. United Health contributed 20 years of its claims records on 150 million people to the project which in turn will be linked to medical records of Mayo and other entities. This opens up new avenues, for instance it is possible to track patients even after they have left Mayo after treatment because claim records follow people even when they move across health systems. This enables tracking long-term outcomes and could provide insights into providing accessible quality health care while keeping the cost reasonable. A demand for data scientists across various domains including medical domain is expected at least for the next few years. Health informatics may need additional specialized skills and an inter disciplinary approach to tap the vast potential. While the vast amount of data offers immense potential, one must be mindful of the pitfalls. Michael I. Jordan, Pehong Chen Distinguished Professor at the University of California, Berkeley in an interview warned of the dangers due to over eagerness in in dealing with big data (Gomes, 2014).

CONCLUSION

Machine learning techniques have been widely used in various applications. In this chapter, an overview of machine learning applications to medical image analysis was provided. While machine learning comprises a useful set of techniques that could be applied to many problems, a good understanding of the strengths and limitations along with awareness of the common pitfalls would equip the individual to make judicious choices about the suitability of a machine learning technique for a particular task.

While challenges in medical image analysis will continue to be present (addressed by machine learning or other methods), increasingly there seems to be a trend towards health informatics. This may partly be due to availability of vast amounts of data and also due to Cloud Computing and Big Data driven technological advancements. Machine learning/data mining could play a key role in this scenario. Health informatics poses its own challenges. Dealing with vast amounts of heterogeneous data continues to present a big challenge. Some of the ongoing efforts in this direction were briefly discussed. While many eminent researchers and practitioners believe that Big Data has immense transformative potential, here too an understanding of the nuances would go a long way in avoiding spurious insights and help realize the potential of the vast amounts of "rich" data.

REFERENCES

Aljabar, P., Wolz, R., & Rueckert, D. (2012). Manifold Learning for Medical Image Registration, Segmentation, and Classification. In K. Suzuki (Ed.), *Machine Learning in Computer-Aided Diagnosis: Medical Imaging Intelligence and Analysis*. IGI Global. doi:10.4018/978-1-4666-0059-1.ch017

BBC News. (2012, May 31). Retrieved from http://www.bbc.com/news/health-18238356

Beckerman, B., Patton, R., Symons, C., McMillan, A., Gleason, S., Kerekes, R., ... Nishikawa, R. (2009). *An Overview of the Data Analytics for Medicine Using Semi-Supervised learning (DAMSEL) Program.* Paper presented at the First Annual ORNL Biomedical Science & Engineering Conference, Chicago, IL.

Bishop, C. M. (2006). *Pattern Recognition and Machine Learning*. Springer.

Breiman, L. (2001). Random forests. *Machine Learning*, *45*(1), 5–32. doi:10.1023/A:1010933404324

Breiman, L., Friedman, J. H., Olshen, R. A., & Stone, C. J. (1984). *Classification and Regression Trees.* Chapman & Hall.

Brimelow, A. (2012). *Trial of "touchless" gaming technology in surgery.* Academic Press.

Brownlee, J. (2013). *A Tour of Machine Learning Algorithms.* Retrieved from http://machinelearningmastery.com/a-tour-of-machine-learning-algorithms/

Bullmore, E., & Sporns, O. (2009). Complex brain networks: Graph theoretical analysis of structural and functional systems. *Nature Reviews. Neuroscience*, *10*(3), 186–198. doi:10.1038/nrn2575 PMID:19190637

Campbell, M. (2012). Kinect imaging lets surgeons keep their focus. *New Scientist.* Retrieved from https://www.newscientist.com/article/mg21428655.200-kinect-imaging-lets-surgeons-keep-their-focus

Carneiro, G., Georgescu, B., & Good, S. (2008). *Knowledge-based Automated Fetal Biometrics.* SIEMENS White Paper.

Chan, T., & Vese, L. (2001). Active contours without edges. *IEEE Transactions on Image Processing*, *10*(2), 266–277. doi:10.1109/83.902291 PMID:18249617

Chapelle, O. A. (Ed.). (2006). *Semi-Supervised Learning.* MIT Press.

Chawla, N. V. (2002). Synthetic Minority Over-sampling Technique. *Journal of Artificial Intelligence Research*, *16*, 321–357.

Cozman, F., & Cohen, I. (2006). Risks of Semi-Supervised Learning. In O. Chapelle, B. Schölkopf, & A. Zien (Eds.), *Semi-Supervised Learning, September 2006.* MIT Press.

Criminisi, A., Robertson, D., Konukoglu, E., Shotton, J., Pathak, S., White, S., & Siddiqui, K. (2013). Regression Forests for Efficient Anatomy Detection and Localization in Computed Tomography Scans. In *Medical Image Analysis (MedIA).* Elsevier.

Crosby, J. (2014). Mayo seeks to dominate with data. *Star Tribune.* Retrieved from http://www.startribune.com/mayo-seeks-to-dominate-with-data/285132621/

Dudoit, S., & Fridyyand, J. (2002). A prediction-based resampling method for estimating the number of clusters in a dataset. *Genome Biology, 3*(7).

Dunn, J. (1974). Well Separated Clusters and Optimal Fuzzy Partitions. *Cybernetics*, *4*(1), 95–104. doi:10.1080/01969727408546059

Fowlkes, E. B., & Mallows, C. L. (1983). A method for comparing two hierarchical clusterings. *Journal of the American Statistical Association*, *78*(383), 553–584. doi: doi:10.1080/01621459.1983.10478008

Freund, Y., & Schapire, R. (1999). A Short Introduction to Boosting. *Journal of Japanese Society for Artificial Intelligence*, *14*(5), 771–780.

Gomes, L. (2014). *Machine-Learning Maestro Michael Jordan on the Delusions of Big Data and Other Huge Engineering Efforts, Big-data boondoggles and brain-inspired chips are just two of the things we're really getting wrong.* IEEE Spectrum.

Hartigan, J. A. (1975). *Clustering Algorithms.* New York, NY: John Wiley & Sons.

Hinton, G., Osindero, S., & Teh, Y. W. (2006). A fast learning algorithm for deep belief nets. *Neural Computation*, *18*(7), 1527–1554. doi:10.1162/neco.2006.18.7.1527 PMID:16764513

Holland, J. H. (1975). *Adaptation in Natural and Artificial Systems.* University of Michigan Press.

Jain, A. K., & Dubes, R. C. (1988). *Algorithms for Clustering Data*. Englewood Cliffs, NJ: Prentice-Hall.

Karaa, W. B. A., Ashour, A. S., Sassi, D. B., Roy, P., Kausar, N., & Dey, N. (2015). MEDLINE Text Mining: An Enhancement Genetic Algorithm based Approach for Document Clustering. In E. Hassanien, C. Grosan, & M. Fahmy Tolba (Eds.), *Applications of Intelligent Optimization in Biology and Medicine: Current Trends and Open Problems* (pp. 267–287). Springer International Publishing.

Karaa, W. B. A., & Dey, N. (Eds.). (2015). *Biomedical Image Analysis and Mining Techniques for Improved Health Outcomes*. Idea Group.

Kaufman, L., & Rousseeuw, P. J. (1990). *Finding Groups in Data: An Introduction to Cluster Analysis*. New York: Wiley. doi:10.1002/9780470316801

Kausar, N., Palaniappan, S., Al Ghamdi, B. S., Samir, B. B., Dey, N., & Abdullah, A. (2015). Systematic Analysis of Applied Data Mining Based Optimization Algorithms in Clinical Attribute Extraction and Classification for Diagnosis of Cardiac Patients. In A. Hassanien, C. Grosan, & M. F. Tolba (Eds.), *Applications of Intelligent Optimization in Biology and Medicine* (Vol. 96, pp. 217–231). Dordrecht: Springer. doi:10.1007/978-3-319-21212-8_9

Krizhevsky, A., Sutskever, I., & Hinton, G. (2012). ImageNet Classification with Deep Convolutional Neural Networks. *Advances in Neural Information Processing Systems*, *25*, 1–14.

Lombaert, H., Criminisi, A., & Ayache, N. (2015). Spectral Forests: Learning of Surface Data, Application to Cortical Parcellation, In *Proceedings of 18th International Conference on Medical Image Computing and Computer-Assisted Intervention (MICCAI)* (LNCS), (vol. 9349, pp. 547-556). Springer. doi:10.1007/978-3-319-24553-9_67

Luo, S., Li, X., & Li, J. (2014). Review on the Methods of Automatic Liver Segmentation from Abdominal Images. *Journal of Computer and Communications*, *2*(02), 1–7. doi:10.4236/jcc.2014.22001

McInerney, T., & Terzopoulos, D. (2008). Deformable Models. In I. Bankman (Ed.), *Handbook of Medical Image Processing and Analysis* (2nd ed.; pp. 145–166). San Diego, CA: Academic Press.

Moghaddam, B., & Yang, M. H. (2002). Learning Gender with Support Faces. *IEEE Transactions on Pattern Analysis and Machine Intelligence*, *24*(5), 707–711. doi:10.1109/34.1000244

Muller, U., Ligges, M., Georgiewa, P., Grnling, C., Kaiser, W. A., Witte, H., & Blanz, B. (2002). How to Avoid Spurious Cluster Validation? A Methodological Investigation on Simulated and fMRI Data. *NeuroImage, 17*, 431–446.

Oktay, O., Schuh, A., Rajchl, M., Keraudren, K., Gomez, A., Heinrich, M. P., & Rueckert, D. et al. (2015). Structured Decision Forests for Multi-modal Ultrasound Image Registration. In *Proceedings of 18th International Conference on Medical Image Computing and Computer-Assisted Intervention (MICCAI)*, (LNCS), (vol. 9349, pp. 363–372). Springer. doi:10.1007/978-3-319-24571-3_44

Osher, S., & Sethian, J. A. (1988). Fronts Propagating with Curvature-Dependent Speed: Algorithms Based on Hamilton-Jacobi Formulations. *Journal of Computational Physics*, *79*(1), 12–49. doi:10.1016/0021-9991(88)90002-2

Park, J. H., Zhou, S. K., Simopoulos, C., & Comaniciu, D. (2008). AutoGate: Fast and Automatic Doppler gate localization in B-mode echocardiogram, In *Proceedings of 11th International Conference on MICCAI* (LNCS), (vol. 5242, pp. 230-237). Springer Verlag Berlin Heidelberg. doi:10.1007/978-3-540-85990-1_28

Power, J. D., Cohen, A. L., Nelson, S. M., Wig, G. S., Barnes, K. A., Church, J. A., & Petersen, S. E. et al. (2011). Functional network organization of the human brain. *Neuron*, *72*(4), 665–678. doi:10.1016/j.neuron.2011.09.006 PMID:22099467

Rand, W. M. (1971). Objective criteria for the evaluation of clustering methods. *Journal of American Statisitics Association*, *66*(336), 846–850. doi:10.1080/01621459.1971.10482356

Roth, H. R., Lu, L., Farag, A., Shin, H., Liu, J., Turkbey, E. B., & Summers, R. M. (2015). DeepOrgan: Multi-level Deep Convolutional Networks for Automated Pancreas Segmentation. In *Proceedings of 18th International Conference on Medical Image Computing and Computer-Assisted Intervention (MICCAI)*, (LNCS), (vol. 9349, pp. 556–564). Springer. doi:10.1007/978-3-319-24553-9_68

Rubinov, M., & Sporns, O. (2011). Weight-conserving characterization of complex functional brain networks. *NeuroImage*, *56*(4), 2068–2079. doi:10.1016/j.neuroimage.2011.03.069 PMID:21459148

Suzuki, K. (Ed.). (2012a). *Machine Learning in Computer-Aided Diagnosis: Medical Imaging Intelligence and Analysis*. Hershey, PA: IGI Global.

Suzuki, K. (2012b). Pixel-based Machine-Learning in Medical Imaging. *International Journal of Biomedical Imaging*. PMID:22481907

Suzuki, K., Abe, H., MacMahon, H., & Doi, K. (2006). Image-processing technique for suppressing ribs in chest radiographs by means of massive training artificial neural network (MTANN). *IEEE Transactions on Medical Imaging*, *25*(4), 406–416. doi:10.1109/TMI.2006.871549 PMID:16608057

Suzuki, K., Li, F., Sone, S., & Doi, K. (2005). Computer-aided diagnostic scheme for distinction between benign and malignant nodules in thoracic low-dose CT by use of massive training artificial neural network. *IEEE Transactions on Medical Imaging*, *24*(9), 1138–1150. doi:10.1109/TMI.2005.852048 PMID:16156352

Vapnik, V. N. (1995). *The Nature of Statistical Learning Theory*. Springer-Verlag. doi:10.1007/978-1-4757-2440-0

Varoquaux, G., Gramfort, A., Poline, J. B., & Thirion, B. (2012). *Markov models for fMRI correlation structure: is brain functional connectivity small world, or decomposable into networks? Journal of Physiology*.

Wernick, M. N., Yang, Y., Brankov, J. G., Yourganov, G., & Strother, S. C. (2010). Machine learning in medical imaging: Drawing conclusions from medical images. *IEEE Signal Processing Magazine*, *27*(July), 25–38. doi:10.1109/MSP.2010.936730 PMID:25382956

Wolterink, J. M., Leiner, T., Takx, R. A., Viergever, M. A., & Isgum, I. (2015). Automatic Coronary Calcium Scoring in Non-Contrast-Enhanced ECG-Triggered Cardiac CT with Ambiguity Detection. *IEEE Transactions on Medical Imaging*, *34*(9), 1867–1878. doi:10.1109/TMI.2015.2412651 PMID:25794387

Xie, Y., & Tao, X. (2011). White Matter Lesion Segmentation Using Machine Learning and Weakly Labeled MR Images, In *Proceedings of SPIE Medical Imaging 2011*, (vol. 7962) doi:10.1117/12.878237

Xu, J. W., & Suzuki, K. (2011). Massive-training support vector regression and Gaussian process for false-positive reduction in computer-aided detection of polyps in CT colonography. *Medical Physics*, *38*(4), 1888–1902. doi:10.1118/1.3562898 PMID:21626922

Zhang, Y., Brady, M., & Smith, S. (2001). Segmentation of brain MR images through a hidden Markov random field model and the expectation-maximization algorithm. *IEEE Transactions on Medical Imaging*, *20*(1), 45–57. doi:10.1109/42.906424 PMID:11293691

Zheng, Y., Liu, D., Georgescu, B., Nguyen, H., & Comaniciu, D. (2015). 3D Deep Learning for Efficient and Robust Landmark Detection in Volumetric Data. In *Proceedings of 18th International Conference on Medical Image Computing and Computer-Assisted Intervention (MICCAI)* (LNCS), (vol. 9349, pp. 565–572). Springer. doi:10.1007/978-3-319-24553-9_69

KEY TERMS AND DEFINITIONS

Big Data: An evolving term generally used to refer to data so large or complex that traditional data processing applications are insufficient. Usually characterized by three Vs, namely volume, variety, velocity. These terms describe the usual challenges associated with big data. Some people add a fourth V, namely veracity as an additional challenge.

CAD: A term that encompasses CADe (Computer -Aided Detection) and CADx (Computer-Aided Diagnosis). Computer-aided detection (CADe) usually focuses on suggesting and marking conspicuous structures. Computer-aided diagnosis (CADx) aims to perform some sort of evaluation similar to diagnosis.

Data Scientist: Usually used as a job title for an employee or consultant who specializes in analyzing data, particularly large amounts of data, with an aim of discovering key insights and/or actionable business intelligence.

Deep Learning: A modern update to Artificial Neural Networks that exploit abundant cheap computation. They are concerned with building much larger and more complex neural networks than traditional Artificial Neural Networks.

Health Informatics: The interdisciplinary study of the design, development, adoption, and application of IT-based innovations in healthcare services delivery, management, and planning. (as defined by the U.S. National Library of Medicine)

Machine Learning: A unified concept subsuming various important problems in statistical methods of automated decision making & modeling and being concerned with: 1) the development of algorithms that quantify relationships within existing data and 2) the use of these identified patterns to make predictions based on new data. (as defined in (Wernick et al., 2010))

PACS: Picture archiving and communication system. A technology for the purpose of short- and long-term storage, retrieval, management, distribution and presentation of medical images.

Supervised Learning: A class of machine learning techniques that relate to situations where labelled data is available i.e. data samples along with corresponding class labels. It includes tasks such as classification.

APPENDIX

A few issues to be aware of while applying machine learning techniques are briefly listed here. A detailed discussion is beyond the scope of this chapter, some of the main points are summarized.

- **Classification Related Issues:**
  - **Overfitting:** Overfitting occurs when a statistical model describes random error or noise instead of the underlying relationship. This generally occurs when a model is excessively complex, such as having too many parameters relative to the number of observations. In classification applications, this manifests in the form of good performance on training set but poor performance on the test set. In practice, one could follow the Occam's razor principle and choose the simpler model that explains the data i.e. if two classifiers yield a similar performance, the "simpler" model should be chosen.
  - **Unbalanced Data (with Respect to Class Distribution):** It is not uncommon to have more samples from one class as compared to others. For instance, if samples are collected as part of a screening procedure it is often the case that a large proportion of samples would belong to one class (normal) since the incidence of a particular abnormality is small among the general population. Care has to be exercised in building a classifier from such training data since many classifiers are either implicitly or explicitly influenced by the proportion of samples in the respective classes. Two commonly used strategies include creating an artificially balanced training set either by undersampling the larger class or oversampling from the smaller class, or cost sensitive learning i.e. training a classifier by assigning different weights to the classes. More sophisticated methods such as SMOTE (Chawla et al., 2002) can also be used. If the imbalance is extremely high, rare event detection techniques may need to be employed.
  - **Performance Evaluation:** In classification, two important related problems are quantifying the performance of a classifier and comparing classifiers. For two class problems with a target class, sensitivity/specificity (or precision/recall) capture the performance on the two classes, accuracy alone could be misleading especially with unbalanced data (suppose there are 1000 test samples, 900 normal and 100 abnormal . A classifier that classifies all the samples as normal achieves an accuracy of 90% even though it fails to correctly identify even one abnormal sample). In a medical scenario ideally 100% sensitivity (all abnormal samples identified correctly) and 100% specificity (all normal samples identified correctly) are desired, usually a classifier provides a trade-off between the two.

Given that in most applications there is finite data available; one has to be careful in building the classifier. Training and testing on the same data gives an overly optimistic estimate of classifier accuracy. Typically multiple train/test splits are created and the measure (accuracy, sensitivity/specificity etc.) is averaged over these multiple test sets. Cross validation is a popular scheme, leave one out testing is a special case of cross validation.

The Receiver Operating Characteristic (ROC) curve is a useful tool for comparing classifiers, since it provides a visualization of the trade-off between sensitivity/specificity for different parameter settings. However if a single score characterizing classifier performance is desired, the Area under the curve (AUC) is a more useful score than accuracy, especially for unbalanced classes. Quantifying classification on medical images involves comparing image segmentation output with a "ground truth". Here too accuracy (number of correct pixels or voxels/total number) can be misleading, appropriate measures are the Dice Similarity Coefficient (DSC), overlap or Jaccard coefficients.

- **Clustering Related Issues:**
  - **Choosing the "Right" Algorithm:** The clustering literature is quite vast and deciding which algorithm is most suitable for a given data is confusing. In general there is no universally good method that works on all data. In practice, it is better to at least run a few clustering algorithms of different flavors. For example, the basic k-means algorithm yields mutually exclusive groupings. Other methods permit a sample to be assigned to multiple clusters (one example if the fuzzy c-means a "soft" variant of the k-means). Hierarchical clustering is useful to examine nested clusters. Another factor that may influence the choice of the algorithm is that some methods require the number of clusters as the input, many others do not.
  - **Choosing the "Right" Number of Clusters:** This is very data dependent and the answer may vary with the clustering algorithm used and the resolution of the data. For a specific dataset and a specific algorithm, if using a clustering algorithm which requires number of clusters as input; a common method is to repeatedly perform clustering by varying the number of clusters and computing a cluster validation index. A variety of cluster validation indices and methods have been proposed in the literature (e.g. (Hartigan, 1975); (Dunn, 1974)).

The author suggests use of silhouette proposed by Kaufman and Rousseeuw (Kaufman & Rousseeuw, 1990) in addition to any of the other internal indices. Roughly speaking, the silhouette for each individual sample is the difference between the dissimilarity to the "closest other cluster" and average within cluster dissimilarity, suitably normalized. One advantage of this method is that it gives a useful visual representation of the quality of the clustering. This is generally far more useful than a single number. Also, the silhouette computation does not make any assumption about data residing in Euclidean space, thus it can be directly applied to clustering methods which use non-Euclidean similarity/distance measures. Another class of methods called resampling methods repeatedly perform clustering by changing the algorithm parameters or using slightly different subsets of data. It is then checked whether the clusters are consistent and reproducible, which would be evidence of structure in the data. One such method is a prediction-based resampling method named Clest (Dudoit & Fridlyland, 2002). Clest automatically estimates the number of clusters, if any, in a dataset.

- **Cluster Validation:** Cluster validation basically addresses how "good" a given clustering result is. Unlike in classification, since no class labels are available, comparing clustering results is far trickier. Various indices have been proposed in the literature. One classification is internal indices and external indices. Internal indices (e.g. Hartigan, Dunn, Davies-Boudlin) try to optimize the clustering result based on the data only; they may for instance try to maximize overall compactness of clusters. Many of the indices implicitly assume that the data resides in a Euclidean space; extensions have been proposed to non-Euclidean spaces. External indices take into account some external information such as some "reference groupings" if available. Well-known external validation indices include the Rand (Rand, 1971), Fowlkes & Mallows (Fowlkes & Mallows, 1983) and Jaccard (Jain & Dubes, 1988) indices. Many approaches use a combination of internal and external validation.

In the author's experience, it may be too ambitious to seek a precise answer in cluster validation. However, one could use the indices above as a guideline to assess whether there is some structure in the data and what is roughly the range of number of clusters i.e. are there a few prominent clusters (say 2-7) or more (say >15). Also if multiple indices yield an answer in the same range, it could be taken as evidence that there is some structure in the data.

It may be a good idea to employ internal validation first followed by external validation. Möller et al. (Möller, 2002) proposed an analysis protocol for cluster validation of clustering results on fMRI data. Their study showed that an insufficient optimization can easily yield a spurious validation result which, in turn, may lead the analyst to a misleading interpretation of the fMRI experiment. On the other hand a careful optimization of clustering results provided the basis for a reliable, adequate characterization of the data. Furthermore, it enabled an adequate evaluation of the validity functions. Based on their results derived from analyses of simulated and real fMRI data they proposed a number of options of how to configure improved clustering tools.

Chapter 3
The Combination of Adaptive Filters to Improve the Quality of Medical Images in New Wavelet Domain

Nguyen Thanh Binh
Ho Chi Minh City University of Technology, Vietnam

Vo Thi Hong Tuyet
Ho Chi Minh City Open University, Vietnam

ABSTRACT

Most of medical images not only have noise but also have blur. This problem reduces the quality of images and influences diagnostic process of medical specialists because a small detail in a medical image is very useful for treatment process. This chapter explores the new generation wavelets, which provides the basic framework for the development of adaptive techniques to improve the quality of medical images. The process of the method for improving medical images includes: decompose of medical images in nonsubsampled contourlet domain and calculate the coefficients of Bayesian thresholding combined with Lucy Richard to reconstruct the medical images. For demonstrating the superiority of the method, the results of the proposed method are compared with the results of the other methods in new generation wavelet domain.

INTRODUCTION

Nowadays, enhancing the quality of medical images becomes a popular topic. There are many factors to affect the quality of medical images such as machine specification, surroundings, etc. Medical images are useful for doctor's treatment. The life of patients depends on the image-based diagnosis. Medical images are taken from many types of technical equipment, such as: X-ray images, ultrasound images, ultrasound - color Doppler, endoscopic image (digestive endoscopy, endoscopic urology, etc), images computerized tomography Scanner (CT image), magnetic resonance imaging (MRI), etc. Each image type

DOI: 10.4018/978-1-5225-0140-4.ch003

gives the information about each different disease, and this information is necessary for the consultation of health professionals. Only the small detail, such as: tumor or unusual point, is the key to detect the disease early and increases the patient's survival chances.

Most of medical images not only have noise but also have blur. This problem reduces the quality of images and causes difficulty for diagnosis. So, denoising and deblurring are necessary for the enhanced medical image processing such as classification, segmentation, etc. The goal of denoising is to extrude noise details from the low quality images. This process is very difficult because it must not only increase the quality of images but also keep edge features. Noise in medical images always leads to the undesirable appearance, but the noise can cover and reduce or lose the visibility of certain features within the image. In many cases, the images are also blur and noise which are combined to each other. Therefore, this problem is harder than denoising. Recently the models of noise in medical images have been proposed by (Gravel, 2004; Ashish, 2005). Practically, the noise in majority of medical images can be represented as some combination of Gaussian additive noise, speckle and impulsive noise.

Wavelet is widely used for denoising, but it suffers from shift, rotation sensitivity and poor in directionality. To improve this drawback, the new generation wavelet transforms such as the ridgelets, curvelets, contourlet transform and nonsubsampled contourlet transform have been proposed. The nonsubsampled contourlet transform (NSCT) is useful for denoising and deblurring because the NSCT comprises two parts: a nonsubsampled pyramid structure which gives multi-scale property and a Nonsubsampled Directional Filter Bank (NSDFB) structure that brings directional property. Both of them are shift - invariant due to nonsubsampled filter banks. This chapter explores the new generation wavelets, which provides the basic framework for the development of adaptive techniques to improve the quality of medical images. The process of the method for improving medical image includes: decompose of medical images in nonsubsampled contourlet domain and calculate the coefficients of Bayesian thresholding combined with Lucy Richard to reconstruct the medical images. For demonstrating the superiority of the method, the results of the proposed method compared with the other methods in new generation wavelet domain such as contourlet, ridgelet, curvelet domain. For performance measure, the authors have used Peak Signal to Noise Ratio (PSNR) and Mean Square Error (MSE) and it has shown that the results of the present method are better than those of the other methods. The contributions of the chapter are:

1. The advantages of new wavelet generation are almost unexplored area, are explored and applied them to solve problems in the image analysis such as: image denoising and image deblurring.
2. The features of new X-let multiscale transforms such as curvelet, ridgelet, contourlet transform, nonsubsampled contourlet transform are also shown.
3. A method for increasing the quality of medical images based on the combination of adaptive filters in new wavelet generation is shown.

RELATED WORK

In the past, there were many methods which were proposed for denoising medical images by Discrete Wavelet Transform (DWT) (Strang, 1989; Tim, 1992; Marcin, 2001). DWT has three serious disadvantages: shift sensitivity, poor directionality and lack of phase information. Several methods have provided solutions for decreasing these disadvantages using new generation wavelet such as: curvelet transform (Zhang, 2008; Donoho, 2000; Starck, 2002), ridgelet transform (Candes, 1998), contourlet transform, nonsubsampled contourlet transform (Arthur, 2005; Arthur, 2006), Laplacian pyramid and direction filter bank in contourlet transform (Minh, 2005). Most of them have the longer time process because of the cost of decomposition and reconstruction, especially the ridgelet and curvelet transform.

Most of transforms need the coefficient to base on the reconstruction of structure of images. Some other methods only base on the thresholdings (Binh, 2013): stationary, cycle-spinning, shiftable, steerable wavelet, Bayesian thresholding, etc. And the combination of transforms and thresholdings are proposed in (Binh, 2010; Ping, 2013; Binh, 2015; Tuyet, 2015). All of the above methods have the difficulties in case of blur combined with noise.

Most of papers (Ashish, 2006; Binh, 2015; Tuyet, 2015) give the ideas to divide the proposed method into two steps: denoising and deblurring in denoising images. In (Ashish, 2006; Binh, 2015; Tuyet, 2015), the ideal of authors is to divides the process into two steps: denoising at first and then is deblurring. The reason of the order is denoising first to remove noise out of pixels. Image denoising is improved in order to make the deblurring process more simple. The deblurring calculates the approximate values, this process gives the good results when the relationship between pixels, and between edges is strong and evident. In recent researches, the denoising for medical images which based on the type of medical images, such as: MRI, CT, etc. (Amira, 2015) uses Cuckoo combined with Logarithm transform for improving the quality of Cuckoo in the past. In this research, the authors set to be 25 nests. Each nest is improved the quality by Lee's algorithm. Although the quality increases, the combination of the filter and thresholding is very complex.

NEW GENERATION WAVELET TRANSFORMS

The Discrete Wavelet Transform (DWT) provides a fast, local, sparse, multiresolution analysis of real-world signals and images. Although DWT is a powerful tool for image analysis, it has three serious disadvantages: shift sensitivity (Selesnick, 2000), poor directionality and lack of phase information (Candes, 1999). To improve this drawback, the new generation wavelet transforms have proposed. In this section, the authors explore some new generation wavelet transforms. Here, new X-let multiscale transforms such as the ridgelets, curvelets, contourlet transform and nonsubsampled contourlet transform have been described.

The Ridgelet Transform

Ridgelets have been recently applied in the image processing application (Starck, 2002; Donoho, 1998; Burns, 1994). It can be adapted to represent objects with curved edges using an appropriate multiscale localization: on a sufficiently fine scale curved edges can be considered as almost straight.

The continuous ridgelet transform may be constructed as a wavelet transform in the Radon domain. All of the forthcoming claims and results are proved in (Candes, 1998).

Donoho (Donoho, 1998) modified the ridgelet construction by essentially replacing the discretization of the angular variable with a periodic wavelet transform resulting in an orthonormal basis. Donoho called these new basis elements as orthonormal ridgelets.

There are two approaches for the localization of ridgelets:

- **Monoscale Ridgelets:** Partitioned into congruent squares of a given fixed sidelength constructs a system of renormalized ridgelets smoothly localized near each such square (Candes, 1999).
- **Multiscale Ridgelets:** Subjected to an infinite series of partitions, based on dyadic scales, where each partition, like in the monoscale case, consists of squares of the given dyadic sidelength. The corresponding dictionary of generating elements is a pyramid of windowed ridgelets, renormalized and transported to a wide range of scales and locations (Starck, 2002).

Orthonormal Ridgelets

The orthonormal ridgelets are indexed using

$$\lambda = \left(j, k, i, l, \varepsilon\right) \quad (1)$$

where:

***j*:** The ridge scale,
***k*:** The ridge location,
***i*:** The angular scale,
***l*:** The angular location, and
***ε*:** A gender token.

The ortho-ridgelets look like pieces of ridgelets which are windowed to lie in discs of radius about 2^i; $\theta_{i,l} = l/2^i$ is roughly the orientation parameter, and 2^{-j} is roughly the thickness.

Relationships between Ridgelet Transform and Radon Transform

The 2-D continuous ridgelet transform in R^2 can be defined as follows. First define a smooth wavelet function $\psi : R \to R$ satisfying the admissibility condition given by

$$\int_{-\infty}^{\infty} \frac{\left|\hat{\psi}(\varepsilon)\right|^2}{\left|\varepsilon\right|^2} d\varepsilon < \infty \quad (2)$$

where $\hat{\psi}$ is the Fourier transform of ψ.

The bivariate ridgelet $\psi_{a,b,\theta} : R^2 \to R^2$ is defined by $\psi_{a,b,\theta}(x,y)$ and the function is constant along the lines $x\cos(\theta) + y\sin(\theta) = const$. The ridgelet values for continuous image $f\left(x,y\right)$ is given by

$$Rf(a,b,\theta) = \iint f(x,y)\psi_{a,b,\theta}(x,y)dxdy \quad (3)$$

The radon transform in continuous terms is defined by

$$Rf(t,\theta) = \int f(x,y)\delta(t - x\cos(\theta) - y\sin(\theta))dxdy \tag{4}$$

where δ denotes the Dirac delta-function. In words, *Rf* is the integral of the continuous image *f*, over the line $L_{t,\theta}$ defined by $t = x\cos(\theta) + y\sin(\theta)$.

In short, the ridgelet transform is the application of a 1-D wavelet transform to the slice of the Radon transform where the angular variable θ is constant and *t* is varying (Starck, 2002). This means the ridgelet coefficients $Rf\left(a,b,\theta\right)$ are given by analysis of the radon transform via,

$$Rf(t,\theta) = \int Rf(t,\theta)a^{-1/2}\psi((t-b)/a)dt \tag{5}$$

where $\psi_{a,b(t)} = a^{-1/2}\psi((t-b)/a)$ is a 1-D wavelet transform.

The ordinary ridgelet transform can be achieved as follows (Donoho, 2000):

1. Compute the 2D Fast Fourier Transform (FFT) of the image.
2. Substitute the sampled values of Fourier transform obtained on the square lattice with sampled values on a polar lattice.
3. Compute the 1D inverse FFT on each angular line.
4. Perform the 1D scale wavelet transform on the resulting angular lines in order to obtain the ridgelet coefficients.

Discrete Curvelet Transform

Curvelets as proposed by Candes (Candes, 1999), constitute a relatively new family of frames that are designed to represent edges and other singularities along curves much more efficiently than the traditional wavelet based transforms.

The idea of curvelets (Candes, 1999) is to represent a curve as a superposition of functions of various lengths and widths obeying the scaling law $width \approx length^2$. This can be done by first decomposing the image into subbands, i.e separating the object into a series of disjoint scales. Then, each scale is analyzed by means of a local ridgelet transform.

Curvelets are based on multiscale ridgelets combined with a spatial bandpass filtering operation to isolate different scales. This spatial bandpass filter nearly kills all multiscale ridgelets which are not in the frequency range of the filter. The bandpass is set so that the curvelet length and width at fine scales. There is a very special relationship between the depth of the multiscale pyramid and the index of the dyadic subbands. The side length of the localizing windows is doubled at every otherdyadic subband, hence maintaining the fundamental property of the curvelet transform which says that elements of length about $2^{-j/2}$ serve for the analysis and synthesis of the jth subband $\left[2^j, 2^{j+1}\right]$

Like ridgelets, curvelets occur at all scales, locations, and orientations. However, while ridgelets have global length and variable widths, curvelets in addition to a variable width have a variable length and so a variable anisotropy.

A few properties of the curvelet transform (Candes, 1999) are:

1. **Tight Frame:** Much like in an orthonormal basis, the authors can easily expand an arbitrary function $f\left(x_1, x_2\right) \in L^2\left(R^2\right)$ as a series of curvelets: the authors have a reconstruction formula

$$f = \sum_{\mu} \left\langle f, \varphi_\mu \right\rangle \varphi_\mu \tag{6}$$

with the equality holding in an L^2 sense and a Parseval relation

$$\sum_{\mu} \left| \left\langle f, \varphi_\mu \right\rangle \right|^2 = \left\| f \right\|^2_{L^2(R^2)}, \quad \forall f \in L^2(R^2) \tag{7}$$

2. **Parabolic Scaling:** The frequency localization of φ_j implies the following spatial structure: $\varphi_j(x)$ is of rapid decay away from a 2^{-j} by $2^{-j/2}$ rectangle with minor axis pointing in the horizontal direction. In short, the effective length and width obey the anisotropy scaling relation

$$length \approx 2^{-j/2}, width \approx 2^{-j} \Rightarrow width \approx length^2 \tag{8}$$

3. **Oscillatory Behavior:** $\hat{\varphi}_j$ is actually supported away from the vertical axis $\xi_1 = 0$ but near the horizontal $\xi_2 = 0$ axis. In a nutshell, this says that $\varphi_j(x)$ is oscillatory in the x_1-direction and lowpass in the x_2-direction. Hence, at scale 2^{-j}, a curvelet is a little needle whose envelope is a specified "ridge" of effective length $2^{-j/2}$ and width 2^{-j}, and which displays an oscillatory behavior across the main "ridge".
4. **Vanishing Moments:** The curvelet template φ_j is said to have q vanishing moments when

$$\int_{-\infty}^{\infty} \varphi_j\left(x_1, x_2\right) x_1^n dx_1 = 0, for\ all\ 0 \le n \le q, for\ all\ x_2 \tag{9}$$

The same property of course holds for rotated curvelets when x_1 and x_2 are taken to be the corresponding rotated coordinates. The integral is taken in the direction perpendicular to the ridge, so counting vanishing moments is a way to quantify the oscillation property mentioned above

5. **Phase-Space Tiling/Sampling:** Curvelets are treated as Heisenberg tiles of minimum volume in phase-space (Candes, 2005). In x, the essential support of φ_μ has size $O(2^{-j} x\ 2^{-j/2})$. In frequency, the support of $\hat{\varphi}_\mu$ has size . The net volume in phase-space is therefore

$$O(2^{-j} \times 2^{-j/2}).O(2^{j/2} \times 2^{j}) = O(1) \tag{10}$$

which is in accordance with the uncertainty principle. The parameters (j,k,l) of the curvelet transform induce a new non-trivial sampling of phase-space, Cartesian in x, polar in ξ, and based on the parabolic scaling.

6. **Complex-Valuedness:** Since curvelets do not obey the symmetry $\hat{\varphi}_\mu(-\xi) = \overline{\hat{\varphi}_\mu(\xi)}$, φ_μ is complex-valued. There exists a related construction for real-valued curvelets by simply symmetrizing the construction (Candes, 2005). The basic process of the digital realization for curvelet transform is given as follows:
   a. **Subband Decomposition:** The authors define a bank of filters $P_0, (\Delta_s, s \geq 0)$. The image f is filtered into subbands with à trous algorithm (Candes, 2005)

$$f \rightarrow (P_0 f, \Delta_1 f, \Delta_2 f, ...) \tag{11}$$

The different subbands $\Delta_s f$ contain details about 2^{-2s} wide.

   b. **Smooth Partitioning:** Each subband is smoothly windowed into "squares" of an appropriate scale

$$\Delta_s f \rightarrow (w_Q \Delta_s f)_{Q \in Q_s} \tag{12}$$

where w_Q is a collection of smooth window localized around dyadic squares

$$Q = \left[\frac{k_1}{2^s}, \frac{(k_1+1)}{2^s}\right] \times \left[\frac{k_2}{2^s}, \frac{(k_2+1)}{2^s}\right] \tag{13}$$

   c. **Renormalization:** Each resulting square is renormalized to unit scale

$$g_Q = \left(T_Q\right)^{-1}\left(w_Q \Delta_s f\right), Q \in Q_s \tag{14}$$

where $\left(T_Q f\right)\left(x_1, x_2\right) = 2^s f\left(2^s x_1 - k_1, 2^s x_2 - k_2\right)$ is a renormalization operator.

   d. **Ridgelet Analysis:** Each square is analyzed in the orthonormal ridgelet system. This is a system of basic elements p_λ making an orthonormal basis for $L^2\left(R^2\right)$:

$$\alpha_\mu = \left\langle g_Q, p_\lambda \right\rangle \tag{15}$$

Curvelets and ridgelets take the form of basic elements which exhibit very high directional sensitivity and are highly anisotropic. In two-dimensions, for instance, curvelets are localized not only in position (the spatial domain) and scale (the frequency domain), but also in orientation. Unlike wavelet transforms, the ridgelet transform processes data by first computing integrals over lines with all kinds of orientations and locations. The curvelet transform, like the wavelet transform, is a multiscale transform, with frame elements indexed by scale and location parameters. Unlike the wavelet transform, it has directional parameters, and curvelet pyramid contain elements with a very high degree of directional specificity. In addition, the curvelet transform is based on a certain anisotropic scaling principle which is quite different from the isotropic scaling of wavelets. All of these properties are very stimulating and have already lead to a range of interesting idealized applications.

The Contourlet Transform

Real valued wavelet transform suffers from three major problems: lack of shift sensitivity, poor directionality and lack of strong edge detection. Do (Do, 2005) proposed a solution to overcome these problems by contourlet transform (CT).

Contourlets constitute a new family of frames that are designed to represent smooth contours in different directions of an image. A contourlet is easily applied in image processing because its representation is a fixed transform (Do, 2005; Binh, 2013). The contourlet not only inherits the main qualities of wavelet transform, such as multi-scale and time-frequency information, but also captures direction characteristics. It holds the geometrical formation of images and implements a true sparse representation of images. The contourlet allows for a different number of directions at each scale and aspect ratio. This feature allows an efficient contourlet-based approximation of a smooth contour at multiple resolutions. The discrete contourlet transform is a multiscale and directional decomposition using a combination of Laplacian pyramid (LP) and directional filter bank (DFB) (Do, 2005; Binh, 2013).

The idea of the contourlet construction (Do, 2005) is: let $a_0(n)$ be the input image, the output after the LP step is I bandpass images $b_i(n)$, i =1, 2,..., I and a lowpass image $a_I(n)$. Each bandpass image $b_i(n)$ is decomposed by an ℓ_i -level DFB into 2^{ℓ_i} bandpass directional images $c_{i,k}^{(l_i)}[n]$, for k = 0, 1,..., 2^{ℓ_i} -1. Figure 1 presents contourlet decomposition.

Figure 1. Contourlet decomposition

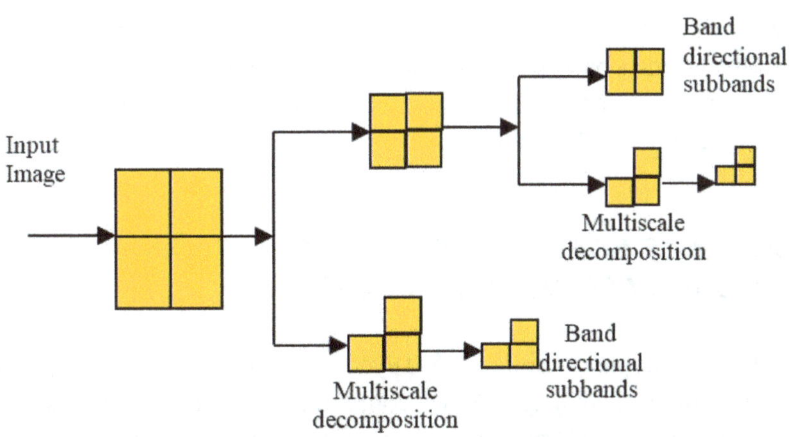

In the discrete contourlet transform, the multiscale and directional decomposition steps are decoupled. Therefore, the authors have different numbers of directions at different scales. Contourlet decomposition proceeds through two main steps: first, LP multiscale decomposition is performed; then directional filter bank decomposition is used to link point discontinuity to linear structures. In more detail, an image is decomposed into a low pass image and bandpass images by the LP decomposition. Each bandpass output is further decomposed by the DFB step. The output of the DFB step consists of smooth contours and directional edges. The authors use each directional subband at each level which consists of 2^n element, where n is a positive integer. Figure 1 shows contourlet decomposition (Binh, 2013). Contourlet transform has the time-frequency-localization and multiscale properties of wavelets. It offers a high degree of directionality and anisotropy. Therefore, the properties of contourlet transform will be useful for denoising and debluring medical images.

Nonsubsampled Contourlet Transform (NSCT)

Arthur (Arthur, 2005) presented clearly about NSCT for denoising images. Nonsubsampled Pyramid (NSP) is similar to Laplacian Pyramid. This algorithm uses two-channel nonsubsampled filter banks and decompostionis realized with level j = 3 stages. The filters of subsequent stages are the result of upsampling filters of the first stage. The subbands are devised into high-pass and low-pass filter. The region of low-pass filter is $\left[-\left(\frac{\pi}{2^j}\right),\left(\frac{\pi}{2^j}\right)\right]^2$, and the complement of the low-pass filter is the high-pass filter which is solved by the region

$$\frac{\left[-\left(\frac{\pi}{2^{j-1}}\right),\left(\frac{\pi}{2^{j-1}}\right)\right]^2}{\left[\left(\frac{\pi}{2^j}\right),\left(\frac{\pi}{2^j}\right)\right]^2}.$$

Directional Filter Bank (DFB) eliminates the down-samplers and up-samplers in each two-channel filter bank that is Nonsubsampled Directional Filter Bank (NSDFB). Arthur (Arthur, 2005) affirms that NSCT is the process that combines NSP and NSDFB. Ping (Ping, 2013) also asserts that NSCT is implemented by two major steps: when multi-scale image multi-scale decomposition is NSP filter to be used in a low-pass subband and a band-pass subband. Then, each level of band pass subbands directional decomposition of band-pass subbands will continue with NSDFB. And image decomposition process is complete with two steps: NSP and NSDFB.

THE COMBINATION OF ADAPTIVE FILTERS TO IMPROVE THE QUALITY OF MEDICAL IMAGES

Blur images always have noise, paper (Binh, 2015; Tuyet, 2015) combined many methods to each other's to remove noise and blur in medical images. When combining methods, the authors (Binh, 2015; Tuyet, 2015) base on the decomposition and transform. In this section, the authors proposed a method for medical image denoising and deblurring using combination of adaptive filters in nonsubsampled contourlet domain. In the proposed method, the medical images are denoised by Bayesian thresholding (BT) and deblurred by Lucy Richard (LR), all of the processes in NSCT domain.

Denoising Images by Thresholding

Filtering threshold is a critical key in denoising and deblurring image. Characteristics of medical images are filtered to the appropriate thresholds to avoid loss, but show better results. Wavelet threshold includes:

- The input image is analyzed into wavelet coefficients.
- Compares the detail coefficients with threshold values given and make the coefficient values closer to 0. This step removes the impact of the existence of medical images.
- Reconstruct the image from the changing coefficients (the inverse wavelet).

In many cases, if the authors use many thresholdings, the result images will give the "too smooth" images and reduce the sharpness because of adaptation to the adjustment of the threshold. The wavelet coefficient is divided into two types: hard-threshold (T_{hard}) and soft-threshold (T_{soft}):

$$T_{hard}\left(\hat{d}_{jk},\lambda\right)=\hat{d}_{jk}I\left(\left|\hat{d}_{jk}\right|>\lambda\right) \tag{16}$$

and

$$T_{soft}\left(\hat{d}_{jk},\lambda\right)=sign\left(\hat{d}_{jk}\right)\max\left(0,\left|\hat{d}_{jk}\right|-\lambda\right) \tag{17}$$

where $\lambda \geq 0$ is parameter wavelet, I is normal parameter value.

Deblurring Images

The blur image is described by equation:

$$g=H\cdot f+n; \tag{18}$$

where g is blur image, H is the PSF value, f is the original image and n is the noise value.

So the blur image has noise value. Therefore, the deblurring process and denoising process are always parallel. The deblurring is the process which searches approximation value based on PSF value. This process is tautologized, again and again, and only stops when the quality of the restored image reaches the quality of the original image. Because of the repetition of deblurring image, the time process is very slow. Most deblurring algorithms base on the value of point-spread function (PSF), then the authors calculated the approximate value to restore the image.

Select a New Generation Wavelet Transform

The DWT is a good tool to provide time - frequency representation of the signal, so its applications appear in many fields. But DWT is not really perfect; it's only good at representing point singularities (Phuong, 2015). If they are lines, edges or textures, DWT has a lot of redundant coefficients and is computationally expensive. Ridgelet transform (Candes, 1999) is proposed with better representation for linear singularities. But most of the real world applications do not show straight - line singularities. Curvelet transform (Cades, 2000) takes its place to solve the problem by partitioning the image then applying ridgelet to each part. The idea is a curve split into many parts which correspond to lines. But curvelet also has two drawbacks: first, not optimal for sparse approximation of curve beyond C^2 singularities and second, highly redundant. Contourlet transform (Do, 2005) is built from a discrete domain first, then extend to the continuous domain, it has lower redundancy and a faster discrete implementation version than curvelet. But contourlet is just multidirectional and multi-scale but not shift - invariant, which causes pseudo-Gibbs phenomena visible on the decoded image by high compression ratio. Nonsubsampled contourlet transform (Cunha, 2006) brings shift - invariance for contourlet with the trade-off of more redundancy. As NSCT is used for contour detection, this redundancy is not a drawback but even gives better results.

The important feature of the proposal bases on object's information and NSCT is chosen to extract the object's information. NSCT belongs to the family of the new generation wavelet transform. The NSCT development through its main predecessors may start at wavelet transform (WT) (Graps, 1995) as in (Ma, 2010; Phuong, 2015).

NSCT comprises two parts: a nonsubsampled pyramid structure which gives multi-scale property and a nonsubsampled directional filter bank (NSDFB) structure that brings directional property. Both of them are shift - invariant due to nonsubsampled filter banks. NSP comprises four filters: $H_0(z)$ and $H_1(z)$ are low and high pass decomposition filters, and $G_0(z)$ and $G_1(z)$ are low and high pass reconstruction filters. In an ideal case, the passband supported by low filter at the jth stage is $\left[-\left(\frac{\pi}{2^j}\right),\left(\frac{\pi}{2^j}\right)\right]^2$ and the corresponding high filter supports the complement region

$$\frac{\left[-\left(\frac{\pi}{2^{j-1}}\right),\left(\frac{\pi}{2^{j-1}}\right)\right]^2}{\left[\left(\frac{\pi}{2^j}\right),\left(\frac{\pi}{2^j}\right)\right]^2}.$$

The filters of first stage are upsampled to obtain filters for next stages, so it gives multi-scale property without any more filter design (Phuong, 2015). NSDFB has filters constructed from fan filter banks. The upsampled fan filters of the second stage which supports checker-board frequency, when combined with first stage filters will give the four directions in frequency decomposition. The properties of NSCT like multi-scale, multi-direction, shift-invariant make it very suitable for denoising and deblurring.

Figure 2. The proposed method

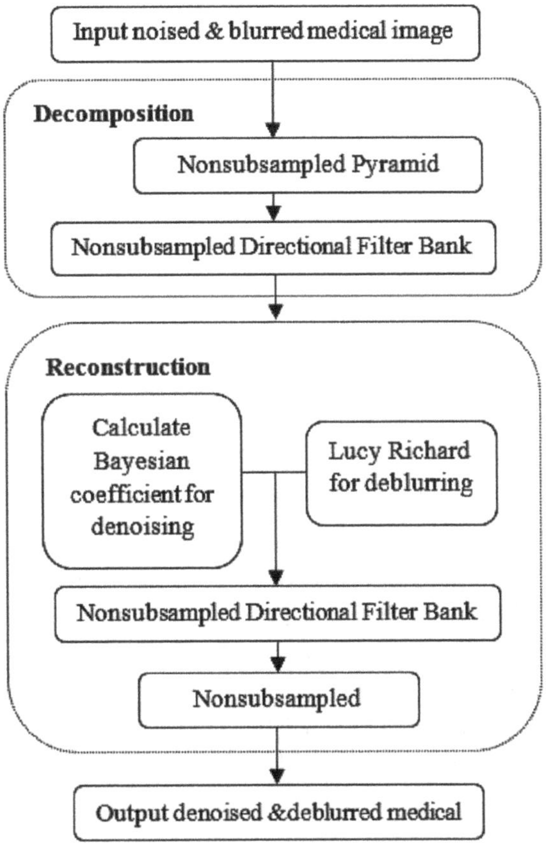

Clarify the Medical Images in Nonsubsampled Contourlet Domain

The proposed method is presented completely in Figure 2. Firstly, the decomposition. The medical images which have blur and noise are the input of the decomposition. In this process, the medical images are decomposed by NSP into subbands. The result subbands include low subbands and high subbands. In low subbands, denoising will remove the first. Each subband is continued by NSDFB with multi-direction. Secondly, the reconstruction. To give the coefficients for denoising and deblurring, the authors calculate the sigmahat value. These values include: the estimate noise variance σ and signal variance σ_s. They can be obtained by equation:

$$\sigma = \left(\frac{median\left(\left| w_{i,j} \right| \right)}{0.6745} \right)^2 \quad (19)$$

$$\sigma_s = \sqrt{\max\left(\sigma_w^2 - \sigma^2, 0 \right)} \quad (20)$$

with

$$\sigma_w^2 = \frac{1}{n^2} \sum\nolimits_{i,j=1}^{n} w^2(i,j) \tag{21}$$

where $w_{i,j}$ is the lowest frequency coefficient after performing transformations.

The proposed threshold which depends σ_s gives better edge preservation. However, the threshold value should go from lower to higher levels. The calculation of the thresholds based on sigmahat:

$$Threshold_{Bayes} = \begin{cases} \frac{\sigma^2}{\sigma_s}, \sigma^2 < \sigma_s^2 \\ \max\{|A_m|\}, \sigma^2 \geq \sigma_s^2 \end{cases} \tag{22}$$

When reconstructing the image based on the Bayesian threshold coefficients, if the value of pixel detail coefficients is less than thresholding then the result is 0. Else the result is array Y, where each element of Y is 1 if the corresponding element of pixel is greater than zero, 0 if the corresponding element of pixel equals zero, -1 if the corresponding element of pixel is less than zero.

In here, the authors choose the Lucy Richard (Maja, 2010) for the deblurring because Lucy Richard bases on the Bayesian framework. Lucy Richard develops an iterative expectation maximization deconvolution and the authors use the multiview fusion. This deblurring method depends on the point spread function (PSF) to compute as an average of the individual correction factors by functions:

$$C^p = \frac{1}{N} \sum_{i=1}^{N} C_i^p \tag{23}$$

$$C_i^p = H_i(-v) * \frac{Y_i(v)}{S_i^p(v)} \tag{24}$$

$$S_i^p(v) = H_i * \hat{X}(-v) \tag{25}$$

where N recordings ($Y_1, \ldots, Y_N$) and the corresponding PSF ($P_1, \ldots, P_N$), the correction factor C is computed for each image Y_i individually. Then the reconstruction of the blur pixels by:

$$\hat{X}^0 = \frac{1}{N} \sum_{i=1}^{N} Y_i^p \tag{26}$$

The result images are reconstructed from each subband in NSDFB with multi-direction reconstruction. Then, continued with NSP in low subbands and high subbands with Bayesian coefficients and Lucy Richard.

EXPERIMENTS AND RESULTS

The authors have given clearly the method in the above section. And the experiments and results are presented in this section. For performance evaluation, the authors test the results of the proposed method and compared the results with the other methods in wavelet domain and new generation wavelet transform such as contourlet, ridgelet and curvelet domain. Experiments are developed in Matlab 2013a and carried out on computer of Intel i7 4700MQ 2.4 GHz CPU and 16 GB DDR3 memory.

Database and Evaluation

The dataset is medical images which are collected in many hospitals. This dataset includes more than 1000 medical images of different sizes: 256x256, 512x512. The medical image types include X-ray images, ultrasound images, images computerized tomography Scanner (CT image) and magnetic resonance imaging (MRI). All of the above methods are done in the same images on the similar scale.

The aim of proposed method is to improve the quality of medical images in case of noise combined with blur. So, the authors use the value of Peak Signal to Noise Ratio (PSNR) and Mean Square Error (MSE) to compare the results (Xiangfei, 2013). The higher the value of PSNR is, the better it is. The smaller the value of MSE is, the better it is. The equation of PSNR is defined as:

$$PSNR = 20\log_{10}\left(\frac{MAX_1}{MSE}\right) \tag{27}$$

where MAX_1 is the maximum pixel value of the image.

And MSE is defined as:

$$MSE = \sqrt{\frac{1}{N \times N}\sum_{i=1}^{N}\sum_{j=1}^{N}\left(x_{i,j} - y_{i,j}\right)^2} \tag{28}$$

where x is the image which has blur and noise, y is the image result and N x N is the size of image.

Experiments and Results Analysis

Recently the models of noise in medical images have been proposed by (Gravel, 2004; Ashish, 2005). Practically, the noise in majority of medical images can be represented as some combination of Gaussian additive noise, speckle and impulsive noise. The CT images are corrupted with blur (Wang, 1998; Jiang, 2003) and their blur can be modeled by Gaussian point spread function (PSF). (Wagner, 1998) suggested a special PSF, called scatter PSF for modeling blur in X-ray image. Ultrasound images can also have a complex nature of blur (Wang, 1996; Taxt, 1997; Michailovich, 2004). Most of the medical images are corrupted by motion blur and Gaussian blur. Analytical models for these blur are given by (Banhan, 1997).

So, the authors test with pairs: motion blur combined with Gaussian noise and Gaussian blur combined with Gaussian noise. The details of the cases are:

- Gaussian blur combined with Gaussian noise.
- Gaussian blur combined with speckle noise.
- Motion blur combined with Gaussian noise.
- Motion blur combined with speckle noise.

The results are given from the testing of more 1000 medical images. In here, the authors present some images in dataset.

Case 1: Denoising and deblurring images in case Gaussian blur combined with Gaussian noise.

Figure 3 shows the denoising and deblurring of blur and noise image which has Gaussian blur combined with Gaussian noise by the proposed method.

Figure 3. Denoising and deblurring images in case of Gaussian blur combined with Gaussian noise by different methods: (a) blur combined with noise in image (PSNR = 18.1851 db); (b) denoised and deblurred image by BT combined LR in Wavelet domain (PSNR = 18.4373 db); (c) denoised and deblurred image by BT combined LR in Contourlet domain (PSNR = 18.7373 db); (d) denoised and deblurred image by BT combined LR in Ridgelet domain (PSNR = 19.8721 db); (e) denoised and deblurred image by BT combined LR in Curvelet domain (PSNR = 23.3561 db); (f) denoised and deblurred image by the proposed method (PSNR = 24.1621 db)

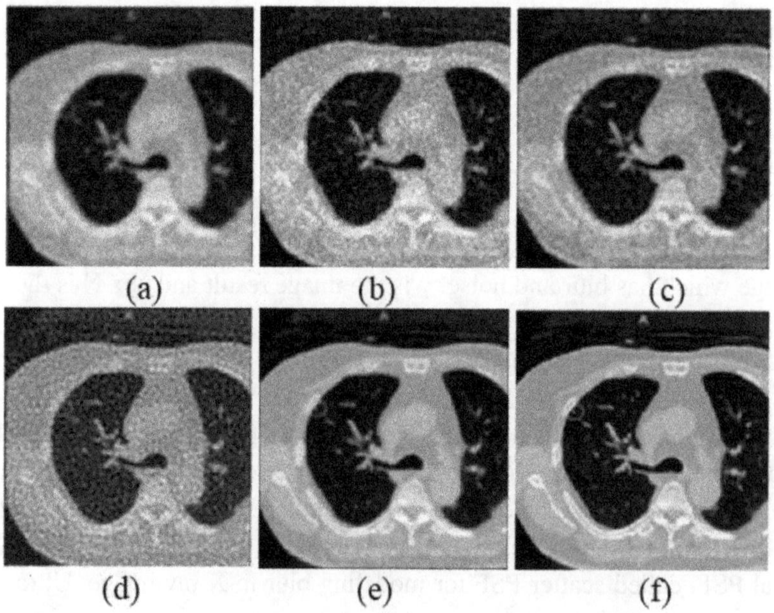

Figure 4. Plot of PSNR values of denoised and deblurred images in case of Gaussian blur combined with Gaussian noise using different methods

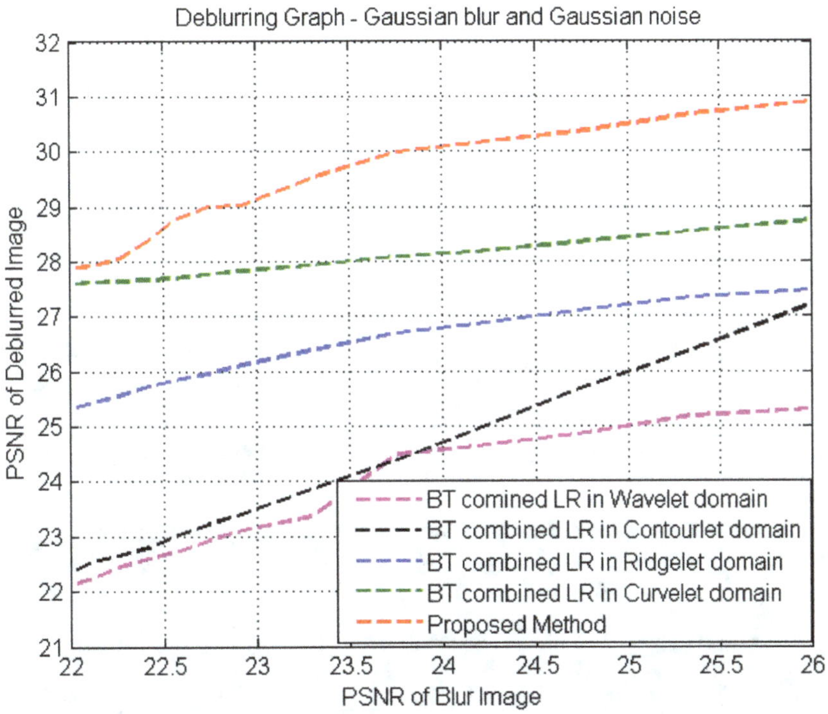

Figure 5. Plot of MSE values of denoised and deblurred images in case of Gaussian blur combined with Gaussian noise using different methods

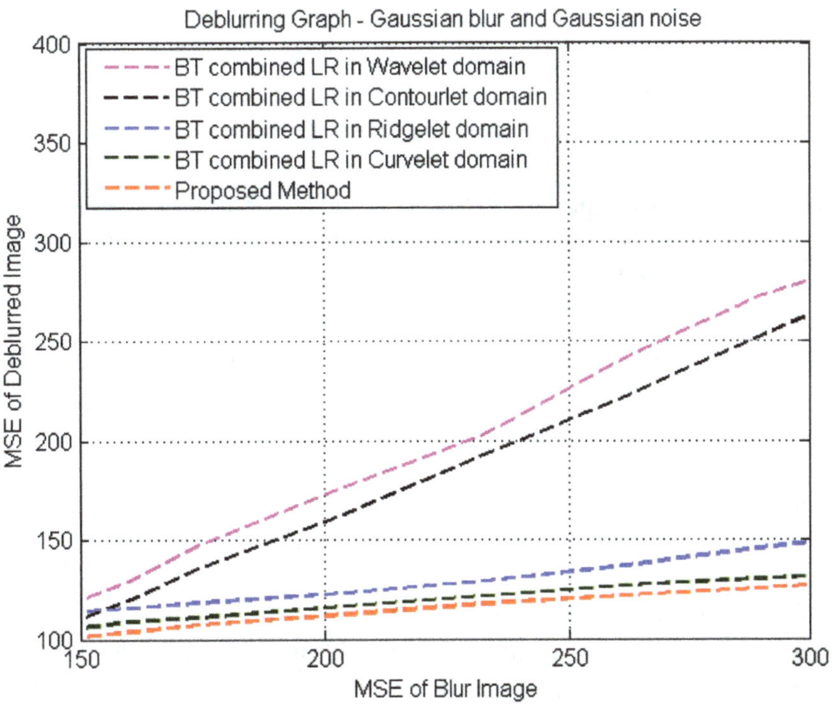

Figure 6. Denoising and deblurring images in case of Gaussian blur combined with speckle noise by different methods: (a) blur combined with noise in image (PSNR = 22.7325 db); (b) denoised and deblurred image by BT combined LR in Wavelet domain (PSNR = 22.4371 db); (c) denoised and deblurred image by BT combined LR in Contourlet domain (PSNR = 22.9371 db); (d) denoised and deblurred image by BT combined LR in Ridgelet domain (PSNR = 23.4501 db); (e) denoised and deblurred image by BT combined LR in Curvelet domain (PSNR = 24.9283 db); (f) denoised and deblurred image by the proposed method (PSNR = 26.0265 db)

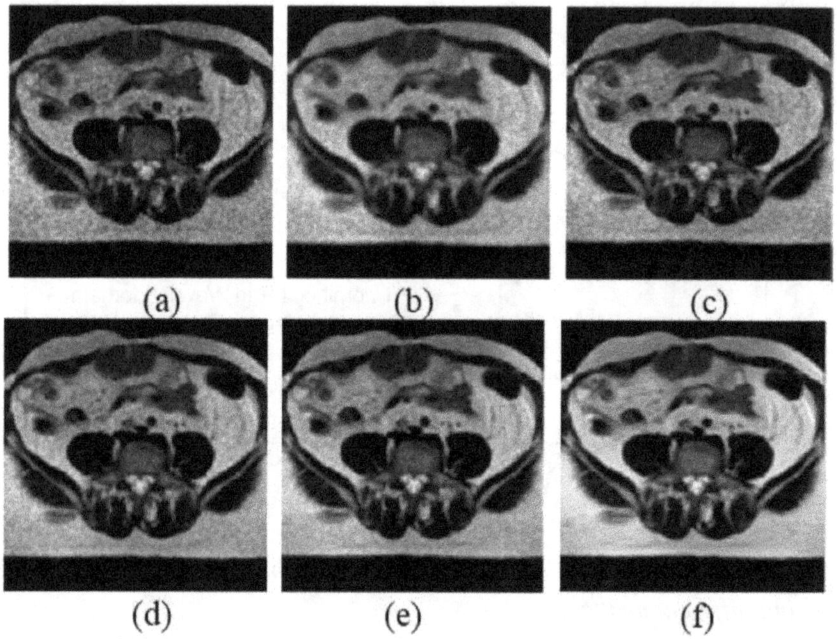

In Figure 3, the result of the proposed method (Figure 3(f)) is better than that of the other methods (Figure 3(b), Figure 3(c), Figure 3(d) and Figure 3(e). Because the PSNR value of Figure 3(f) is higher than the PSNR value in the rest figures.

Figure 4 and Figure 5 show the plot of PSNR, MSE values of different methods in denoising and deblurring corrupted in case of Gaussian blur combined with Gaussian noise. The results of the proposed methods are better than those of the other methods.

Case 2: Denoising and deblurring images in case Gaussian blur combined with speckle noise.

Figure 6 shows the denoising and deblurring of blur and noise image which has Gaussian blur combined with speckle noise by the proposed method.

In Figure 6, the result of the proposed method (Figure 6(f)) is better than that of the other methods (Figure 6(b), Figure 6(c), Figure 6(d) and Figure 6(e)). Because the PSNR value of Figure 6(f) is higher than the PSNR value in the rest figures.

Figure 7 and Figure 8 show the plot of PSNR, MSE values of different methods in denoising and deblurring corrupted in case of Gaussian blur combined with speckle noise. The results of the proposed methods are better than those of the other methods.

Figure 7. Plot of PSNR values of denoised and deblurred images in case of Gaussian blur combined with speckle noise using different methods

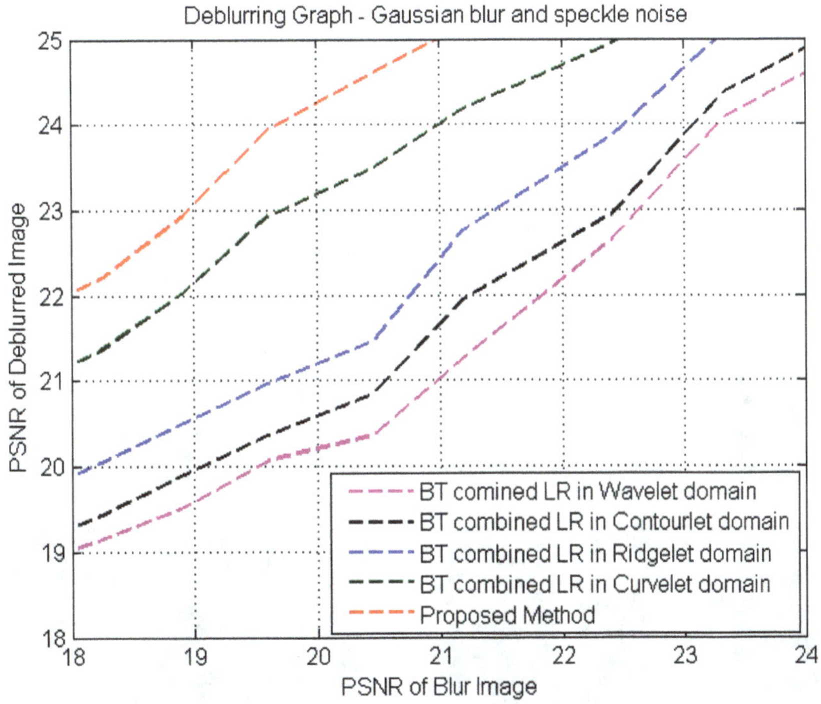

Figure 8. Plot of MSE values of denoised and deblurred images in case of Gaussian blur combined with speckle noise using different methods

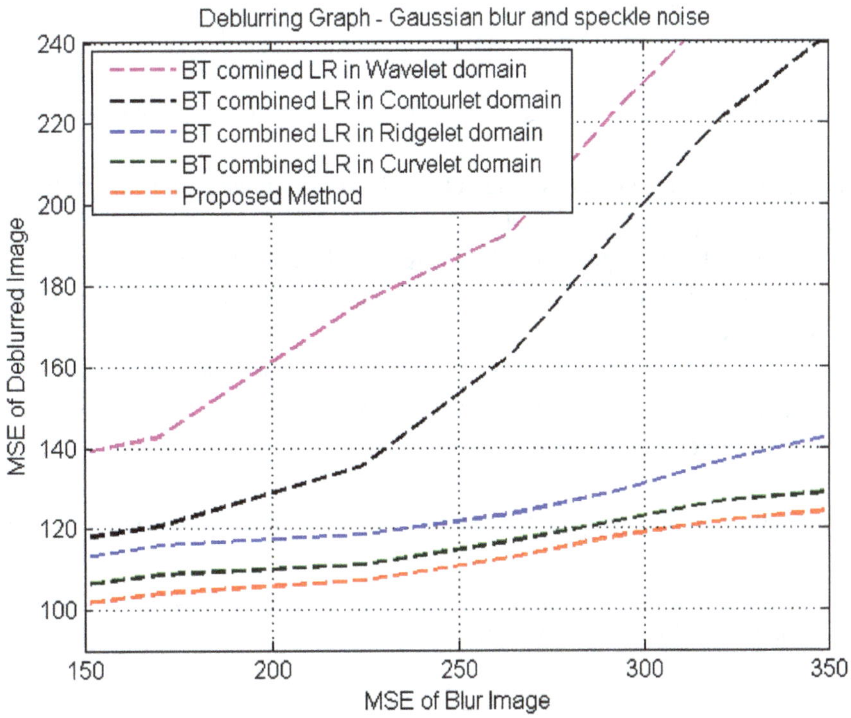

Figure 9. Denoising and deblurring images in case of motion blur combined with Gaussian noise by different methods: (a) blur combined with noise in image (PSNR = 19.2844 db); (b) denoised and deblurred image by BT combined LR in Wavelet domain (PSNR = 17.5256 db); (c) denoised and deblurred image by BT combined LR in Contourlet domain (PSNR = 17.8256 db); (d) denoised and deblurred image by BT combined LR in Ridgelet domain (PSNR = 21.1117 db); (e) denoised and deblurred image by BT combined LR in Curvelet domain (PSNR = 24.5251 db); (f) denoised and deblurred image by the proposed method (PSNR = 25.1516 db)

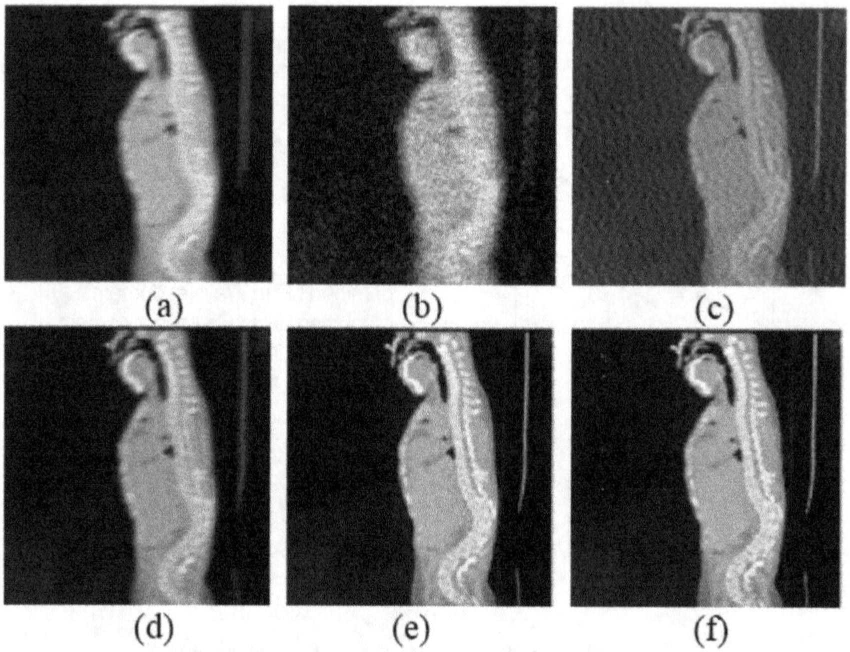

Case 3: Denoising and deblurring images in case motion blur combined with Gaussian noise.

Figure 9 shows the denoising and deblurring of blur and noise image which has motion blur combined with Gaussian noise by the proposed method.

In Figure 9, the result of the proposed method (Figure 9(f)) is better than the other methods (Figure 9(b), Figure 9(c), Figure 9(d) and Figure 9(e)). Because the PSNR value of Figure 9(f) is higher than the PSNR value in the rest figures.

Figure 10 and Figure 11 show the plot of PSNR, MSE values of different methods in denoising and deblurring corrupted in case of motion blur combined with Gaussian noise. The results of the proposed methods are better than the other methods.

Case 4: Denoising and deblurring images in case motion blur combined with speckle noise.

Figure 12 shows the denoising and deblurring of blur and noise image which has case motion blur combined with speckle noise by the proposed method.

Figure 10. Plot of PSNR values of denoised and deblurred images in case of motion blur combined with Gaussian noise using different methods

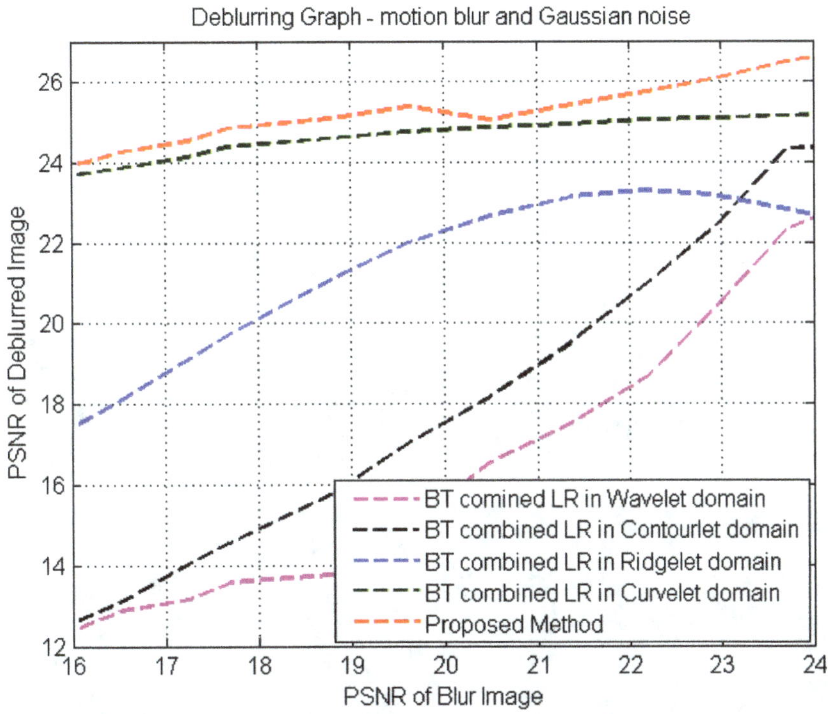

Figure 11. Plot of MSE values of denoised and deblurred images in case of motion blur combined with Gaussian noise using different methods

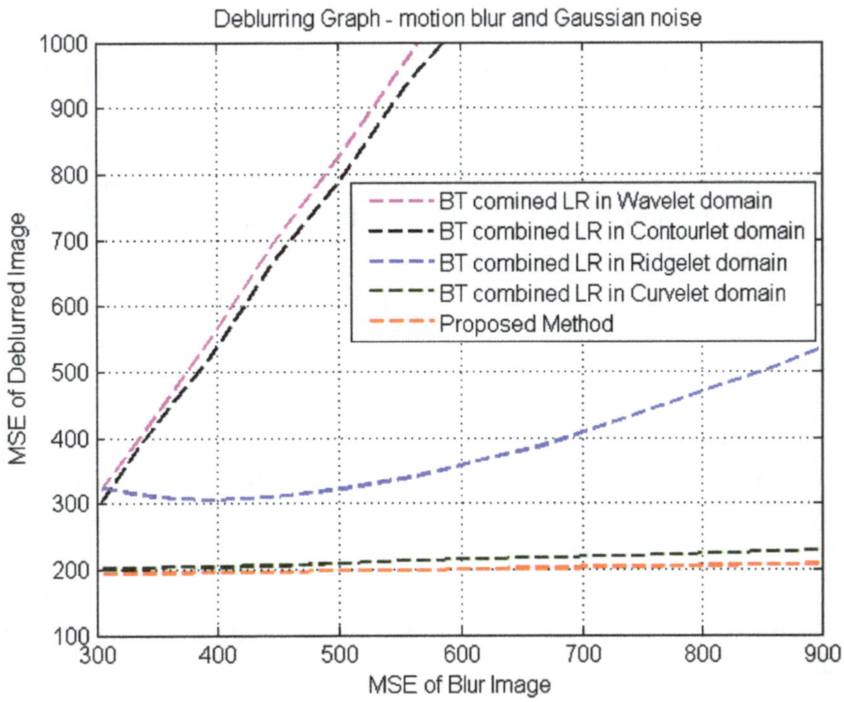

Figure 12. Denoising and deblurring images in case of motion blur combined with speckle noise by different methods: (a) blur combined with noise in image (PSNR = 19.0272 db); (b) denoised and deblurred image by BT combined LR in Wavelet domain (PSNR = 19.9272 db); (c) denoised and deblurred image by BT combined LR in Contourlet domain (PSNR = 20.7713 db); (d) denoised and deblurred image by BT combined LR in Ridgelet domain (PSNR = 21.4850 db); (e) denoised and deblurred image by BT combined LR in Curvelet domain (PSNR = 21.9936 db); (f) denoised and deblurred image by the proposed method (PSNR = 24.7218 db)

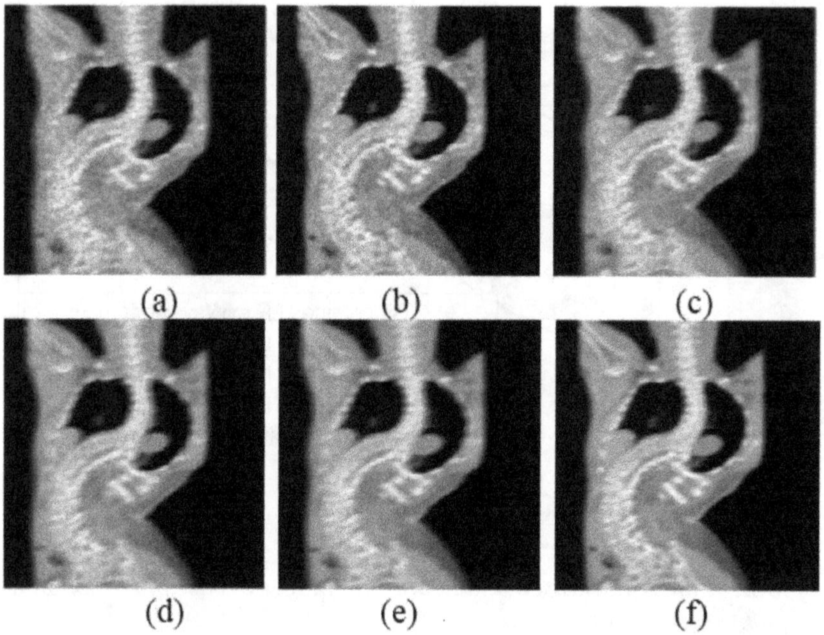

In Figure 12, the proposed method (Figure 12(f)) is better than the other methods (Figure 12(b), Figure 12(c), Figure 12(d) and Figure 12(e)). Because the PSNR value of Figure 12(f) is higher than the PSNR value in the rest figures.

Figure 13 and Figure 14 show the plot of PSNR, MSE values of different methods in denoising and deblurring corrupted in case of motion blur combined with speckle noise. The results of the proposed methods are better than the other methods.

DISCUSSION

As mentioned in the above, most of medical images not only have noise but also have blur. Clarification of medical images is hard work. This process is very difficult because it must not only increase the quality of images but also keep edge features. The NSCT uses the nonsubsampled Laplacian pyramid filter bank and the nonsubsampled directional filter bank to replace the old Laplacian pyramid and the directional filter bank in contourlet transform. The NSCT uses a double filter bank structure. So, most of the above cases from Figure 3 to Figure 14, the results of the proposed method are better than those of the other methods.

Figure 13. Plot of PSNR values of denoised and deblurred images in case of motion blur combined with speckle noise using different methods

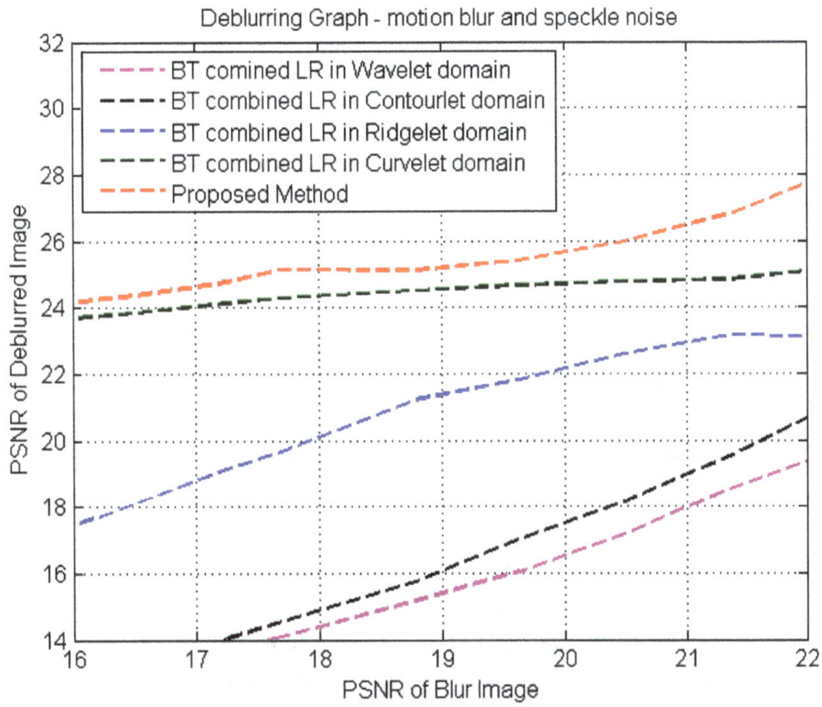

Figure 14. Plot of MSE values of denoised and deblurred images in case of motion blur combined with speckle noise using different methods

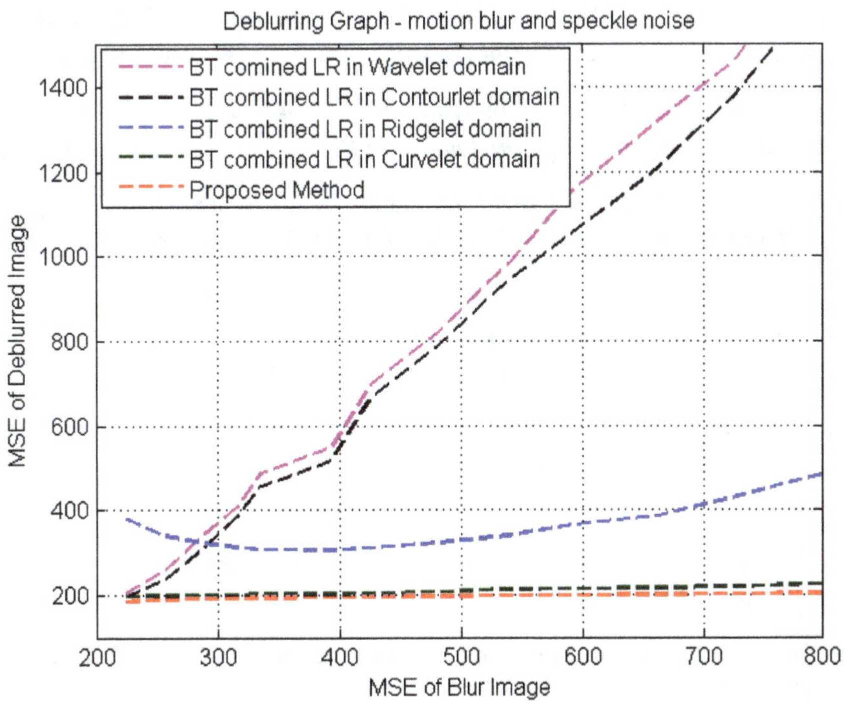

CONCLUSION

This chapter explores the new generation wavelets, which provides the basic framework for the development of adaptive techniques for medical image denoising and deblurring. Medical imaging has significantly contributed to improving the accuracy, timeliness and efficiency of diagnosis. Medical images are collected from many types of technical equipment. Each image type gives the information about each different disease and this information is necessary for the consultation of health professionals. So, the quality of medical images is very important and useful. It is necessary to increase the quality of medical images for treatment process. The quality depends on the environment, capture devices, technician's skills, etc. Most of medical images have blur combined with noise. Removing noise and blur in medical images is not easy. The goal of denoising and debluring is to remove noise and blur details from the corrupted image while maintaining edge features. In this chapter, the authors propose a new method to remove blur and noise in medical images. The proposed method includes two steps: decomposition and reconstruction. The construction is given by the value of Bayesian thresholding to remove noise and Lucy Richard to remove noise and blur again, and all of them are realized in nonsubsampled contourlet domain. The proposed method is tested with the dataset collected in many hospitals. The authors test the results of the proposed method in cases: motion blur combined with Gaussian noise and Gaussian blur combined with Gaussian noise. The authors compared the results with the other methods in wavelet domain and new generation wavelet transform such as ridgelet, curvelet and contourlet domain. The results of the proposed method are better than those of the other methods. In medical image field, the thresholding must be chosen carefully which must keep the information of images.

REFERENCES

Abramovich, T. S., & Silverman, B. W. (1998). Wavelet thresholding via a Bayesian approach. *Journal of the Royal Statistical Society. Series B. Methodological*, *60*(4), 725–749. doi:10.1111/1467-9868.00151

Al-Ameen, Sulong & Johar. (2012). Fast Deblurring Method for Computed Tomography Medical Images Using a Novel Kernels Set. *International Journal of Bio-Science and Bio-Technology*, *4*(3), 9–20.

Amira, S. A., & Sourav, S. (2015). Computed Tomography Image Enhancement Using Cuckoo Search: A Log Transform Based Approach. *Journal of Signal and Information Processing*, *6*(03), 244–257. doi:10.4236/jsip.2015.63023

Arthur, L, Zhou, & Do. (2005). Nonsubsampled Contourlet Transform: Theory, Design, and Applications. *IEEE Transactions on Image Processing*, *159*(10), 3089–3101. PMID:17022272

Arthur, L., Zhou, J., & Do Minh, N. (2006). Nonsubsampled Contourlet Transform: Filter design and applications in denoising. In *Proceedings of the 12th IEEE International Conference on Image Processing*, (pp. 749–752). IEEE.

Banhan, M., & Katsaggelos, A. K. (1997). Digital image restoration. *IEEE Signal Processing Magazine*, *14*(2), 24–41. doi:10.1109/79.581363

Bharath, A. (1998). Steerable filters from Erlang functions. *Proc. 9th British Machine Vision Conference*, (pp. 144–153).

Binh, N. T., & Dien, T. A. (2013). Object Detection and Tracking in Contourlet Domain. *Context-Aware Systems and Applications*, *109*, 192–200. doi:10.1007/978-3-642-36642-0_20

Binh, N. T., & Khare, A. (2010). Multilevel threshold based image denoising in curvelet domain. *Journal of Computer Science and Technology*, *25*(3), 632–640. doi:10.1007/s11390-010-9352-y

Binh, N. T., & Khare, A. (2013). *Image Denoising, Deblurring and Object Tracking, A new Generation wavelet based approach*. Lap Lambert Academic Publishing.

Binh, N. T., Tuyet, V. T. H., & Vinh, P. C. (2015). Increasing the quality of medical images based on the combination of filters in ridgelet domain. *Nature of Computation and Communication, Springer*, *144*, 320–331. doi:10.1007/978-3-319-15392-6_30

Burns, T., Rogers, S., Ruck, D., & Oxley, M. (1994). Discrete, spatiotemporal, wavelet multiresolution analysis method for computing optical flow. *Optical Engineering (Redondo Beach, Calif.)*, *33*(7), 2236–2247. doi:10.1117/12.172250

Candeș, E. J. (1998). *Ridgelets: Theory and Applications*. Stanford University.

Candes, E. J. (1998). *Ridgelets: Theory and Applications*. (PhD thesis). Department of Statistics, Stanford University.

Candes, E. J. (1999). *Monoscale ridgelets for the representation of images with edges. Dept. Statist., Stanford Univ*. Stanford, CA: Technical Representation.

Candes, E. J., Demanet, L., Donoho, D. L., & Ying, L. (2006). Fast Discrete Curvelet Transforms. *Multiscale Modeling & Simulation*, *5*(3), 861–899. doi:10.1137/05064182X

Candes, E.J. & Donoho, D.L (1999). Ridgelets: a Key to Higher- Diemensional Intermittency?. *Philosophical Transactions of the Royal Society A: Mathematical, Physical & Engineering Sciences, 357*(1760), 2495-2509

Candes, E. J., & Donoho, D. L. (2000). Curvelets - A Surprisingly Effective Nonadaptive Representation for Objects with Edges. In *Curves and Surface Fitting* (pp. 105–120). Saint-Malo: Vanderbilt University Press.

Candes, J., & Demanet, L. (2005). The curvelet representation of wave propagators is optimally sparse. *Communications on Pure and Applied Mathematics*, *58*(11), 1472–1528. doi:10.1002/cpa.20078

Candes & Donoho. (1999). *Curvelets: A surprisingly effective nonadaptive representation of objects with edges* (pp. 123–143). Nashville, TN: Vanderbilt University Press.

Chui, M. Feng, Wang, Li & Xu. (2012). Image Denoising Method with Adaptive Bayes threshold in Nonsubsampled Contourlet Domain. American Applied Science Research Institute, 1, 512 – 518.

Clonda, J.-M. L., & Goulard, B. (2004). Complex Daubechies wavelets: Properties and statistical image modeling. *Signal Processing*, *84*(1), 1–23. doi:10.1016/j.sigpro.2003.06.001

Cunha, L. D., Zhou, J., & Do, M. N. (2006). The Nonsubsampled Contourlet Transform: Theory, Design, and Applications. *IEEE Transactions on Image Processing*, *15*(10), 3089–3101. doi:10.1109/TIP.2006.877507 PMID:17022272

Do, M. N., & Vetterli, M. (2005). The Contourlet Transform: An Efficient Directional Multiresolution Image Representation. *IEEE Transactions on Image Processing*, *14*(12), 2091–2106. doi:10.1109/TIP.2005.859376 PMID:16370462

Donoho, D. L., & Duncan, M. R. (2000). Digital curvelet transform: Strategy, implementation and experiments. Rpoc. *SPIE*, *4056*, 12–29.

Donoho, L. (1998). *Orthonormal ridgelets and linear singularities. Tech. Report*. Department of Statistics, Stanford University.

Edwards (1992*). Discrete Wavelet Transforms: Theory and Implementation*. Academic Press.

Ghofrani. (2015). Comparing Nonsubsampled Wavelet, Contourlet and Shearlet Transforms for Ultrasound Image Despkeckling. *International Journal of Image, Graphics and Signal Processing*, 15-22.

Graps, A. (1995). An Introduction to Wavelets. *IEEE Computational Science & Engineering*, *2*(2), 50–61. doi:10.1109/99.388960

Gravel, P., Beaudoin, G., & DeGuise, J. A. (2004). A method for modeling noise in medical images. *IEEE Transactions on Medical Imaging*, *23*(10), 1221–1232. doi:10.1109/TMI.2004.832656 PMID:15493690

Jiang, M., Wang, G., Skinner, M. W., Rubinstien, J. T., & Vannier, M. W. (2003). Blind deblurring of spiral CT images. *IEEE Transactions on Medical Imaging*, *22*(7), 837–845. doi:10.1109/TMI.2003.815075 PMID:12906237

Jiang & Sha. (2013). Image De-Nosing Based on Non-Subsampled Contourlet Transform Domain in Multi-Bessel K Form Model. Research Journal of Applied Sciences. *Engineering and Technology*, *6*(18), 3400–3403.

Khare, A., & Tiwary, U. S. (2005). Soft-thresholding for denoising of medical images –A multiresolution approach. *International Journal of Wavelets, Multresolution, and Information Processing*, *3*(4), 477–496. doi:10.1142/S021969130500097X

Khare & Tiwary. (2006). Symmetric Daubechies Complex Wavelet Transform and its application to denoising and deblurring. *WSEAS Transactions on Signal Processing, 2*(5), 738 - 745.

Khare & Tiwary. (2006). A new method for deblurring and denoising of medical images using complex wavelet transform. Engineering in Medicine and Biology Society, IEEE.

Khare & Uma. (2006). A new method for deblurring and denoising of medical images using complex wavelet transform. *27th Annual International Conference of the Engineering in Medicine and Biology Society*, (pp. 1897 – 1900).

Lina, M. (1997). Image processing with complex Daubechies wavelets. *Journal of Mathematical Imaging and Vision*, *7*(3), 211–223. doi:10.1023/A:1008274210946

Lina, M., & Mayrand, M. (1995). Complex Daubechies Wavelets. *Journal of Applied and Computational Harmonic Analysis*, *2*(3), 219–229. doi:10.1006/acha.1995.1015

Ma, J., & Plonka, G. (2010). The Curvelet Transform a Review of recent Applications. *IEEE Signal Processing Magazine*, *27*(2), 118–133. doi:10.1109/MSP.2009.935453

MajaTemerinac, O. (2010). *Tile-based Lucy-Richardson Deconvolution modeling a spatially-varying PSF for Fast Multiview Fusion of Microscopical images*. Teachnical Report 260.

Marcin, K., Materka, Strzelecki, & Szczypinski. (2001). Discrete Wavelet transform – derived features for digital image texture analysis. *Proc. Of International Conference on Signals and Electronic Systems*, (pp. 163 -168).

Michailovich, O., & Adam, D. (2004). Phase unwrapping for 2-D blind deconvolution of ultrasound images. *IEEE Transactions on Medical Imaging*, *23*(1), 7–25. doi:10.1109/TMI.2003.819932 PMID:14719683

Phuong, L. T., & Binh, N. T. (2015). Human Object Classification Based on Nonsubsampled Contourlet Transform Combined with Zernike Moment. *4th EAI International Conference on Context-Aware Systems and Applications*. Springer.

Selesnick, I. W., & Sendur, L. (2000). Iterated oversampled filter banks and wavelet frames. Wavelet Applications VII. *Proceedings of the Society for Photo-Instrumentation Engineers*, 733–744. doi:10.1117/12.408663

Sitara, K., & Remya, S. (2012). Image deblurring in bayesian framework using template based blur estimation. *The International Journal of Multimedia & Its Applications*, *4*(1), 137–153. doi:10.5121/ijma.2012.4112

Stanley, H. (2011). An Augmented Lagrangian Method for Total Variation Video Restoration. *IEEE Transactions on Image Processing*, *20*(11), 3097–3111. doi:10.1109/TIP.2011.2158229 PMID:21632302

Starck, L., Candès, E. J., & Donoho, D. L. (2002). The Curvelet Transform for Image Denoising. *IEEE Transactions on Image Processing*, *11*(6), 670–684. doi:10.1109/TIP.2002.1014998 PMID:18244665

Strang. (1989). Wavelets and dilation equations: A brief introduction. *SIAM Review, 31*(4).

Taxt, T. (1997). Comparison of cepstrum - based methods for radial blind deconvolution of ultrasound images. *IEEE Transactions on Ultrasonics, Ferroelectrics, and Frequency Control*, *44*(3), 666–674. doi:10.1109/58.658327

Tuyet, V. T. H., & Binh, N. T. (2015). Reducing impurities in medical images based on curvelet domain. *Nature of Computation and Communication, Springer*, *144*, 306–319. doi:10.1007/978-3-319-15392-6_29

Wagner, F. C., Macovski, A., & Nishimura, D. G. (1988). A characterization of the scatter point-spread function in terms of air gaps. *IEEE Transactions on Medical Imaging*, *7*(4), 337–344. doi:10.1109/42.14517 PMID:18230487

Wang, G., Vannier, M. W., Skinner, M. W., Cavalcanti, M. G. P., & Harding, G. (1998). Spiral CT image deblurring for cochlear implantation. *IEEE Transactions on Medical Imaging*, *17*(2), 251–262. doi:10.1109/42.700737 PMID:9688157

Wang, X., Ritchie, C. J., & Kim, Y. (1996). Elevation direction deconvolution in three-dimensional ultrasound imaging. *IEEE Transactions on Medical Imaging*, *15*(3), 389–394. doi:10.1109/42.500148 PMID:18215920

Xiangfei, K., Kuan, L., Qingxiong, Y., Liu, W., & Ming, H. Y. (2013). A New Image Quality Metric for Image Auto-Denoising. *IEEE International Conference on Computer Vision*, (pp. 2888-2895). IEEE.

Zhang, J. M. F., & Starck, J. L. (2008). Wavelets, ridgelets and curvelets for poisson noise removal. *IEEE Transactions on Image Processing*, *17*(7), 1093–1108. doi:10.1109/TIP.2008.924386 PMID:18586618

Zhang, W., Yu, F., & Hong-mi, G. (2009). Improved adaptive wavelet threshold for image denoising. *Control and Decision Conference, Chinese*. IEEE. doi:10.1109/CCDC.2009.5195268

KEY TERMS AND DEFINITIONS

Contourlet Transform: A new two-dimensional transform method for image representations which has properties of multiresolution, localization, directionality, critical sampling and anisotropy.

Curvelet Transform: A higher dimensional generalization of the wavelet transform designed to represent images at different scales and different angles.

Discrete Wavelet Transform: A special case of the wavelet transform that provides a compact representation of a signal in time and frequency that can be computed efficiently.

Mean Square Error (MSE): Equal to the square of the bias plus the variance of the estimator.

Nonsubsampled Contourlet Transform: A fully shiftinvariant version of contourlet transform. It is based on a nonsubsampled pyramid structure and nonsubsampled directional filter banks.

Nonsubsampled Directional Filter Banks: A shift-invariant version of the critically sampled directional filter bank inthe contourlet transform.

Nonsubsampled Pyramids: Provide multiscale decomposition.

Peak Signal-to-Noise Ratio (PSNR): An expression for the ratio between the maximum possible value of a signal and the power of distorting noise that affects the quality of its representation.

Ridgelet Transform: Allows representing edges and other singularities along lines in a more efficient way compared to wavelet transform.

APPENDIX: TABLES

Table 1. PSNR values (db) of different denoised and deblurred images with Gaussian blur combined with Gaussian noise

Test Image	Blur and Noise Image	BT Combined LR in Wavelet Domain	BT Combined LR in Contourlet Domain	BT Combined LR in Ridgelet Domain	BT Combined LR in Curvelet Domain	The Proposed Method
1	21.9551	22.0886	22.2635	25.2925	27.5851	27.8651
2	22.1225	22.2447	22.5432	25.4436	27.6260	27.9231
3	22.2553	22.4534	22.6744	25.5623	27.6416	28.0476
4	22.4200	22.5970	22.9647	25.7279	27.6727	28.3748
5	22.5599	22.7166	23.0428	25.8310	27.7031	28.7523
6	22.7435	22.9340	23.2424	25.9556	27.7614	28.9915
7	22.9195	23.1097	23.4097	26.1129	27.8289	29.0289
8	23.2956	23.3615	23.8738	26.3840	27.9276	29.5229
9	23.7509	24.4852	24.3859	26.6923	28.0844	29.9844
10	24.1763	24.6278	24.9229	26.8494	28.1616	30.1401
11	24.7159	24.8509	25.6932	27.1021	28.3408	30.3429
12	25.3421	25.1876	26.3895	27.3429	28.5368	30.6666
13	26.0773	25.3132	27.3161	27.4898	28.7644	30.9152
14	27.0030	25.5200	27.1208	27.6189	29.1284	31.2111
15	27.4680	25.9635	27.4268	27.9916	29.3674	31.9127

Table 2. PSNR values (db) of different denoised and deblurred images with Gaussian blur combined with speckle noise

Test Image	Blur and Noise Image	BT Combined LR in Wavelet Domain	BT Combined LR in Contourlet Domain	BT Combined LR in Ridgelet Domain	BT Combined LR in Curvelet Domain	The Proposed Method
1	16.9551	17.1886	17.2517	17.5886	18.5851	18.8613
2	17.1225	17.8428	17.9372	18.2447	18.9261	19.4231
3	17.2553	18.2534	18.6525	18.9533	19.2516	19.9476
4	17.4200	18.5970	18.9970	18.9970	20.3728	20.9748
5	17.5599	18.8166	19.0166	19.6166	20.9033	21.7523
6	18.2435	19.1340	19.4340	20.0434	21.3614	22.1915
7	18.9195	19.5097	19.9092	20.5097	22.0289	22.9289
8	19.5956	20.0615	20.3613	20.9615	22.9279	23.9229
9	20.4509	20.3522	20.8552	21.4522	23.4844	24.5844
10	21.1763	21.2278	21.9270	22.7278	24.1611	25.1401
11	22.4159	22.6509	22.9505	23.8509	24.9408	26.9429
12	23.3421	24.0876	24.3892	25.0876	25.8366	26.9666
13	24.5773	25.0132	25.3142	25.9132	26.7656	27.9152
14	25.8003	26.1291	26.5270	27.2291	28.1110	29.2111
15	26.3891	26.8383	26.9182	27.5719	28.4894	29.9423

Table 3. PSNR values (db) of different denoised and deblurred images with motion blur combined with Gaussian noise

Test Image	Blur and Noise Image	BT Combined LR in Wavelet Domain	BT Combined LR in Contourlet Domain	BT Combined LR in Ridgelet Domain	BT Combined LR in Curvelet Domain	The Proposed Method
1	15.8363	12.2024	12.4021	17.2438	23.6217	23.9257
2	16.1698	12.5903	12.7800	17.6511	23.7351	24.0129
3	16.5096	12.8389	13.0920	18.0945	23.8461	24.2564
4	17.2470	13.1725	14.0534	19.1103	24.1311	24.5321
5	17.6881	13.2745	14.5703	19.7393	24.3803	24.8330
6	18.7852	13.9873	15.7520	21.0841	24.5912	25.0811
7	19.6209	15.8484	17.0190	21.9878	24.7435	25.3650
8	20.4853	16.5509	18.7838	22.6720	24.8542	25.0412
9	21.3479	17.4969	19.8333	23.1315	24.9343	25.4032
10	22.1843	18.6751	20.9328	23.2809	25.0401	25.7401
11	22.8801	20.2703	22.4525	23.1789	25.0825	26.0512
12	23.7053	22.3346	24.3363	22.8175	25.1279	26.4789
13	24.8021	23.3706	24.3673	22.2733	25.1947	26.8917
14	25.2021	23.9754	24.6322	22.5346	25.4589	27.6613
15	25.8021	23.9994	24.8327	23.8463	25.9542	27.9524

Table 4. PSNR values (db) of different denoised and deblurred images with motion blur combined with speckle noise

Test Image	Blur and Noise Image	BT Combined LR in Wavelet Domain	BT Combined LR in Contourlet Domain	BT Combined LR in Ridgelet Domain	BT Combined LR in Curvelet Domain	The Proposed Method
1	15.8363	12.2021	12.4048	17.2438	23.6217	24.0257
2	16.1698	12.5800	12.7381	17.6511	23.7351	24.2129
3	16.5096	12.8920	13.0478	18.0945	23.8461	24.3564
4	17.2470	13.7534	14.3731	19.1103	24.1311	24.7321
5	17.6881	14.0703	14.5384	19.6393	24.2803	25.1233
6	18.7852	15.1520	15.7520	21.1841	24.4912	25.0811
7	19.6209	16.0190	17.0190	21.7878	24.6435	25.3650
8	20.4853	17.1509	18.1272	22.5720	24.7542	25.9412
9	21.3479	18.4969	19.4373	23.1315	24.8343	26.8032
10	22.1843	19.5751	20.9751	23.0809	25.1401	27.9401
11	22.8801	20.4703	21.2958	23.1789	25.0005	28.7512
12	23.7053	21.6346	22.6378	22.7175	25.1089	29.4789
13	24.8021	22.5706	23.4782	22.7330	25.2047	29.8917
14	25.5891	22.8948	23.8938	22.9328	25.5921	29.9910
15	26.9392	23.9328	24.6163	23.8478	26.9989	30.6781

Table 5. MSE values of different denoised and deblurred images with Gaussian blur combined with Gaussian noise

Test Image	Blur and Noise Image	BT Combined LR in Wavelet Domain	BT Combined LR in Contourlet Domain	BT Combined LR in Ridgelet Domain	BT Combined LR in Curvelet Domain	The Proposed Method
1	129.6527	129.6754	126.6527	112.5092	100.4562	095.3152
2	144.9713	115.8291	105.7628	113.6351	104.4389	099.8541
3	160.4551	129.7835	120.7154	115.9038	108.7739	103.9567
4	174.1348	147.3876	135.6323	118.4373	111.0471	107.0821
5	203.9480	176.5497	162.6307	123.2613	116.6487	112.5410
6	232.5486	202.6411	192.6949	129.0343	121.6020	117.7920
7	261.6603	241.7006	221.7573	136.6586	126.7080	121.7215
8	289.2192	272.1109	252.1306	145.5433	129.9827	125.2477
9	317.0187	292.9837	279.9598	152.3246	133.2157	129.4109
10	345.7267	338.7994	308.7854	165.0138	137.0709	133.6238
11	372.4618	371.5771	341.4907	173.8953	139.8947	136.5534
12	398.8666	391.8614	361.9214	185.6629	141.4060	139.8650
13	420.8848	409.9848	374.9389	195.5350	162.2364	153.9636
14	450.1353	418.3749	385.1335	207.1940	178.3092	169.3562
15	486.1332	432.7409	399.5754	221.5284	192.7547	180.4356

Table 6. MSE values of different denoised and deblurred images with Gaussian blur combined with speckle noise

Test Image	Blur and Noise Image	BT Combined LR in Wavelet Domain	BT Combined LR in Contourlet Domain	BT Combined LR in Ridgelet Domain	BT Combined LR in Curvelet Domain	The Proposed Method
1	109.6527	129.6527	126.6823	112.5092	100.4562	95.3152
2	134.9710	135.7683	115.7628	110.6351	104.4389	99.8541
3	170.4551	142.7389	120.7154	115.9038	108.7739	103.9567
4	224.1348	175.9373	135.6323	118.4373	111.0471	107.0821
5	263.9480	192.6736	162.6307	123.2613	116.6487	112.5410
6	292.5486	222.9082	192.6949	129.0343	121.6020	117.7920
7	321.6603	249.0019	221.7576	136.6586	126.7080	121.7215
8	365.2192	272.9390	252.1306	145.5433	129.9827	125.2477
9	392.0187	299.9381	279.9597	152.3246	133.2157	129.4109
10	425.7267	358.0037	308.7994	165.0138	137.0709	133.6238
11	472.4618	391.5895	341.4907	173.8953	139.8947	136.5534
12	498.8666	421.8938	361.9214	185.6629	141.4060	139.8650
13	520.6888	453.4894	380.8947	201.4784	173.5636	150.3818
14	545.3529	475.8489	402.4672	230.4003	199.5454	170.4434
15	576.3741	499.4673	435.3501	253.4741	228.4236	197.4673

Table 7. MSE values of different denoised and deblurred images with motion blur combined with Gaussian noise

Test Image	Blur and Noise Image	BT Combined LR in Wavelet Domain	BT Combined LR in Contourlet Domain	BT Combined LR in Ridgelet Domain	BT Combined LR in Curvelet Domain	The Proposed Method
1	240.5859	199.3631	190.3631	385.2574	198.0095	190.0705
2	277.044	249.6745	239.6425	339.8808	199.6001	191.6611
3	307.5838	330.0825	310.1105	322.5789	201.1268	193.1328
4	335.0175	399.5232	385.5002	312.7464	201.6291	194.7601
5	365.4463	478.6311	458.5512	307.7112	204.7150	195.2320
6	393.2294	549.4841	519.4841	305.4876	203.7372	195.6815
7	445.4134	694.6912	664.1966	309.9549	205.3902	196.3409
8	501.7824	830.9802	790.8802	322.5217	208.4466	197.4916
9	558.5589	979.8377	939.7111	339.6479	213.2577	198.2002
10	612.2898	1155.3000	1055.8120	364.5995	215.8121	199.6580
11	662.1546	1296.6124	1206.6000	385.5235	217.3992	201.3215
12	733.8379	1473.7000	1333.6132	428.4344	220.3930	203.3135
13	860.1225	1819.4000	1729.4134	506.6031	225.9913	206.9231
14	989.4599	2197.7000	1987.1764	596.5529	235.5765	210.5619
15	1038.3838	2392.8378	2010.3533	604.7382	276.5240	225.8573

Table 8. MSE values of different denoised and deblurred images with motion blur combined with speckle noise

Test Image	Blur and Noise Image	BT Combined LR in Wavelet Domain	BT Combined LR in Contourlet Domain	BT Combined LR in Ridgelet Domain	BT Combined LR in Curvelet Domain	The Proposed Method
1	220.5859	199.9473	190.3631	385.2574	198.0422	185.0705
2	257.0440	259.9345	239.6725	339.8808	199.8777	189.6611
3	287.5838	340.8681	310.0825	322.5789	201.5261	191.1328
4	315.0175	405.6483	385.5232	312.7464	201.9657	192.7601
5	335.4463	488.6311	458.6311	307.7112	204.5391	193.2320
6	393.2294	549.5345	519.4841	305.4876	203.7544	194.7372
7	425.4134	694.4284	664.1966	309.9549	205.0946	195.3409
8	481.7824	820.9721	790.9802	322.0557	208.8958	196.4466
9	538.5589	979.8395	939.8377	339.6479	213.8937	197.2577
10	592.2898	1155.3000	1055.3987	364.5995	215.1111	198.6580
11	662.1546	1316.6784	1206.6654	385.5235	217.6301	199.3992
12	723.8379	1453.7364	1373.7763	428.4344	220.3874	201.3930
13	830.1225	1849.4674	1729.4566	506.6031	225.9444	202.9231
14	899.4599	2297.7958	1997.7452	596.5529	235.9241	203.5765
15	968.5335	2300.3784	2090.4322	605.4352	267.4321	240.4904

Section 2

Filtering and Thresholding for Medical Image Quality Improvement

Chapter 4
Intensity-Based Classification and Related Methods in Brain MR Images

Luminita Moraru
Dunarea de Jos University of Galati, Romania

Simona Moldovanu
Dunarea de Jos University of Galati, Romania & Dumitru Motoc High School, Romania

Anjan Biswas
Delaware State University, USA & King Abdulaziz University, Saudi Arabia

ABSTRACT

Today, medical image processing and analysis are highly active research fields boosted by rapid technical developments in medical imaging field. This chapter describes common procedures such as thresholding methods and clustering algorithms (both non-hierarchical and hierarchical approaches) used for digital image processing, with specific reference to brain magnetic resonance images. These techniques represent starting points for other sophisticated methods such as segmentation and classification. The results, which are an outcome of these methods, are used for classification of neurodegenerative diseases such as Alzheimer, Pick's, Huntington's or cerebral calcinosis. A number of applications together with the code listing are provided with the aim to make the subject accessible and practical. The MATLAB software will help the readers to identify and choose the best solution for a particular problem.

INTRODUCTION

Images contain plenty of objects and patterns that are actually embedded with valuable information essential for medicine, biology, photo or video areas. In image analysis, inputs are images and outputs are measured data or information extracted from those images. The final goal of image analysis is to take action or to make sense of gathered data through recognized or classified objects (or classes or attributes).

DOI: 10.4018/978-1-5225-0140-4.ch004

Basically, segmentation means to separate an image into regions by finding contours that correspond to objects embedded in the image. These regions are segmented either based on some common features or on differences between edges at objects' boundaries. One of the most difficult tasks in image processing is the fully automatic segmentation. The quality of segmentation will guarantee the accuracy of objects recognition, feature extraction or classification.

The main goal of this chapter is to provide advanced methods and algorithms in the area of intensity-based image segmentation and classification. In this context, thresholding methods based on histogram and binarization techniques are presented. *K*-means, *c*-means clustering and dendrograms as hierarchical methods for classification and their applications mainly for medical image segmentation are also discussed. In order to explain some concepts in image processing and analysis, two threshold methods are presented. One is based on adaptive thresholding and global binarization and the other is based on dendrograms. They are the starting point for the classification process based on clustering analysis. The cluster validity and classification accuracy are evaluated by using the Euclidean distance as a similarity measure between clusters.

Thresholding is an important approach in image segmentation. Some binarization methods for segmentation, via thresholds, based on the distribution of pixel properties such as intensity values, are presented. Also, cluster technique as another way of determining the optimal threshold is discussed. Optimal threshold for classification allows differentiating classes of objects between them.

Classification assigns particular objects to the existing groups of objects into image. These groups were obtained through clustering operations. In this context, clustering can be interpreted as a form of classification. Generally, classification techniques include supervised and unsupervised classification. Unsupervised classification provides outcomes based on the software analysis without any human implication. It allows an objective classification but it takes no advantage of previous information known to the user. Unlabeled objects are assigned to a group or cluster by using a model developed based on *a priori* knowledge on the relevant characteristics of the objects that already belong to that group. In supervised classification, the user can select certain features or qualitative descriptors that are representative for objects in order to build the training sets for classification. Also, the user can impose the number of clusters or groups for classification. Hierarchical clustering is one of the most common unsupervised classification methods. Its graphical representation is a dendrogram or a tree structure. Various supervised classification algorithms such as naïve Bayes derived from Bayesian classifiers, C4.5 derived from classification tree, K-nearest neighbors, multilayer perceptron, neural networks or logistic regression have found many application in medical imaging.

The evaluation of cluster validity and classification accuracy is done by two approaches. The first technique assesses the extent to which a cluster contains objects belonging of a single class. The second approach uses the Euclidean distance to measure the distance between clusters as a similarity measure between clusters.

In this study, 2D MRI images that belong to the Harvard Medical School database are used. They are freely available at http://www.med.harvard.edu/AANLIB/home.html. For comparison purposes, the same test image is used across this work. MATLAB programming language is used to demonstrate some practical image processing techniques. The operations have been implemented using the Wavelets and Image Processing tools for MATLAB R2014a software. Some examples of code listing of MATLAB algorithms for image manipulation are presented.

BACKGROUND

Thresholding is the simplest procedure for image segmentation as it separates objects and background into non-overlapping sets. Thresholding converts a grayscale input image to a binarized image by using binary arithmetic and an optimal threshold (Sahoo et al., 1988; Sezgin & Sankur, 2004). All pixels that are below threshold are turned to zero and all pixels about the threshold to one. It is called bi-level thresholding. Multilevel thresholding outputs more than one threshold and these thresholds are used to divide the whole range of gray values into several sub ranges (Liang & Cuevas, 2013; Arora et al., 2006). Through the thresholding operations, there are extracted those pixels from an image which represent an object. Two types of thresholding algorithms exist: (i) global thresholding algorithms, when a single threshold for all the image pixels is used; (ii) local or adaptive thresholding algorithms when different threshold values for different local areas are used. Global thresholding is more appropriate for images with uniform contrast distribution of background and foreground. When important background noise or variation in contrast and illumination exist, the pixels classification as foreground or background is hampered. Here, binarization, with local thresholding, is more appropriate. In many practical applications, thresholding techniques utilize shape information of the histogram of the image to determine the appropriate threshold (Gonzalez & Richard, 2002; Nakib et al., 2007; Moldovanu et al., 2010; Bibicu et al., 2013; Bibicu et al., 2015).

Depending on the application, the binarization techniques for grayscale images are grouped into two broad categories: global binarization and local binarization.

The most common method is Otsu's thresholding method which utilizes discriminant analysis to find the maximum separability of classes (Otsu, 1979). It belongs to global binarization methods and pixels are divided into two classes and the threshold is calculated by using total mean and the between-classes variance. The optimum threshold can be determined by optimizing the average pixel classification error rate based on the histogram of the image (Kittler & Illingworth, 1986). Also, thresholding can be regarded as a clustering problem (Kwon, 2004; Kwon et al., 2008). This involves both pixels' probability distribution and the information on their spatial distribution. This evaluation optimizes intra-class similarity to achieve most similar classes and inter-class similarity to conclude that every cluster is clearly separate. Arifin & Asano (2006) proposed a method for image thresholding based on hierarchical cluster organization. In order to obtain a clear separation between object and background, they developed a dendrogram of gray levels in the histogram of an image, based on similarity measure and merging criteria by involving the inter-class variance and the intra-class variance of the clusters.

The local binarization techniques estimate the threshold individually, for each pixel, according to the gray scale information of neighboring pixels (Moldovanu et al., 2015). The methods of Niblack (1986), Sauvola (2000) or Bernsen (1986) belong to this category. Niblack's method is a local variance-based method and computes the optimum threshold according to the local mean, standard deviation and the size of a sliding mask. Sauvola et al. (2000) proposed an improved method that provides better results for images containing inhomogeneity. Bernsen's method is a local adaptive method based on image contrast. The threshold is set as the mean of the minimum and maximum gray values within a local window.

Cluster analysis belongs to unsupervised learning. It handles several objects or variables, examines how much variance these objects/variables share, and groups them together to same class based on the similarity of their responses to several measurements or based on relevant features. Here, the "similarity" addresses to pair of objects and is interpreted as an average global measure over the whole set of characteristics. Cluster analysis is concerned to a pre-classification stage. It provides only the existence of clusters where the dependent objects/variables form a group. In order to find some relationship between the objects, the degree of similarity relative to the group can be analyzed by using similarity or dissimilarity coefficients. Clustering procedures could be divided into two broad categories:

- Hierarchical methods provide a hierarchy of clusters, look for relative relation between them to create high order cluster and then allow drawing dendrograms (or vector graphs);
- Non-hierarchical methods use cluster without looking at relationship between objects.

Objects classification in medical imaging such as lesions, organs or patterns that belong to specific diseases represents a challenging task. In image processing field, classification aims to identify features, patterns, structures or objects into an image and then, assigns them to a particular class (Jia et al., 2014; Lu & Ba, 2010; Bui & Taira (eds) 2010; Dai & Ji, 2014; Amiri et al., 2013; Collins et al., 2002). The steps to be followed in unsupervised classification are:

1. Generate clusters; and
2. Assign classes.

In supervised classification, the user selects representative samples and generates the training sets. Then, the image classification software uses these training sets to identify the classes of interest in the analyzed images. The image classification algorithms establish each class on what it resembles most in the training set. The steps to be followed in supervised classification are:

1. Choose the training sets and their associated class labels;
2. Generate the relevant patterns;
3. Classify.

One of the simplest ways of defining a classifier is to use the minimum distance between defined classes. Here, the Euclidian distance computed in the feature space is the most common approach. It works as a similarity/dissimilarity measure and groups similar feature using a constant threshold. By calculating the linear distance between pair of analyzed classes it is possible to classify a feature class.

K-means clustering divides objects/variables of a dataset into non-overlapping clusters and is based on the iterative relocation of data points between clusters (MacQueen, 1967). It is used to produce groups of cases/variables with a high degree of similarity within each group and a low degree of similarity between groups (Hastie et al., 2009; Ng et al., 2006). Also, *K*-means clustering algorithm reduces the complexity of the data. Clustering is a form of classification (i.e. unsupervised classification) since it labels an object through the label of cluster where this object is assigned. In order to classify a given data set, a certain number of clusters (i.e. *K* clusters) is fixed *a priori* by defining the corresponding *k* centroids. The efficacy of the method strongly depends on the position of these centroids. Different locations will cause different results. It is highly recommended using as few clusters as possible, placed as far away from each other as possible and, to capture all statistically important clusters. The next step consists of assigning each object/variable of a given data set to the nearest center. When all objects have been assigned, the first iteration is completed and a clustering is done. A new relocation of centroids of the clusters, resulting from the previous step, is necessary through re-association the same data set points and the nearest new centroid. During this iterative process, the *k* centroids change their location until no more changes are done. In order to calculate the similarity between objects, particular cases of the Minkowski distance $\Delta_{MKW} = \sqrt[\lambda]{\sum_{i}^{k} \left|y_i - x_i\right|^{\lambda}}$ are used. Here y is the cluster center, x is the analyzed case/object, i is the dimension of instances x and y being compared, k is the total number of dimensions and λ the order of the Minkowski metric. $\lambda = 1$ corresponds to the Manhattan distance $\Delta_1 = \sum_{i}^{k} \left|y_i - x_i\right|$ and $\lambda = 2$ to the Euclidean distance $\Delta_2 = \sqrt{\sum_{i}^{k} \left(y_i - x_i\right)^2}$. The Euclidian distance is the most used (Morissette & Chartier, 2013). $\Delta_3 = \sum_{i}^{k} \left(y_i - x_i\right)^2$ is the Euclidean Squared distance. These three distances are metric similarity functions and indicate the magnitude of difference between attributes of two vectors. A valid distance measure is symmetric and, in case of identical vectors, its minimum value is zero. The vector cosine angle distance $\Delta_4 = \frac{\left(\sum_{i}^{k} y_i \cdot x_i\right)}{\left(\sqrt{\sum_{i}^{k} y_i^2} \cdot \sqrt{\sum_{i}^{k} x_i^2}\right)}$ is a nonmetric similarity function and gives a measure of how similar attributes of vectors are, but with no regard to magnitude (Qian et al., 2002).

To be able to successfully use *K*-means algorithm it is necessary to know how many clusters are present in the dataset. Generally, this information is not available and for this reason it needs to be noted that the *K*-means algorithm does not necessarily find the most optimal configuration, corresponding to the global objective function minimum. Another limitation of the *K*-means clustering technique is the outliers' issue. There is a variety of outlier detection techniques (Laurikkala et al., 2000; Tang et al., 2001; Hodge & Austin, 2004, Moldovanu et al., 2015). Outlier detection looks for those data that do not conform to expected behavior or is deviate largely from the expected pattern. In the case of MR images, outlier detection shouldn't be interpreted as noise removal techniques. They are complementary techniques. The outlier detection techniques determine the outliers with *no prior* knowledge of the data (similar to unsupervised clustering) or can work analogous to supervised classification but require pre-labeled data, tagged as normal or abnormal. Also, semi-supervised outlier detection techniques exist and assume that only the normal class is labeled. Different approaches are suitable for different types of data. Recently, the cluster analysis has been employed for determination of optimal threshold (Kwon, 2004; Arifin & Asano, 2006).

Dendrograms are useful for validating classification models and are based on hierarchical cluster analysis (Murtagh & Legendre, 2014; Dou et al., 2007; Moldovanu et al., 2014). They are a tree-like diagram which displays the cluster-subcluster relationship and the dynamic of clusters merging. First, the algorithm computes the distances between each pair of classes, and then it iteratively merges the closest pair of classes until the classes are all merged. The distances at which the signatures of classes are merged are used to construct a dendrogram. The height at which two clusters are merged is the distance between the two clusters. The following operations are performed in order to plot the hierarchical clustering groups as a tree:

- The distance between two objects $p[y_i]$ and $q[x_i]$ is computed using the Euclidean metric $\Delta_2 = \sqrt{\sum_i^k (y_i - x_i)^2}$ (Liu et al., 2005);
- The metric data are clustered according to the linkage criterion $d(r,s) = \frac{1}{n_r n_s} \sum_{i=1}^{n_r} \sum_{j=1}^{n_s} dist(x_{ri}, x_{sj})$. This criterion for choosing which pairs of class to merge at each step is the average distance that computes the average distance between the pairs of points for any two clusters *r* and *s* with n_r and n_s items;
- At the final stage, all items are assigned to a single cluster. This allows the determination of the stopping group mergers.
- By using dendrograms it is possible to evaluate the efficacy of hierarchical clustering approach on various types of data and to compare to *K*-means results.

THRESHOLDING

Often, it is necessary to examine the foreground and /or background of images because they divide an image into regions that correspond to the objects. This is straightforward matter and is called image segmentation based on thresholding.

Simple Thresholding

For a grayscale input image $f(x,y)$ the thresholded image $g(x,y)$ for a global threshold *T* is:

$$g(x,y) = \begin{cases} 1, & if\ f(x,y) \geq T \\ 0, & if\ f(x,y) < T \end{cases}$$

The thresholding segmentation method along with its inputs and outputs images is shown in Figure 1. The first module is the original image and the second is the resulted binary image for a selected threshold *T*.

The above description can easily be implemented in MATLAB. Given an *m* × *n* image, *f*, the following code fragment provides the image *g* with the same size, in binary format.

Figure 2 shows the effect of the Code Listing 1 on input image.

Figure 1. Illustration of the thresholding segmentation pipeline

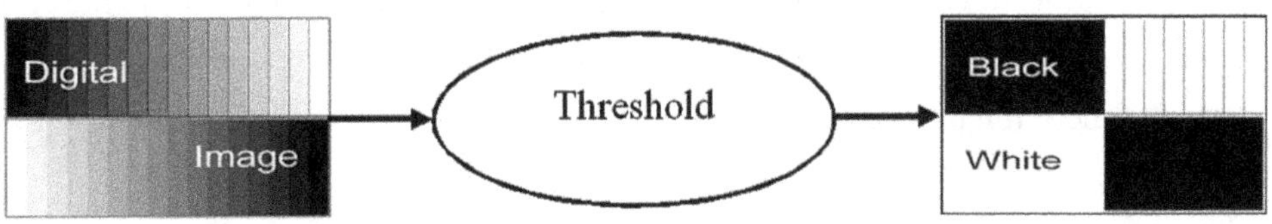

Code Listing 1. A very simply thresholding

```
f = propsSynthesizeImage;
figure, imshow(f)
T=150;
g = f > T;
figure,imshow(g);
```

Figure 2. (a) The input grayscale image; (b) result of global thresholding with T = 150

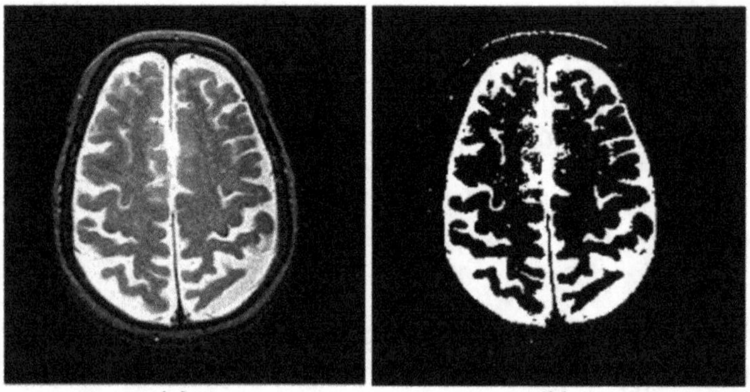

(a) (b)

Adaptive Thresholding

Non-uniform illumination due to image acquisition technologies may dramatically change the histogram, so it becomes impossible to segment an image based on a single threshold value. Adaptive thresholding segmentation separates the foreground and background based on non-uniform illumination. Apart for the global threshold method, the adaptive thresholding computes the individual threshold values for small regions of the image (Bradley, 2007; Gorgolewski et al., 2012). It examines the intensity values of local neighborhood of each pixel based on the mean of the local intensity distribution and median statistic functions. The next code includes the default functions of MATLAB software: imfilter (that filters multidimensional images with an average multidimensional filter), fspecial (that creates predefined 'average' filter, in the presented example), medfilt2 (performs median filtering of an image in two dimensions), im2bw (converts original image to binary image), imcomplement (computes the complement of an image). The combination of these functions in the Code Listing 2 detects a threshold for binarization (Figure 3).

Histogram Thresholding

Image histograms are tools to visualize the distribution of grayscale intensity values in the entire image. The histogram of an image *f* with *m* lines and *n* columns and the gray levels in the range $\left[0, L-1\right]$ is given by a discrete function *h* having the following properties:

Figure 3. Binary image with adaptive thresholding

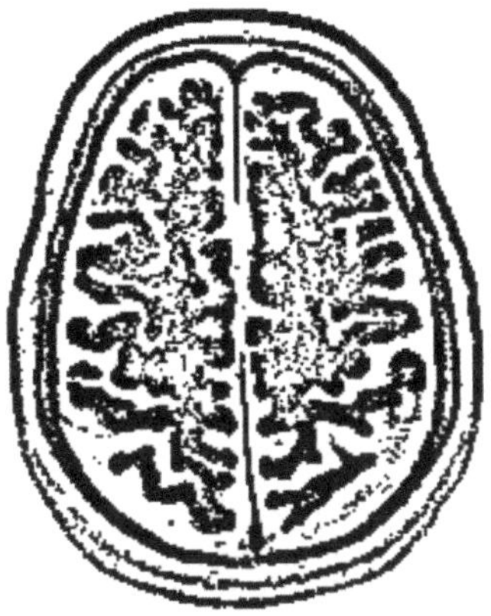

Code Listing 2. Adaptive thresholding

```
d=11;% ws is the local window size
% s is 0 or 1, a switch between mean and median
%C is the threshold
 g=imread('mri.bmp');
 f=mat2gray(g);
if s==0
    IM=imfilter(f,fspecial('average',d),'replicate');
else
    IM=medfilt2(f,[d d]);
end
SIM=IM-f-C;
bw=im2bw(SIM,0);
bw=imcomplement(bw);
figure,imshow(bw);
```

$$h\left(i\right)=\frac{1}{MN}\sum_{m=0}^{M-1}\sum_{n=0}^{N-1}\delta\left(i,f\left(m,n\right)\right), i=0,\ldots,L-1 \text{ and } \sum_{i=0}^{L-1}h\left(i\right)=1$$

where $\delta\left(x,y\right)=\begin{cases}1 & if \quad x=y\\ 0 & if \quad x\neq y\end{cases}.$

Image histogram includes peaks and valleys and the valley point can be used as the threshold so that the image is separated into a number of objects. Figure 4 shows the corresponding histogram and two binary images obtained for two threshold values. The peaks and valleys are examined and the thresholds were chosen in two ways. First, binary image corresponds to the thresholds chosen as maximum (the higher number of pixels at this value) or minimum (the lower number of pixels at this value) gray-level values. It has to be noted that these values do not necessary correspond to the background or foreground

Figure 4. (a) The image histogram with the manually detected threshold highlighted; (b) binarization at the highest threshold value; (c) binarization at the threshold value manually determined

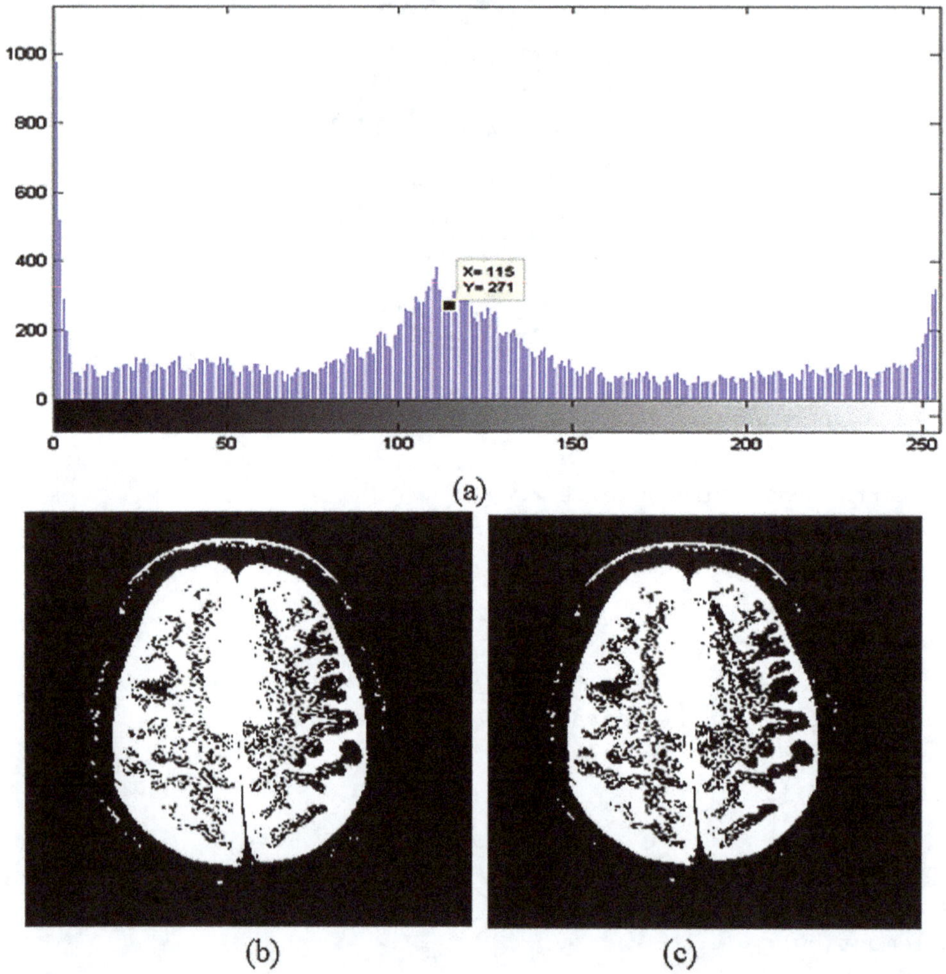

Code Listing 3. Histogram thresholding based on the highest threshold

```
I=imread('mri.bmp');
figure, imshow(I);
H=imhist(I);
[counts,x] = imhist(H);
T=max(counts)% T=highest peak does not correspond to the background
g = I >= T;
figure,imshow(g)
```

(see Figure 4b, where the binary image is obtain for the highest T, and Code Listing 3). The second approach uses a threshold value that was manually determined as the minimum value (or valley) that separates the two peaks (see Figure 4c and Code Listing 4).

Code Listing 4. Histogram thresholding based on threshold manually detected

```
I=imread('mri.bmp'');
figure, imshow(I);
g = I >= 110;
figure,imshow(g);
```

However, for real applications, the threshold value should be determined automatically, via computer programs, by using algorithms based on discriminant analysis or unsupervised classification methods.

Methods to automatically separate objects in an image will be discussed below. Binarized images can be further used to determine various properties/features in an image such as area, diameter, shape, convexity, eccentricity, etc.

Otsu's Binarization

Otsu's thresholding technique is based on a discriminant analysis which partitions an image into two classes $C_0 = \{0,1,2,\ldots,t\}$ and $C_1 = \{t+1, t+2,\ldots, L-1\}$ at the gray level *t*. Here, *L* represents the total number of the gray levels in image. Let the number of pixels at the *i*th gray level be n_i, and *n* is the total number of pixels in a given image. The probability of occurrence of gray level *i* is $p_i = n_i/n$. C_0 and C_1 correspond to the object and the background, respectively, and the probabilities of the two classes are $\omega_0 = \sum_{i=0}^{t} p_i$ and $\omega_1 = \sum_{i=t+1}^{L-1} p_i$. Also, the means of the two classes are $\mu_0(t) = \sum_{i=0}^{t} ip_i/\omega_0(t)$ and $\mu_1(t) = \sum_{i=t+1}^{L-1} ip_i/\omega_1(t)$. Now, let σ_B^2 and σ_T^2 be the variance in between classes and total variance, respectively. An optimal threshold t^* can be computed by maximizing the between-class variance $t^* = Arg\left\{\max_{0\le i\le L-1}\left(\sigma_B^2 / \sigma_T^2\right)\right\}$ where $\sigma_B^2 = \omega_0(\mu_0 - \mu_T)^2 + \omega_1(\mu_1 - \mu_T)^2$ and $\sigma_T^2 = \sum_{i=0}^{L-1}(i - \mu_T)^2$. μ_T denotes the total mean of the whole image and it is defined as $\mu_T = \sum_{i=0}^{L-1} ip_i$.

According to Otsu's method (Otsu, 1979) an equivalent, but simpler formula for obtaining optimal threshold t^* is as follows:

$$t^* = Arg\left\{\max_{0\le i\le L}\left(\omega_0\left[\mu_0 - \mu_T\right]^2 + \omega_1\left[\mu_1 - \mu_T\right]^2\right)\right\}$$

Figure 5 shows the binarized image of the test image. In MATLAB application the function graythresh detects the global image threshold by using the Otsu's method and im2bw converts the original image to binary image (see Code Listing 5).

Figure 5. Thresholded image with Otsu's method

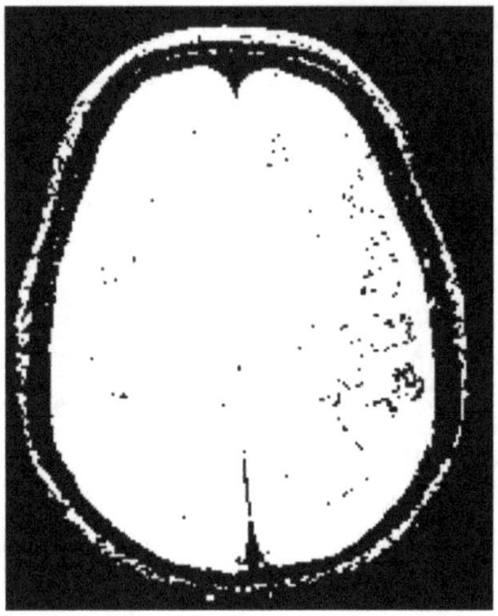

Figure 6. Thresholded image using Bernsen's local thresholding method

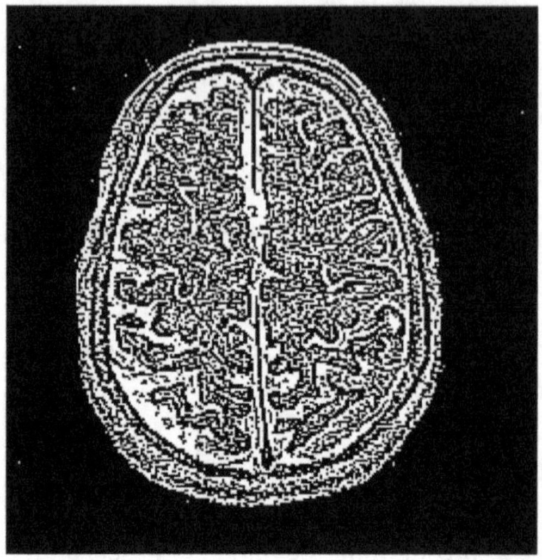

Bernsen's Method

The Bernsen's local thresholding method is used when different parts of an image show large variation between background and foreground, especially as a result of darkness or shadow (Bernsen, 1986). Let $f(x,y)$ denotes the gray level value in a point (x,y) in the original image. For a $\left(2\omega+1\right)\times\left(2\omega+1\right)$ mask centered at point (x,y), the threshold $T(x,y)$ characteristic to image is (Talab, 2014):

$$T\left(x,y\right)=0.5\times\left(\max_{\substack{-\omega\leq m\leq\omega\\-\omega\leq n\leq\omega}} f\left(x+m,y+m\right)+\min_{\substack{-\omega\leq m\leq\omega\\-\omega\leq n\leq\omega}} f\left(x+m,y+m\right)\right)$$

It has to be noted that the main drawback of the Bernsen's method is related to mask size. It is necessary that mask size to be adapted to the size of the existing objects so, some *a priori* information on the objects' size are required.

Code Listing 5. Otsu's thresholding method

```
I = imread('mri.bmp');
level = graythresh(I);
BW = im2bw(I,level);
imshow(BW)
```

Code Listing 6. Bernsen's method

```
I=imread('mri.bmp');
figure, imshow(I);
% Convert to double
J = double(I);
% w size window
% computing of mean value
mean = averagefilter(J, w, padding);
% detecting of the of local contrast
T = maxfilt(J, w) - minfilt(J, w);
% Initialize the output
output = zeros(size(J));
% Whenever contrast in the window w is low assume homogenous area
mask = local_contrast < T;
output(mask & J>=5)=1;
figure, imshow (J);
```

The Code Listing 6 contains sequence of the MATLAB code that implements this method and the processed test image is presented in Figure 6. Here, and for the next codes, listing numbered 7 and 8, the averagefilter, maxfilt, minfilt functions will be defined by the users. The MATLAB functions double (converts to double precision) and zeros (creates array of all zeros) are predefined.

Niblack's Method

Niblack's algorithm is a local thresholding method that adapts the threshold's value based on the local mean and local standard deviation, respectively, over a specific rectangular window around each pixel location (Niblack, 1986). The threshold $T(x,y)$ is defined as:

$$T\left(x,y\right)=m\left(x,y\right)+k\sqrt{\frac{\sum_{i} p_i^2}{NP}-m\left(x,y\right)^2}=m\left(x,y\right)+k\sqrt{std\left(x,y\right)}$$

where NP represents the number of pixels in the gray image, m and std denote the mean and standard deviation values, respectively, of the pixels p_i. The parameter k is fixed by the users to the value of -0.2 (Khurshid, 2009). The values of k and window size can be changed to improve the results of segmentation based on local thersholding. A balance between the denoising efficacy and the preservation of local details should be maintained. The Code Listing 7 contains sequence of the MATLAB code that implements this method and the processed test image is presented in Figure 7.

Figure 7. Thresholded image with Niblack's method

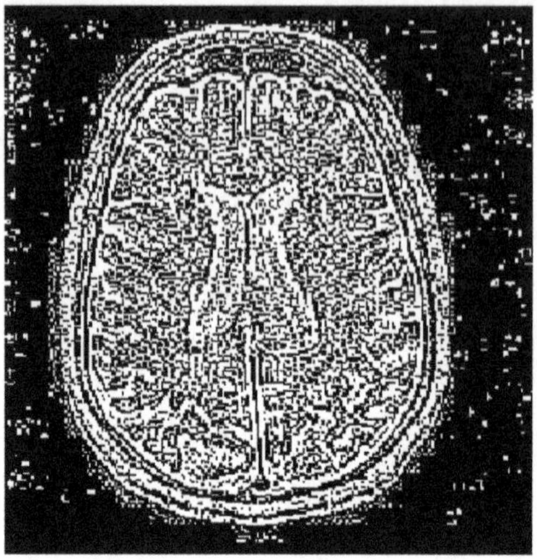

Code Listing 7. Niblack's method

```
I=imread('mri.bmp');
figure, imshow(I);
% Convert to double
J = double(I);
mage = double(image);
 % Mean value
mean = averagefilter(J, w, padding);
 k=-0.2
% Standard deviation
meanSquare = averagefilter(J.^2, w, padding);
std = (meanSquare - mean.^2).^0.5;
% Initialize the output image
output = zeros(size(J));
% Niblack method
T=mean + k * std - offset
out(J >T)=1;
figure, imshow(out);
```

Sauvola's Method

Sauvola's method claims to improve Niblack's method for images that contain both small and large objects. It computes the threshold by using the dynamic range of standard deviation (Sauvola & Pietikainen, 2000). For a gray scale image (with 256 gray levels) and a local pixel (x,y), the Sauvola's algorithm establishes the threshold $T(x,y)$ by computing the mean $m(x,y)$ and standard deviation $std(x,y)$ of a local window $w \times w$ centered at pixel (x,y):

Code Listing 8. Sauvola's method

```
I=imread('mri.bmp');
figure, imshow(I);
% Convert to double
J = double(I);
% w size window
% Convert to double
J = double(I);
% Mean value
mean = averagefilter(J, w, padding);
% Standard deviation
meanSquare = averagefilter(J.^2, w, padding);
std = (meanSquare - mean.^2).^0.5;
% Sauvola's Method
R = max(std(:));
T= mean.*(1 + k * (std / R-1));
out = (J > T);
figure, imshow(out);
```

Figure 8. Thresholded image with Sauvola's method

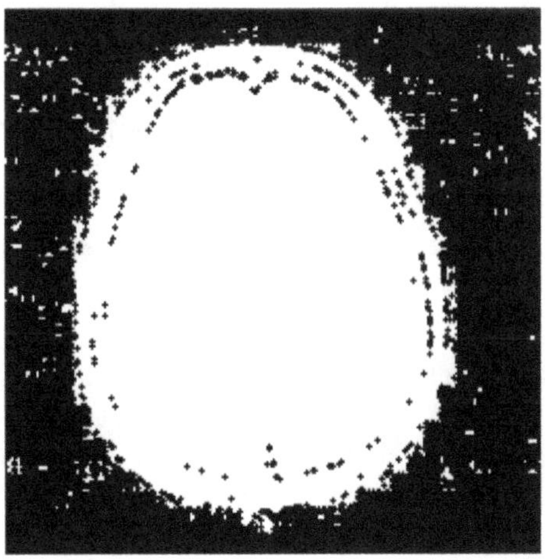

$$T(x,y) = m(x,y)\left[1 + k\left(\frac{std(x,y)}{R} - 1\right)\right]$$

where k is a parameter that ranges from 0.2 to 0.5. R is the maximum value of standard deviation, and according to (Shafait et al., 2008) has the value of 128 for a gray scale image. This method has several limitations: the windows size should be carefully established to fit to the objects in the image and, it is not robust to images with low contrast. The Code Listing 8 provides the main sequence of the algorithm and the processed test image is displayed in Figure 8.

CLUSTER ANALYSIS

Cluster analysis is used in situations where little prior knowledge on the raw data exists. Often, clustering is used for the segmentation of images and might be implemented using various features extracted from textured images. These selected features are grouped into clusters corresponding to different classes. The distance between classes is the main criterion of separation and the similarity of the data into the cluster is the building criterion of one cluster. Various algorithms have offered from cluster analysis. Here, two algorithms namely *K*-means clustering and fuzzy *c*-means clustering are presented. MATLAB software provides good clustering with high intra-class similarity and low inter-class similarity.

K-Means Clustering

The image segmentation based on *K*-means clustering algorithm is one of the most widely used methods. It is an unsupervised clustering algorithm that performs the partition of an image into *k* clusters using the distance between multiple classes existing in image (Jumb et al., 2014; Chandhok et al., 2012; Tatiraju & Mehta, 2011).

The distance $V=\sum_{i=1}^{k}\sum_{x_j\in S_i}\left(x_j-\mu_j\right)^2$ between analyzed points (observations or features) that clusters around centroids μ_i, $\forall i=\overline{1,k}$ is minimized and allows the clustering operation. Here *k* is the number of cluster and μ_i is the centroid of all the points $x_j \in S_i$. The iterative algorithm works as follows:

1. Compute the histogram of a digital image as a distribution of its discrete intensity levels.
2. Initialize *k* class centers randomly.
3. Cluster the points/features using distance minimization relation:

$$c^{(i)} := \arg\min_{j}\left\|x^{(i)}-\mu_j\right\|^2$$

4. Recalculate the new position of centroids:

$$\mu_i = \frac{\sum_{i=1}^{m}\left\{c_{(i)}=j\right\}x^{(i)}}{\sum_{i=1}^{m}\left\{c_{(i)}=j\right\}}$$

5. Repeat steps 3 and 4 until the cluster labels of the image does not change.

The *K*-means algorithm for image segmentation is sensitive to the initially selected centroids and to the number of clusters. In order to overcome this drawback, it is strongly recommended to run multiple times the algorithm. The initial centroids are randomly chosen as distinct points for different number of clusters. The algorithm has been repeated as many times MATLAB program required.

Code Listing 9. K-means clustering method

```
I = imread('mri.png');
[nrows,ncols]=size(I);
ab = double(I(:,:,2:3));
nColors=1;
% K-mean algorithm
[cluster_idx, cluster_center] = kmeans(ab,nColors,'distance',
'sqEuclidean','Replicates',2,3);
% Label Every Pixel in the Image Using the Results from KMEANS
J = reshape(cluster_idx,nrows,ncols);
imshow(J);
```

The Code Listing 9 uses two important predefined functions, kmeans (partitions the points of a $n \times p$ matrix into k clusters) and reshape (reshapes an array). The segmented images for two and three clusters are shown in Figure 9.

Fuzzy c-Means Clustering

Fuzzy c-means clustering algorithm is mainly used in medical image processing for pattern texture exploration, anomalies detection or salient features identification (Zhang, 2009; Xin-bo & Jiang, 2009). This clustering approach allows that some data belong to two or more clusters with different values of the membership coefficient. It is an iterative method based on minimization of the functional (Dunn, 1973; Bezdek, 1981; Kwon, 1998) called c-means functional:

$$J_{FCM} = \sum_{k=1}^{n} \sum_{i=1}^{c} \left(u_{ik}\right)^p d^2\left(x_k, v_i\right)$$

Figure 9. K-means clustering result: (a) original image; (b) two clusters (c = 2); c) three clusters (c = 3)

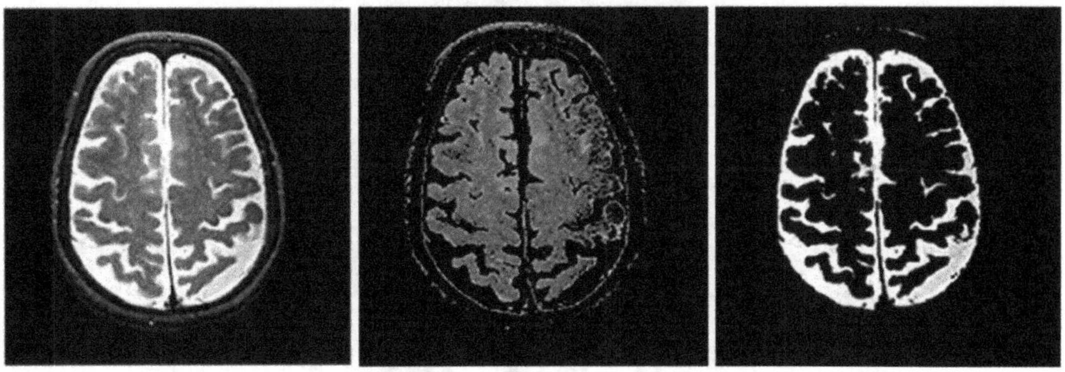

(a) (b) (c)

Code Listing 10. Fuzzy c-means clustering method

```
I = imread('mri.png');
data=reshape(I,[],1);
[c,m]=fcm(data,3);
[center,cidx]=sort(center);
m=m';
m=m(:,cidx);
[maxm,label]=max(m,[],2);
%  s is 0 or 1, a switch of cut-off position.
if s==0    level=(max(data(label==1))+min(data(label==2)))/2;
else     level=(max(data(label==2))+min(data(label==3)))/2;
end
J=im2bw(I,level);
imshow(J);
```

According to Yang (2007) $X = \{x_1, x_2, \ldots, x_n\} \subseteq \Re^p$ is data set in the *p*-dimensional vector space, *c* is the number of the clusters and *n* is number of data items $(2 \le c \le n)$, u_{ik} is the fuzzy partition of x_k in the ith cluster, v_i is a cluster prototype (or center), $d^2(x_k, v_i)$ is distance measure between object x_k and cluster center v_i. The cluster center v_i has to be determined.

In the Code Listing 10 the following MATLAB default functions are used: reshape (reshapes an array), fcm (fuzzy c-means clustering), sort (sorts array elements), min (finds the smallest elements in array), max (finds the largest elements in array), im2bw (converts image to binary image, based on threshold). The result of algorithm is shown in Figure 10.

It has to be note that *c*-means functional allows the fuzzy *c*-means algorithm to converge to a local minimum. As consequence, different initializations may provide different results. Also, the number of cluster *c* is an important parameter. It is necessary to make hypothesis without any *a priori* information

Figure 10. Fuzzy c-means clustering

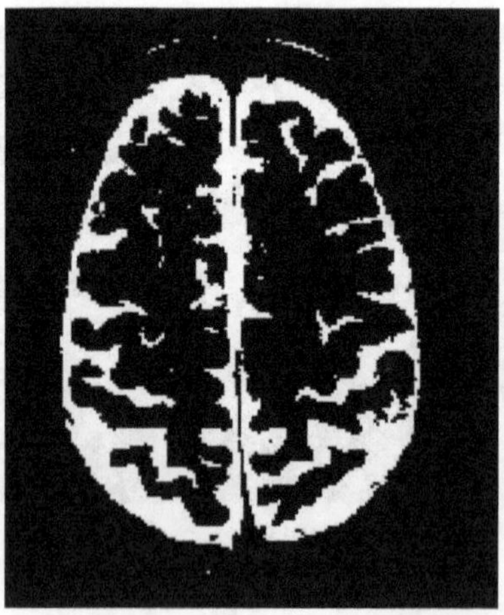

Figure 11. a) Hierarchical association or dendrogram of histogram bins via average linkage method; b) zoom into a specific 'between the main clusters' region of interest to highlight the computed threshold.

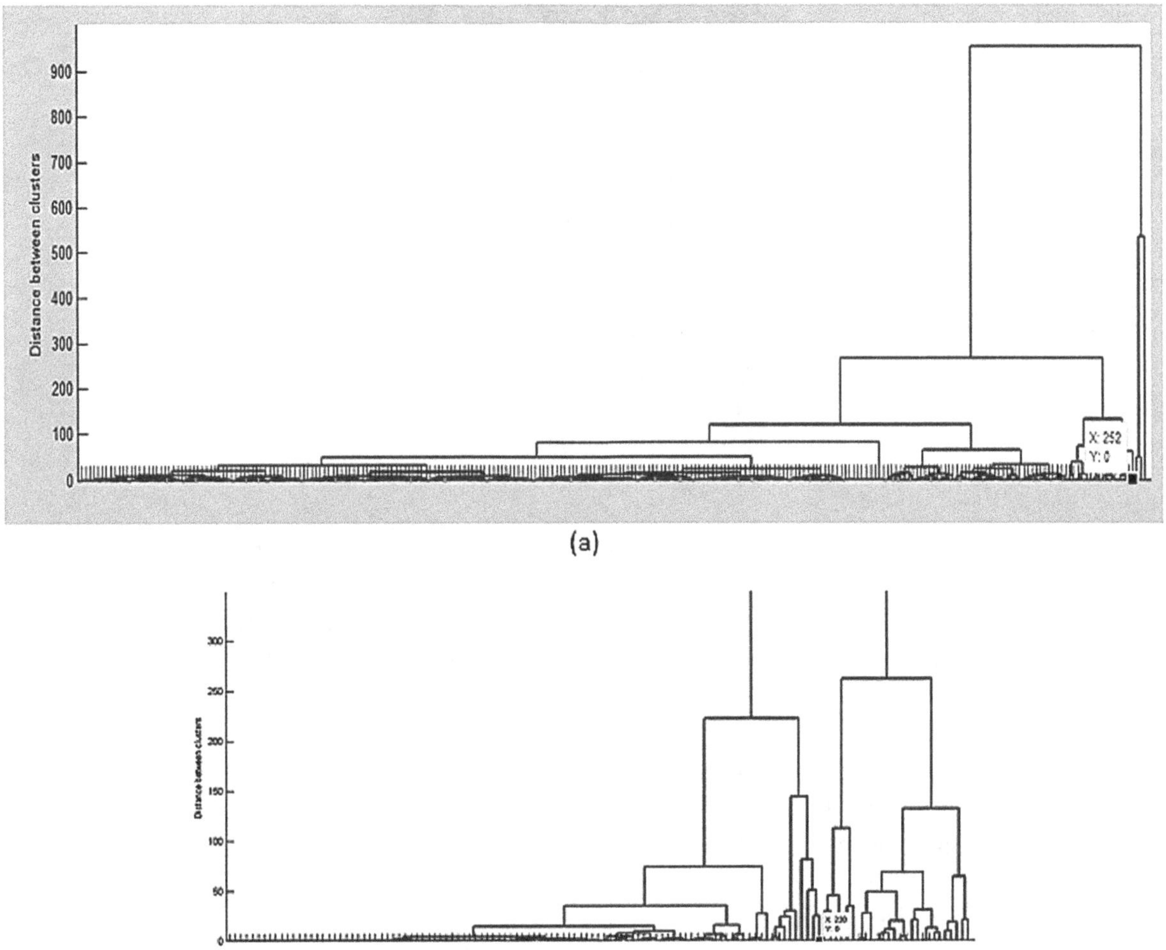

(a)

(b)

on the structure of the analyzed data. The algorithm will search for the indicated number of clusters even if this does not correspond to a real situation. In order to overcome this drawback, the validity measures such as the Xie-Beni index (Xie & Beni, 1991), Know index (Know, 1998) or cluster merging approach should be carried out.

Image Binarization by Dendrograms

Clustering methods are important in the classification of various types of data extracted from the brain MR images because these images have various types of histograms correlated to their informational content. Dendronic image analysis is a robust technique that provides the optimal threshold values. The applicability of this method is demonstrated by using an algorithm that computes the hierarchies associated to the histogram bins in order to create dendrograms (Figure 11a). The result of the hierarchical

Figure 12. Image binarization by dendrogram

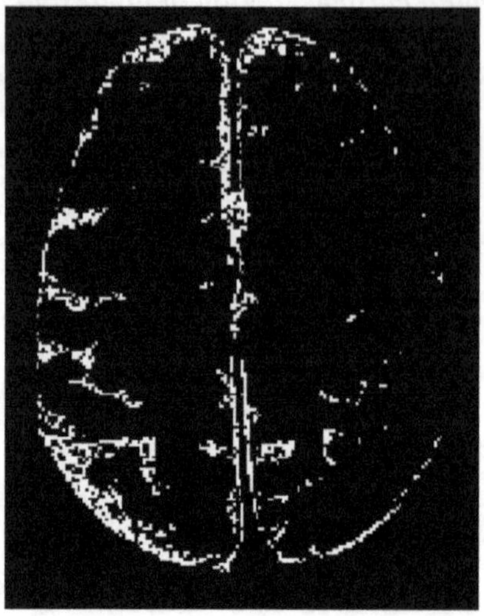

clustering is a tree-like graph. The heights of the branches indicate how different the clusters are. Longer vertical lines indicate that the clusters below are very different. In this case, the optimal threshold is chosen, based on visual assessment, as being placed between the main clusters as being the 'deep valley' of the dendrogram (Figure 11b). The dendrograms algorithm consists of the following steps:

1. Read the input image;
2. Compute the histogram of the image;
3. Detect the values of the bins;
4. Show the dendrogram from the bins' values detected in step 3.

The values of the estimated threshold are used for binarization. The result of binarization is shown in Figure 12. The following MATLAB functions are used in Code Listing 11: rgb2gray (converts RGB image or colormap to grayscale), imhist (generates the histogram of an image data), linkage (computes

Code Listing 11. Thresholding by dendrogram

```
I = imread('mri.jpg');
I=rgb2gray(I1);
J=imhist(I);
% x is an array that contain the values of the bins histogram
tree1 = linkage(J,'average');
H=dendrogram(tree1,0);
f = clustergram(x)
figure, imshow(f)
T=252;
g = f > T;
figure,imshow(g);
```

Figure 13. Flowchart of the proposed method; the following notations were used: ED-Euclidian distance between histograms images; H - healthy patients' class; PiD - Pick's disease class; AD - Alzheimer's disease class; CCD - cerebral calcinosis disease class; T - range of variation of threshold values

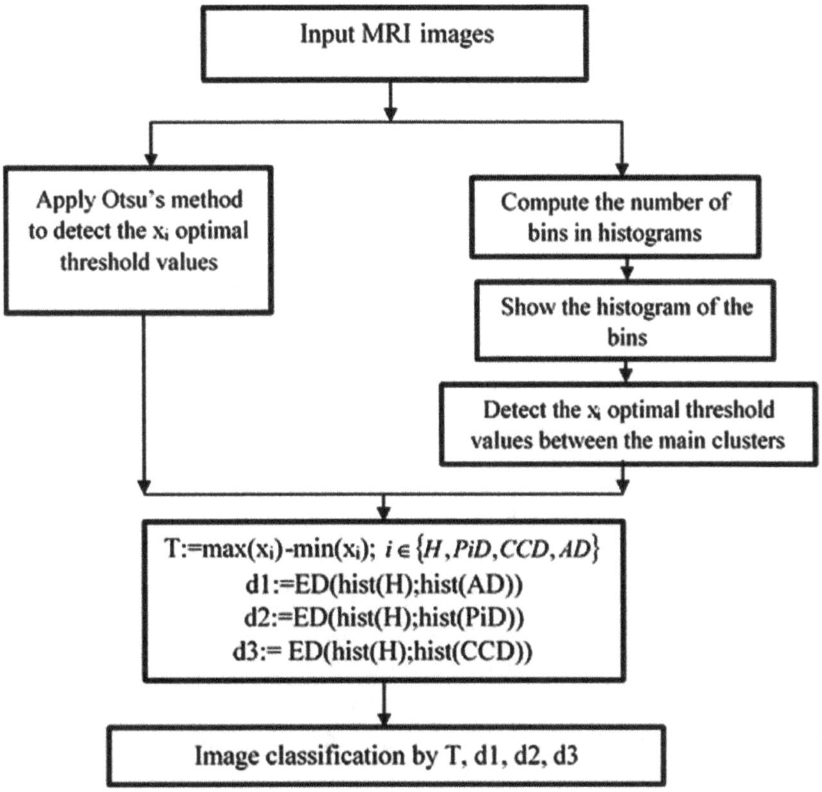

the agglomerative hierarchical cluster tree), clustergram (displays clustergram and dendrograms of clustergram object). In this example, average linkage namely the average distance between two sets of bins has been set.

APPLICATIONS

Neurodegenerative MR Image Classification with Binary Threshold Method

Medical images classification can be performed by a wide variety of methods and features involved in this operation. One of most common approach is based on thresholding, which, in turn, can be performed by using binarization methods (Otsu's method is the most wide used) or by dendrograms based method.

Usually, classification divides an image into distinct domains containing pixels showing similar characteristics. Classification is meaningful for neurodegenerative MR image analysis when the objects or features of interest are accurate depicted.

In order to provide a practical example of classification, a database containing 80 brain MRI images has been utilized. It comprises 20 images of healthy patients and 60 patients with neurodegenerative diseases: Alzheimer (20 images), Pick's (20images) and cerebral calcinosis (20 images). The 2D MRI images have been acquired as T2w and PD (proton density) sequences. They belong to the Harvard Medical School database and are freely available at http://www.med.harvard.edu/AANLIB/home.html.

The contextual classification exploits the computed threshold values specific to each image type (PD and T2w) and each patient class (namely, Alzheimer's disease, Pick's disease, cerebral calcinosis and healthy patients). This example will demonstrate the applicability and efficacy of both kinds of approaches: thresholding and hierarchical cluster analysis methods. The Otsu's method detects global image threshold and another way to detect the optimal threshold is based on dendrograms. The flowchart of the proposed method is presented in Figure 13.

The proposed method consists of the next steps.

Step 1: The inputs for the algorithm consist of 80 brain MRI images belong to four main classes of diseases.

Step 2: Detect the global image threshold using the Otsu's method.

Step 3: Find the optimal number of bins in histograms. The bin-width has been set to $1/\sqrt{n}$ where n = 256 gray levels.

Step 4: Display the histogram of the bins and select the optimal threshold as the value placed between the main clusters.

Step 5: Compute the range of variation of threshold values T that characterize each analyzed class. Clustering is done according to these values.

Step 6: Compute the Euclidean distance between the histograms of the bins of analyzed disease classes in order to assess the cluster validity and classification accuracy. Euclidean distance works as a similarity measure and validates the range of variation of threshold T. The test class is the healthy patients' class.

Step 7: Brain MRI images classification.

The range of variation of threshold values, namely the absolute difference between the maximum and minimum values, was obtained using the both approaches. The larger variation in threshold range indicates important variability of both uniformity measure of pixels (i.e. the degree of spread of intensity from the mean) and shape measure of pixels (the gradient value of every pixel or the distance between the determined threshold value and the gray value of the neighboring pixels). The best threshold value is correlated to the larger variability. For the proposed application, the results were visualized by using horizontal charts (Figures 14 and 15).

The threshold range variation (T) determined using the Otsu's method, for each image type and each disease class, has the values as follows: healthy patients, $T = 0.036$ (PD) and $T = 0.043$ (T2w); Pick's disease, $T = 0.055$ (PD) and $T = 0.053$ (T2w); cerebral calcinosis disease, $T = 0.084$ (PD) and $T = 0.041$ (T2w); Alzheimer's disease, $T = 0.096$ (PD) and $T = 0.094$ (T2w). As observed in Figure 14, the Otsu's method provides results that can be summarized as follows: (i) the smaller variation in threshold range is obtained for healthy patients (PD type images) and the larger one is for Alzheimer disease (PD type images); (ii) PD images show a larger variation in threshold values in comparison with that of T2w images; the healthy patients class is the exception; (iii) the larger variation in threshold range exists for Alzheimer's diseases.

Figure 14. The computed threshold value range and its variation by using the Otsu's method, for all experimental conditions

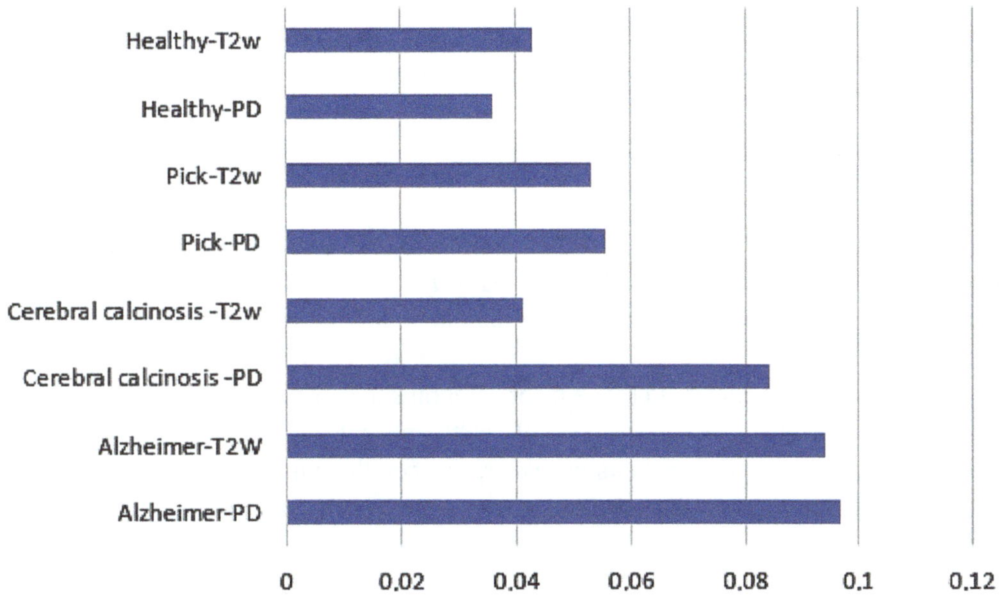

Figure 15. The computed threshold value range and its variation by using dendrograms, for all experimental conditions

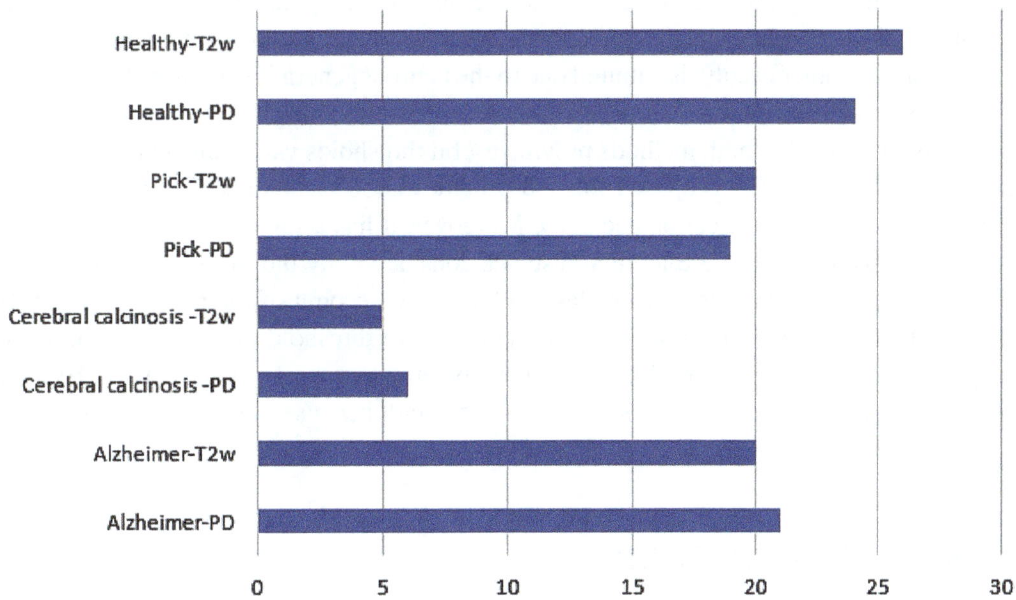

Another tool for assessing the optimal threshold values and to classify the images is based on dendrograms. The optimal threshold is placed between the main clusters. The required condition is to obtain a good separation between clusters. The threshold range variation (T) determined for each image type and each disease class by using dendrograms has the values as follows: for healthy patients, $T = 24$ (PD)

Table 1. Mean ± deviation standard of the Euclidian distance between the histograms of the bins of analyzed classes

	Euclidian Distance		
	ED(hist(H);hist(AD))	ED(hist(H);hist(PiD))	ED(hist(H);hist(CCD))
PD image	0.301±0.026	0.117±0.085	0.192±0.013
T2w image	0.182±0.018	0.115±0.101	0.096±0.025

and $T = 26$ (T2w); for Pick's disease, $T = 19$ (PD) and $T = 20$ (T2w); for cerebral calcinosis disease, $T = 6$ (PD) and $T = 5$ (T2w); and for Alzheimer's disease, $T = 21$ (PD) and $T = 20$ (T2w). In Figure 15, the range of variation of threshold values is shown and the following remarks are done:

1. The smaller variation in threshold range is for cerebral calcinosis;
2. The larger variation characterizes the class of healthy patient;
3. The range of variation of threshold values is larger when the number of narrow bins exceeds the number of wider bins. This indicates a higher precision as in the area of narrower bins the signal reduces the noise.

The resulting threshold value range and its variation for each analyzed class allow the image classification because there are important differences between these values. The classification results provided by the proposed algorithm were validated through similarity analysis based on Euclidian distance. From the quantitative results displayed in Table 1, it can see that the computed distances between adjacent clusters of analyzed diseases are clearly different and the clusters are exclusive. On the other hand, the cluster membership is rather evenly distributed due to the neurodegenerative disease characteristics and a high intra-class similarity exists.

These results illustrate that both methods provide useful thresholds values and classify the analyzed neurodegenerative diseases. The proposed method provides good results and Euclidean distance is a good metric to assess the classification accuracy. Moreover, it has a low complexity. However, there are limitations of this method. The Euclidian distance considers only the mean of distribution of features specific to the studied instance into a class and takes no account of their statistical distribution. With an option to choose how much information is lost due to threshold operation, the best choice is the dendrograms method because it performs a better separation among analyzed classes. However, the recommendation of a specific algorithm is particularly difficult because the choice depends mainly on the characteristic of the data.

FUTURE RESEARCH DIRECTIONS

The theme presented here indicated a huge variety of solutions and this opens a variety of research directions. However, the main goal of image processing and analysis is to provide reliable, accurate and fast algorithms as a way to simplify and improve the automatic analysis methods. These algorithms do not intent to replace the professional physician expertise, but, instead come as a complementary tool supporting the diagnosis. E-Health applications or remote diagnosis can be developed based on these automatic analysis methods.

CONCLUSION

In this chapter, some thresholding methods have been presented. There are two popular approaches: global thresholding algorithms, and local or adaptive thresholding algorithms. The selected threshold values are used in binarization operations. The binarization techniques for grayscale images are grouped into two broad categories: global binarization and local binarization. Also, binarization has been performed using dendrograms. Two classification approaches were implemented based on optimal threshold values determined using Otsu's method and dendrograms.

REFERENCES

Amiri, S., Movahedi, M. M., Kazemi, K., & Parsaei, H. (2013). An automated MR image segmentation system using multi-layer perceptron neural network. *Journal of Biomedical Physics & Engineering*, *3*(4), 115–122. PMID:25505757

Arifin, A. Z., & Asano, A. (2006). Image segmentation by histogram thresholding using hierarchical cluster analysis. *Pattern Recognition Letters*, *27*(13), 1515–1521. doi:10.1016/j.patrec.2006.02.022

Arora, S., Acharya, K., Verma, A., & Panigrahi, P. K. (2006). Multilevel thresholding for image segmentation through a fast statistical recursive algorithm. *Pattern Recognition Letters*, *29*(2), 119–125. doi:10.1016/j.patrec.2007.09.005

Bernsen, J. (1986). Dynamic thresholding of gray level images. In *Proceedings of the 8th International Conference on Pattern Recognition*, (pp. 1251– 1255). Paris, France.

Bezdek, J. C. (1981). *Pattern recognition with fuzzy objective function algorithms*. New York, NY: Plenum Press. doi:10.1007/978-1-4757-0450-1

Bibicu, D., Moraru, L., & Biswas, A. (2013). Thyroid nodule recognition based on feature selection and pixel classification methods. *Journal of Digital Imaging*, *26*(1), 119–128. doi:10.1007/s10278-012-9475-5 PMID:22546981

Bibicu, D., Moraru, L., & Biswas, A. (2015). Efficient segmentation using active contours embedded in an image feature. *Journal of Medical Imaging and Health Informatics*, *5*(2), 241–247. doi:10.1166/jmihi.2015.1379

Bradley, D., & Roth, G. (2007). Adaptive thresholding using the integral image. *Journal of Graphics, GPU, and Game Tools*, *12*(2), 13–21. doi:10.1080/2151237X.2007.10129236

Bui, A. A. T., & Taira, R. K. (Eds.). (2010). *Medical imaging informatics*. New York: Springer. doi:10.1007/978-1-4419-0385-3

Chandhok, C., Chaturvedi, S., & Khurshid, A. A. (2012). An approach to image segmentation using k-means clustering algorithm. *International Journal of Information Technology*, *1*(1), 11–17.

Collins, M., Schapire, R. E., & Singer, Y. (2002). Logistic regression, AdaBoost and Bregman distances. *Machine Learning*, *48*(1/3), 253–285. doi:10.1023/A:1013912006537

Dai, W., & Ji, W. (2014). A MapReduce implementation of C4.5 decision tree algorithm. *International Journal of Database Theory and Application*, *7*(1), 49–60. doi:10.14257/ijdta.2014.7.1.05

Dou, W. B., Ruan, S., Chen, Y. P., Bloyet, D., & Constans, J. M. (2007). A framework of fuzzy information fusion for the segmentation of brain tumor tissues on MR images. *Image and Vision Computing*, *25*(2), 164–171. doi:10.1016/j.imavis.2006.01.025

Dunn, J. C. (1973). A fuzzy relative of the ISODATA process and its use in detecting compact well-separated clusters. *Journal of Cybernetics*, *3*(3), 32–57. doi:10.1080/01969727308546046

Gonzalez, R. C., & Richard, E. (2002). *Woods digital image processing* (2nd ed.). Upper Saddle River, New Jersey: Prentice Hall.

Gorgolewski, K. J., Storkey, A. J., Bastin, M. E., & Pernet, C. R. (2012). Adaptive thresholding for reliable topological inference in single subject fMRI analysis. *Frontiers in Human Neuroscience*, *6*(245), 1–14. PMID:22936908

Hastie, T., Tibshirani, R., & Friedman, J. (2009). *The elements of statistical learning: Data mining, inference and prediction*. New York, NY: Springer-Verlag. doi:10.1007/978-0-387-84858-7

Hodge, V. J., & Austin, J. (2004). A survey of outlier detection methodologies. *Artificial Intelligence Review*, *22*(2), 85–126. doi:10.1023/B:AIRE.0000045502.10941.a9

Jia, W., Hu, R., Lei, X., Zhao, Y. K., & Gui, J. (2014). Histogram of oriented lines for palmprint recognition. *IEEE Transactions on Systems, Man, and Cybernetics. Systems*, *44*(3), 385–395.

Jumb, V., Sohani, M., & Shrivas, A. (2014). Color image segmentation using k-means clustering and Otsu's adaptive thresholding. *International Journal of Innovative Technology and Exploring Engineering*, *3*(9), 72–76.

Khurshid, K., Siddiqi, I., Faure, C., & Vincent, N. (2009). Comparison of Niblack inspired binarization methods for ancient documents, *Proceedings SPIE 7247. Document Recognition and Retrieval, XVI*, 72470U, 72470U-9. doi:10.1117/12.805827

Kittler, J., & Illingworth, J. (1986). Minimum error thresholding. *Pattern Recognition*, *19*(1), 41–47. doi:10.1016/0031-3203(86)90030-0

Kwon, S. H. (1998). Cluster validity index for fuzzy clustering. *Electronics Letters*, *34*(22), 2176–2177. doi:10.1049/el:19981523

Kwon, S. H. (2004). Threshold selection based on cluster analysis. *Pattern Recognition Letters*, *25*(9), 1045–1050. doi:10.1016/j.patrec.2004.03.001

Kwon, S. H., Jeong, H. C., Seo, S. T., Lee, I. K., & Son, C. S. (2008). Histogram equalization-based thresholding. *Journal IEICE - Transactions on Information and Systems Archive, E91-D(11)*, 2751-2753.

Laurikkala, J., Juhola, M., & Kentala, E. (2000). Informal identification of outliers in medical data. In *Fifth International Workshop on Intelligent Data Analysis in Medicine and Pharmacology* (vol.1, pp. 20-24). Berlin, Germany: IOS Press.

Liang, Y.-C., & Cuevas, J. R. (2013). An automatic multilevel image thresholding using relative entropy and meta-heuristic algorithms. *Entropy*, *15*(6), 2181–2209. doi:10.3390/e15062181

Liu, J., Udupa, J. K., Odhner, D., Hackney, D., & Moonis, G. (2005). A system for brain tumor volume estimation via MR imaging and fuzzy connectedness. *Computerized Medical Imaging and Graphics*, *29*(1), 21–34. doi:10.1016/j.compmedimag.2004.07.008 PMID:15710538

Lu, F., & Ba, Q. (2010). A refined weighted K-Nearest Neighbors algorithm for text categorization. In *Proceedings of International Conference on Intelligent Systems and Knowledge Engineering* (pp. 326-330). Hangzhou, China: IEEE.

MacQueen, J. B. (1967). Some methods for classification and analysis of multivariate observations. In *Proceedings of 5-th Berkeley Symposium on Mathematical Statistics and Probability* (vol. 1, pp. 281-297). Berkeley, CA: University of California Press.

Moldovanu, S., Moraru, L., & Nicolae, M. C. (2010). Comparative analysis of ultrasound image using gray level. *Annals of Dunarea de Jos University. Fascicle II*, *2*(33), 145–151.

Moldovanu, S., Obreja, C., & Moraru, L. (2014, November). *Threshold selection for classification of MR brain images by clustering method.* Paper presented at the meeting of the TIM 2014 Physics Conference, Timisoara, Romania.

Moldovanu, S., Punga Visan, M., & Moraru, L. (2015). Evaluation of outliers in acquired brain MR images. *Journal of Physics: Conference Series*, *574*, 012121. doi:10.1088/1742-6596/574/1/012121

Moldovanu, S., Moraru, L., & Biswas, A. (2015). Robust skull stripping segmentation based on irrational mask for magnetic resonance brain images.Journal od Digital Imaging, 28(6) 738-747 PMID:25733013

Morissette, L., & Chartier, S. (2013). The k-means clustering technique: General considerations and implementation in mathematic. *Tutorials in Quantitative Methods for Psychology*, *9*(1), 15–24.

Murtagh, F., & Legendre, P. (2014). Ward's hierarchical agglomerative clustering method: Which algorithms implement Ward's criterion? *Journal of Classification*, *31*(3), 274–295. doi:10.1007/s00357-014-9161-z

Nakib, A., Oulhadj, H., & Siarry, P. (2007). Image histogram thresholding based on multiobjective optimization. *Signal Processing*, *87*(11), 2516–2534. doi:10.1016/j.sigpro.2007.04.001

Ng, H. P., Ong, S. H., Foong, K. W. C., Goh, P. S., & Nowinski, W. L. (2006). Medical image segmentation using k-means clustering and improved watershed algorithm. In *Proceedings of the Symposium on Image Analysis and Interpretation* (pp. 61-65). Denver, CO: IEEE. doi:10.1109/SSIAI.2006.1633722

Niblack, W. (1986). *An introduction to digital image processing*. Denmark: Prentice Hall.

Otsu, N. (1979). A threshold selection method from gray-level histograms. *IEEE Transactions on Systems, Man, and Cybernetics*, *9*(1), 62–66. doi:10.1109/TSMC.1979.4310076

Qian, G., Sural, S., & Pramanik, S. (2002). A comparative analysis of two distance measures in color image databases. In *Proceedings of the International Conference on Image Processing* (vol. 1, pp. I-401 - I-404). New York, NY: IEEE doi:10.1109/ICIP.2002.1038045

Sahoo, P. K., Soltani, S., & Wong, A. K. C. (1988). A survey of thrsholding technique. *Computer Vision Graphics and Image Processing*, *41*(2), 133–260. doi:10.1016/0734-189X(88)90022-9

Sauvola, J., & Pietikainen, M. (2000). Adaptive document image binarization. *Pattern Recognition*, *33*(2), 225–236. doi:10.1016/S0031-3203(99)00055-2

Sezgin, M., & Sankur, B. (2004). Survey over image thresholding techniques and quantitative performance evaluation. *Journal of Electronic Imaging*, *13*(1), 146–165. doi:10.1117/1.1631315

Shafait, F., Keysers, D., & Breuel, T. (2008). Efficient implementation of local adaptive thresholding techniques using integral image. In *Proceedings of the 15th Document Recognition and Retrieval Conference* (vol. 6815, pp. 651–660). San Jose, CA: SPIE.

Talab, A. M. A., Huang, Z., & Junfei, W. (2014). An enhanced Bernsen algorithm approaches for vehicle logo detection. *International Journal of Signal Processing. Image Processing and Pattern Recognition*, *7*(4), 203–210. doi:10.14257/ijsip.2014.7.4.20

Tang, J., Chen, Z., Wai-chee Fu, A., & Cheung, D. (2001). A robust outlier detection scheme for large data sets. In *The 6th Pacific-Asia Conference on Knowledge Discovery and Data Mining* (vol. 1, pp. 6-8). London, UK: Springer-Verlag.

Tatiraju, S., & Mehta, A. (2011). Image Segmentation using k-means clustering, EM and Normalized Cuts. In *ICIAP'11 Proceedings of the 16th International Conference on Image Analysis and Processing* (vol. 2, pp. 229-240). Genova, Italy: Springer-Verlag.

Xie, X., & Beni, G. (1991). A validity measure for fuzzy clustering. *IEEE Transactions on Pattern Analysis and Machine Intelligence*, *13*(8), 841–847. doi:10.1109/34.85677

Xin-bo, Z., & Jiang, L. (2009). An image segmentation algorithm based on fuzzy c-means clustering. *Digital Image Processing*, *1*, 22–26.

Yang, Y. (2007). Image Segmentation by fuzzy c-means clustering algorithm with a novel penalty term. *Computing and Informatics*, *26*, 17–31.

KEY TERMS AND DEFINITIONS

Binarization: Converts a gray-scale image to only black and white. The pixels into image have only two values '0' (for black) and '1' (for white).

Clustering: Allows grouping a set of objects/variables or features together to same class or group based on the similarity of their responses to several measurements or based on relevant features. The objects belong to the same group (called a cluster) are more similar to each other than to those in other groups (or clusters).

Dendrogram: A branching diagram that shows the relationships of similarity among a group of entities based on attribute distances between each pair of sequentially merged classes.

Image Histogram: The tonal distribution in a digital image or a graphical representation counting how many pixels are at each gray level.

Magnetic Resonance Images (MRI): A diagnostic imaging procedure that uses radio waves, a magnetic field, and a computer to generate images of the body.

Segmentation: Performs partitions an image into groups of pixels which are homogeneous with respect to some characteristics. Another definition states that image segmentation is the process of partitioning an image into homogeneous and non-convergent domains.

Thresholding: A technique dealing with pixels classification into object or background classes.

Chapter 5
GPU-Based Level Set Method for MRI Brain Tumor Segmentation using Modified Probabilistic Clustering

Ram Kumar
National Institute of Technology Silchar, India

Abahan Sarkar
National Institute of Technology Silchar, India

Sweta Rani
Nobel Medical College and Teaching Hospital, Nepal

Fazal Ahmed Talukdar
National Institute of Technology Silchar, India

ABSTRACT

The level set method (LSM) has been widely used in image segmentation due to its intrinsic nature which allows handling complex shapes and topological changes easily. We propose a new level set algorithm, which is based on probabilistic c mean objective function which incorporates intensity inhomogeneity in image and robust to noise. The computational complexity of the proposed LSM is greatly reduced by using highly parallelizable lattice Boltzmann method (LBM). So the proposed algorithm is effective and highly parallelizable. The proposed LSM is implemented using Experimental results demonstrate the performance of the proposed method.

RESEARCH OBJECTIVE

The goals of the research are to

1. The accurate segmentation of brain tumor with different size and shape in presence of intensity inhomogeneity and noise.
2. Automatic segmentation of brain tumor with high speed.

DOI: 10.4018/978-1-5225-0140-4.ch005

INTRODUCTION

Accurate image segmentation plays a vital role for anatomic structures inspection, disease identification as well as tracking of its progress in the field of biomedical image processing. It is also used for surgical planning and simulation. Now a day's Image processing is used to identify the brain tumor. According to the WHO, more than 500,000 people undergo brain tumor treatment in a year. Tumors may appear at different places with distinct intensity. It may differ in size, shape, and location. There are two major types of brain tumor: First one is called benign type which does not spread and second one is known as Malignant which spread from any part of the body to the brain. Since brain are very complicated structure, therefore a precise segmentation is needed for detecting tumors, edema and necrosis tissue. Based on MRI technique, the study of the main cerebral tissues such as white matter, gray matter and CSF is carried out. In such studies, segmentation step is required whose aim is partitioning the intra-cranial volume into potentially overlapping parts such as WM, GM and CSF. MR images are one of the common ways to visualize brain structure. MRI image segmentation is very helpful for research and clinical study. The MRI scan is more reliable than CT scan for diagnosis because it does not affect the human body as it does not use any kind of radiation. MRI shares a common advantage with CT of high spatial resolution images but without ionizing radiation exposure. It possesses good contrast resolution for different tissues.

Various techniques related to brain tumor inspection are proposed by many researchers in recent past. The domain of automated inspection for brain tumor is found to be populated mostly by level set image Segmentation. The level set technique is a general framework for tracking dynamic interfaces and shapes. It was first developed as a way to model fluid boundaries, such as a flame front. In computer vision and pattern recognition the level set method (LSM) had been widely used for segmentation. The attractive advantage of the LSM is its ability to extract complex contours and to automatically handle topological changes, such as splitting and merging (S. Balla-Arabe, et al. 2013). The LSM belongs to the active contours model (ACMs) which is based on the Eulerian framework, i.e., the geometric representation of the active contour instead of the parametric representation which is based on the Lagrangian framework.

A huge literature is devoted to brain segmentation from MRI data. Simulated charged fluid framework governed by Poisson's equation as a deformable model is used by Chang and Valentino (H Chang and D. Valentino, et al. 2006). in order to perform general segmentation. Later Chang et al. proposed a new deformable model CFM for T2MRI brain tumor segmentation. Ho et al. (H Chang and D. Valentino, et al. 2008) introduced an improved method in which blobby-shaped brain tumors are automatically segmented in MR images (S. Ho, et al. 2006). A knowledge-based detection and segmentation algorithm based on registered brain model for finding abnormal tissues is proposed by Prastawa et al. (M. Prastawa, et al. 2004). Edema with tumor in unusual region can be determined by MR images. Geometric active contour was applied to detect the outlier pixel in normal brain tumor. Region–based deformation model is described by Li et al. (C. Li, et al. 2008) for segmenting the MRI of brain. Both data fitting energy i.e. contour and two fitting functions are addressed by Li et al. For energy minimization, a curve evolution equation was derived from regularization term which is included in the level set formulation. To ensure accurate computation, the regularity of the level set function was preserved intrinsically by the level set regularization term while avoiding expensive initialization of the evolving level set function. A local intensity clustering property and a local clustering function for neighborhood points is proposed by Li et al. (C. Li, et al. 2007:16). Integrating the local clustering criterion over neighborhood center, they define energy functional which was converted to level set formulation. This minimization of the energy was gained by an interleaved process of level set evolution along with estimation of the bias field. A hybrid level set segmentation approach is presented by Xie et al. (K. Xie, et al. 2005) in which, the evolution of curve is driven by region and provide the boundary information at the same time. Region information and boundary information are served as propagation force and stopping functional respectively. ROI followed by LSM is used to segment the tumor. Lefohn et al. (A. Lefohn, et al. 2003) proposed a semi-automatic method in which tumor Segmentation process is repeated after visual inspection by tuning the level set parameters. Cobzas (D. Cobzas, et al. 2007) and Popuri (K. Popuri, et al. 2009) proposed a vibrational method for brain tumor segmentation. In this approach, templates and atlases form which are fully integrated is used as prior knowledge for the appearance of anatomical structures in the normal brain (Nelly Gordillo Vol 31) (D. Jayadevappa, et al. 2011). Fuzzy external force is used to stop the level set function on objects boundary by Balla. (S Balla-Arabe, et al. 2012). As the FCM uses the probabilistic constraint that the memberships of a data point across must sum to 1, it avoids the trivial solution of all memberships being equal to 0. Due to this constraint this membership is interpreted as degrees of sharing, but not as degrees of possibility of a point belonging to a class .The another deficiency of the FCM it is sensitive to noise. To overcome the existing drawbacks, we proposed a new energy function using modified probabilistic clustering. Finite difference, volume or element approximations and explicit computation of curvature are used to solve LSE with high CPU time. To reduce the CPU time, LBM is a substitute method used in recent days.

The GPU recognized as one of the most promising techniques to accelerate scientific computations. The GPU architecture favors dense data and local computations because the communications between microprocessor is time consuming. Since the majority of LBM is local, it is thus suitable for GPU-based computation (S. Balla-Arabe, et al. 2013). In this paper, the proposed algorithm is accelerated using an NVIDIA graphics processing units.

The current chapter is organized as follows. A background on the research domain including the proposed algorithm discussion. Afterwards, the proposed system is introduced followed by the Results and Discussions. Finally, the conclusion is introduced.

BACKGROUND

Active Contour is one of the most powerful methods that have been applied to the image segmentation. The basic idea is to evolve a curve around the object to be detected, and the curve moves toward its interior normal and stops on the true boundary of the object based on the minimization energy. The active contour method can be classified as the snake or parametetric active contour (M. Kass, et al. 1987) and level set methods or geometric active contour proposed by Osher and Sethian (M. O. Berger, et al. 1990).

Parametric Active Contour

Parametric active contour also called Snake is a semi-automatic method based on an energy minimizing deformable model guided by the external constraint forces and pulled by image forces toward the contours of the ROI (M. Kass, et al. 1987). The ability of parametric deformable models is to segment images of an anatomic structure with a deductive knowledge about their location, size, and shape of these structures.

Let us define a contour '*C*' parameterized by arc length'*s*' as

$$C(s) = \left\{ \left(x(s), y(s) \right) : 0 \le s \le L \right\} : R \to \Omega \tag{1}$$

where L denotes the length of the contour 'C' and 'Ω' denotes the entire domain of an image $I(x,y)$. An energy function $E(C)$ can be defined on the contour such as

$$E(C) = E_{\text{int}} + E_{ext} \tag{2}$$

where E_{int} and E_{ext} represents the internal and external energies respectively. The internal energy function determines the smoothness of the contour. The internal energy is a quadratic function given by

$$E_{\text{int}} = \int_0^1 \left[\alpha \left| C'(s) \right|^2 + \beta \left| C''(s) \right|^{"2} \right] ds \tag{3}$$

Here 'α' controls the tension of the contour and 'β' controls the rigidity of the contour. The external energy term that determines the criteria of contour evolution depending on the image $I(x,y)$ can be defined as

$$E_{\text{int}} = \int_0^1 E_{data} \left(C(s) \right) ds \tag{4}$$

$E_{data}(x,y)$ denotes a scalar function defined on the image plane, so that local minimum of $E_{data}(x,y)$ attracts the snakes to edges. A common edge indicator is a function of the image gradient and is given by

$$E_{data}(x,y) = \int_0^1 \frac{1}{1 + \left\| \nabla (G_\sigma * IC(s)) \right\|} ds \tag{5}$$

where G denotes the Gaussian smoothing filter with standard deviation 'σ', 'λ' is the controlling parameter and '*' is the convolution operator. To find the contour 'C' that minimizes the total energy 'E' that uses Greedy algorithm with the help of a given set of weights 'α' and 'β', we need to solve the problem of snakes.

Berger (M. O. Berger, et al. 1990) introduced the first utilization of parametric models in 2D medical image segmentation. However, this classic snake model provides an accurate location of the edges only if the initial contour is close to edges. This limitation indicates that, traditional snake model alone cannot perform the purpose of accurate segmentation and they require further modifications.

Cohen (L. D. Cohen, et al. 1991) has incorporated an expansion force in the original snake model (M. Kass, et al. 1987) and the contour curve is treated as a balloon that is expanded in order to avoid local minima solutions i.e., the curve passes over edges and is stopped only if the edge is strong. However, it does not work image with weak edges.

In order to make the snake less sensitive to initial conditions, Cohen and Cohen (L. D. Cohen, et al. 1993) uses an internal inflation force to expand the snake's model past spurious edges towards the real edges of the structure. But it suffers with poor capture range.

Poon *et al.* (C. S. Poon, et al. 1994) proposed active contour models using simulated annealing to minimize the energy. This method improves the capture range but in noisy image it can lead to boundary discontinuities or inaccurate region.

Xu and Prince (C. Xu, et al. 1998) introduced gradient vector flow as an external force by utilizing region based attribute, which significantly improves the capture range. But this technique requires the prior knowledge of the object. However this difficulty is removed in modified GVF.A novel interpolation scheme is proposed by Sum and Chung (K. W. Sum, et al. 2007) which can reduce the computational requirement significantly.

Snake models have been widely used for its sensitivity in searching the boundary of brain tumors. In fact, the sensitivity of the boundary found by the snake is better than the conventional edge detection methods. Luo et al. (S. Luo, et al. 2000) implemented two of these improved methods for tumor segmentation on 2D T1 brain MRI: the balloon model, and the Gradient Vector Flow snake (GVF). The improvement provided by these methods is that the balloon model permits to enlarge the snake's capture range and the GVF uses a vector diffusion of the gradient of an edge map of the image, instead of using image gradients as an external force. Later in (S. Luo, et al. 2006), Luo et al. extended their approach to 3D.

Law et al. (A. Law, et al. 2002) presented a modified deformable region model for the extraction of brain tumor boundary in 2D MR images. The model used a point sampling technique in order to reduce the number of boundary points processed. The time required for the extraction of brain tumor boundary in MR image was greatly reduced compared with traditional active contour models. In some applications, the initial position of the model needs to be manually placed close enough to the desired boundary to avoid converging to wrong boundaries. Khotanlou et al. (H. Khotanlou, et al. 2009) proposed an automatic method for brain tumor segmentation in which the brain tumor is initially segmented on the basis of fuzzy clustering or symmetry analysis of the brain. After that segmentation refinement is performed with the help of parametric deformable model. This method provides an accurate estimation of the boundaries of any type of brain tumors on T1 MRI.

The major issues with the Snake method are its sensitivity towards the initial conditions and the difficulties faced with the topological changes for the merging and splitting of the evolving curve.

Geometric Deformable Models or Level Set

LSM was suggested by Osher and Sethian to implement active contours. In this method, the contour implicitly is represented via a 2D Lipschitz-continuous function $(x, y)\Omega \rightarrow R$ which is specified on image plane. The function $\Phi(x,y)$ is known as level set function. The zero level of $\Phi(x,y)$ is defined as the contour which is expressed as

$$Z(s) = \left\{(x, y) : \Phi(x, y) = 0\right\} : \forall(x, y) \in \Omega \quad (6)$$

where Ω denotes the entire image plane.

In this Zero level set, curvatures and normals may be easily evaluated, topological changes occur in a natural manner, and the technique extends trivially to three dimensions.

Figure 1. Level set representation

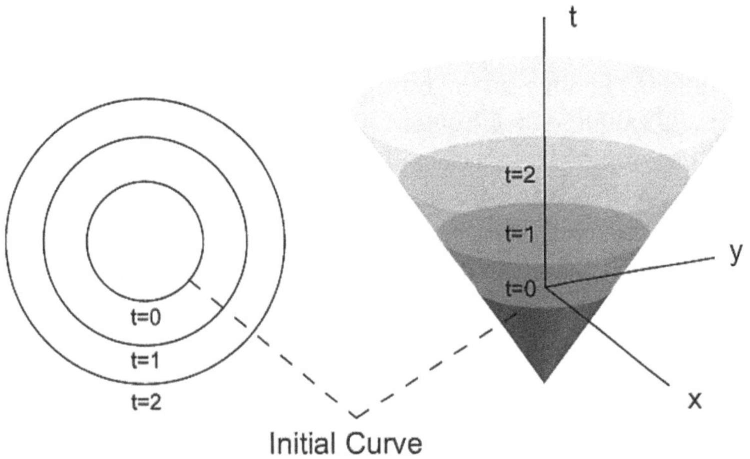

Figure 1 shows the Level set representation where Initial contour is defined by the set $\{(x,y):\Phi(0,x,y)\}$. The value of Φ is negative and positive when it is inside the object region and when it is outside the region of interest respectively. Level set equation is defined by the evolution of the curve Z is in normal direction with a speed F and is given by

$$\frac{\partial \phi}{\partial t}+F\left|\nabla \phi\right|=0 \tag{7}$$

LSM depends on energy minimization to implicitly signify the evolution curves as compared to parametric deformable model. The LSM does not depend on the parameterization of the surface (J. A. Sethian, et al. 1999). Due to this, LSM becomes quite attractive and flexible in image segmentation. The whole segmentation is totally automatic after setting initial zero level. Due to the tuning of numerous parameters and difficulties in using level sets, this method is not useful in some circumstances.

Edge-based methods and region-based methods are the two existing LSM. Edge-based methods stop the evolving contours by applying an image gradient.

First level set implemented active contour model with stopping function is discussed by Caselles et al. The speed function is shown in Equation (8).

$$\frac{\partial \phi(x,y)}{\partial t}=g(I(x,y))(K(\Phi((x,y))+\nu)\left|\nabla \Phi(x,y))\right| \tag{8}$$

where $g(\bullet)$ shows the stopping function, which is a positive and decreasing function of the image gradient.

$$g(I(x,y))=\frac{1}{1+\left|\nabla I(x,y)\right|^{n}} \tag{9}$$

These models are possessed of an edge-based stopping term and a force term to control the movement of the contour.

Local edge information to draw the active contour toward the target is used by Edge based model. It is sensitive to initial conditions and often suffers from serious boundary leakage problems in images with weak object boundaries. Geodesic Active Contour (GAC) model (V. Caselles, et al. 1995) is the most popular Edge based model proposed by Caselles et al. (V. Caselles, et al. 1993). To derive ESE, image gradient is used in this method. It consists of a simplified snake model without second order smoothness.

Based on the principle of the classic dynamic systems, solving the active contour problem is equivalent to finding a path of minimal distance, called geodesic curve (V. Caselles, et al. 1997) given by

$$\frac{\partial C}{\partial t} = (g(I(x,y))k(\Phi(x,y)) - \nabla g(I(x,y)) \cdot N)N \tag{10}$$

where N denotes the inward unit normal is given by

$$N = -\frac{\nabla \Phi}{\left\| \nabla \Phi \right\|}$$

and Gradient driven term that adjusts the position of the contour when close to the real object boundaries. Some active contour models become very difficult to design when they introduce the balloon forces which are use either to compress or expand the contour. The large balloon force causes the contour to pass through the weak edges of the object. If, however, the balloon force is not large enough, the contour cannot pass through the narrow part of the object. The disadvantage of the edge-based model is the failure to detect the boundaries when the initial contour is far from the desired object boundary. There are several advantages of using Region-based models over the edge-based models. For example in Region-based models, each ROI is identified using a certain region descriptor to guide the motion of the active contour. These models utilize the statistical information inside and outside the contour to handle the evolution of the curve, and are independent of edge information. Therefore, these models have better performance over the images that have weak edge boundaries, and it is also less sensitive to the initial position of the contours. The popular region-based method active contour models, (G. Sapiro et al. 1997) depend on the intensity homogeneity in each of the regions to be segmented.

In medical imaging, intensity inhomogeneity occurs due to technical limitations or artifacts introduced by an object being imaged. At radio-frequency, a magnetic resonance images is generated due to the non-uniformity of the magnetic fields produced by coils and is responsible for causing intensity inhomogeneity. The segmentation of such MR images normally needs an intensity inhomogeneity correction. One of the most popular region-based models is the C–V model (T. Chan, et al. 2001) (V. Caselles, et al. 1993), which is based on the Mumford–Shah segmentation techniques (D. Mumfort, et al. 1985) and has been applied successfully to image segmentation.

The CV model is powerful method which is able to segment many type of images and is used widely in the medical image analysis. This method is formulated independent of the gradient information. The model is to minimize the energy.

$$E_1(C) + E_2(C) = \int_{inside(C)} \left|\mu_0(x) - C_1\right|^2 dxdy + \int_{outside(C)} \left|\mu_0(x) - C_1\right|^2 dxdy \tag{11}$$

where $\mu_0(x)$ the image and C_1 and C_2 are closed segmentation curve, and the constants depending on, are the averages of inside and respectively outside. The C–V method can detect all the contours, irrespective of where the initial contours begin within the image. Compared to the GAC method, GAC can only segment the objects when the initial contour close to the boundary of the object.

LBM

The LBM is firstly designed to simulate Navier-Stokes equations for an incompressible fluid (M. Y. Zhao, et al. 2007). A precise and extremely parallelizable multiphase Entropy-Based Level Set Algorithm is designed by Balla et al. (S. Balla-Arabe, et al. 2013). This method is applied for Image Segmentation of MR breast images using LBM. Balla et al. (S. Balla-Arabe, et al. 2012) proposed an adaptive image multi-thresholding by incorporating LBM with localized LS algorithm. This technique is used to detect the best thresholds values for some known initial values. Less computational time is the focal advantages of this proposed technique due to histogram domain analysis rather than pixel domain. The performance of the proposed method is revealed by experiment on real world, man made, and medical images.

Level set region based image segmentation applying LBM is discussed by Balla et al. (S. Balla-Arabe, et al. 2011) which can identify and proficiently stop the contour the weak blurred edges.

The Figure 2 represents the D2Q9 LBM lattice structure.

The evolution equation of LBM is

$$f_i(\vec{r} + \vec{e_1}, t+1) - f_i(\vec{r}, t) = \Omega \tag{12}$$

Figure 2. Spatial structure of D2Q9 LBM lattice

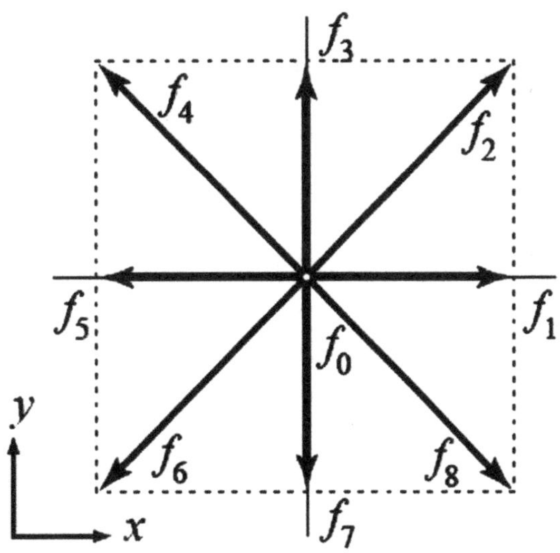

$$\Omega = \frac{1}{\tau}\left[f_i^{eq}(\vec{r},t) - f_i(\vec{r},t)\right] + \frac{2\tau - 1}{2\tau} \cdot \vec{F} \cdot \vec{e_i} \tag{13}$$

The local equilibrium particle distribution which can be expressed as follows when modeling typical diffusion phenomenon,

$$f_i^{eq}(\rho) = \rho A_i \text{ with } \rho = \sum f_i \tag{14}$$

Literature survey reveals that LBM is helpful to solve LSE due to parallelizable in nature.

Possibilistic C-Mean Clustering

Clustering technique has been extensively used in image processing and computer vision. Clustering is used to classify the objects into portions. FCM is a common clustering method which is used to detect hyper-volume clusters. The summation of memberships of a data point across it is 1 (Krishnapuram R, et al. 1996). Due to this constraint this membership is interpreted as degrees of sharing, but not as degrees of possibility of a point belonging to a class. A major disadvantage of FCM's use in imaging applications is that it does not incorporate information about spatial context causing it to be sensitive to noise. To mitigate such an effect, Krishnapuram and Keller throw away the constraint of memberships in FCM and propose the Possibilistic C-Means (PCM) algorithm.

In the case of PCM it incorporates the spatial context also due to this its noise filtering capability is better than FCM.

Let L be the set of Possibilistic c partition, which is defined by

$$L = \left\{ T \in R^{cX_n} t_{ij} \in [0,1] \forall i, j; n \geq \sum_{j=1}^{n} T_{ij} \geq 0, \forall i, j; T_{ij} \geq 0 \exists i \right\} \tag{15}$$

Objective Function of PCM is defines as

$$P(T,V,X) = \sum_{j=1}^{l}\sum_{i=1}^{C} t_{ij}^{m} \left\| x_j - v_i \right\|^2 + \sum_{i=1}^{C} n_i \sum_{j=1}^{l} \left(1 - t_{ij}\right)^m \tag{16}$$

where n_i is a suitable possible number and n_i can be obtained from the average possibilistic intra-cluster distance of cluster i as

$$n_i = \frac{K \sum_{j=1}^{l} t_{ij}^{m} \left\| x_j - v_i \right\|}{\sum_{j=1}^{l} t_{ij}^{m}} \tag{17}$$

Typically K is chosen to be 1 and we set K a constant with the value 1 in this paper. The new membership update equation is:

$$t_{ij} = \frac{1}{1 + \left(\frac{\left\| x_j - v_i \right\|^2}{n_i} \right) \frac{1}{m-1}} \tag{18}$$

The prototype update equation for this version of the PCM can be written as

$$v_i = \frac{\sum_{j=1}^{l} t_{ij}^m x_i}{\sum_{j=1}^{l} t_{ij}^m} \tag{19}$$

PROPOSED LEVEL SET METHOD

Energy Function Design

Let's revise objective function of PCM by introducing parameter with respect to each training data. The aim is to reduce influence of noise. So, we obtain the following objective function:

$$P(T,V,X) = \sum_{j=1}^{l} \sum_{i=1}^{C} t_{ij}^m \left\| x_j - v_i \right\|^2 + \sum_{i=1}^{C} n_i \sum_{j=1}^{l} (\lambda_j - t_{ij})^m \tag{20}$$

where $\lambda_j \geq 0$ correspondingly, the set of possibilistic 'C' partition is as follows

$$L = \left\{ T \in R^{cX_n} \middle| t_{ij} \in [0,1], \forall i, j; \sum_{j=1}^{n} T_{ij} \geq 0, \forall i, j; T_{ij} \geq 0, \exists i \right\} \tag{21}$$

Similar to PCM, we derive membership and prototype from objective function

$$n_i = \frac{K \sum_{j=1}^{l} t_{ij}^m \left\| x_j - v_i \right\|}{\sum_{j=1}^{l} t_{ij}^m}$$

$$t_{ij} = \psi(\alpha) = \frac{\lambda_j}{1 + \left(\frac{\left\| x_j - v_i \right\|^2}{n_i} \right) \frac{1}{m-1}} \tag{22}$$

$$v_i = \frac{\sum_{j=1}^{l} t_{ij}^m x_i}{\sum_{j=1}^{l} t_{ij}^m}. \tag{23}$$

It can be seen that too many parameters are determined each iteration in PCM. In order to simplify computation and improve clustering speed, using reformulation theorem (Kaili, et al. 2003) with *P(T,V,X)* we derive

$$P_R\left(V, X\right) = \sum_{j=1}^{l} \sum_{i=1}^{c} \left(\frac{\lambda_j}{1 + \left(\frac{x_j - v_i^2}{n_i} \right)^{\frac{1}{m-1}}} \right)^{m-1} x_j - v_i^2$$

$$P_R(V, X) = \sum_{j=1}^{l} \sum_{i=1}^{C} \left(\frac{\lambda_j}{1 + \left(\frac{\left\| x_j - v_i \right\|^2}{n_i} \right)^{\frac{1}{m-1}}} \right)^{m-1} \left\| x_j - v_i \right\|^2 \tag{24}$$

According to reformulation theorem $\psi(\alpha^*)\alpha^*$ globally minimizes *P*

$$Z_{ij}(v, x, a) = \left(\frac{\lambda_j}{1 + \left(\frac{\left\| x_j - v_i \right\|^2}{n_i} \right)^{\frac{1}{m-1}}} \right)^{m-1} \tag{25}$$

where $a = [n_i, m, \lambda_j]^T$ so P_R becomes

$$P_R\left(V, X\right) = \sum_{j=1}^{l}\sum_{i=1}^{c} z_{ij} \left\|x_j - v_i^2\right\| \tag{26}$$

$$v_i = \frac{\sum_{j=1}^{l} Z_{ij}^m x_i}{\sum_{j=1}^{l} Z_{ij}^m} \tag{27}$$

λ_j is calculated as

$$\lambda_j = \sum_{i=1}^{C} \exp\left\{-\alpha\left\|x_j - v_i\right\|\right\}^2 \tag{28}$$

In a continuous form, the aforementioned criterion can be written as

$$P\left(T, V, Y, B\right) = \sum_{i=1}^{C} \int_{\Omega} Z^m_i(x, y) \left\|X(x, y) - v_i\right\|^2 dxdy \tag{29}$$

Consider the two-phase level set although the method can be easily extended to more than two phases [37]. The image domain Ω is segmented into two disjoint regions Ω1 and Ω2, i.e., C=2. In this case, we can introduce a level set function as follows:

$$\begin{aligned} P\left(Z, V, Y, B, \phi\right) = \int_{\Omega} Z_1^m\left(x, y\right) X\left(x, y\right) - v_1^2 H\left(\phi\right) dxdy \\ + \int_{\Omega} Z_2^m\left(x, y\right) X\left(x, y\right) - v_2^2 \left(1 - H\left(\phi\right)\right) dxdy \end{aligned} \tag{30}$$

where ϕ is a signed distant function. The aforementioned term $P(T,V,Y,B,\phi)$ is used as the data link in our energy functional which is defined as follows:

$$E(Z, V, Y, B, \phi) = P(Z, V, Y, B, \phi) + v(C) \tag{31}$$

where $\nu\left|C\right|$ is a regularization term with $\nu>0$ being a fixed parameter and C being a given curve which is represented implicitly as the zero level of ϕ and $\left|C\right|$ is the length of C and can be expressed by the following equation.

$$\left|C\right| = \int_{\Omega} \left|\nabla H(\phi)\right| dxdy \tag{32}$$

By using the gradient descent method, the level set equation can be recovered from the above defined energy functional

$$\frac{\partial \phi}{\partial t} = -\frac{\partial \varepsilon}{\partial \phi}$$

where $\partial \varepsilon / \partial \phi$ is the Gateaux derivative of ε.

$$+\nu\delta\left(\phi\right) div\left(\frac{\nabla \phi}{\left|\nabla \phi\right|}\right)$$

$$\frac{\partial \phi}{\partial t} = \partial(\phi)\left(Z_1^m(x,y)\left\|X(x,y) - v_1\right\|^2\right) - Z_2^m(x,y)\left\|X(x,y) - v_2\right\|^2 + v\partial(\phi) div\left(\frac{\nabla \phi}{\left|\nabla \phi\right|}\right) \quad (33)$$

$$v_i = \frac{\int_\Omega Z_i^m(x,y)X(x,y)dxdy}{\int_\Omega Z_i^m(x,y)dxdy} \quad (34)$$

$$B(x,y) = Y(x,y) - \frac{\sum_{i=1}^{C} Z_i^m(x,y)v_i}{\sum_{i=1}^{C} Z_i^m} \quad (35)$$

$$\frac{\partial \Phi}{\partial t} = \left(Z_1^m(x,y)\left\|X(x,y) - v_1\right\|^2\right) - Z_2^m(x,y)\left\|X(x,y) - v_2\right\|^2 + v div(\nabla \phi) \quad (36)$$

$$\frac{\partial \Phi}{\partial t} = \gamma div(\nabla \phi) + F \quad (37)$$

The gradient projection method [14] allows us to replace $\partial \phi$ by $\mid \nabla \varphi \mid$ and as φ is a signed distance function (SDF) we have $\mid \nabla \varphi \mid = 1$.

Body force *F* is expressed as:

$$F = \beta\left(Z_1^m(x,y)\left\|X(x,y) - v_1\right\|^2\right) - Z_2^m(x,y)\left\|X(x,y) - v_2\right\|^2 \quad (38)$$

β is positive parameter and suitable choice of the parameter m can be the value of two, which is therefore used in our experiments.

EXPERIMENTAL RESULTS AND DISCUSSION

In this section, we carried out several experiments using various kinds of test images in order to demonstrate the performance of the proposed method. The proposed method is compared subjectively and objectively, in terms of speed and effectiveness.

Figure 3 shows the segmentation results of a brain tumor of 256 × 256 size. Figure 3(a) is the original image. When the proposed method is applied to the original image, the contour begins and search for the targeted object. Figure 3(b) shows the starting of the contour in the 16th iteration. The contour

Figure 3. Segmentation of brain tumor images: (a) represents original image, (b-e) represent result of proposed method

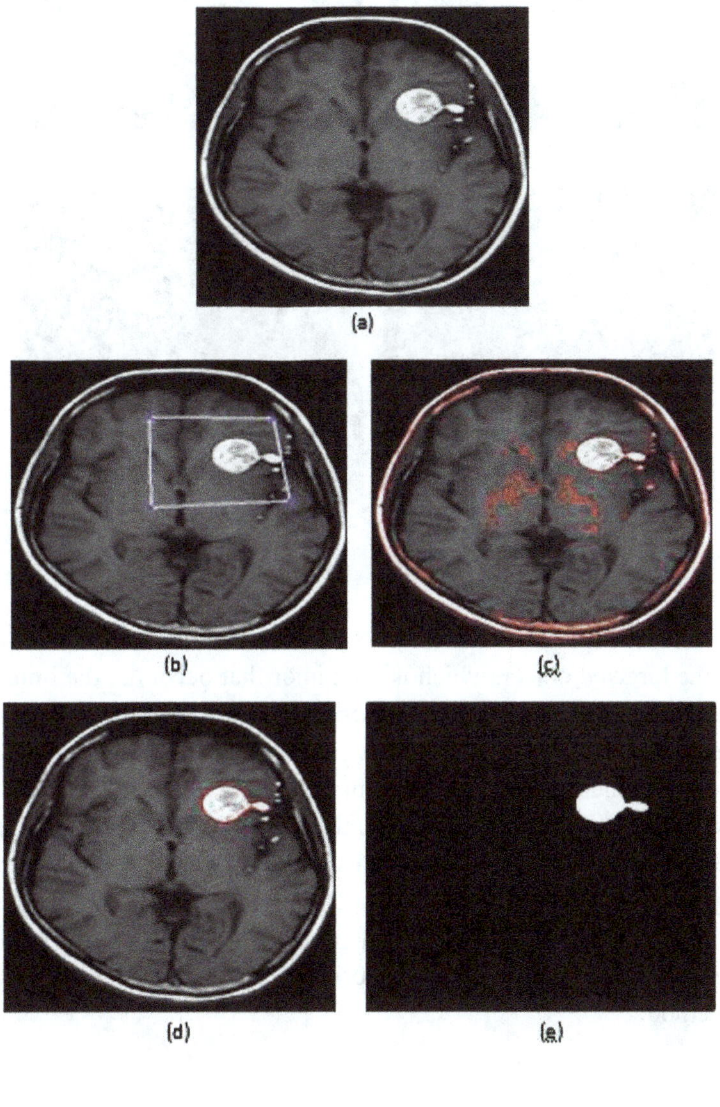

Figure 4. Segmentation of brain tumor Images. (a) represents original image, (b-e) represent result of proposed method

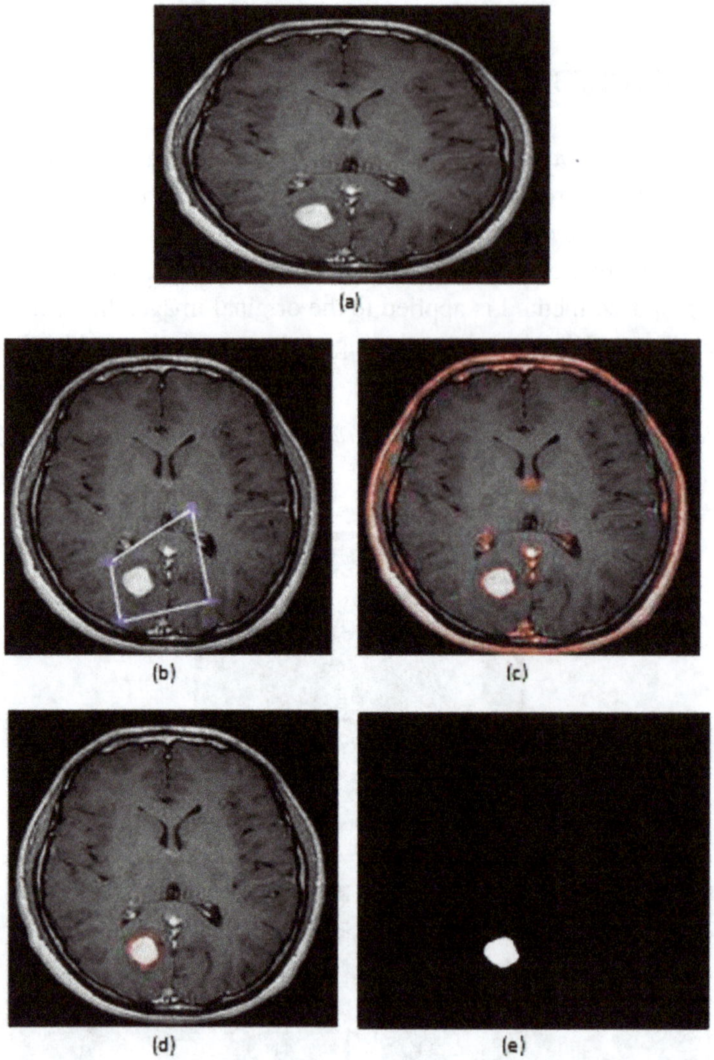

is attracted gradually toward the object and it covers the different objects. In this iteration, the contour stops and surrounds the targeted object, which is the tumor that occurs in the brain. Figure 3(d) is the image obtained in binary form from the proposed algorithm. Figure 3(e) shows the binary image obtained from the proposed method.

Figure 4 shows the segmentation results of a brain tumor of 256 × 256 size. Figure 4(a) is the original image. When the proposed method is applied to the original image, the contour begins and search for the targeted object. Figure 4(b) shows the starting of the contour in the 10th iteration. The contour is attracted gradually toward the object and it covers the different objects. In this iteration, the contour stops and surrounds the targeted object, which is the tumor that occurs in the brain. Figure 4(d) is the image obtained in binary form from the proposed algorithm. Figure 4(e) shows the binary image obtained from the proposed method.

Figure 5. Segmentation of light intensity brain tumor Images. (a) represents original image, (b-e) represent result of proposed method

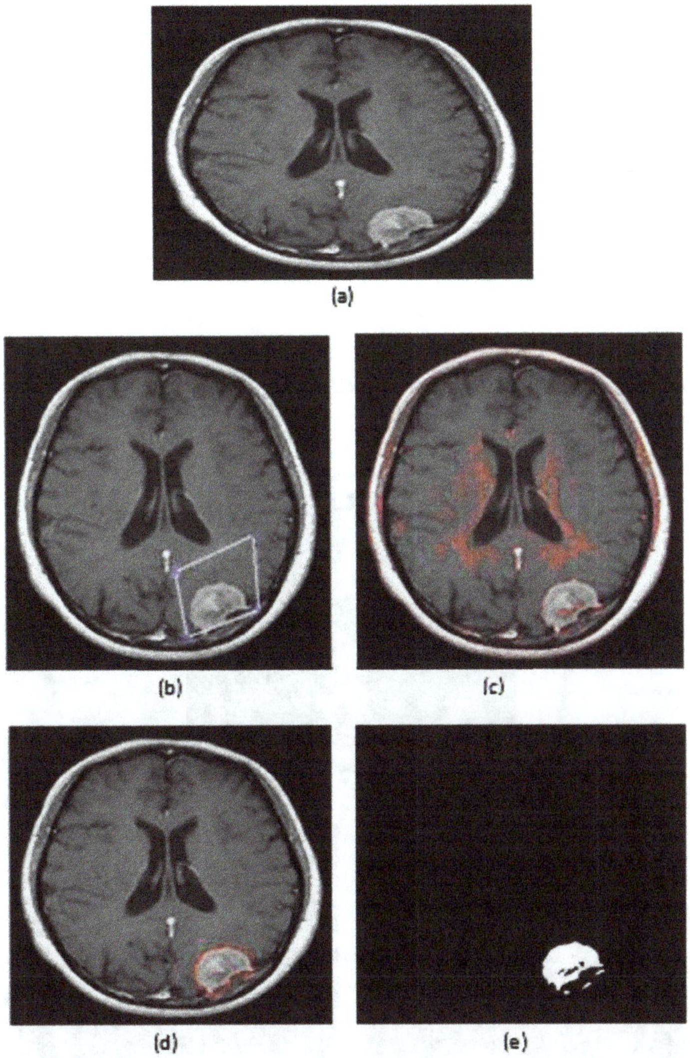

When the proposed method is applied to the original image, the contour begins and search for the targeted object. Figure 5(b) shows the starting of the contour in the 24th iteration. The contour is attracted gradually toward the object and it covers the different objects. In this iteration, the contour stops and surrounds the targeted object, which is the tumor that occurs in the brain. Figure 5(d) is the image obtained in binary form from the proposed algorithm. Figure 5(e) shows the binary image obtained from the proposed method.

Figure 6 shows the segmentation results of a brain tumor of 256 × 256 size. Figure 6(a) is the original image. When the proposed method is applied to the original image; the contour begins and search for the targeted object. Figure 6(b) shows the starting of the contour in the 17th iteration. The contour is attracted gradually toward the object and it covers the different objects. In this iteration, the contour stops and surrounds the targeted object, which is the tumor that occurs in the brain. Figure 6(d) is the image obtained in binary form from the proposed algorithm. Figure 6(e) shows the binary image obtained from the proposed method.

Figure 7 shows the segmentation results of an irregular shape brain tumor of 256 × 256 size. Figure 7(a) is the original image. When the proposed method is applied to the original image, the contour begins and search for the targeted object. Figure 7(b) shows the starting of the contour in the 14th iteration. The contour is attracted gradually toward the object and it covers the different objects. In this iteration, the contour stops and surrounds the targeted object, which is the tumor that occurs in the brain. Figure 7(d) is the image obtained in binary form from the proposed algorithm. Figure 7(e) shows the binary image obtained from the proposed method.

Figure 6. Segmentation of multiple brain tumor images: (a) represents original image, (b-e) represent result of proposed method

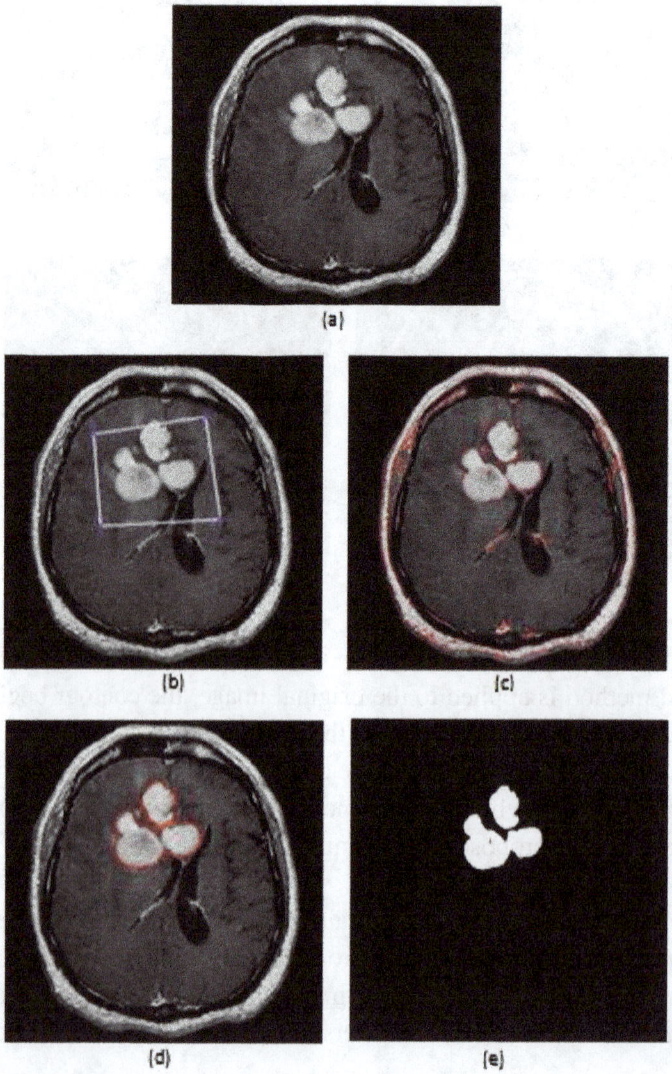

Figure 7. Segmentation of irregular shaped brain tumor images: (a) represents original image, (b-e) represent result of proposed method

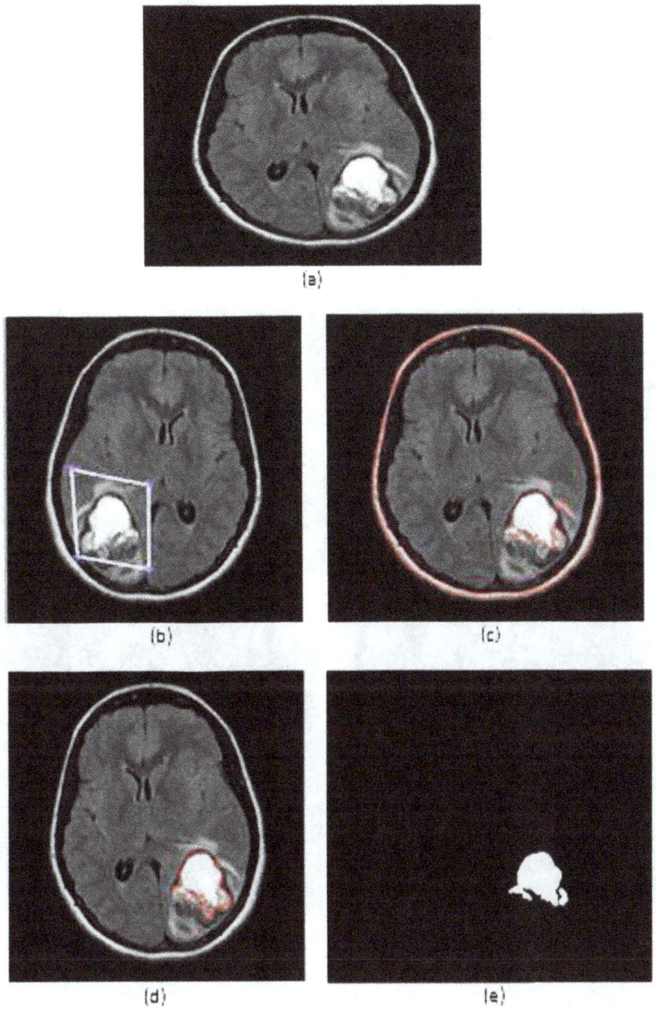

Figure 8 shows the segmentation results of a light intensity brain tumor of 256 × 256 size. Figure 8(a) is the original image. When the proposed method is applied to the original image, the contour begins and search for the targeted object. Figure 8(b) shows the starting of the contour in the 18th iteration. The contour is attracted gradually toward the object and it covers the different objects. In this iteration, the contour stops and surrounds the targeted object, which is the tumor that occurs in the brain. Figure 8(d) is the image obtained in binary form from the proposed algorithm. Figure 8(e) shows the binary image obtained from the proposed method.

Figure 8. Segmentation of brain tumor Images. (a) represents original image, (b-e) represent result of proposed method

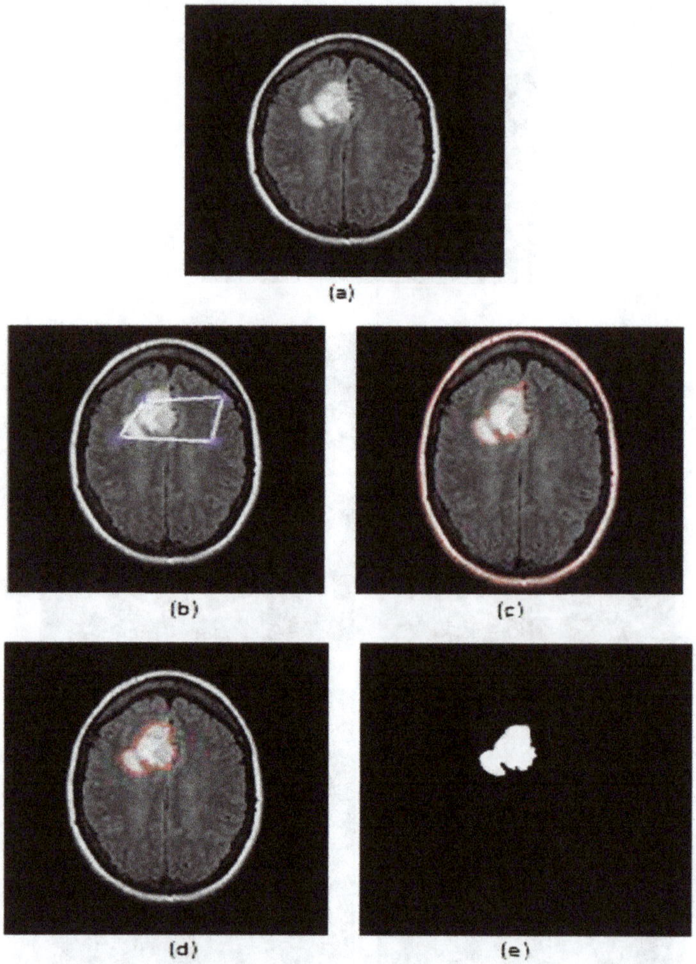

Segmentation Analysis Validation

In this section we analysis and validate the results of brain tumor segmentation over six MR images for the proposed method. Figs. show the segmentation results from the proposed method on some of the test images. In this paper, two validation techniques were applied for quantitative study of the different methods. Let Q_M denote the tumor voxels in the manual segmentation and Q_A denote the tumor voxels obtained from the different method.

The proposed method used the Jaccards measure and Dice coefficient, for an objective analysis of the proposed method, Caselles, Chan & Vese, Chunming Li and Lankton methods. Table shows the value calculated for the Jaccards measure, and dice coefficient, values for the proposed, Caselles, Chan & Vese, Chunming Li and Lankton methods. Figure 9 shows the graphical representation of those values. The proposed technique achieved improved result than the other methods. When graphs of Figure were

Figure 9. Graphical comparisons in terms of the Jaccards measures, dice from Tables 1 and 2

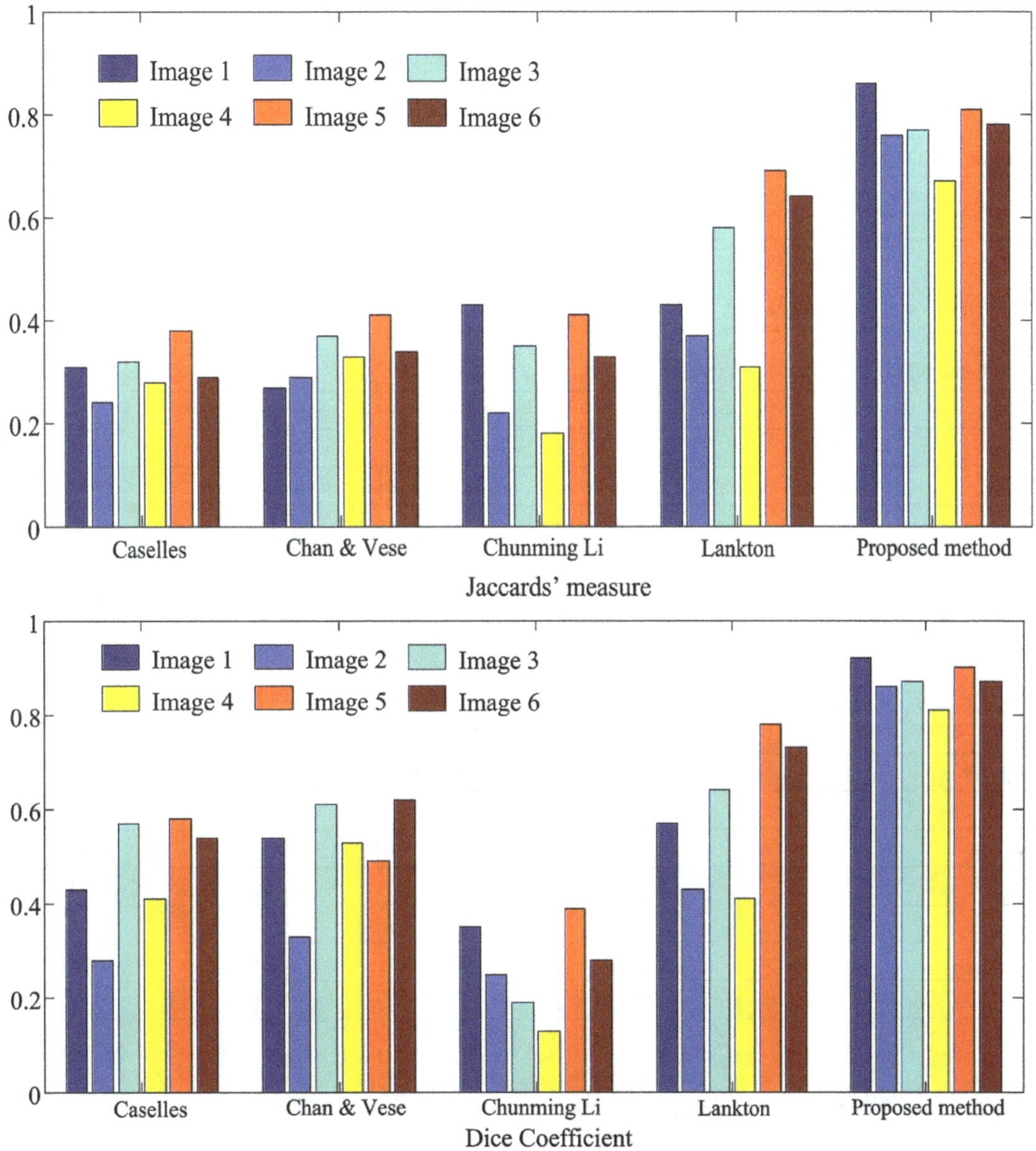

compared, the proposed technique shows the better performance than Caselles, Chan & Vese, Chunming Li and Lankton methods according to the these two validation techniques. Therefore, the proposed method is better than the other four methods in terms of accuracy and speed.

Jaccards' Measure

The special overlap between the pair of segmentations defined by Q_M and Q_A can be measured by using Jaccards coefficient. It can also expressed as a ratio in percentage as exhibited below where Q_M and Q_A are arrays of tumor which are segmented manually and by different methods respectively.

Table 1. Comparative analysis between existing used methods

Author	Year	Method used	Advantage	Disadvantage
Caselles	1995	Geodesic active contour	changes in geometry of contours are handled automatically,	less prone to variation on the edges
Chan & Vese	2001	Active contour without edge	Good for discrete pixel cluster	Sensitive to noise
Chunming Li	2008	Region based Active contour	It can detect weak edge	Suffers from Intensity homogeneity
Lankton	2008	Localized active contour	Accuracy for segmenting heterogeneous image	Large tuning parameter is required

Table 2. Jaccards' measure

Image Index	Caselles	Chan & Vese	Chunming Li	Lankton	Proposed Method
Image 3	0.31	0.27	0.43	0.43	**0.86**
Image 4	0.24	0.29	0.22	0.37	**0.76**
Image 5	0.32	0.37	0.35	0.58	**0.77**
Image 6	0.28	0.33	0.18	0.31	**0.67**
Image 7	0.38	0.41	0.41	0.69	**0.81**
Image 8	0.29	0.34	0.33	0.64	**0.78**

Table 3. Dice coefficient

Image Index	Caselles	Chan & Vese	Chunming Li	Lankton	Proposed Method
Image 3	0.43	0.54	0.35	0.57	**0.92**
Image 4	0.28	0.33	0.25	0.43	**0.86**
Image 5	0.57	0.61	0.19	0.64	**0.87**
Image 6	0.41	0.53	0.13	0.41	**0.81**
Image 7	0.58	0.49	0.39	0.78	**0.90**
Image 8	0.54	0.62	0.28	0.73	**0.87**

Jaccards' measure and is calculated by

$$JM = \frac{\left|Q_M \cap Q_A\right|}{\left|Q_M \cup Q_A\right|} \tag{39}$$

Dice Coefficient

Dice Coefficient measures the similarity between one set to another. This is one of a number of measures of the degree of spatial intersection between the two binary images. This coefficient is widely used in validating the performance of image segmentation and its value ranges from zero to one, where zero indicates no overlap and one denotes perfect agreement.

Table 4. Total time taken to run the algorithm in seconds

Image Index	Li Method	Proposed Method		
		CPU	GPU	TOTAL
Figure 3	123	.029	.24	.269
Figure 4	109	.024	.22	.244
Figure 5	92	.021	.20	.221
Figure 6	73	.018.	.17	.188
Figure 7	81	.020	.21	.230
Figure 8	69	.017	.16	.177

Dice coefficient is calculated by

$$DC = \frac{2\left|Q_M \cap Q_A\right|}{\left|Q_M\right|\left|Q_A\right|} \quad (40)$$

where Q_M and Q_A are the tumor voxels segmented manually and the different methods respectively.

In this section, we carried out several experiments using various kinds of images in order to demonstrate the performance of the proposed method. The proposed method is compared subjectively and objectively, in terms of speed and effectiveness.

CONCLUSION

In this contemporary period, countless category of diseases are discovered by mankind whose diagnosis require a precise technique. And in the medical science, Image segmentation method is one of such method. Image-segmentation method defined region of an image which are partition into different segment. Due to increase in death rate because of mistaken diagnosis done by manual method, image segmentation method is preferred over manual diagnosis. Therefore, doctors favor image segmentation method for efficiently drawing out the information of the infected region of an affected patient so that speedy and successful treatment can be achieved. Because of this features, this proposed method is recommended as one of the best approach for pulling out the statistics of brain tumor from the MR images.

A set of algorithms are used for extracting brain tumors from MR images are presented in this thesis along with the proposed algorithm whose main target is to segment the tumor from the brain picture. The proposed method exploit the region based technique who's only focused is to segment the chosen entity.

The key dominance of this approach over other is that it extract information disregarding where the contour developed. Whatever is its origin, the contour tends to advance toward the entity, making it swell/shrink inside and outside of the chosen object segment.

Chances of misdiagnosis is reduced in this method as manual calculation is not involved. Even for images having diverse region can employed this proposed method. Here experimental results of both subjective and quantitative analysis are discussed and compared and found that both shows extremely good performance. Hence, it is suitable to say that the proposed method is best suited for logically extracting tumor from the drain image.

In this paper, various MRI brain tumor detection techniques using active contour have been discussed and an overview of all related image segmentation techniques has been shown. Segmentation techniques have been given according to the characteristics that allow distinguishing tumors from normal tissues. Active contour method plays a consequential role in Medical image segmentation and it delivers a bright future as the universal segmentation algorithm and has become the focal point of contemporary research.

ACKNOWLEDGMENT

I am very thankful to Dr. Shubhash Choudhry, Radiology department Silchar medical college, Silchar, Assam (India) who help and motivate me to work on this area of biomedical. I am also very much thankful to Dr. Sweta Rani, Nobel medical college research and hospital, Nepal who work with us and help in understanding the medical area.

REFERENCES

Balla-Arabe, S., & Gao, X. (2012). Image multi-thresholding by combining the lattice Boltzmann model and a localized level set algorithm. *Neurocomputing*, *93*, 106–114. doi:10.1016/j.neucom.2012.04.019

Balla-Arabé, S., & Gao, X. (2013). A multiphase entropy-based level set algorithm for MR breast image segmentation using lattice boltzmann model. In *Proc. Sino, Foreign, Interchange Workshop Intell. Sci. Intell. Data Eng*. doi:10.1007/978-3-642-36669-7_2

Balla-Arabé, S., Gao, X., & Wang, B. (2012). A fast and robust level set method for image segmentation using fuzzy clustering and lattice Boltzmann method. *IEEE Transactions on Systems, Man, and Cybernetics. Part B, Cybernetics*, *99*, 1–11. PMID:23076068

Balla-Arabe, S., Gao, X., & Wang, B. (2013). GPU Accelerated Edge-Region Based Level Set Evolution Constrained By 2D Gray-scale Histogram. *IEEE Transactions on Image Processing*, *10*(1), 1–11. PMID:23549895

Balla-Arabé, S., Wang, B., & Gao, X.-B. (2011). Level set region based image segmentation using lattice Boltzmann method. In *Proc. 7th Int. Conf. Comput. Intell. Security*. doi:10.1109/CIS.2011.257

Berger, M. O. (1990). Snake Growing. In *Computer Vision Proc. First European Conference on Computer Vision (ECCV'90)*.

Caselles, V., Catte, F., Coll, T., & Dibos, F. (1993). *A geometric model for active contours*. Numerische Mathematik.

Caselles, V., Catte, F., Coll, T., & Dibos, F. (1993). *A geometric model for active contours in image processing*. Numerical Math.

Caselles, V., Kimmel, R., & Sapiro, G. (1997). Geodesic active contours. *International Journal of Computer Vision, No.*, *1*(1), 61–79. doi:10.1023/A:1007979827043

Caselles, V., Kimmel, R., & Sapiro, G. (1995). Geodesic active contours. In *Proceedings of IEEE international conference on computer vision*. doi:10.1109/ICCV.1995.466871

Chan, T., & Vese, L. (2001). Active contours without edge. *IEEE Transactions on Image Processing*, *10*(2), 266–277. doi:10.1109/83.902291 PMID:18249617

Chang, H., & Valentino, D. (2006). Image segmentation using a charged fluid method. *Journal of Electronic Imaging*, *15*(2).

Chang, H., & Valentino, D. (2008). An electrostatic deformable model for medical image segmentation. *Computerized Medical Imaging and Graphics*, *32*(1), 22–35. doi:10.1016/j.compmedimag.2007.08.012 PMID:17933492

Cobzas, D., Birkbeck, N., Schmidt, M., Jagersand, M., & Murtha, A. (2007). *3D variational brain tumor segmentation using a high dimensional feature set*. Computer Vision. doi:10.1109/ICCV.2007.4409130

Cohen, L. D. (1991). On Active Contour Models and Balloons. *CVGIP. Image Understanding*, *53*(2), 211–218. doi:10.1016/1049-9660(91)90028-N

Cohen, L. D., & Cohen, I. (1993). Finite Element Methods for Active Contour models and Balloons for 2D and 3D Images. *IEEE Transactions on Pattern Analysis and Machine Intelligence*, *15*(11), 1131–1147. doi:10.1109/34.244675

Gordillo, N., Montseny, E., & Sobrevilla, P. (2013, October). State of the art survey on MRI brain tumor segmentation. *Magnetic Resonance Imaging*, *31*(8), 1426–1438. doi:10.1016/j.mri.2013.05.002 PMID:23790354

Ho, S., Bullitt, E., & Gerig, G. (2002). *Level set evolution with region competition: automatic3-D segmentation of brain tumors*. Int Conf Pattern Rec.

Jayadevappa, D., Srinivas Kumar, S., & Murty, D. S. (2011). Medical Image Segmentation Algorithms using Deformable Models: A Review. *IETE Technical Review*, *28*(3), 248. doi:10.4103/0256-4602.81244

Kaili & Huang. (2003). A modified PCM clustering algorithm. In *Proceedings of the Second International Conference on Machine Learning and Cybernetics*.

Kass, M., Witkin, A., & Terzopoulos, D. (1987). Snakes: Active contour models. *Int Comput Vis*, *1*(4), 321–331. doi:10.1007/BF00133570

Khotanlou, H., Colliot, O., Atif, J., & Bloch, I. (2009). 3D brain tumor segmentation in MRI using fuzzy classification, symmetry analysis and spatially constrained deformable models. *Fuzzy Sets and Systems*, *160*(6), 1457–1473. doi:10.1016/j.fss.2008.11.016

Krishnapuram, R., & Keller, J. (1996). The possibilistic c means algorithm: Insights and recommendations. *IEEE Transactions on Fuzzy Systems*, *4*(3), 385–393. doi:10.1109/91.531779

Law, A., Lam, F., & Chan, F. (2002). *A fast deformable region model for brain tumor boundary extraction*. Int Conf EMBS. doi:10.1109/IEMBS.2002.1106273

Lefohn, A., Cates, J., & Whitaker, R. (2003). Interactive GPU-based level sets for 3D brain tumor segmentation. Technical Report. University of Utah.

Li, C., Huang, R., Ding, Z., Gatenby, C., Metaxas, C., & Gore, J. (2011). A level set method for image segmentation in the presence of intensity in homogeneities with application to MRI. *IEEE Transactions on Image Processing*, *20*(7), 2007–2016. doi:10.1109/TIP.2011.2146190 PMID:21518662

Li, C., Kao, C., Gore, J., & Ding, Z. (2008). Minimization of region-scalable fitting energy for image segmentation. *IEEE Transactions on Image Processing*, *17*(10), 1940–1049. doi:10.1109/TIP.2008.2002304 PMID:18784040

Luo, S. (2006). Automated medical image segmentation using a deformable surface model. *Int J Comput Sci*, *6*(5), 109–115.

Luo, S., Li, R., & Ourselin, S. (2000). A new deformable model using dynamic gradient vector flow and adaptive balloon forces. In *APRS Workshop on Dig Image Comp.*

Mumford, D., & Shah, J. (1985). Boundary detection by minimizing functional. In *Proc. of IEEE Conference on Computer Vision and Pattern Recognition*. IEEE.

Osher, S., & Sethian, J. A. (1988). Fronts propagating with curvature-dependent speed algorithm based on Hamilton–Jacobi formulations. *Journal of Computational Physics*, *79*(1), 12–49. doi:10.1016/0021-9991(88)90002-2

Poon, Braun, Fahrig, Ginige, & Dorrell. (1994). Segmentation of Medical Images using an Active Contour Model Incorporating Region-based Images Features. In *Robb*, (pp. 90-97).

Popuri, K., & Cobzas, D. (2009). *3D variational brain tumor segmentation on a clustered feature set.* SPIE Med Imaging.

Prastawa, M., Bullitt, E., Ho, S., & Gerig, G. (2004). A brain tumor segmentation framework based on outlier detection. *Medical Image Analysis*, *8*(3), 275–283. doi:10.1016/j.media.2004.06.007 PMID:15450222

Sapiro, G. (1997). Color snakes. *Computer Vision and Image Understanding*, *2*(2), 247–253. doi:10.1006/cviu.1997.0562

Sethian, J. A. (1999). *Level set methods and fast marching methods: evolving interface sin geometry, fluid mechanics, computer vision and materials science* (2nd ed.). Cambridge University Press.

Sum, K. W., & Cheung, Y. S. (2007). Boundary Vector Field for Parametric Active Contours. *Pattern Recognition*, *40*(6), 1635–1645. doi:10.1016/j.patcog.2006.11.006

Xie, Yang, Zhan, & Zhu. (2005). Semi-automated brain tumor and edema segmentation using MRI. *Eur J Radiol*, *56*.

Xu, C., & Prince, J. L. (1998). Generalized Gradient Vector Flow External Force for Active Contours. *Signal Processing*, *71*(2), 71–79. doi:10.1016/S0165-1684(98)00140-6

Zhao, M. Y. (2007, May). Lattice Boltzmann based PDE solver on the GPU. *The Visual Computer*, *24*(5), 323–333. doi:10.1007/s00371-007-0191-y

Section 3

Classification and Clustering of Magnetic Resonance Imaging

Chapter 6
Classification of Magnetic Resonance Image and Segmentation of Brain Tissues for Tumor Detection

Manjula Pushparaj
Jeppiaar Engineering College, India

Arokia Renjith J
Jeppiaar Engineering College, India

Mohan Kumar P
Jeppiaar Engineering College, India

ABSTRACT

Advancing techniques in image processing has led to many inventions and provides valuable support especially in medical fields to identify and analyze the diseases. MRI images are chosen for detection of brain tumor as they are used in soft tissue determinations. Brain tumor is one of the severe diseases in the field of medicine. Early identification of disease increases the chances for successful treatment. Classification and Segmentation plays a vital role in identifying the disease. First, image Pre-processing is used to enhance the image quality. Subsequently, Decomposition is performed using Dual-Tree Complex Wavelet Transform to analysis texture of an image and features are extracted using Gray-Level Co-Occurrence Matrix. Then, Neuro-Fuzzy and Neural Network can be used to categorize the types of Brain Tumor such as normal, benign and malignant. Finally, tumor region is detected using Kernel weighted clustering method by segmenting the brain tissues and also to find the size of the tumor.

INTRODUCTION

Classification and segmentation plays an important role in medical imaging. Classification used to classify the MRI image into Normal, Benign and Malignant. Segmentation segments the brain tissues to detect tumor region. The objective of this work is to classify the MRI image and identify the tumour region. In

DOI: 10.4018/978-1-5225-0140-4.ch006

order to correctly classify the image, it is necessary to analysis texture using Dual- Tree Complex Wavelet Transform and to extract features from multiple sub- bands. Using Neuro- fuzzy technique, accurately classify the MRI image into Benign, Malignant and Normal image. Then, segmentation algorithm further segments the brain tissues of enhanced image into white matter, Gray matter and cerebrospinal fluid (CSF) to detect the tumor region.

Manual classification of tumor is done by technician by looking at Magnetic resonance image which leads to incorrect prediction of tumor and suggesting wrong medicine to patients. It is a time consuming and needs expert persons to identify the tumor. Classification deals with human life which should be accurate. We used two techniques for accurate classification such as Neural Network and Adaptive neuro-fuzzy inference system. If both classification results are same, then it should be given to segmentation step. New input MR image would be taken, if results are not same.

El-Dansham et al. (2010) have proposed three steps; they are feature extraction, dimensionality reduction, classification. Here, features are extracted from MR image using DWT. Features are selected by principal component analysis and classification is done by using artificial neural network and k-nearest neighbour. The limitation of this work is that it requires fresh training when there is an increase in image database. Jianzhong Wang et al. (2008) describe a modified fuzzy-c means algorithm for image segmentation. Modified fuzzy-clustering means outperforms than standard FCM. This algorithm is computationally expensive and it is not suitable to apply for large 3D data. Wushuai jian et al. (2012) proposed a technique to detect tumor in MR Image which consists of two steps such as feature extraction and classification. Features are extracted based on DT-CWT and classification using SVM. DT-CWT achieved accuracy of 96% when classified normal and abnormal images.

Salim lahmiri et al. (2013) presents an automatic feature extraction and classification from MR image. Features are extracted using DWT and classification is done by SVM. Ze-xuan ji et al. (2011) presented a modified method for improve accuracy with respect to noise and intensity in-homogeneity. Results show that the proposed method is more robust for different level of noise and more accuracy for both 2D and 3d brain MR image segmentation. A segmentation technique for segmenting the Magnetic resonance image into multiple clusters using multi objective fuzzy clustering technique presented in (Mukhopadhyaya et al., 2011).

Forouzanfar et al. (2010) proposed a technique to detect the tumor from magnetic resonance image. Genetic algorithm and particle swarm optimization to calculate the value of neighbourhood attraction includes location and features of neighbouring pixels. An automatic brain image segmentation method is presented in (Demirhan et al. and Guler, 2011). It consists of preprocessing, feature extraction, segmentation and evaluation stages. Statistical wavelet transform is used for feature extraction and Self-organization map is used for segmentation.

A hierarchical FCM algorithm, based on template matching techniques was suggested in (Kwon et al., 2003). But its main problem is a need to an exact framework. A combination of anisotropic diffusion model for enhancing the image quality, and k-means clustering technique for extracting the cancerous tissue was used in (Ahmed and Mohamad, 2008).

Murugavalli and Rajamani (2007) described a neuro-fuzzy segmentation process was used to detect various tissues such as white matter, gray matter and cerebrospinal fluid. Singhai and Ladhake (2013) presented a technique to detect tumor using watershed segmentation algorithm which is termed as the most effective algorithm for segmentation. Awe and Philips (2001) deals with the minimum error thresholding and the FCM for the MRI brain image segmentation. Distribution matching approach was used to detect the tumor in the image found in (Njeh et al., 2012).

Nathan Moon et al. (2002) presented brain segmentation using Expectation Maximization algorithm based on Probability Density Function for the detection of Brain Tumor. Jain and Mishra (2012) presents the artificial neural network approach namely Back propagation network (BPNs) and probabilistic neural network (PNN). It is used to classify the type of tumor in MRI images of different patients with Astrocytoma type of brain tumor.

Iftekharuddin et al. (2003) demonstrate effectiveness of fractal features in segmenting brain tumor tissue. Considering intricate pattern of tumor texture, regular fractal based feature extraction techniques appear rather homogeneous. Among feature based techniques, Lee et al. (2005) proposed brain tumor segmentation using Discriminative Random Field (DRF) method. The authors exploit a set of multi-scale image-based and alignment-based features for segmentation. However, the proposed framework does not allow training and testing the proposed models across different patients.

Corso et al. (2007) discussed Conditional Random Field (CRF) based hybrid discriminative generative model for segmentation and labelling of brain tumor tissues in MRI. The CRF model employs cascade of boosted discriminative classifier where each classifier uses a set of about one thousand features. Cobzas et al. (2007) studied textons and level set features with atlas-based priors to build statistical models for tissues. Such level set techniques are very sensitive to initialization and known to suffer from boundary leaking artefacts.

Intensity, intensity gradient and Haar-like features in a Markov Random Field (MRF) method that combines probabilistic boosting trees and graph cuts for tumor segmentation used in (Wels et al., 2008). Overall, these methods of incorporating spatial dependencies in classification using DRF/CRF/MRF demand very careful tumor characterization for convergence. Bauer et al. (2012) exploits patient-specific initial probabilities with non-local features to capture context information. The authors use a standard classification forest (CF) as a discriminative multi-class classification model. The techniques used in this paper are combined random forest (RF) classification with hierarchical CRF regularization as an energy minimization scheme for tumor segmentation.

Geremia et al. (2012) introduced a symmetry feature and RF classification for automated tumor segmentation. Hamamci and Unal (2012) proposed a multi-modal modified tumor cut method for tumor and edema segmentation. The proposed method needs user interaction to draw maximum diameter of the tumor.

Raviv et al. (2012) presented a statistically driven level-set approach for segmentation of subject-specific MR scans. The technique is based on latent atlas approach, where common information from different MRI modalities is captured using spatial probability. However, this method also requires manual initialization of tumor seed and boundary for effective segmentation.

T. Wang et al. (2009) proposed a parametric active contour model that facilitates brain tumor detection in MRI. The proposed model makes rather simplistic assumption that there is a single continuous region associated with tumor. Prastawa et al. (2003) developed a tumor segmentation and statistical classification of brain MR images using an atlas prior. There are few challenges associated with atlas-based segmentation. Atlas based segmentation requires manual labelling of template MRI. In addition, the elastic registration of template MRI with distorted patient images due to pathological processes is non-trivial. Combined elastic atlas registration with statistical classification to mask brain tissue from surrounding structures described in (Warfield et al., 2000).

MATERIALS AND METHODS

In this section, we give the materials, brain MR Image datasets and methods used to perform brain MR Image Classification and Segmentation algorithm. Architecture of the proposed method is illustrated in Figure 1. It consists of six major steps, i.e., image pre-processing, decomposition, feature extraction, classification, segmentation and post processing.

Image Pre-Processing

Magnetic Resonance Brain image is taken as the original image to perform the pre-processing process. MRI does not cause any radiation so it is desirable for medical imaging. There are various methods which come under this step; we will be dealing with only resizing and gray scale conversion. Input image is resized and converted into gray scale image. The forthcoming steps use only the gray scale image for the process.

Figure 1.

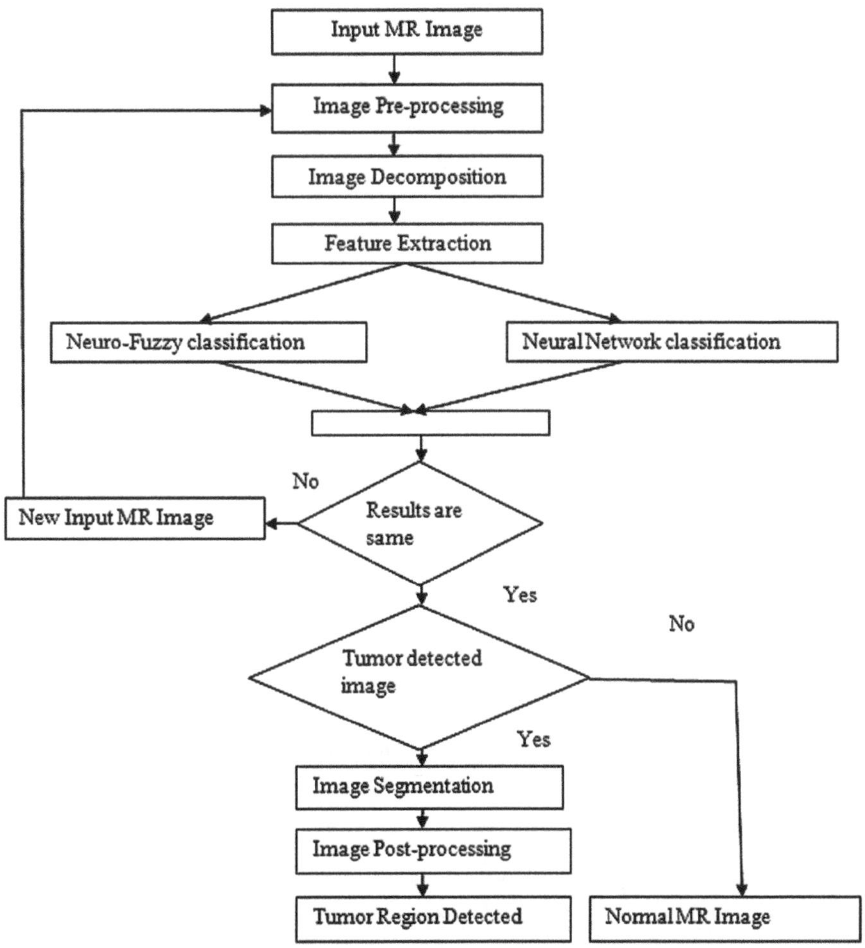

Image Decomposition

We utilized Dual-tree complex wavelet transform to decompose the image into multiple sub-images for analysis texture of an image has been proposed in (Kingsbury, 1998; Selesnick et al., 2005). It has eight high frequency and four low frequency coefficients. High frequency coefficient includes texture and edge details, low frequency sub-band have slight variations in pixels. Accurate classification is possible with more high-frequency subbands which are satisfied by DT-CWT (Eight high frequency sub-images).

Feature Extraction

We used GLCM to extract features from the decomposed image that will be given as input to neural network and neuro-fuzzy technique. Four Haralick features are extracted from eight high frequency sub-image. We construct thirty two features for each input image.

The algorithm for feature extraction is as follows:

1. Create gray-level co-occurrence matrix (http://in.mathworks.com/help/images/gray-level-co-occurrence-matrix-glcm.html) from each high-frequency sub-band image.

Calculate properties of GLCM such as Contrast, Correlation, energy and homogeneity as shown in Equations 1, 2, 3, 4.

$$\sum_{m,n} \left| m - n \right|^2 p(m,n) \tag{1}$$

$$\sum_{m,n} \frac{(m - \beta m)(n - \beta n)p(m,n)}{\alpha_i \alpha_j} \tag{2}$$

$$\sum\nolimits_{m,n} p(m,n)^2 \tag{3}$$

$$\sum_{m,n} \frac{p(m,n)}{1 + \left| m - n \right|} \tag{4}$$

where m, n indicates the pixel pairs, p(m,n) is joint probability occurrence of pixel pairs.

Find mean values of each feature from eight high frequency sub-bands as shown in Equation 5.

$$Total\ value = \left[mean(f1)mean(f2)mean(f3)mean(f4)\right] \quad (5)$$

where f1, f2, f3, f4 indicates contrast, correlation, energy and homogeneity value for eight high- frequency co-efficient.

4. Save the features.

Neural Network and Neuro-Fuzzy Classification

We used neural network presented in (Hiran & Doshi, 2013) and adaptive neuro-fuzzy inference system (Hemanth et al., 2010; Barisci & Hardalac, 2007) for classifying the type of tumor. Extracted features from GLCM are given as input to Training phase, based on that image has been classified into three stages of brain tumour- Normal, Benign and Malignant. There are two phases- training and testing. In training, we have to train feature set generated from feature extraction. In testing, image has been given to trained network, we got classified image. Finally based on kernel weighted clustering method, the tumour location is detected and visually represented in the MATLAB software.

The algorithm for training phase is as follows:

1. Get the training samples in JPEG format.
2. Decompose image I, using Dual-tree complex wavelet transform.
3. Compute the texture features for each sub bands of the wavelet decomposition and obtain the feature vector f.
4. Repeat steps (1), (2), (3) for all training images of each class.

The algorithm for testing phase is as follows:

1. Get the unknown MR image.
2. Decompose an unknown MR image with the DT-CWT.
3. Compute the texture features for each co-efficient of the wavelet decomposition and obtain a feature vector f_m.
4. Compare the feature vector f and f_m using Neural network and neuro- fuzzy technique
5. Assign a class to unknown MR image

Segmentation

Segmentation segments the image into multiple clusters for detecting tumor region (Zhanpeng Zhang et al., 2012). Image segmentation is an indispensable process in outlining boundaries of organs and tumors and in the visualization of human tissues during clinical analysis. Therefore segmentation of medical images is very important for clinical research, diagnosis, and applications leading to requirement of robust, reliable and adaptive segmentation techniques.

Kernel weighted clustering method is used for segmentation. It segments the brain tissues into Gray-matter, White matter, Cerebro-spinal fluid for detecting tumor location. Fuzzy clustering method is based on objective function which leads to some drawback such as not suitable for non linear data and mostly depends on edges. Here, Kernel weighted clustering method is based on weighting and applies kernel function at the same time presented in (Santhosh Kumar & James Albert, 2014). It leads to higher clustering accuracy when compared to previous algorithms.

Post-Processing

Segmentation is segmenting the cluster which shows the predicted tumor at the Kernel weighted clustering output. The extracted cluster is given to the thresholding process. It applies binary mask over the entire image. In threshold coding, each transform coefficient is compared with a threshold. If it is less than the threshold value then it is considered as zero. If it is larger than the threshold, it will be considered as one. Binary decision is to define the value of the particular pixel in an output binary image 'k'. Post-processing is done by Morphological operations such as opening, fill the holes in image, removes small object in binary image.

$$k(n) = \begin{cases} 0 & if\ f(n) \geq T \\ 1 & if\ f(n) < T \end{cases} \tag{6}$$

The algorithm for post-processing the image is as follows:

1. Convert segmented image to binary image based on the threshold.
2. Create morphological structuring element.
3. Performs morphological open operation which is an erosion followed by dilation, using the same structuring element for both operations.
4. Fills holes in the binary image.
5. Identify number of connected objects found in binary image.
6. Measure area for each connected objects in the binary image.
7. Subtract lesser area component from major area connected component.
8. Removes all connected component from a binary image that have fewer than above subtracted value in Step 7, producing another binary image.
9. Trace the exterior boundaries of object in post-processed image.
10. Plot the boundary in pre-processed image for locating tumor region.
11. Calculate the number of white points(w) in image.

$$\text{Number of white pixels, } P = \sum_{W=0}^{255} \sum_{h=0}^{255} [f(0)] \tag{7}$$

where f(0)=white pixel(digit 0), P=number of white pixels

12. Calculate the size of tumor using the formula

$$size\ of\ tumor = \left[\left(\sqrt{w}\right) * 0.264\right] mm^2 \tag{8}$$

where w indicates the number of white points

13. Display the size of tumor in mm^2.

Evaluation Method

Performance evaluation is made to compare the developed system against the evaluation of a trained expert. The accuracy of the classification is obtained by calculating sensitivity and specificity values. The outcome of the classification can be demonstrated in (Heston & Thomas, 2011). They are True positive, False positive, True negative, False negative.

- **True Positive (TP):** An image predicted to be in class Cj, and actually in it.
- **False Positive (FP):** An image predicted to be in class Cj, but is actually not in it.
- **True Negative (TN):** An image not predicted to be in class Cj, but is actually not in it.
- **False Negative (FN):** An image not predicted to be in class Cj, but is actually in it. From the above classes we can calculate the values of accuracy, specificity and sensitivity as follows:

$$sensitivity = \frac{TP}{(TP + FN)} \tag{9}$$

$$specificity = \frac{TN}{(TN + FP)} \tag{10}$$

$$accuracy = \frac{TP + TN}{(TP + TN + FP + FN)} \tag{11}$$

RESULTS AND DISCUSSION

The proposed technique is implemented on a real human brain images. Training database consists of 15 images. They are 5 Normal, 5 Benign and 5 malignant images. Testing database consists of 7 unknown images. Magnetic Resonance Brain image is taken as the original image to perform the pre-processing process. MRI does not cause any radiation so it is desirable for medical imaging. Original image is re-sized and converted into grayscale image which is shown in Figure 2. The forthcoming steps use only the

Figure 2.

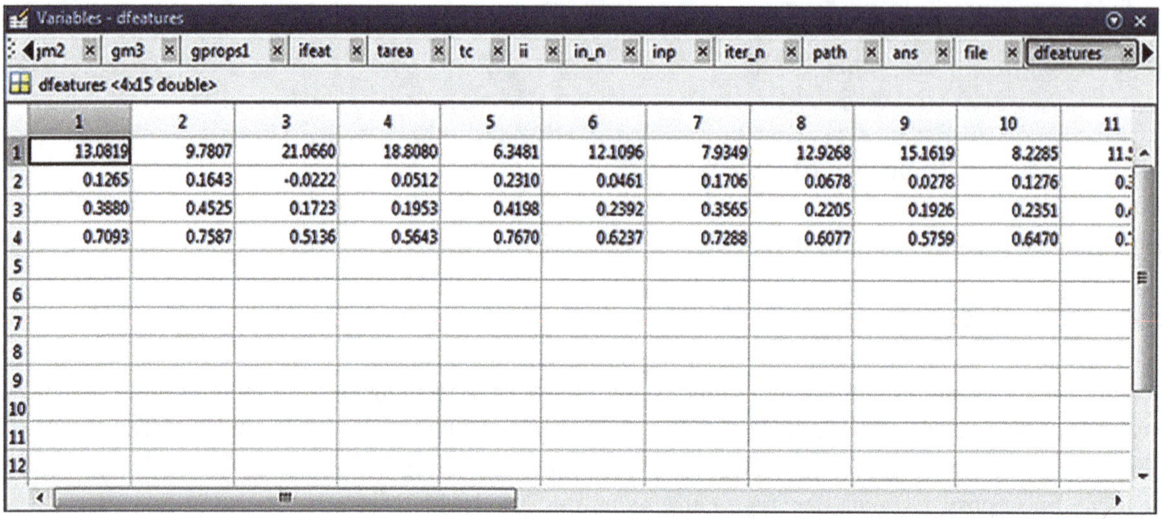

	1	2	3	4	5	6	7	8	9	10	11
1	13.0819	9.7807	21.0660	18.8080	6.3481	12.1096	7.9349	12.9268	15.1619	8.2285	11.
2	0.1265	0.1643	-0.0222	0.0512	0.2310	0.0461	0.1706	0.0678	0.0278	0.1276	0.
3	0.3880	0.4525	0.1723	0.1953	0.4198	0.2392	0.3565	0.2205	0.1926	0.2351	0.
4	0.7093	0.7587	0.5136	0.5643	0.7670	0.6237	0.7288	0.6077	0.5759	0.6470	0.
5											
6											
7											
8											
9											
10											
11											
12											

grayscale image for the process. Image decomposition decomposes the image into multiple sub-bands for analysis texture of an image. It has eight high frequency and four low frequency coefficients as shown in Figure 3. High frequency coefficient constitutes the detail of image such as texture, edge.

Figure 3.

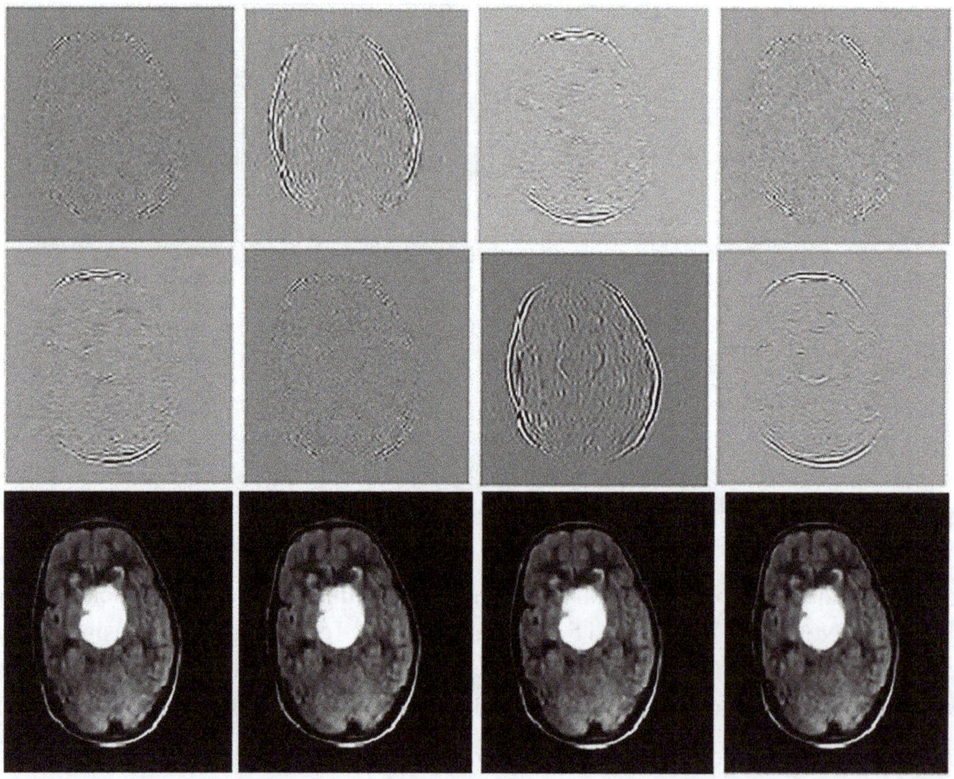

Figure 4.

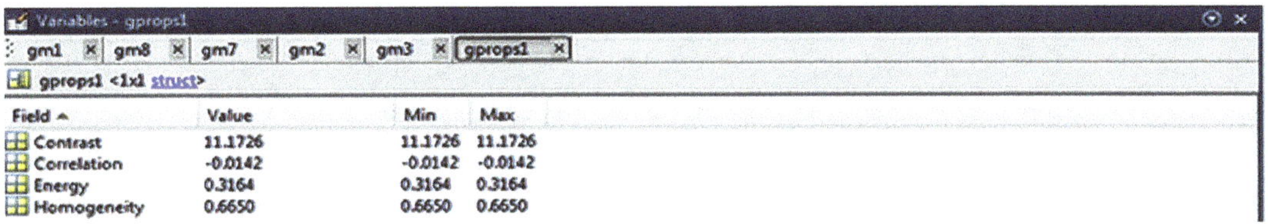

Figure 5.

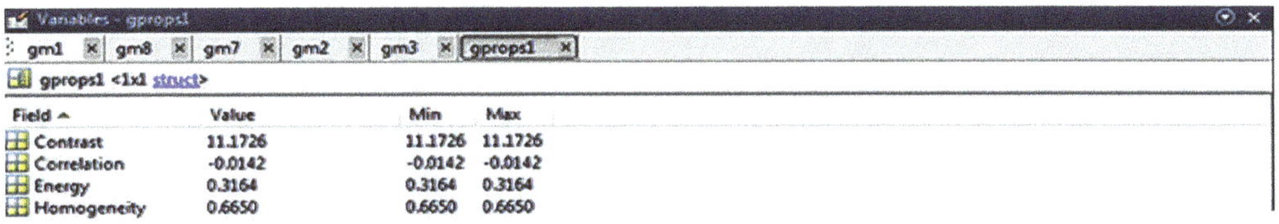

Figure 6.

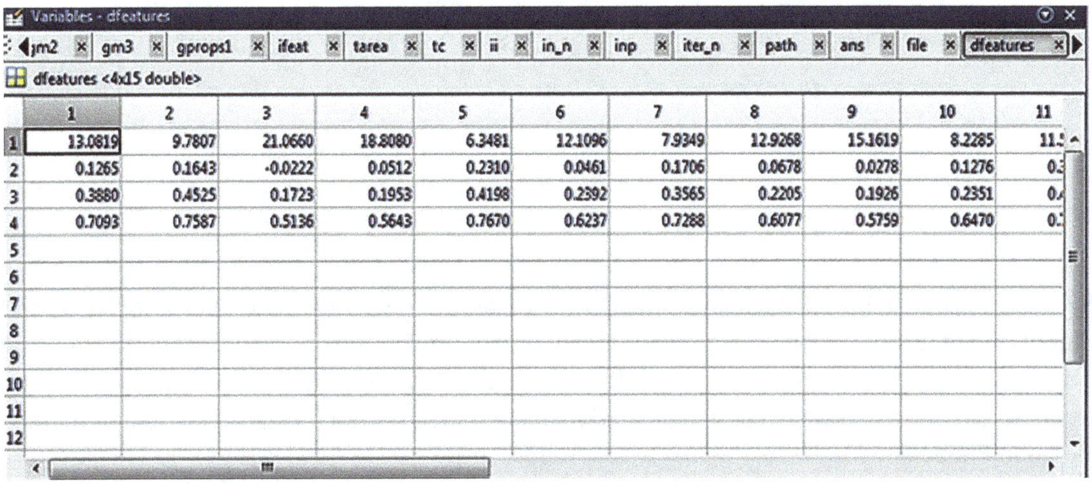

In Figure 4, Gray-level co-occurence matrix is created for each high frequency sub-bands. Features such as contrast, correlation, energy and homogenity are calculated from GLCM shown in Figure 5. In Figure 6 features are extracted from fifteen training samples. Mean features are obtained from testing image as shown in Figure 7.

Neural network and neuro-fuzzy is used to classify whether the image is normal or abnormal. The extracted features from the reference images containing both normal and abnormal are given to a Network in order to train it. Classification classifies the MR Image into types of brain tumor such as normal, benign and malignant. Here, we use two classifications such as Neuro-fuzzy and neural Network classification. The following screenshots describe that final result of classification showing that the sample is normal or abnormal as shown in Figure 8.

Figure 7.

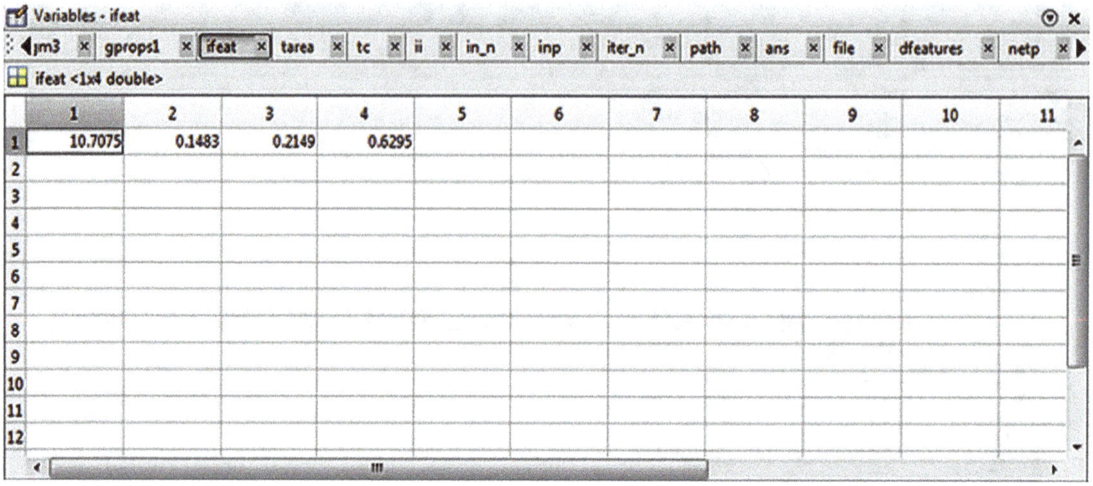

Figure 8.

Command Window
Classifier Results
Neural network Classifier Result
Malignant Case
ANFIS Classifier Result
Malignant Case

Segmentation of MRI brain image is mainly based on clustering method. Clustering is a process for classifying objects or patterns in which samples of the same group are more similar to one another than samples belonging to different groups. Kernel weighted clustering algorithm segments the brain tissues into four clusters namely Grey matter, white matter, cerebrospinal fluid (CSF) and tumor region as shown in Figure 9.

In Figure 10(a), converts grayscale image into binary image by binarization technique. Then, Morphological operation such as opening, filling is performed as shown in Figure 10(b-d). Also, size of the segmented MRI brain tumor is calculated by number of white points in the image as shown in Figure 10(e). Tumor is located by trace the exterior boundary of object as shown in Figure 10(f). Area calculation calculates size of tumor in mm^2 and Number of defect cell from malignant.

Table 1 shows the values of various features like contrast, correlation,energy, homogenity for the sample input of 15 images which are both normal and abnormal. Based on the below values the sample input is identified as normal or abnormal using neuro-fuzzy and neural network technique.

A set of 15 test images are taken for analysis. It is seen that out of 15 images, the trained network predicts 14 samples correctly and 1 sample incorrectly. With these values the accuracy of the classifier is calculated. Table 2 shows the confusion matrix for the test samples using Neural Network from which the classification accuracy is calculated.

Figure 9.

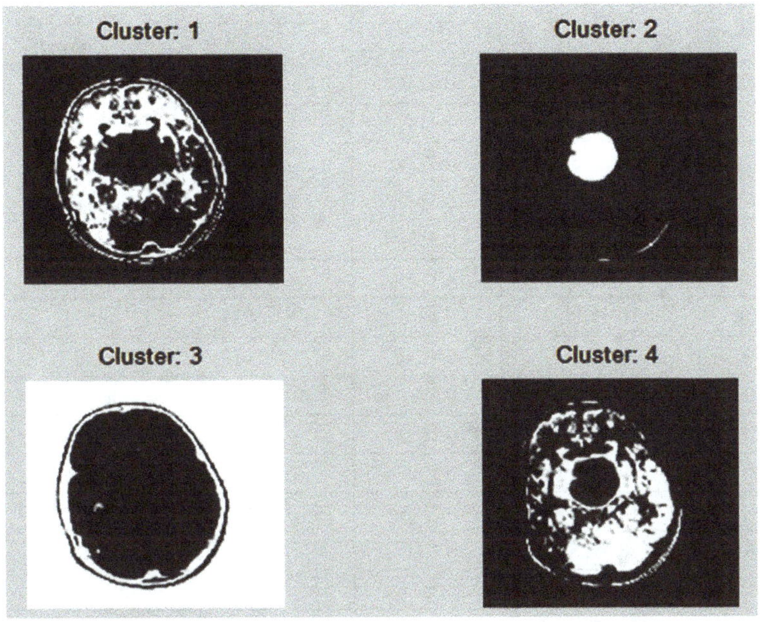

Figure 10.

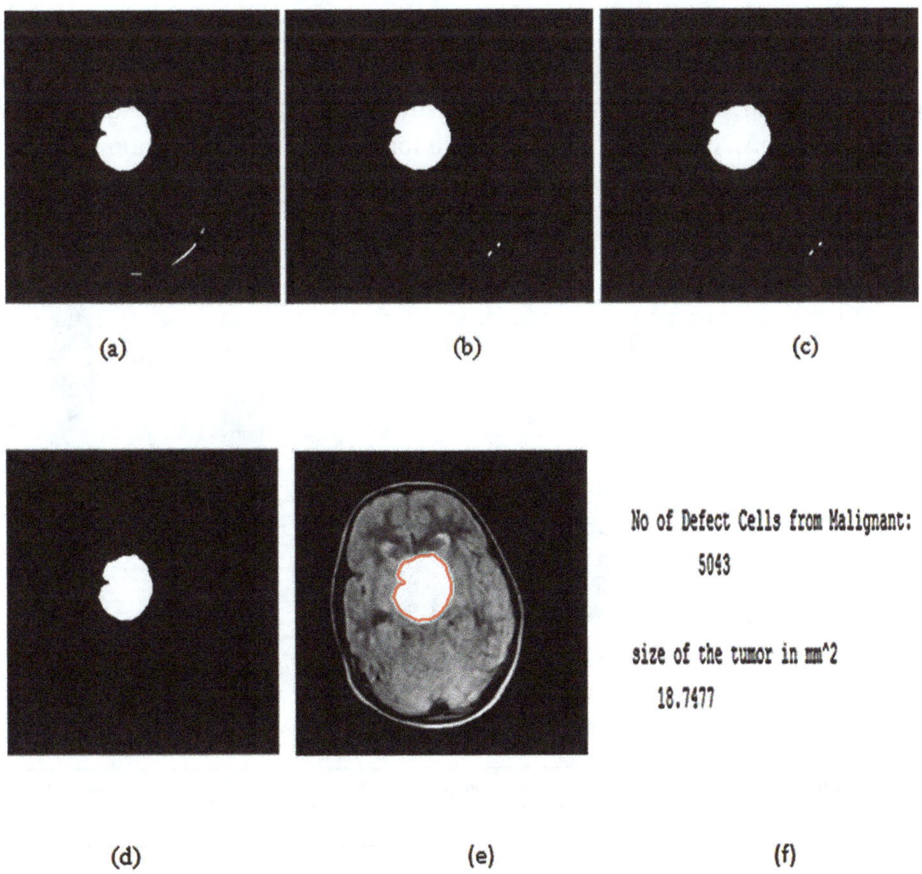

Table 1. Features of sample input images

Image	Contrast	Correlation	Energy	Homogenity	Neuro-Fuzzy Result	Neural Network Result
1	15.6212	0.1346	0.1745	0.5806	Malignant	Malignant
2	10.7075	0.1483	0.2149	0.6295	Benign	Benign
3	7.7909	0.1905	0.3789	0.7404	Benign	Benign
4	13.0819	0.1265	0.3880	0.7093	Normal	Normal
5	7.9349	0.1706	0.3565	0.7288	Benign	Benign
6	21.0660	-0.0222	0.1723	0.5136	Normal	Normal
7	15.1619	0.0278	0.1926	0.5759	Benign	Benign
8	4.7509	0.2336	0.4759	0.8018	Normal	Normal
9	5.0340	0.2339	0.4387	0.7857	Normal	Normal
10	20.5538	-0.1045	0.1560	0.4882	Normal	Normal
11	14.6727	0.0536	0.2515	0.6213	Malignant	Benign
12	12.7322	0.0973	0.2125	0.6187	Benign	Benign
13	12.63684	0.0675	0.2292	0.6202	Malignant	Benign
14	10.6982	0.1231	0.3517	0.7045	Benign	Malignant
15	13.4279	0.0532	0.2172	0.6063	Malignant	Normal

The various parameters like accuracy, senstivity, specificity that have been calculated for neural network technique shown in Table 3. Figure 11 shows the comparison of classification accuracy of the proposed system against the existing system. The classification accuracy of the Neuro-fuzzy system is 100%. Hence this is a robust classifier that can be used for identifying brain tumor.

Figure 11.

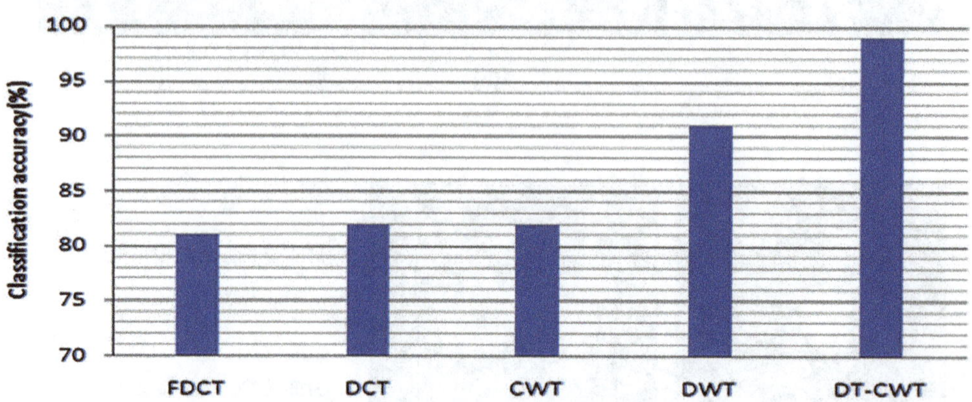

Table 2. Confusion matrix of neural network system

Actual/Predicted	Abnormal	Normal
Abnormal	10	1
Normal	0	5

Table 3. Performance calculation of neural network

Accuracy	93.75
Sensitivity	90.90
Specificity	100

Table 4. Performance calculation of neuro-fuzzy network

Accuracy	100
Sensitivity	99.88
Specificity	100

Performance of Neuro-fuzzy network is calculated based on accuracy, sensitivity, specificity shown in Table 4. It shows Neuro-fuzzy technique better performed when compared to Neural network.

Accuracy of designed neuro-fuzzy technique is as follows:

$$accuracy = \frac{TP + TN}{TP + TN + FP + FN} = \frac{11 + 5}{11 + 5 + 0 + 0} = 0.10$$

Accuracy of designed Neural network technique is as follows:

$$accuracy = \frac{TP + TN}{TP + TN + FP + FN} = \frac{10 + 5}{10 + 5 + 0 + 1} = 0.9375$$

CONCLUSION

In this study, we proposed a new approach to Classification and Segmentation technique for detecting and locating brain tumour. MR Images are taken from 22 patients suffering from the brain tumour are used. We used DT-CWT to decomposes MR image into multiple sub bands for analyzes texture of an image. We performed GLCM to extract features from decomposed sub bands that will be used as input to the neural network and Neuro-Fuzzy Technique. Classification operation is performed by Neuro-Fuzzy and Neural network technique for detecting type of brain tumour such as benign, malignant and normal. We presented Segmentation using kernel weighted clustering method for locating brain tumour. We used Sensitivity, Specificity and Accuracy to estimate the performance of the developed algorithm. Performance Comparison of the developed algorithm for classification and segmentation to the existing algorithm showed that our technique outperforms than other methods. The proposed integrated image processing algorithm implemented using MATLAB. However, simulation results using this algorithm showed its clarity in the proposed classification, its computational time were much less than its corresponding algorithms. In this proposed classification it has to undergo various steps for the final classification of the images. In future, the steps taken for the classification can be reduced.

REFERENCES

Ahmed, M. M., & Mohamad, D. B. (2008). Segmentation of brain MR images for tumor extraction by combining C-means clustering and Perona-Malik anisotropic diffusion model. *International Journal of Image Processing*, *2*(1), 27–34.

Awe, J.-H., Philips, W., Pizunca, A., & Lemahieu, I. (2001). A Novel Method for Adaptive Enhancement and unsupervised Segmentation of MRI Brain Image. *International Conference on Accoustics, speech and signal processing(ICASSP)*. IEEE.

Barisci, N., & Hardalaç, F. (2007). Application of an adaptive neuro-fuzzy inference system for classification of behcet disease using the fast Fourier transforms method. *Expert Systems: International Journal of Knowledge Engineering and Neural Networks*, *24*(2), 123–130. doi:10.1111/j.1468-0394.2007.00424.x

Bauer, S., Fejes, T., Slotboom, J., Weist, R., Nolte, L. P., & Reyes, M. (2012). Segmentation of brain tumor images based on integrated hierarchical classification and regularization. *Proceedings MICCAI-BRATS*.

Cobzas, D., Birkbeck, N., Schmidt, M., Jagersand, M., & Murtha, A. (2007). 3D variational brain tumor segmentation using a high dimensional feature set. *IEEE 11th International Conference on Computer Vision*.

Corso, J. J., Yuille, A. L., Sicotte, N. L., & Toga, A. W. (2007). Detection and segmentation of pathological structures by the extended graph shifts algorithm. *Medical Image Computing and Computer Aided Intervention*, *1*, 985–994. PMID:18051154

Demirhan, A., & Guler, I. (2011). Combining stationary wavelet transform and self-organizing maps for brain MR image segmentation. *Engineering Applications of Artificial Intelligence*, *24*(2), 358–367. doi:10.1016/j.engappai.2010.09.008

El-Dansham, Hosny, & Salem. (2010). Hybrid intelligent techniques for MRI brain images classification. *Digital Signal Processing, 20*, 433–441.

Forouzanfar, M., Forghani, N., & Teshnehlab, M. (2010). Parameter optimization of improved fuzzy c-means clustering algorithm for brain MR image segmentation. *Engineering Applications of Artificial Intelligence*, *23*(2), 160–168. doi:10.1016/j.engappai.2009.10.002

Geremia, E., Menze, B. H., & Ayache, N. (2012). Spatial decision forest for glioma segmentation in multi-channel MR images. *Proceedings MICCAI-BRATS*.

Hamamci, A., & Unal, G. (2012). Multimodal brain tumor segmentation using the tumor-cut method on the BraTS dataset. *Proceeding MICCAI-BRATS*.

Heston, T. F. (2011). Standardizing predictive values in diagnostic imaging research. *Journal of Magnetic Resonance Imaging*, *33*(2), 505. doi:10.1002/jmri.22466 PMID:21274995

Hiran & Doshi. (2013). An Artificial Neural Network Approach for Brain Tumor Detection Using Digital Image Segmentation. *IJETTCS*, *2*(5).

Iftekharuddin, K. M., Jia, W., & March, R. (2003). Fractal analysis of tumor in brain MR images. *Machine Vision and Applications*, *13*(5-6), 352–362. doi:10.1007/s00138-002-0087-9

Ivan Selesnick, W., Richard Baraniuk, G., & Nick Kingsbury, G. (2005). 2005. The Dual-Tree Complex Wavelet Transform. *IEEE Signal Processing Magazine*, *22*(nov), 123–150. doi:10.1109/MSP.2005.1550194

Jain, S., & Mishra. (2012). Automated Brain Tumor Detection and Identification Using Image Processing and Probabilistic Neural Network Techniques. *International Journal of Image Processing and Visual Communication, 1*(2).

Ji, Sun, & Xia. (2011). A modified possibility fuzzy c-means clustering algorithm for bias field estimation and segmentation of brain MR image. *Computerized Medical Imaging and Graphics, 35*, 383–397.

Jian, Sun, & Luo. (2012). Computer-aided diagnosis of breast microcalcifications based on dual-tree complex wavelet transform. *Biomedical Engineering Online*.

Jude Hemanth, D., Kezi Selva Vijila, C., & Anitha, J. (2010). Application of Neuro-Fuzzy Model for MR Brain Tumor Image Classification. *Biomedical Soft Computing and Human Sciences, 16*(1), 95–102.

Kingsbury, N.G. (1998). The dual-tree complex wavelet transform: a new technique for the shift invariance and directional filters. *IEEE Digital Signal Processing Workshop.*

Kwon, M., Han, Y., Shin, I., & Park, H. (2003). Segmentation of brain MR image using template matching and hierarchical fuzzy C-means. *Proc. of the Int. Society for Magnetic Resonance in Medicine*, *11*, 904.

Lahmiri & Boukadoum. (2013). Hybrid discrete wavelet transform and gabor filter banks processing for feature extraction from biomedical images, Hindawi Publishing Corporation. *Journal of Medical Engineering*.

Lee, C. H., Schmidt, M., Murtha, A., Bistritz, A., Sander, J., & Greiner, R. (2005). Segmenting brain tumor with conditional random fields and support vector machines. *International Conference on Computer Vision*. doi:10.1007/11569541_47

Mukhopadhyaya, A., & Maulik, U. (2011). A multiobjective approach to MR brain image segmentation. *Applied Soft Computing*, *11*(1), 872–880. doi:10.1016/j.asoc.2010.01.007

Murugavalli, S., & Rajamani, V. (2007). An improved implementation of brain tumor detection using segmentation based on neuro fuzzy technique. *Journal of Computer Science*, *3*(11), 41–846.

Njeh, I., Ayed, I. B., & Hamida, A. B. (2012). A distribution-matching approach to MRI brain tumor segmentation. *9th IEEE International Symposium on Biomedical Imaging (ISBI)*. doi:10.1109/ISBI.2012.6235908

Prastawa, M., Bullitt, E., Moon, N., Van Leemput, K., & Gerig, G. (2003). Automatic brain tumor segmentation by subject specific modification of atlas priors. *Academic Radiology*, *10*(12), 1341–1348. doi:10.1016/S1076-6332(03)00506-3 PMID:14697002

Pratik & Ladhake. (2013). Brain Tumor Detection Using Marker Based Watershed Segmentation from Digital MR Images. *International Journal of Innovative Technology and Exploring Engineering, 2*(5).

Raviv, T. R., Leemput, K. V., & Menze, B. H. (2012). Multi-modal brain tumor segmentation via latent atlases. *Proceeding MICCAIBRATS*.

Santhosh Kumar, S., & Albert. (2014). Medical Image Segmentation using Kernel Weighted Fuzzy Clustering (KWFC) Algorithm. *International Journal of Inventions in Computer Science and Engineering, 1*(9).

Wang, T., Cheng, I., & Basu, A. (2009). Fluid vector flow and applications in brain tumor segmentation. *IEEE Transactions on Bio-Medical Engineering, 56*(3), 781–789. doi:10.1109/TBME.2009.2012423 PMID:19174335

Wang, Kong, Lu, Qi, & Zhang. (2008). A modified FCM algorithm for MRI brain image segmentation using both local and non-local spatial constraints. *Computerized Medical Imaging and Graphics, 32*, 685–698

Warfield, S., Kaus, M., Jolesz, F., & Kikinis, R. (2000). Adaptive template moderated spatially varying statistical classification. *Medical Image Analysis, 4*(1), 43–55. doi:10.1016/S1361-8415(00)00003-7 PMID:10972320

Wels, M., Carneiro, G., Aplas, A., Huber, M., Hornegger, J., & Comaniciu, D. (2008). A Discriminative model-constrained graph cuts approach to fully automated pediatric brain tumor segmentation in 3-D MRI. *Lecture Notes in Computer Science, 5241*, 67–75. doi:10.1007/978-3-540-85988-8_9 PMID:18979733

Zhang, Z., Zhu, Q., & Xie, Y. (2012). MRI Segmentation of Brain Tissue Based on Spatial Prior and Neighboring Pixels Affinities. *21st International Conference on Pattern Recognition (ICPR 2012)*. Retrieved from http://in.mathworks.com/help/images/gray-level-co-occurrence-matrix-glcm.html

Chapter 7
Analysis and Comparison of Developed 2D Medical Image Database Design using Registration Scheme, Retrieval Scheme, and Bag-of-Visual-Words

Swarnambiga Ayyachamy
SACS MAVMM Engineering College, India

ABSTRACT

There is certain to be a significant increase in the use of registration, retrieval and registration based retrieval of medical images in healthcare. But there is a related major concern that these initiatives are narrowly policy or technology led rather than evidence based or case based reasoning. Or else, either they will be based on old paradigm structures without considering the new paradigms that they create. It is planned to look at the image registration and retrieval from a unified perspective based on their performance for clinical diagnosis and treatment. It is concluded with an experiment carried out on histopathology and five types of anatomic (radiology) images. The results showed that this approach works better with more images from the Bag-Of-Visual words and Affine with B-Spline registration based retrieval for modality and histopathological images. Bag-of-Visual Words is more suitable for histopathological images than registration based retrieval techniques.

INTRODUCTION

Medical imaging refers to several different technologies that are used to view the human body in order to diagnose, monitor, or treat for various critical medical conditions. Each type of technology gives different information about the area of the body being studied or treated, related to possible disease,

DOI: 10.4018/978-1-5225-0140-4.ch007

injury, or the effectiveness of medical treatment either based on evidence based and case based reasoning (Swarnambiga Ayyachamy & Vasuki S, 2013; Swarnambiga Ayyachamy, 2014). The view carried by physicians' and radiologists' is that actual medical imaging techniques are not yet precise enough for an effective clinical diagnosis and treatment.

The recent trend in computerization and interconnection of medical devices and systems are computerization of medical devices as a natural consequence for the need to rapidly acquire, process, and present an ever-increasing quantity and variety of healthcare information (Huang HK, 2004). Combined, these trends will increasingly move us away from the traditional clinical care set up hospitals and physician's offices and move us toward their virtual successors.

A user friendly front end database design is lagging for routine clinical use. The results of the various experiments done under this work have found to vary with the clinical results. To be used as a diagnostic aid, the perfect database as a tool is needed by both the physicians' and radiologists'.

Overall the last decade, automatic methods for intrasubject registration and intersubject registration methods of high resolution anatomical images have been widely developed. The registration, retrieval and registration based retrieval for medical imaging expertise is possible with Mathematical programming and algorithm design. The designs are made possible by 2D analysis and geometry editing operations, feature extraction, object segmentation and image registration. The treatment planning includes geometric applications, CAD (Computer Aided Diagnosis) applications, surgical guides, database design. The information management includes, patient lifecycle data management, visualization solution with markup and annotation support.

Content Based Medical Image Retrieval (CBMIR) is valuable to radiologists in assessing medical images by identifying similar images in large archives that could assist with decision support. Radiology images pose specific challenges compared with images in the consumer domain; they contain varying, rich, and often subtle features that need to be recognized in assessing image similarity.

Radiology images pose specific challenges compared with images in the consumer domain; they contain varying, rich, and often subtle features that need to be recognized in assessing image similarity. BOW (Bag-of- Visual –Words) is the histogram representation, based on the independent Features.

A combined perspective of semi-automatic and computer assisted clinical decision-making to integrate a larger system using registration based retrieval is designed and proposed. The major contribution of this chapter is focused on developing an entire system framework for Medical image registration based retrieval for Computer assisted clinical diagnosis. The usefulness of this activity resides in offering new elements for computer assisted diagnosis in order to improve and facilitate the physicians' and radiologists' activities. This chapter has a strong interdisciplinary character that comes from the necessity to establish the new elements for validating the results of registration techniques and retrieval techniques.

The novel work focused in this chapter is justification of the obtained results using exact medical terms and also technical discussions are carried out for scientific merit. This entire proposed system is developed and practically implemented in clinical care settings to obtain and analyze the real clinical usage effectively. Both qualitative and quantitative measures are given equal importance for supporting in real time clinical diagnosis. This developed system is certified as an immediate effective assistance for clinical diagnosis by Radiologists and Physicians. Also a unique contribution from this research for computer assisted clinical diagnosis is this framework consist of integrated database including both X-ray, CT (Computed Tomography) and MRI (Magnetic Resonance Imaging) image modalities of five various anatomical organs. But, the combination of various modalities in a single database has not been proposed so far (Maintz 1998; Quddus 2011 and Diez 2011). The objectives of this proposed work are, ultimately, diagnosis and treatment will take place at an earlier stage, with less impact on the patient's lifestyle, and with more effect in healthcare. This system is completely created in an interoperable manner for day to day clinical care settings. The time is a critical requirement in diagnosis to prove its effectiveness. Hence both registration and retrieval can be effectively dealt within few minutes. The proposed strategy can be easily extendible to perform generalized registration based retrieval. An obvious extension is for computer assisted clinical diagnosis without a bottleneck in creating the dataset.

BACKGROUND OFFERED

Registration of images is the process of finding a transformation that will align images in a more comparable way. With the current advanced possibilities in medical imaging, images can be collected from each patient, using different modalities or using the same modality and different acquisition methods. Content Based Medical Image Retrieval is valuable to radiologists in assessing medical images by identifying similar images in large archives that could assist with decision support.

Computer assisted diagnosis has been proposed to support clinical decision making, and also supporting for evidence based and case based reasoning. The information gained from two images acquired in the clinical track of events is usually of complementary nature. An example of registration concerns radiotherapy treatment, where both CT and MR can be employed. The former is needed to compute the radiation dose accurately, while the latter is usually better suited for delineation of tumor tissue. The major work by most of the researcher's is focused on computer aided image guidance (Huang HK, 2004; Muller H, 2004; Haux R, 2006). The registration brings high resolution information in to operating room to prove more realistic informatics about patient's anatomy is suggested by (Antonie Maintz, JB & Max Viergerer, A, 1998).

Diagnostic decision-making has consistently involved using evidence from a patient's data with the physician's prior experiences (Diagnostic knowledge in rare cases) or similar cases, Thus, the acceptance of image similarity has important applications in the medical domain (P.A. Van Den Elsen; Pol E.J.D & Viergever M.A 1993; Muller H et.al., 2004; Holt A et.al., 2005; Haux R, 2006; Doi K, 2007; Cai TW et.al., 2008; Long LR et.al.,2009; Zaidi H et.al., 2009; Marcus C et.al., 2009; Muller H et.al., 2010; Akgul C et.al., 2011; Sedghi S et.al., 2012) had given classification of Image registration has given a more detailed and augmented version of classification based on nine basic criteria.

Regmentation leads to a new classification scheme for segmentation and registration methods (Lowe D, 2004). This involves segmentation, registration approaches and atlas Problems in the analysis of functional and structural imaging data, data transport, boundary identification, volume estimation, three-dimensional reconstruction and display, surface and volume rendering, shape analysis, and image overlay were dealt. The accuracy for registration of structural MRI images was in the range of 75 to 150 μm (Babu, G & Sivakumar R, 2013). Indexing the medical reports using the proposed model which combines between the textual description and visual description and reduced by latent semantic is reported by (Riadh Bouslimi, et.al, 2013).

The use of medical literature is needed in the design of CBIR which requires investigation. Disease staging and classification schemes in cancer provide contextual information that can be used to optimize medical CBIR systems rather than based on ground truth and especially based by the guidelines used by physicians (Detterbeck FC et.al., 2009; Edge SB et.al., 2010). Majority of CBIR research is evaluated purely in nonclinical environments. Collaboration between physicians and computer scientists is generally limited to sharing data (Muller H et.al. 2010).

(Antani S et.al., 2011; Depursinge A et.al.,, 2012;) implemented three clinical workflows to assist students, radiologists, and physicians in the diagnosis of interstitial lung disease using a hybrid detection-CBIR diagnosis system and the implementation of CBIR research as integral components of the clinical workflow, as opposed to regular stand-alone applications, facilitate its adoption in routine clinical diagnosis. Imaging is having great significance or value in modern medicine and is used widely for diagnosis, treatment planning and assessing response to treatment.

Image annotation (Salton et.al, 1975) is considered a most trivial task for the management of image database (Wang.Y & Feng.D 2009). Finding objects in images (Sivicand & Zisserman, 2003) and matching images are generally carried directly using local features computed on the images (Kim et.al. 2011; Erdt et.al., 2012). The objective functions were evaluated by genetic algorithm (GA) using normalized correlation, mutual information and mean square error method (Shanmugapriya et.al., 2014). Multimodality medical image registration has poor robust and accuracy, hence a registration method based on contour mutual information was proposed and shows more accurate registration results, which is applicable only to nonlinear registration in multimodality medical image (Ying Qian et.al., 2014). (Surka, 2004 & Nowak, 2006; Yang et.al., 2007, Gou HJ, 2010; Ravishekhar & Jawahar CV, 2012) presented a document retrieval which is highly independent and scalable system based on Bag-of –Visual- Words (BoVW) (Chen.X, 2009; Kim S & Kim.D, 2009).

In BoW model, the following several procedures must be taken in to consideration, First step involves to choose methods to detect key points (Van De Sande, Gevers & Snoek, 2011) and describe local patches around key points (Wu. M, 2007; Lu Z, 2009). Quantize local descriptors into 'Visual words' is the second step followed by (Agarwal A & Triggs.B, 2006; Lazebnik S, et.al., 2006 & Marszalek M & Schmid C, 2006) indexing and search. For domains such as evidence-based medicine or case-based reasoning, it is essential to supply relevant, similar cases for comparison.

Building on the background offered, a new framework for registration based retrieval is designed. The problem overcome by this research is, so far registration and retrieval is performed separately, but in this framework, after performing registration, on the registered image the retrieval of medical image is processed. To retrieve medical images content based medical image retrieval and visual bag of words is implemented and analyzed. The registration based retrieval is implemented and the applicability is checked with five different anatomical images. To be used as a diagnostic aid, the techniques proved their performance and they have been accepted by the physicians' and radiologists' as a useful tool. It has been found that the proposed system is capable of producing accurate and highly consistent retrieval rate in an interoperable manner for clinical diagnosis.

METHODOLOGY

The ever increasing number of medical images in clinics and research centers urges on the need for generic and very effective real time content based image retrieval systems for healthcare providers. In general, image registration is performed as a preprocessing step when a new image is entered into the database or if a query image would be submitted. The images are registered to a common global coordinate system to ensure that subtle pathologies apparent in the query image are matched to a correct region of a database image of similar pathology. To integrate and assemble all these together with the processing center would be an arduous and complex task due to the problem of interoperability between subsystems and require combine efforts from different disciplines. For domains such as evidence-based medicine or

Figure 1. Preliminary design of module

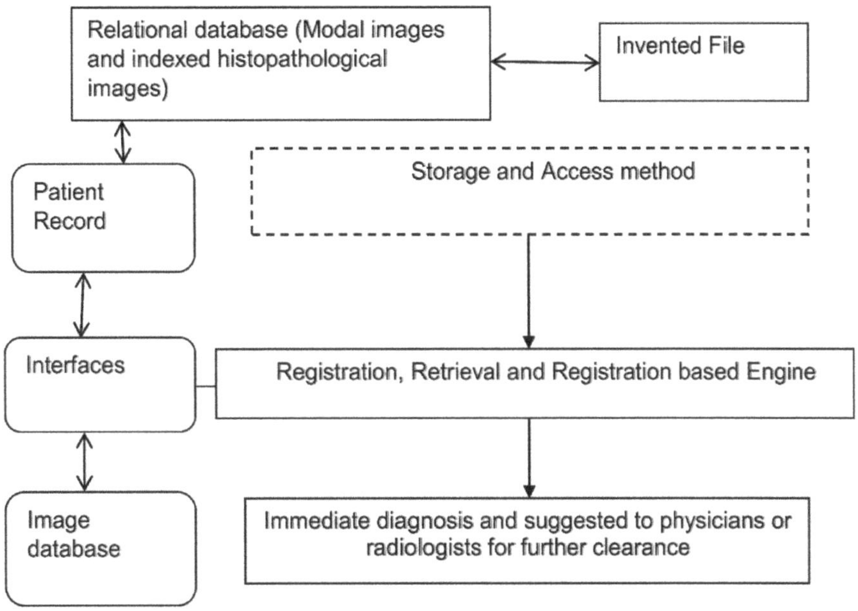

case-based reasoning, it is essential to supply relevant, similar cases for comparison. Such registration based retrieval need special visual features that model the visual detection of a clinical diagnosis using as much domain knowledge as possible and is depicted in the Figure 1. Another idea is the creation of databases. This is even more natural compared to the normal work flow in medicine where the first requirement is to find out whether the case is similar or not. Dissimilarity could be combined without highlighting regions in the registration based retrieved image. Such a technique can help to find cases that might otherwise be missed. This is the general proposed model of this chapter.

Figure 1 explains how the most clinical research departments have computerized information system in which patient images and reports are to be stored, and they can be handled in two ways, the integrated report and review applications (Web reference, Diagnostic and interventional Radiology). The report involves retrieving and viewing images, processing, interpretation and annotation of the diagnosis, composition of final diagnostic multimedia report and storage in the database. The content based image retrieval system is based on primitive features, derived attributes and abstract attributes for radiological images.

Registration based retrieval need special visual features that model the visual detection of clinical diagnosis using as much domain knowledge as possible and is depicted in detail in Figure 2. Affine, Demons and Affine with B-Spline is implemented for registration technique, Distance, Transform and CBMIR is implemented for Retrieval technique. The metrics used are Euclidean, Manhattan, Mahalanobis, Canberra, Bray-Curtis, Squared Chord and Chi-Squared using energy as a feature. The second technique implemented is transform based retrieval. Though transform has served as an engine to convert from the spatial domain (Monay, 2006) the frequency domain, they can also be served as a tool for retrieval of images by extracting the features from them. DFT, DCT, DWT, CWT, RCWF and Curvelet are applied Azhar Quddus & Otman Basir, 2008). The transform which has lesser performance is combined with higher performance, to check the applicability of the results. The combination of transform which has lesser performance is combined with higher performance to check the applicability of the results.

Figure 2. Combined system architecture

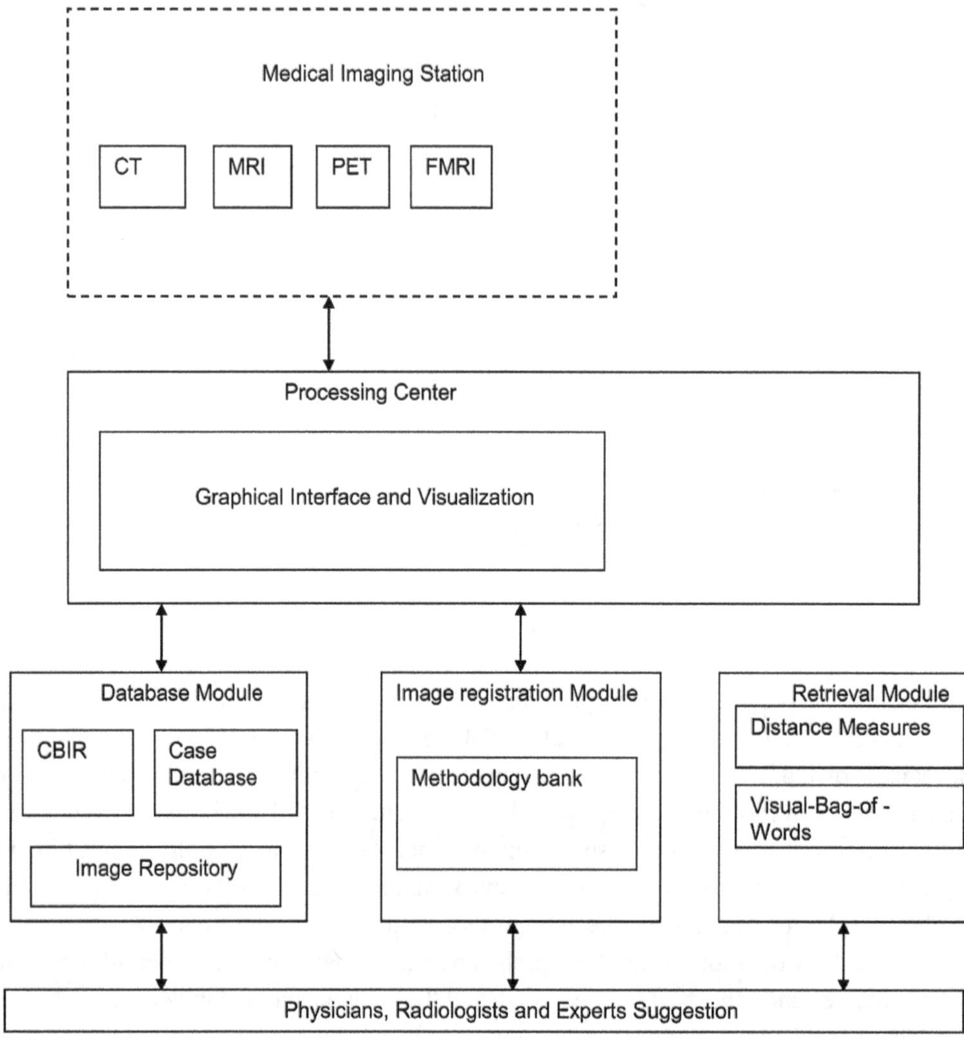

Certain transform technique does not perform well in the retrieval system. But, certain transform techniques do perform well due to their inherent features. It is already proved that DCT and Curvelet found to have lesser retrieval rate. CWT and DWT found to have higher retrieval rate. So, the combination of DCT+CWT, DCT+DWT and Curvelet+ DWT have been implemented.

The third technique implemented is content based medical image retrieval. Texture and shape based retrieval techniques are also applied. GLCM, LBP and GLCM with LBP are used for texture based retrieval. Shape based retrieval is processed using canny edge with the Otsu method. The multifeature based technique (Canny edge with Otsu) is also applied and analyzed. For Visual-Bag-of-Words, Harris Affine is the key point detector used and Speeded up Robust Features (SURF) is the local descriptor used. Due to constraints in space the Equation part is not discussed, the methodology, issues and solutions are highly focused. The purpose of local invariant features is to provide a representation that allows to efficiently matching local structures between images which is very important in registration and for geometric stability. It defines key points to be "points that have locally maximal self-matching precision under translational least-squares template matching". It is observed that, the computational complexity is less in Harris Affine. By using SURF the descriptors obtained from different images can be well recognized and best matching pairs can be found which speeds up the process.

- **Experimental Database:** Determining the ground truth by database, on what basis retrieval is performed and performance is measured is most important. To ensure the quality of research it is necessary to select a proper dataset as it plays an important role in the CBMIR performance and BOVW. A short summary of the database system is discussed here. The database is created with 10 sets of databases. Each database set includes Brain images, Chest, Liver, Knee and Spine images comprising of 100 images with each 5 sets with a total of 1000 images.

This medical image system design is constructed by considering the two layer system, the database with front end and back end relies on design concept. Back end system embodies higher end programs than that of the front end system. The front end design is image information, which connects with the back end design in registration, retrieval, BOVW and registration based retrieval for improving retrieval precision and recall. The back end design includes the techniques used for feature extraction and retrieval Schema for effective retrieval. The system is the most simple and the basis, also extracts information from diagnosis report. The image description and diagnosis results from radiologists are taken as an explanation and conclusion on images. This layer offers assistant description information. The images used to form the database are Brain, Chest, Liver, Knee and Spine images and their specific criteria considered for justifying the results are given below. Throughout this experiment for registration, retrieval, BOVW and registration based retrieval the same set of database is used. The web reference database and personally collected images are used as images in the database.

After performing registration and retrieval separately, registration based retrieval is implemented. The registered images are made as a separate database. Now these images are applied for retrieval. The applicability of various methods is checked and evaluated for achieving better performance in terms of the retrieval rate. The thing has to be cleared here is though registration changes the alignment of images in the application of clinical diagnosis and by applying this in the retrieval system does not affect the retrieval rate but, it gradually increases the performance. The alignment of images differs after performing registration. Hence, while combining retrieval with registration, when compared with the query image, these registered images may show some variations. This could affect the retrieval rate. But, the framework developed using the conventional techniques increases the retrieval rate. This has the added advantage of both registration and retrieval. This framework is linked to the database to the files in the folder containing all information about the patients, helping with immediate clinical reference serving for clinical diagnosis, treatment and surgical planning and is depicted in Figure 3 and Figure 4

Figure 3. Patient record details

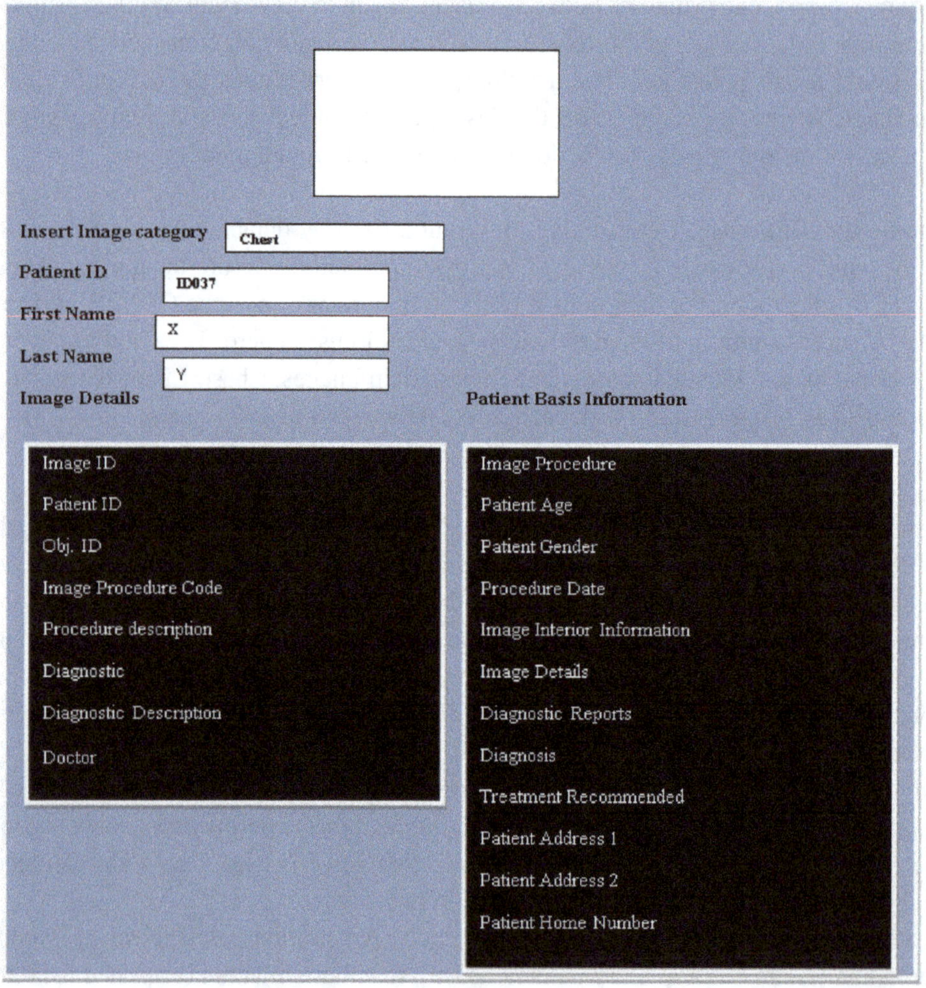

PERFORMANCE EVALUATION

The performance of the medical image retrieval system techniques is analyzed by the following measures.

The level of retrieval accuracy which is achieved by a system is important to establish its performance illustrated by (Muller et al. 2004). In CBMIR, precision-recall is the most widely used measurement methods to evaluate the retrieval accuracy. Precision P is defined as the ratio of the number of retrieved relevant images r to the total number of retrieved images n. Precision measures the accuracy of the retrieval and it is given in Equation (1).

$$P = \frac{Number\ of\ relevant\ images\ retrieved}{Total\ number\ of\ relevant\ images\ in\ retrieved} = \frac{r}{n} \quad (1)$$

Figure 4. Proposed diagnosis system using medical image registration based retrieval framework

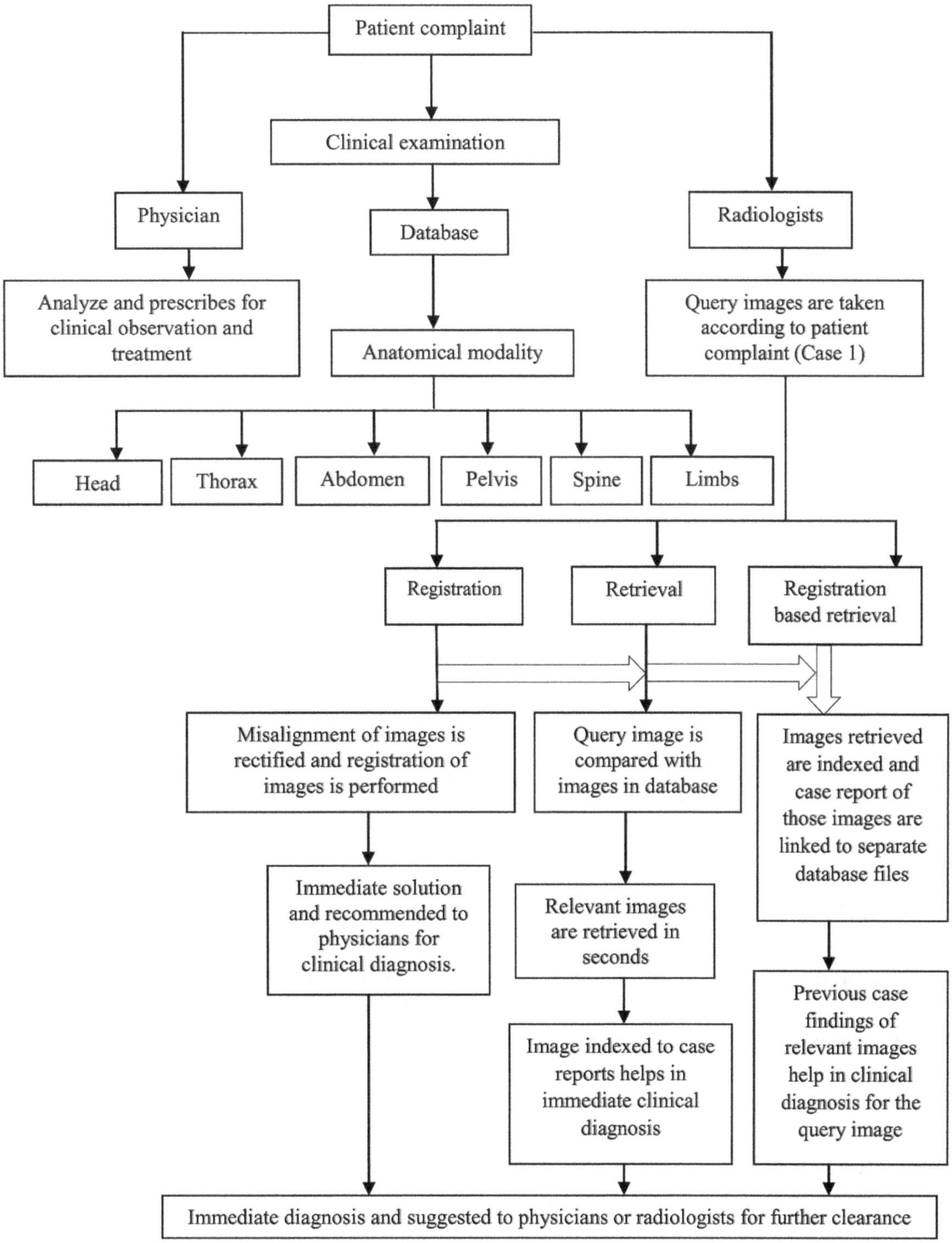

Table 1. Measured performance parameters using affine, demons and affine with b-spline based registration for brain, liver and knee images

Performance Parameters	Before Registration	After Registration		
		Affine Based Registration	Demons Based Registration	Affine with B-Spline Based Registration
Registration of Brain Image				
SSD	123.1011	135.7515	131.4718	98.5715
MI	1.7181	1.9301	1.6598	1.902
Registration of Liver Image				
SSD	240.5798	240.299	247.8	124.0495
MI	0.02015	0.2172	0.0434	0.2872
Registration of Knee Image				
SSD	248.57	230.85	187.61	186.06
MI	0.0658	0.2002	0.2052	0.2019

The recall is defined by (Muller et al. 2004) and is denoted as R which is the ratio of the number of retrieved relevant images r to the total number of relevant images in the whole database (m). Recall measures the robustness of the retrieval and is given in Equation (2).

$$R = \frac{Number\ of\ relevant\ images\ retrieved}{Total\ number\ of\ relevant\ images\ in\ database} = \frac{r}{m} \tag{2}$$

Generally, the precision value falls with increases in the recall values. A retrieval system can be called 'ideal' if both the precision and recall values remain high. However, in reality, no such image retrieval systems have yet been found. Precision-recall pair is a good standard of performance evaluation.

RESULTS AND DISCUSSION

From the overall analysis it is clear that Affine with B-Spline performs well in registration of medical images than Affine and Demons and the results are depicted in Table 1. The reason is, while performing Affine transform the entire image is subjected to translation, rotation and scaling. This leads to a change in the orientation and hence while selecting control points more care should be given. The Demons uses a diffusing model concept. Hence this leads to lesser disorientation of details present in the image. This can be easily identified by the Observers' group and qualitatively by metrics SSD and MI. Here comes the reason for the better performance of Affine with B-Spline, as it is already known that a combination will always provide a good result. Here Affine is chosen because, though it gives orientation changes but, when it is combined with B-Spline which uses basis function with their intimate property of smoothness and multi resolution strategy could overcome it. This is the reason for Affine with B-Spline to perform well in monomodal registration of medical images (see Table 2).

Table 2. Overall best analyzed results from medical image registration based retrieval system using distance, transform, texture, shape and multi feature techniques

Type	Results of Affine		Results of Demons		Results of Affine + B-Spline	
	Methods with (Precision/ Recall)	**Image with (Precision/ Recall)**	**Methods with (Precision/ Recall)**	**Image with (Precision/ Recall)**	**Methods with (Precision/ Recall)**	**Image with (Precision/ Recall)**
Distance	Bray-Curtis (90/45)	Brain (70/35)	Squared Chord &Chi-Squared (90/35)	Brain (74/37)	Bray-Curtis (73/37)	Brain (73/36)
Transform	CWT (72/43)	Brain (56/33)	DFT (83/50)	Liver (53/32)	DFT (78/47)	Liver (60/36)
Texture	GLCM (93/47)	Knee (100/50)	GLCM, GLCM+LBP (100/50)	Brain (100/50)	GLCM, GLCM+LBP (100/50)	Knee (100/50)
Shape	Canny edge with Otsu (60/30)	Knee (80/40)	Canny edge with Otsu (87/43)	Brain (100/50)	Canny edge with Otsu (87/43)	Brain and Knee (100/50)
Multi-feature	GLCM+ Canny edge with Otsu method (87/43)	Knee (100/50)	GLCM+ Canny edge with Otsu method (93/47)	Liver and Knee (100/50)	GLCM+ Canny edge with Otsu method (100/50)	Brain (100/50) Liver (100/50) Knee (100/50)
Bag-Of-Visual Words	Harris Affine &SURF (53/32)	Brain (20/10) Knee (20/10)	Harris Affine &SURF (100/50)	Brain (100/50) Liver (100/50) Knee (100/50)	Harris Affine &SURF (100/50)	Brain (100/50) Liver (100/50) Knee (100/50)

Since, registration of images will make a drastic change in the pixel distribution and orientation of the image. On comparing the retrieval of images without registration, for distance metrics, the retrieval rate is found to be decreased. For transform based retrieval, the retrieval rate is found to be increased for all three registration based retrieval techniques from (47/28)% to (72/43)%, (83/50)% and (78/47)% of (APR/ARR) and is depicted in Figure 5 and 6 graphically. This proves that registration of images, which makes several transformation (Affine, Demons and Affine with B-Spline) based on control points selection serves with double advantage of registration and retrieval by increasing the retrieval rate.

Using texture based techniques, the retrieval rate is found to be more similar for retrieval without registration and registration based retrieval. This confirms that, change in the gray level distribution before and after registration will not affect the retrieval rate. Thus, confirming that only the orientation change will affect the retrieval rate. The features used in shape based retrieval search for exact size and shape which is not possible in medical images because of their difference in orientation. But when care is given during the selection of control points while applying the transformation, using shape based techniques, the retrieval rate is found to be increased from (60/30) % of (APR/ARR) to (87/43) % of (APR/ARR) for Demons and Affine with B-Spline registration based retrieval. Edge details are preserved by maximizing the separability of clusters in gray level, where the transformation does not affect the image distribution and orientation. Hence using multifeature techniques, both retrieval and registration based retrieval have same APR and ARR. The above analysis provides the detail analysis of results. By using registration based retrieval, the retrieval rate for transform based techniques and shape have found to be increased. Texture based techniques and multifeature based techniques perform similar for registration based retrieval and retrieval without registration. Moreover the performance of Affine with B-Spline is

Figure 5. Overall best analyzed results (precision) from medical image registration based retrieval system using distance, transform and CBMIR

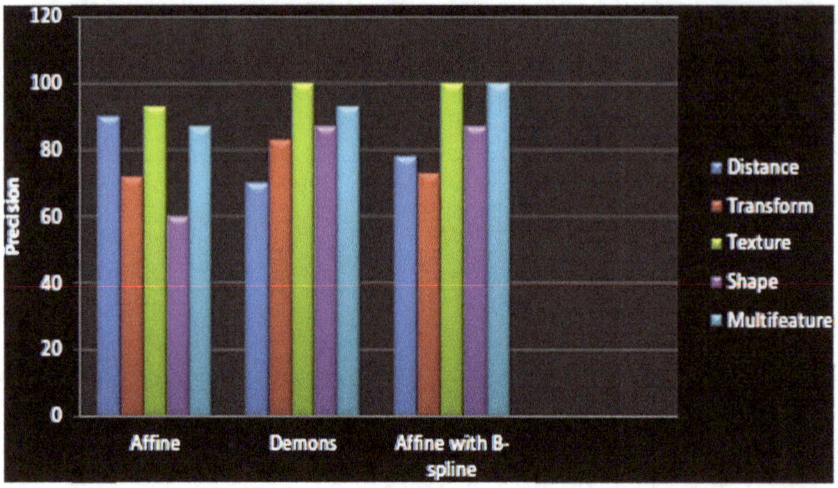

better than Affine registration. Demons perform equally similar to Affine with B-Spline registration. Hence, here comes the conclusion that both retrieval and registration based retrieval, has its unique advantage and carry out the process. So the techniques for images could be selected and preceded based on the above analysis for clinical diagnosis and treatment planning. This advantage is also proved from the Observers' certification of the physicians' and radiologists'.

The proposed experimentation helps in the analysis for selecting the appropriate technique for appropriate images. The overall conclusion is that registration of images does not decrease the retrieval rate at all circumstances. It depends on the appropriate transformation chosen for registration and technique

Figure 6. Overall more relevant retrieved images from medical image registration based retrieval systemusing distance metrics

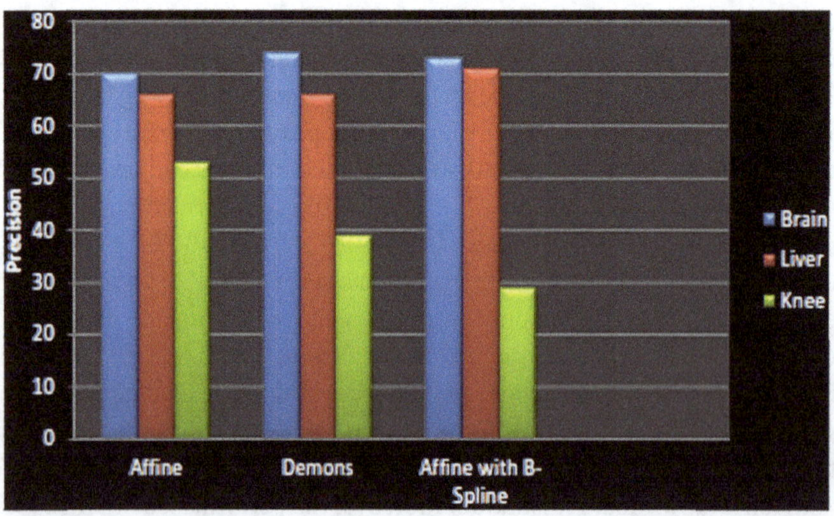

chosen for retrieval. The results for retrieval without registration and registration based on retrieval both have the unique advantage of itself. Though registration based retrieval has an added advantage of both registration and retrieval leading to the double advantage in clinical diagnosis.

The detected affine-invariant regions may still differ in their rotation and illumination, hence it is observed that, BOVW cannot perform better in Affine based image registration based retrieval. Harris affine region points tend to be small and numerous. Small regions are less likely to be occluded but have a smaller chance of overlapping neighboring regions. SURF shows its stability and fast speed in the experiments. SURF creates a "stack for higher levels in the pyramid resulting in images of the same resolution. Their repeatability score increases as the overlap threshold is increased hence perform well with Surf while combined performing with higher accuracy (100/50) for all images and with Demons and Affine with B-Spline

From registration based retrieval, Affine with B-Spline performs well by increasing the retrieval rate and the next better performances are given by Demons and Affine registration. The best of registration based retrieval is given by Demons and Affine with B-Spline registration based retrieval using Bag-of-visual-words (100/50) %. Based on more relevant retrieved images, Brain (100/50) % and Knee (100/50) % observed to have more relevant retrieved image. From the developed system, images can be retrieved automatically based on the objects of anatomical interest and diagnosis can be performed automatically using visual features by incorporating appropriate domain knowledge, visual observance, and reasoning of Observers'. From, overall analysis, it is finally concluded that $\pm$ 5% of $\left(\frac{P}{R}\right)$ variation is found for Bag-of-Visual words than content based retrieval.

FUTURE RESEARCH DIRECTIONS

In existing work present a new way of medical image categorization, registration and retrieval system. The system shows initial capabilities in image categorization for clinical diagnosis. This proposed method is a first step towards similarity based categorization that has a major clinical importance in computer aided diagnostics. The proposed system can be tuned to achieve high accuracy in medical image classification and retrieval.

This work can be further extended to analyze the registration based retrieval for multimodal registration. From the multimodal domain can explore much diagnostic information compared to the existing techniques. The development of open toolboxes is another important factor for successful applications. It is clear that new tools and methods are needed to manage the increasing amount of visual information that is produced in medical institutions.

CONCLUSION

It is now time to create medical applications for clinical decision-making. The results from experimental analysis done under this work have found to coincide with the Observers' results confirming for clinical diagnosis. Practitioners have given their opinion on the usability and the applicability of the technologies.

Since their acceptance is needed to be gained before they can be used in daily practice. Such acceptance with the system, improves the interface quality when good feedback is delivered. This decision support system enhances case based reasoning.

From the extreme conclusion of the retrieval result, can identify the suitable technique which particularly suits for each image. The retrieved patient images with files reveal the patient history. This provides the effective way for clinical diagnosis and treatment planning. From the condensed analysis it is observed that Affine with B-Spline registration when combined with Bag-of-Visual-Words found to be performing best in registration based retrieval.

REFERENCES

Agarwal, A., & Triggs, B. (2006). *Hyperfeatures - Multilevel local coding for visual recognition*. Paper presented at the Conference on Computer Vision. doi:10.1007/11744023_3

Akgul, C., Rubin, D., Napel, S., Beaulieu, C., Greenspan, H., & Acar, B. (2011). Content-based image retrieval in radiology: Current status and future directions. *Journal of Digital Imaging*, *24*(2), 208–222. doi:10.1007/s10278-010-9290-9 PMID:20376525

Akgül, C. B., Rubin, D. L., Napel, S., Beaulieu, C. F., Greenspan, H., & Acar, B. (2011). Content-based image retrieval in radiology: Current status and future directions. *Journal of Digital Imaging*, *24*(2), 208–222. doi:10.1007/s10278-010-9290-9 PMID:20376525

Antani, S., Xue, Z., Long, L. R., Bennett, D., & Ward, S. Thoma and G.R. (2011): *Is there a need for biomedical CBIR systems in clinical practice: Outcomes from a usability study*. Paper presented at the SPIE. doi:10.1117/12.878268

Antonie Maintz, J. B., & Max Viergerer, A. (1998). A survey of medical image registration. *Medical Image Analysis*, *2*(1), 1–36. doi:10.1016/S1361-8415(01)80026-8 PMID:10638851

Babu, G.R. & Sivakumar. (2013). Automatic 3D Brain Image Registration - Survey. *International Journal of Innovation. Management and Technology*, *4*(5), 502–505.

Bouslimi, R., Messaoudi, A., & Akaichi, J. (2013). Using a bag of words for automatic medical image annotation with a latent semantic. *International Journal of Artificial Intelligence & Applications*, *4*(3), 51–60. doi:10.5121/ijaia.2013.4305

Cai, T. W., Kim, J., & Feng, D. D. (2008). *Content-based medical image retrieval in Biomedical Information Technology*. Burlington: Academic Press.

Caputo, B., Muller, H., Syeda-Mahmood, T., Duncan, J., Wang, F., & Kalpathy-Cramer, J. (Eds.). Medical Content-Based Retrieval for Clinical Decision Support, Vol. 5853 of Lecture Notes in Computer Science. Berlin: Springer. doi:10.1007/978-3-642-11769-5

Caputo, B., Syeda-Mahmood, T., & Wang, F. (2010). *Overview of the first workshop on medical content-based retrieval for clinical decision support*. MICCAI 2009.

Cauvin, J. M. (2003). Computer-assisted diagnosis system in digestive endoscopy. *IEEE Transaction on Information Technology in Biomedicine*, *7*(4), 256-262.

Chen, X., Hu, X., & Shen, X. (2009). *Spatial weighting for bag-or-visual-words and its application in content-based image retrieval.* Paper presented at the Pacific-Asia Conference on Knowledge Discovery and Data Mining. doi:10.1007/978-3-642-01307-2_90

Comaniciu, D., Meer, P., & Foran, D. J. (1999). Image-guided decision support system for pathology. *International Journal of Machine Vision and Applications.*, *11*(4), 213–224. doi:10.1007/s001380050104

Csurka, G., Dance, C., Fan, L., Willamowski, J., & Bray, C. (2004). *Visual categorization with bags of keypoints.* Paper presented at the ECCV'04 workshop on Statistical Learning in ComputerVision.

Depeursinge, A., Vargas, A., Gaillard, F., Platon, A., Geissbuhler, A., Poletti, P.A., et al (2012). Case-based lung image categorization and retrieval for interstitial lung diseases: Clinical workflows. *International Journal of Computer Assisted Radiology Surgery, 7*(1), 97–110.

Derek Hill, L. G., & Philipp Batchelor, G. (2001). Medical image registration. *Physics in Medicine and Biology*, *46*(3), R1–R45. doi:10.1088/0031-9155/46/3/201 PMID:11277237

Detterbeck, F. C., Boffa, D. J., & Tanoue, L. T. (2009). The new lung cancer staging system. *Chest, 136*(1), 260–271. doi:10.1378/chest.08-0978 PMID:19584208

Diagnostics and Interventional Radiology. (n.d.) *Computational Environment for Radiotherapy Research.* Retrieved from http://www.cerr.info

Doi, K. (2007). Computer-aided diagnosis in medical imaging: Historical review, current status and future potential. *Computerized Medical Imaging and Graphics*, *31*(4–5), 198–211. doi:10.1016/j.compmedimag.2007.02.002 PMID:17349778

Edge, S. B., Byrd, D. R., Compton, C. C., Frtiz, A. G., Greene, F. L., & Trotti Eds, A. (2010). *AJCC Cancer Staging Manual and Handbook.* New York: Springer.

Erdt, M., Steger, S., Sakas, G., & Fraunhofer, I. G. D. (2012). Regmentation: A New View Of Segmentation and Registration Germany, Technical University Darmstadt, Darmstadt, Germany. *Journal of Radiation Oncology Informatics, 4*(1), 1-23.

Fitzpatrick, J. M. (2010). The role of registration in accurate surgical guidance. Proceedings of the institution mechanical engineering Part H. *Journal of Engineering in Medicine*, *224*(5), 607–622. doi:10.1243/09544119JEIM589 PMID:20718266

Gao, J., Zhou, M. C., & Zhang, C. (2001). 2D and 3D medical image database design. *Proceedings of the IEEE international conference on systems, man, and cybernetics* (vol. 3, pp. 2011-2015). IEEE.

Gletsos, M. (2003). A computer-aided diagnostic system to characterize CT focal liver lesions: design and optimization of a neural network classifier. *IEEE Transaction on Information Technology on Biomedicine*, *7*(3), 153–162.

Gou, H.U., Douze, M., & Schmid, C. (2010). Improving bag-of-features for large scale image search. *International Journal of Computer Vision, 87*(3), 316–336.

Haux, R. (2006). Health Information systems-Past, present, future. *International Journal of Medical Informatics*, *75*(3–4), 268–281. doi:10.1016/j.ijmedinf.2005.08.002 PMID:16169771

Holt, A., Bichindaritz, I., Schmidt, R., & Perner, P. (2005). Medical applications in case-based reasoning. *The Knowledge Engineering Review*, *20*(03), 289–292. doi:10.1017/S0269888906000622

Huang, H. K. (2004). PACS and Imaging Informatics: Basic Principles and Applications. New York: Wiley. doi:10.1002/0471654787

Kim, S., & Kim, D. (2009). Scene classification using PLSA with visterm spatial location. *Proceedings of the 1st ACM International Workshop on Interactive Multimedia for Consumer Electronics (IMCE '09)*, (pp. 57–66). doi:10.1145/1631040.1631050

Kumar, Cai, & Feng. (2011). Multi modal Content Based Image Retrieval in Multi-modal Healthcare. Current Applications and Future Challenges.

Kwak, D. M. (2003). Content-based ultrasound image retrieval using a coarse to fine approach. *Annals of the New York Academy of Sciences*, 212–224. PMID:12594091

Lazebnik, S., Schmid, C., & Ponce, J. (2006). Beyond bags of features: spatial pyramid matching for recognizing natural scene categories. *Proceedings of the IEEE Computer Society Conference on Computer Vision and Pattern Recognition (CVPR '06)*. doi:10.1109/CVPR.2006.68

Loeckx, D., Slagmolen, P., Maes, F., Vandermeulen, D., & Suetens, P. (2006). *Automated non-rigid intra-patient image registration using B-Splines.* Paper presented at the Information Processing in Medical Imaging.

Long, L. R., Antani, S., Deserno, T. M., & Thoma, G. R. (2009). Content-based image retrieval in medicine: Retrospective assessment, state of the art, and future directions. *International Journal of Healthcare Information Systems and Informatics*, *4*(1), 1–16. doi:10.4018/jhisi.2009010101 PMID:20523757

Lowe, D. (2004). Distinctive image features from scale-invariant keypoints. *International Journal of Scale Invariant Computer Vision*, *60*(2), 91–110.

Lu, Z., & Ip, H. S. S. (2009). Image categorization by learning with context and consistency. *Proceedings of the IEEE Computer Society Conference on Computer Vision and Pattern Recognition (CVPR '09).*

Maintz, J. B. A., & Viergever, M. A. (1998). A survey of medical image registration. *Medical Image Analysis*, *2*(1), 1–36. doi:10.1016/S1361-8415(01)80026-8 PMID:10638851

Marcus, C., Ladam-Marcus, V., Cucu, C., Bouché, O., Lucas, L., & Hoeffel, C. (2009). Imaging techniques to evaluate the response to treatment in oncology: Current standards and perspectives. *Critical Reviews in Oncology/Hematology*, *72*(3), 217–238. doi:10.1016/j.critrevonc.2008.07.012 PMID:18760935

Marszałek, M., & Schmid, C. (2006). Spatial weighting for bag-of- features. *Proceedings of the IEEE Computer Society Conference on Computer Vision and Pattern Recognition (CVPR '06).*

Muller, H., Michoux, N., Bandon, D., & Geissbuhler, A. (2004). A review of content- based image retrieval systems in medical applications - Clinical benefits and future directions. *International Journal of Medical Informatics*, *73*(1), 1–23. doi:10.1016/j.ijmedinf.2003.11.024 PMID:15036075

Muller, H., Zhou, X., Depeursinge, A., Pitkanen, M., Iavindrasana, J., & Geissbuhler, A. (2007). Medical visual information retrieval: State of the art and challenges ahead. *Proceedings of the IEEE International Conference on Multimedia and Expo*. doi:10.1109/ICME.2007.4284742

Nowak, E., Jurie, F., & Triggs, B. (2006). *Sampling strategies for bag-of-features image classification* ECCV'06: 9th European Conference on Computer Vision: workshop on statistical Learning in Computer Vision.

Quddus, A., & Basir, O. (2008). *Wavelet-based medical image registration for retrieval applications*. Paper presented at the International Conference on Biomedical Engineering and Informatics. doi:10.1109/BMEI.2008.257

Rahman, M., Wang, T., & Desai, B., C (2003). Medical image retrieval and registration: towards computer assisted diagnostics approach. *Proceedings of the fourth international workshop on design of reliable communication networks*.

Salton, G., Wong, A., & Yang, C. S. (1975). A Vector Space model for automatic indexing. *Model Communication of ACM., 18*(11), 613–620. doi:10.1145/361219.361220

Sedghi, S., Sanderson, M., & Clough, P. (2012). How do health care professionals select medical images they need? *Aslib Proceedings, 64*(4), 437–456. doi:10.1108/00012531211244815

Shanmugapriya, Poonguzhali, & Umamaheshwari. (2014). An intensity-based medical image registration using genetic algorithm, signal & Image Processing. *Signal & Image Processing: An International Journal, 5*(3), 197–206.

Shekhar & Jawahar. (2012). *Word Image Retrieval using Bag of Visual Words* 10th IAPR Paper presented at the International Workshop on Document Analysis Systems IEEE Computer Society.

Shyu, C. R., Brodley, C. E., Kak, A. C., Kosaka, A., Aisen, A. M., & Broderick, L. S. (1999). ASSERT: A physician-in-the-loop content-based image retrieval system for HRCT image databases. *Computer Vision and Image Understanding, 75*(2), 111–132. doi:10.1006/cviu.1999.0768

Shyu, C. R., Kak, A., Brodley, C., & Broderick, L. S. (1999). Testing for human perceptual categories in a physician-in-the-loop CBIR system for medical imagery. *Proceedings of the IEEE Workshop on Content-based Access of Image and Video Libraries (CBAIVL)*. doi:10.1109/IVL.1999.781132

Sivicand, A., & Zisserman. (2003). *Video Google: A text retrieval approach to object matching in videos*. ICCV'05: 10th IEEE International Conference on Computer Vision.

Toews, M., & Arbel, T. (2007). A statistical parts-based model of anatomical variability. *IEEE Transactions on Medical Imaging, 26*(4), 497–508. doi:10.1109/TMI.2007.892510 PMID:17427737

Van De Sande, K. E. A., Gevers, T., & Snoek, C. G. M. (2011). Empowering visual categorization with the GPU. *IEEE Transactions on Multimedia, 13*(1), 60–70. doi:10.1109/TMM.2010.2091400

Van Den Elsen, Pol, & Viergever. (1993). Medical image matching: a review with classification. *IEEE Engineering in Medicine and Biology, 12*(1), 26-39.

Wang, J. Z. (2000). Pathfinder: Multiresolution region based searching of pathology images using IRM. *Proceedings of the AMIA Symposium, 2000*, 883–887. PMID:11080011

Wang, Y., & Feng, D. (2009). Image Registration for Biomedical Information Integration. In Data Mining and Medical Knowledge Management: Cases and Applications (pp. 122-136). Hershey, PA: IGI Global. doi:10.4018/978-1-60566-218-3.ch006

Wu, L. M., Li, Z., Ma, W.Y., & Yu, N. (2007). Visual language modeling for image classification. *Proceedings of the 9th ACM SIG Multimedia International Workshop on Multimedia Information Retrieval (MIR '07)*. doi:10.1145/1290082.1290101

Yang, J., Jiang, Y. G., Hauptmann, A., & Ngo, C. W. (2007). *Evaluating bag-of-visual-words representations in scene classification*, MIR'07. International workshop on Multimedia Information. doi:10.1145/1290082.1290111

Ying, Q. M. L., Wei, Q., & Ren, X. (2014). A Registration Method for Multimodal Medical Images Using Contours Mutual Information. *International Journal of Advanced Research in Artificial Intelligence*, *3*(4), 2014.

Zaidi, H., Vees, H., & Wissmeyer, M. (2009). Molecular PET/CT imaging- guided radiation therapy treatment planning. *Academic Radiology*, *16*(9), 1108–1133. doi:10.1016/j.acra.2009.02.014 PMID:19427800

ADDITIONAL READING

Swarnambiga Ayyachamy, Vasuki, S Manivannan (2013). Medical image registration based retrieval using distance metrics. International Journal of Imaging Systems and Technology. vol. 23, pp. 360-371. (Impact factor: 0.639)

Swarnambiga Ayyachamy (2014). Affine with B-Spline registration based retrieval using Distance metrics. Applied medical Informatics: 34(2); 41-52. (Journal)

Ayyachamy, S., & Mannivannan, V. (2013). Content Based Medical Image Retrieval for Histopathological, CT and MRI Images. *Applied Medical Informatics*, *33*(3), 33–45.

Diez, Y., Oliver, A., Llado, X., Freixenet, J., Marte, J., Vilanova, J. C., & Marti, R. (2011). Revisiting intensity based image registration applied to mammography. *IEEE Transactions on Information Technology in Biomedicine*, *15*(5), 716–725. doi:10.1109/TITB.2011.2151199 PMID:21550890

Yang Song, Weidong Cai, Yun Zhou, Lingfeng Wen & Feng, DD (2013). Pathology-centric medical image retrieval with hierarchical contextual spatial descriptor'. Proceedings of the IEEE 10th International Symposium on biomedical imaging (ISBI), techniques San Francisco, CA. pp. 198-201.

Young Rui & Thomas Huang, S. (1999). Image retrieval: Current techniques, promising directions and open issues. *Journal of Visual Communication and Image Representation*, *10*, 39–62.

Zhengwei Yang, , & Cohen, F. S.Zhengwei Yang & Fernand Cohen. (1999). Image registration and object recognition using affine invariants and convex hills. *IEEE Transactions on Image Processing*, *8*(7), 934–946. doi:10.1109/83.772236 PMID:18267506

Zhiyong Xie, , & Farin, G. E.Zhiyong Xie & Gerald Farin. (2004). Image registration using hierarchical B-Splines. *IEEE Transactions on Visualization and Computer Graphics*, *10*(1), 85–94. doi:10.1109/TVCG.2004.1260760 PMID:15382700

Zitova, B., & Flusser, J. (2003). Image registration methods: A survey'. *Image and Vision Computing. Elsevier*, *21*(11), 977–1000. doi:10.1016/S0262-8856(03)00137-9

KEY TERMS AND DEFINITIONS

Bag-of-Visual Words: A bag of visual words is a vector of occurrence counts of a vocabulary of local image features.

Clinical Diagnosis: A diagnosis made on the basis of medical signs and patient-reported symptoms, rather than diagnostic tests.

Content-Based Image Retrieval: The term "content" in this context refers to colors, shapes, textures, or any other information that can be derived from the image itself while retrieval.

Database: A collection of information that is organized so that it can easily be accessed, managed, and updated.

Framework: Broad overview of interlinked item which support a particular system to a specific objective.

Image Registration: Registration is the determination of a geometrical transformation that aligns points in one view of an object with corresponding points in another view of that object or another object.

Image Retrieval: A computer system for browsing, searching and retrieving images from a large database of digital images.

Image: Image is a visual representation of something in information technology, idea produced by the imagination. "To copy or imitate".

Performance Evaluation: The systematic evaluation of the performance and its outcomes.

APPENDIX

The certification furnished in Figure 7 is based on Observers' classification as described in the earlier chapters 3 and 4. The Observer states the usefulness of this medical image registration, retrieval and registration based system for effective clinical diagnosis thus confirming the qualitative analysis of this system. The Observer is under the category of orthopedic surgeon and Bone specialists with Twenty seven years of experience.

Figure 7. Observer's certification

Dr. A. CHINNA DURAI, M.S., (Ortho), D.Ortho — Cell : 94433 53822
BONE SPECIALIST

Arunodhaya Hospital
22-A, Gokhale Road, (Near Malligai Sweets),
Chinna Chokkikulam,
Madurai - 625 002.
Ph : 0452 - 2528358

Arunodhaya Hospital
20, Madha Koil Main Road,
K. Pudur,
Madurai - 625 007.
Ph : 0452 - 2563212

OBSERVERS CERTIFICATION

I Dr.A.Chinnadurai Consultant orthopedic surgeon, with 27 years of clinical experience, hereby certify that I personally observed and evaluated medical image registration based retrieval done by Ms.A.Swarnambiga (Ph.D) and found that this particular modality is clinically very useful in the following ways.

1. Quick and easy retrieval of records of the particular patient in the front office.

2. From an query image given by registration based retrieval we can get back all the similar cases so far and able to analyze the various forms of treatment given for such cases.

3. From the collection of the similar cases the various kinds of treatment or variations of treatment given can be analyzed in the case of such similar cases. Likewise we can analyze the prognosis of similar cases for a period of time and able to analyze the results in the retrospective manner also.

4. Finally this system is very useful clinically by serving the expected results within a short spell of time. We can get all the ideas about the similar cases treated so far, thereby we can improvise the treatment in future cases.

I appreciate this work of "Medical image registration based retrieval". I feel it is very useful tool for my practice as well as for all clinicians. I hope it will be appreciated by everybody and every clinical practitioner will make use of this work.

Observer's category: Orthopedic surgeon
Observers Name and Address: Dr. A.Chinnadurai, M.S., (Ortho), D.Ortho, M.Ch(ortho),
Arunodaya Hospital,
22-A, Gokahle road, Chinna Chokkikulam,
Madurai-625002.

Specialization: Bone and Joint specialist and orthopedic surgeon
Years of Experience: 27 years
Observers Approval: A Chinnadurai 14.9.13

DR. A. CHINNADURAI. M.S (Ortho)
ORTHOPAEDIC SURGEON
ARUNODAYA MEDICAL CENTER
22-A. GOKALAE ROAD
CHINNA CHOKKIKULAM. MADURAI

Section 4
Medical Image Retrieval

Chapter 8
Multimodal Indexing and Information Retrieval System Based on Mammographic Image Analysis:
Gabor Model in Digital Learning

Sahbi Sidhom
University of Lorraine, France

Noureddine Bourkache
University of Mouloud Mammeri, Algeria

Mourad Laghrouche
University of Mouloud Mammeri, Algeria

ABSTRACT

In this chapter, we propose a new indexing approach on medical "image scanner" databases combining the analysis process of the texture characteristics with the descriptive information. The proposed model is based on the digital image components using the characteristics vector. This vector represents the morphological processing result on image texture. It is linked to image semantic attributes using the annotations of medical professionals. Our application context is based on "Mammographic Image Analysis" (MIAS) in databases. The first aspect concerning the morphology processing on images called the "numerical signature" vector. In this approach, the texture analysis of the image is based on the Gabor Wavelets (or Filters) Theory. In offline processing for each image in MIAS databases, the Gabor Wavelets determine all numerical signatures: image characteristics as multi-index vectors. In online, the query processing by image in real-time defines the query signature (or image-query vectors) and determines all similarities by multi-index matching with images in databases. The similarities are built between the image-query and images in MIAS databases using the same Gabors' algorithms implementation. In order to evaluate the robustness of our system (based on multi-index, semantic attributes, query and information retrieval by image), we experiment with a controlled database of 320 mammographies. The efficient results show a set of successful criteria in image representations based on the Gabor's Wavelets, semantic attributes and significant ratios in the system recall and precision. The objective is to design an intelligent application to assist medical professionals in the decision-making on tumor dignosis based on mammography scanner.

DOI: 10.4018/978-1-5225-0140-4.ch008

INTRODUCTION

The development of imagery electronic devices in various forms has contributed to the creation of trillions of stored images on the internet and new needs have been expressed for image analysis in medical contexts especially in medicine. Actually, the medical field generates significant billions of images for therapeutic interest. In the medical context, images come mainly from x-rays (or scanner), magnetic resonance image (or MRI), ultrasonic imagery, microscopic nuclear medicine imagery (Singh & Mazumdar, 2010),(Zheng, Kuai, Liu, Teng, & Zhang, 2011). This dynamic in information sources comes from practical variability with extreme difficulty to analyze and to exploit images in quantitative, qualitative and objective ways (Sivakamasundari, Kavitha, Natarajan, & Ramakrishnan, 2014),(Candemir et al., 2014).

In this referring works to medical image, a lot of implemented systems were based on text representation of images (Text-Based Image Retrieval: TBIR). For these kind of systems, the image indexing process is based only on text descriptors (as significant words in text, index terms using specific thesaurus in the domain, keywords in descriptions or annotations, user or expert semantic tags, semantic terms in bibliographic records, etc.). Today, this way of image processing is the case of major search engines in the Web. However, it was proved that these processes in image indexing are not sufficient particularly concerning the indexing of significant images in sensitive areas like medicine, mechanical engineering, biometrics, photo-satellites, etc. other than those found in social networks. Especially since our objective is to design an intelligent application to assist medical professionals in decision-making on tumor dignosis from mammography scanner (Oussalah, 2008),(Sinha, Ahmed, & Greenspan, 2014),(Zhang, Zhang, Yao, Pu, Knudson, Weinstock, & Krol, 2005),(Wang, Wang, Li, Liu, Li, & Zhang, 2007). Therefore, it will be a significant contribution to develop other kinds of systems based on digital components and numerical characteristics of images. Since the 90s, scientific communities started implementations of image indexing systems based on query by contents (Content-Based Image Retrieval System: CBIR system) (Akgül, Rubin, Napel, Beaulieu, Greenspan, & Acar, 2011),(Florea, Rogozan, Bensrhair, Dacher, & Darmoni, 2005),(De Oliveriaa, Machadob, & Chaveza, 2010),(Ramos, Kockelkorn, Ramos, Ramos, Ginneken, Viergever, Campilho, & Grutters, 2015), (Rajalakshmi & Minu, 2014).

Today, we find some kinds of CBIR Systems which make the information retrieval from images over the web possible. As examples, we can list *tineye (*www.tineye.com*), cydral (*www.cydral.fr*), gazopa (*www.gazopa.com*),* etc. These image recognition systems using the web of images make it possible to carry out an information image search by URL or by a direct remote loading of an image query stored in a local machine. Several indexing techniques and information image search approaches were elaborated (Harbaoui, Ghenima, & Sidhom, 2009),(Sidhom & David, 2007). However observations in this type of image representation show limits to remain faithful to the analyzed image (Rangayyan, Mudigonda, & Desautels, 2000),(Tong, Xie, & Weng, 2014),(Marino & Tarchi, 2014). Certainly an image file contains a set of digital components characterized by sets of colors, textures and forms (Ravani, Mirali, & Baniasadi, 2010), instead of text representations. For some of these reasons, the indexing systems and image-query (or query by image) engines have been under the study since the 90s (Ravani, Mirali, & Baniasadi, 2010),(Giro-i-Nieto, Ventura, Jordi Pont-Tuset, & Marques, 2010).

We begin the chapter with a review in scientific literature on content-based image retrieval (CBIR), contrasting their respective technologies and applications, and following with related work to present a set of approaches, as the approach using the text semantic attributes and as the approach using the numerical signature on image processing. Specifically, the theoretical aspects of the Gabor Model approach will be detailed at the presentation of the image indexing process.

Related Works

This overview gives an introduction to content-based / text-based image retrieval (CBIR/ TBIR) system and some aspects of the associated technologies. Nowadays, the information retrieval (IR) domain and specifically using image has been an extremely active research area over the last three decades together with mutation technology around multimedia and Internet. The first research papers on methodology in image databases and processing had appeared in the early 80's (Eakins, Boardman, & Graham, 1998). The scientific community in this field of image processing (Hunter, 2008) had given in details a set of descriptions in image archives, indexing approaches and searching needs, based on text retrieval using annotated images. Others in scientific communities had given an overview in this research topic in 90's as the future of research over the image processing and image retrieval. We had to note that is important to explain all alternatives in image retrieval methods and to discuss the future progress in technics and methodologies improvements. As a definition utility, "image retrieval is the process of browsing, searching and retrieving images from a large database of digital images" (Prasad, Gupta, Toong, & Madnick, 1987). The advanced technology progress in image storage and acquisition had enabled the progress in big-data, cloud computing of image databases. In order to deal with high quality information in image, it will be necessary to develop appropriate CBIR systems to efficiently manage these image datasets in stored collections.

In these recent years with tera-bytes data storing of medical images, the main need expressed is: "How to develop efficient methods of indexing, searching and retrieval in image databases?". In CBIR systems, image processing is used to extract information that represents a set of properties such as color, texture, shape, etc. These properties are the morphologic aspects as low-level attributes in the image. In these systems, it is possible to retrieve similar images according to image-query. By this way, the text-based image retrieval (TBIR) systems can give main advantages to CBIR by completing processing on annotations or descriptive texts as high-level attributes (or semantic patterns) in image. A brief recapitulation for any CBIR system, it involves in four main steps:

Step 1: Feature extraction and indexing of images in the database according to the chosen visual features, which form the perceptual feature space, e.g., color, shape, texture or any combination of the above; This forms the indexing part of the CBIR;

Step 2: Feature extraction of query as image (like in step 1); This forms the query-attributes part of the CBIR;

Step 3: Matching the query-image to the most similar images in the database according to some similarity measure. This forms the search-matching part of the CBIR;

Step 4: End-user and feedback which governs the display of the outcomes, their ranking, the type of the user-interaction with possibility of refining (in step 1 or 2) the search process through some automatic or manual preferences. This forms the relevance feedback (or refining) part of the CBIR.

The CBIR system distinguishes the different regions present in an image based on their similarity in color, texture, shape, etc. (as low-level attributes in patterns) and determines the similarity between two images by reckoning the closeness of these different patterns. Thus, we overcome the difficulties present in TBIR system because in morphology features in image can be automatically extracted by CBIR system and to some extent it index the image with better specifications compared to the text-based approach.

Most of the methods used for image indexing (CBIR) are adopted from text indexing research (TBIR). As definition utility, "text-based image indexing is achieved by assigning (manually or automatically) descriptive metadata in the form of keywords, subject headings or classification codes to each image, and then use these as retrieval key-descriptors" (Datta, Joshi, Li, & Wang, 2008). However the complexity and subjectivity of TBIR have been reported by many researchers.

In order to deal with morphology features (and/or key-descriptors) in CBIR (and/or TBIR) applications, it is necessary to develop appropriate approaches in image clustering that depends on similarities. Image clustering is often developed by computing the similarity measurement. This process is restricted to images in big-databases that belong to the nearest classes as predicted for the query. The logical further in testing, the image retrieval process becomes skewed: categorization in clustering and similarity measurement become the retrieval process.

Finally, the semantic aspects in image are still in rumination. Efforts in defining appropriate vocabulary (patterns, metadata, attributes, descriptors or ontologies) and language to represent the different objects in image are still a challenging task for both information retrieval (applying image processing) and CBIR/TBIR communities. The progress of multimedia semantics from MPEG-7 to Web3.0 and W3C community (description framework in RDF and XML for metadata) will be ongoing image research in many prototypes of CBIR systems in different context applications (medicine, astronomy, remote sensing in geographical information systems, media, social networks, etc.) (Camargo, Caicedo, & Gonzalez, 2013).

Research Work

Our objective in this research work is to represent and combine both approaches, as the informational approach using semantic attributes (or TBIR) and as the numerical approach using the digital vector signature (or CBIR). For testing methodology, we used the "Mammographic Image Analysis" (or MIAS) databases containing 320 mammographies. All mammographic images were diagnosed by medical specialists and all of them are completed by a set of notes (like bibliographic records) describing the pathological case of the disease. In the first step of analysis and development, we carry out, in offline processing, the semantic indexing of all images in MIAS sources based on medical specialist notes. Next, we extend semantic representations by the aspect of numerical characteristics by calculating the Gabor Wavelets of the image: all numerical signatures are determined as image characteristics or multi-index vectors (Clausi & Jernigan, 1999). This last process is based on the extraction of texture parameters in a mammography. In the second step of development, our system computes in online (or real-time processing) three possible types of treatment:

- Search for the semantic content of the image: semantic descriptors in notes;
- Search for the digital content of the image: Gabor Wavelet vectors on image processing;
- Search by combining the two last approaches: Gabor Wavelet vectors and semantic descriptors.

For each case of implementation, specific algorithms have been written to serve the concerned processes with an adapted optimization to the time-machine computation, ensuring appropriate responses to the user interface.

BACKGROUND

The construction details such as the image indexing by the semantic descriptors, the image content indexing (or numerical signature) using the texture parameters and the Gabor Filter analysis, are shown as follows.

Image Indexing by Semantic Descriptors

Like the image representations on the Web, the image indexing process is generally in automatic run applying the “indexing robots” into research engines. The image location is determined by examining the HTML code: in the web page where the image is linked. More specifically, the SRC-tag contains the image URL and the image-file name followed by its format (.jpg, .png, .gif, .bmp, etc.), as: <img src=”*URL*”> and like src=”http://www.mias.com/dbmammo/mammo_0001.gif’. The descriptive text about the concerned image is generally included in the ALT-tag: it is often not annotated but is supposed to provide descriptive information of the image, as: <img alt=”*text*”> and use alt=“*mammography mammo_0001 can find only advanced tumor in (x,y)=122,225 and r=52*”. Several difficulties can be encountered during this process:

- Processing time is considerable and proportional to the number of indexed images;
- Diversity of description levels and image interpretations;
- Fitness problem during indexing process with user aspirations (subjectivity).

However, these difficulties have been examined to be nearly attenuated in our case of study: specific and homogeneous image databases (Akgül, Rubin, Napel, Beaulieu, Greenspan, & Acar, 2011),(Suapang, Puttanakit, & Yimman, 2013),(Costa Oliveira & Raniery Ferreira, 2013), (Ingole & Kulat, 2012). In this case, the indexing methodology is more oriented using the concepts: a set of limited number of key-words suggested by professionals or specialists in medicine. These selected key-words from professional notes in image databases are in the search using with the concepts of the users. The Figure 1 presents the standard architecture of this kind of indexing process. Other linked processes are used for matching in the information search phase to determine similarities between image concepts and user concepts.

Image Content Indexing or Digital Signature

In such systems, images are represented by the characteristic vectors in the space of numeric attributes as low level descriptors. Then the similarity measure between images is defined by a set of distances in the same defined space (Das & Kundu, 2012),(Lu, He, & Li, 2012). As illustration cf. Figure.2, the standard architecture of such approach based on image content (or numerical signature) in indexing and searching (Eschler, O’Leary, Kendall, Ralston, & Pratt, 2015),(Lanata, Valenza, Nardelli, Gentili, & Scilingo, 2015),(Jai-Andaloussi, Lamard, Cazuguel, Tairi, Meknassi, Cochener, & Roux, 2010).

This architecture represents the principal steps of indexing and image search using its own digital components. In our case study, this approach was experimented in the process of image retrieval. The implemented system operates in two principal steps:

Figure 1. Standard image indexing system based on semantic descriptors

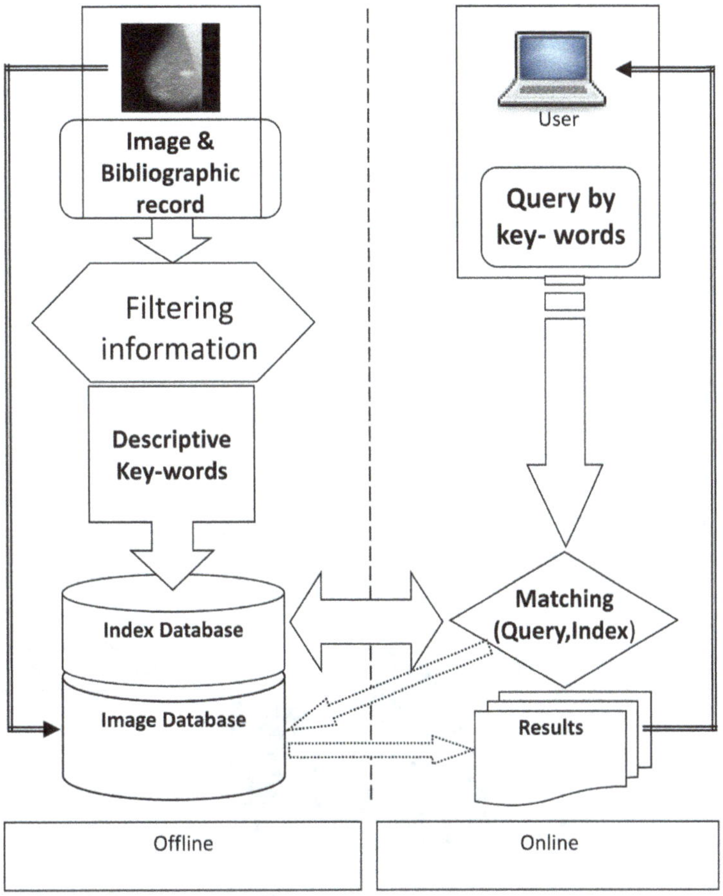

- **Indexing Step:** In offline process, the system extracts image characteristics from image-database using the Gabor Model (or digital vectors). The vector-index of the image is stored in the index-database. The image characteristics using Gabor vector representations can be retrieved efficiently and formally queried using the database management system (DBMS) and the MySQL query language.
- **Image Retrieval Step:** In online process, the system uses a query as image, extracts its numerical signature applying Gabor Model and measures the distance from image-query signature to all the images-signatures in index-database (indexing step).

During experiments, content image retrieval system had many problems. Most of them had a lack in semantic aspects to index the image as well as in image retrieval aspects. Such weakness could be overcome in the hybrid process using semantic descriptors and digital signatures of image. In this hybrid approach, comparative results will be discussed later in this chapter.

Figure 2. Standard image indexing and information retrieval subsystems based on image characteristics (or numerical signature)

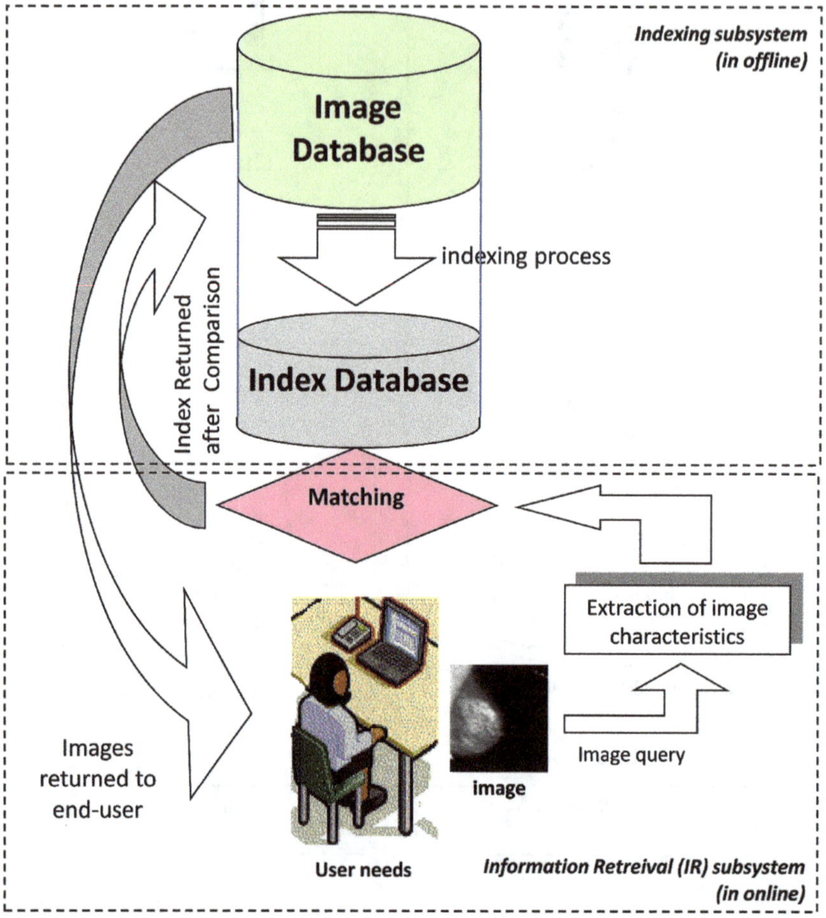

Image Texture Parameters

We noted the effectiveness of the image content using its texture. As a first approach, we had chosen to study this type of parameter to be able to construct the digital component of images (Chen, Lu, & Han, 2000).

In the literature (Rao & Raju, 2010),(Bloch, Gousseau, Maître, Matignon, Schmitt, Sigelle, & Tupin, 2005),(Yuan, Li, & Meng, 2015),(Regniers, Bombrun, Guyon, Samalens, & Germain, 2015) the first definition given in this context is that "a texture is a field of the image which seems a coherent and homogeneous field". In our study, the coherence of required texture is coded in the form of numerical signatures which will make possible to carry out comparisons between a query-image signature and images in databases (Haralick, Shanmugam, & Dinstein, 1973),(Kim & Park, 1999),(Zhuang, Yu, & Haralick, 1984),(Mundy et al., 1992),(Costianes & Plock, 2010),(Choi, Choi, & Park, 2004),(Costianes & Plock, 2010).

Subsequently, the data from the texture will be collected in the form of a vector, called "texture vector" or "digital signature" (He, Zhuo, Zhao, Yin, & Chen, 2015),(Cheng, Han, Guo, Liu, Bu, & Ren, 2015),(Pham, Mercier, & Michel, 2015). This one should be not sensitive to image transformations to leave unchanged texture in particular for translation and rotation of the image. For this important reason, we have chosen in our study the coding by Gabor wavelets in our study.

Gabor Filter Analysis Based on Texture

In theoretical studies, the Gabor wavelet (or filter) proves to be an interesting tool for texture analysis applied to image (Bhatt, Rusiya, & Birchha, 2014),(Mohammed & Squire, 2013) and it is largely adopted in in performance measures (Alzu'bi, Jaber, & Amira, 2014),(Raina, Roshi, Chauhan, & Goudar, 2014). Formally, the texture parameters are given by computing the average and the standard deviation of the gray levels of the image filtered by the Gabor model (Li, Duan, & Zhong, 2015),(Al-Marzouqi & Al Rebig, 2014),(Anju & Chandy, 2014). The various computed values are combined into a single vector called: characteristics vector.

For an image *I(x, y)* having dimensions *MxN*, its conversion into discrete Gabor Wavelet (Agarwal & Maheshwari, 2012),(Chen, Lu, & Han, 2000) is given by the following convolution formula:

$$G_{mn}(x,y) = \sum_{s}\sum_{t} I(x-s, y-t)\psi^{*}_{mn}(s,t) \quad (1)$$

where *s and t* represent the mask of analysis window (using dimensions *3x3, 5x5, 7x7*, etc.); *m and n* parameterize respectively the scales (frequencies) and the orientations with: m=0,1,...E-1; *n =0,1,...O-1*; *E and O* are respectively the total number of scales and orientations; Ψ * is the combined of $\Psi(x,y)$ such as the formula:

$$\psi(x,y) = \frac{1}{2\pi\sigma_x\sigma_y}\exp\left[-\frac{1}{2}\left(\frac{x^2}{\sigma_x^{\ 2}}+\frac{y^2}{\sigma_y^{\ 2}}\right)+j2\pi\cdot f\cdot x\right] \quad (2)$$

$\Psi(x,y)$ function is related to Gabor 2D. It takes the shape of a sinusoid in the complex form with frequency *f*, modulated by *Gaussian 2D*. The standard deviation of the Gaussian envelope according to *x and y* are respectively σ_x *and* σ_y. The 2D Gabor wavelets are obtained starting from the Gabor function (Agarwal & Maheshwari, 2012),(Clausi & Jernigan, 1999),(Bhatt, Rusiya, & Birchha, 2014),(Khan, Deep, Li, Kumar, Shaikh, & Hasan, 2014). The two formulas are written as follow:

$$\psi_{f,\theta}(x,y) = \frac{f}{\sqrt{2\pi}k} e^{-\left(f^2/8k^2\right)\cdot\left(4x'^2+y'^2\right)} \times \left[e^{j\left(xf\cos\theta+yf\sin\theta\right)} - e^{-k^2/2}\right] \quad (3)$$

where:

***θ*:** is wavelet orientation; θ=nπ/*O*.
***f*:** *is* the radial frequency;
***k*:** *constant* (≈π for a band-width of *1.0* octaves and 2.5 for 1.5 octaves);

x' and *y'* are given as follows:

$$x' = a^{-m}(x\cos\theta + y\sin\theta) \tag{4}$$

$$y' = a^{-m}(-x\sin\theta + y\cos\theta) \tag{5}$$

For optimum formulation, Manjunath and Ma (Agarwal & Maheshwari, 2012),(Clausi & Jernigan, 1999) proposed a new representation such as the function (3) becomes:

$$\psi_{mn}(x,y) = a^{-m}\psi(x',y') \tag{6}$$

such as: *a*>1, θ=nπ/*O*, with:

$$a = \left(U_k / U_t\right)^{\frac{1}{E-1}} et\ f_{m,n} = a^m U_t \tag{7}$$

In our implementation as used in the theoretical foundation, we use the following values for the constants: $U_k = 0,4$; $U_t = 0,05$;
Starting from function (1), the following Fourier transform will be:

$$G\left(u,v\right) = e^{\left(-\frac{1}{2}\left[\frac{\left(u-f\right)^2}{\sigma_u^2} + \frac{v^2}{\sigma_v^2}\right]\right)} \tag{8}$$

where:

$$\sigma_u = \frac{1}{2\pi\sigma_x} et\ \sigma_v = \frac{1}{2\pi\sigma_y} \tag{9a}$$

$$\sigma_{x,m,n} = \frac{(a+1)\sqrt{2\ln 2}}{2\pi a^m (a-1)U_l} \tag{9b}$$

$$\sigma_{y,m,n} = \frac{1}{2\pi \tan\left(\frac{\pi}{2N}\right)\sqrt{\frac{U_h^2}{2\ln 2} - \left(\frac{1}{2\pi\sigma_{x,m,n}}\right)^2}} \tag{9c}$$

Gabor Filter Algorithm in Image Processing

After applying the Gabor filter to the image with various orientations and levels of filtering, we get two computed formula of σ_{mn} (average) and μ_{mn} (standard deviation):

$$\mu_{m,n} = \frac{E\left(m,n\right)}{MxN} \tag{10}$$

with

$$E\left(m,n\right) = \sum_x \sum_y \left|G_{m,n}\left(x,y\right)\right| \tag{11}$$

$$\sigma_{m,n} = \frac{\sqrt{\sum_x \sum_y \left(\left|G_{m,n}\left(x,y\right)\right| - \mu_{m,n}\right)^2}}{M \times N} \tag{12}$$

The values of σ_{mn} and μ_{mn} represent the components of the characteristics vector (*V*). Thus, for four orientations and five scales, this vector *V* had the following formula:

$$V = \left(\mu_{0,0}, \sigma_{0,0}, \mu_{0,1}, \sigma_{0,1}, \ldots, \mu_{4,3}, \sigma_{4,3}\right) \tag{13}$$

In this example (13), there are forty elements for calculating the twenty values of average (σ_{mn}) and the twenty values of standard deviation (μ_{mn}).

In image processing using Gabor filtering, the main algorithm is based on the extraction of texture characteristics applying multiple steps, in the following:

- **Energy Computing:** The energy computing in our case study corresponds to the sum of the gray levels of the whole pixels in the image according to a given orientation and a given scale. After applying the Gabor filter to the image with various orientations and scales, the obtained results are all values of "magnitude" in Formula (11) as described previously.
- **Average and Standard Deviation Computing:** Both parameters of the Gabor transform are used to represent the "texture" of areas or the "homogeneous zones" in the image, as follows:
    - The average (μ_{mn}) characterizes the "light intensity" of the image corresponding to the average gray level of the whole pixels of the image, as described in Formula (10);

Figure 3. Flowchart of the main algorithm for image indexing applying the Gabor (filter) model

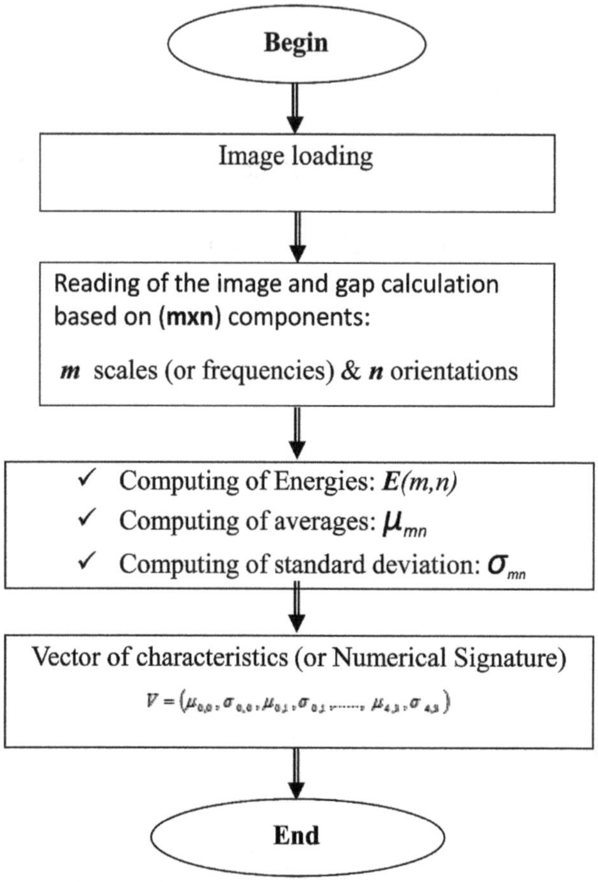

- The standard deviation (σ_{mn}) characterizes the variation of the "average intensity" of the whole pixels. It corresponds to the "*contrast change*s" of the image, as described in Formula (12).

The Figure 3 illustrates the key steps of the indexing algorithm based on Gabor Filter Model to extract the digital/numeric signature of the image.

MAIN FOCUS OF THE CHAPTER

This chapter focuses on constructing an effective system for medical image analysis with the aspects of image modeling, indexing and information retrieval with robust criteria in evaluating results. In this work, we experimented with three aspects of indexing and information retrieval on the medical image databases. We used three approaches to search by

1. Semantic attributes or professional keywords, by
2. Image content or image texture, and by
3. A combination of semantic attributes and textures. This last approach is called "intermodal search".

Figure 4. Annotations in a mammography scanner from MIAS databases

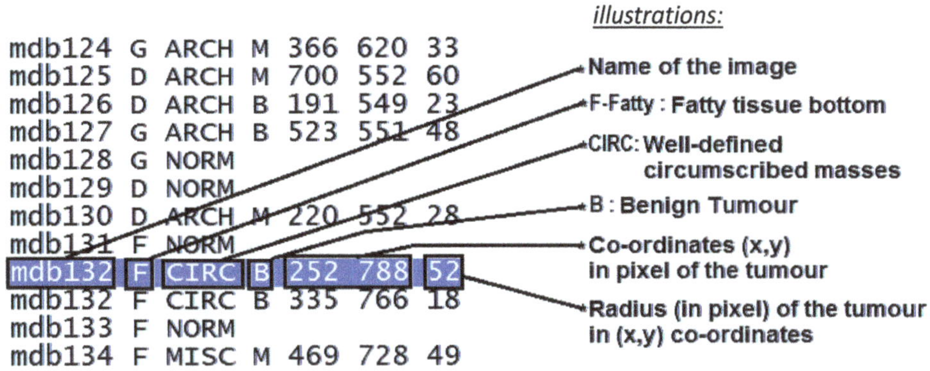

Analysis, Indexing, and Searching by Semantic Attributes

Our application was tested in a learning database on medical mammography images. It concerns the MIAS (Mammagrophic Image Analysis Society [MIAS], 2015),(Sampat, Markey, & Bovik, 2005),(Rangayyan, Ayres, & Desautels, 2007) database containing 320 mammographies with added diagnosis by specialists' radiologists and pathologists. Each MIAS's image is represented by the snapshot/image scanner and the description note of its pathological case. The Figure 4 illustrates an outline example of this description note of a mammography. The significant data represent the description of the semantic attributes and location data of a tumor.

From left to right in Figure 4, we read the name of the mammography image (ex. mdb132), the tissue type bottom (ex. F), the tumor shape (ex. CIRC), the pathology case of tumor (ex. B), the tumor xy-coordinates in pixels (ex. 252:788) and the tumor radius in pixel (ex. 52).

In the first approach on semantic attributes indexing, we are more interested in pathology descriptions and particularly the "tissue type", the "tumor shape", the "pathology case", etc. These three semantics attributes (or AS_i) will be indexed (in offline) by our system into the databases.

In matching (in online), the query is formulated using user keywords or suggestions of our system. Responses are built on the foundations of the formulated query according to the model in Figure 5. This model enables to formulate correctly and precisely the user-query and avoids redundancies in system results.

In logical sequence, the Figure 6 shows the answers to a formulated query using two semantic attributes: in this query, the specification concerns only the "tissue type" (F: fatty) and the "tumor type" (CIRC). While supposing that doctor had noted in a new mammography (during diagnosis) that the "tissue type" is fatty (in major cases) and a well-defined circumscribed masses (less easy to locate with the eye naked). These two reports enable us to carry out a query in the databases by injecting them like attributes. The results of the benign and malignant cases existing in the databases cannot help the doctor to make his decision. We need to extend the attributes with the morphological characterizations of images (Zhuang, Yu, & Haralick, 1984),(Mundy et al., 1992),(Costianes & Plock, 2010),(Choi, Choi, & Park, 2004),(Costianes & Plock, 2010). Thus we observe that the component exploitation on the digital image signature is more than necessary.

Figure 5. Interdependence model applied to semantic attributes: AS_1: "tissue type", AS_2: "tumor shape", AS_3: "pathology case"/ $\bar{A}_i$= neg(A_i), ∧=and

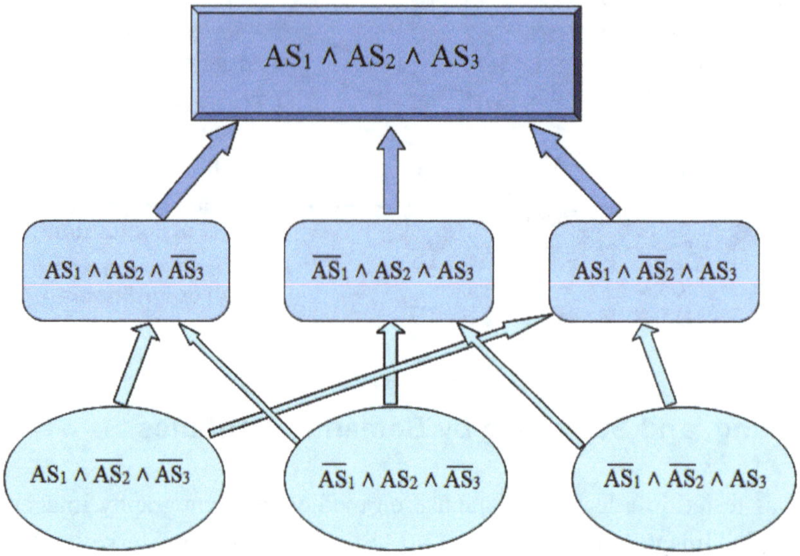

Figure 6. Example of a formulated query using two semantic attributes: "tissue type" (F: fatty) and "tumor type" (CIRC)

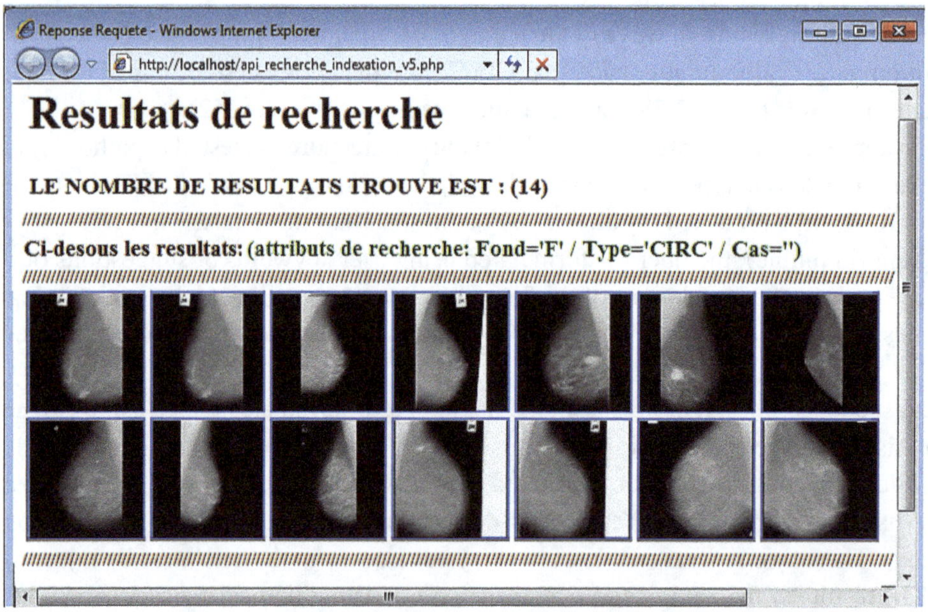

Figure 7. Principal steps of the Information Retreival (IR) process by image content: application of the Gabor Filter model

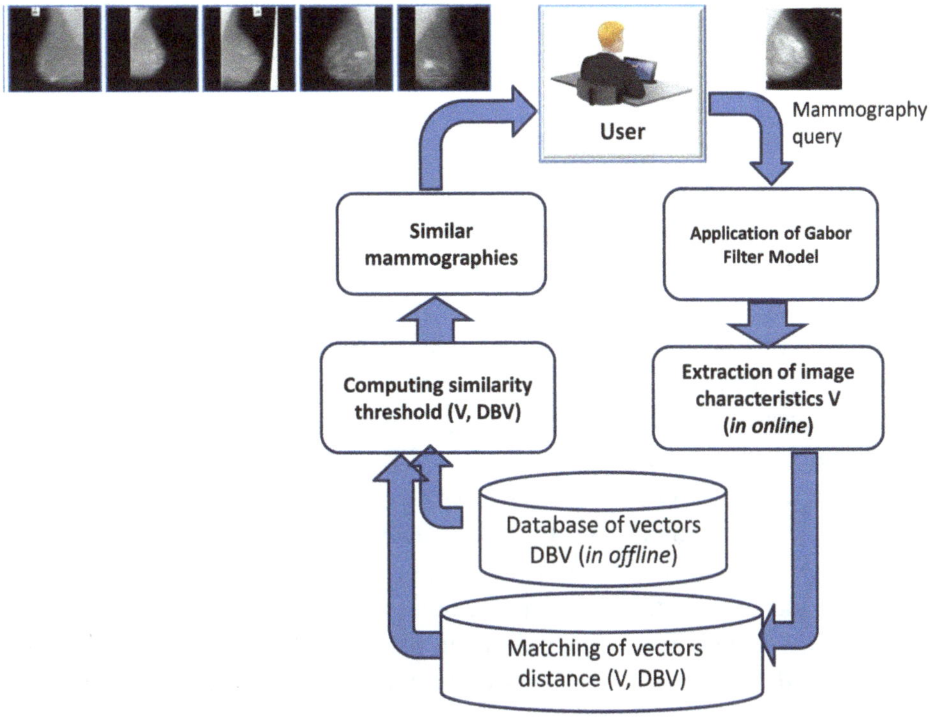

Analysis, Indexing, and Searching by Gabor Signatures

In the system implementation, we carry out the mammography indexing according to the architecture depicted in the Figure 2. The indexing algorithm characterizes each image analysis by a vector with dimensions "scale x orientation" applying the Gabor filter parameters. Its formula (1) is used in the algorithm processing: where "scale" represents the total number of filtering levels, parameterized with "m"; and "orientation" represents the total number of orientations, parameterized by "n". Thus, each vector component represents two values determined by the "average" and the "standard deviation" parameters: for each "scale" and for each "orientation", the system determines the values (μ, δ) of the processed image $I(x, y)$ having dimensions $m \times n$.

Searching Step

The Figure 7 illustrates the various steps of the search process. The extraction of image characteristics is always carried out by the Gabor Filter Model applied to the mammography query.

In system processing to seek (in search process) similar mammographies $T_{i/(i=1..n)}$ compared to a mammography-query Q, the indexing process applying the Gabor Filter Model is required in order to extract the signature vector from the mammography-query. The similarities are computed with the query Q and the targets (mammographies) T using for each vector values the distance $D(Q,T)$ (Agarwal & Maheshwari, 2012),(Kekre & Mishra, 2010), using the formula:

$$D(Q,T) = \sum_{m}\sum_{n} d_{mn}(Q,T) \tag{14}$$

where

$$d_{mn} = \sqrt{\left(\mu_{mn}^{Q} - \mu_{mn}^{t}\right)^{2} + \left(\sigma_{mn}^{Q} - \sigma_{mn}^{T}\right)^{2}} \tag{15}$$

This distance *D(Q,T)* represents the variations of "*average*" and "*standard deviation*" between two signatures corresponding to the image-(Q)uery and the image-(T)arget in MIAS-database.

A suitable weight must be calculated during the computing of this entity *D(Q,T)*. However, we noted both in our experiments as in other studies that the variation in "*average*" is much higher than the variation in "*standard deviation*". The figure.8 shows the results of an example using the query by image content. The mammographic query presents a precise pathology case. In fact, we took in this example the same case as previously (well-defined circumscribed masses: CIRC) in order to better evaluate the two results.

The first mammographies given by our system interface are shown in descending order (from left to right) corresponding to the high level in similarity values. These mammographies in output are very close to the mammography-query, as from the aspect of textures as from the aspect of semantic attributes. However, it should be noted that the mammographies located in the last system responses are less similar in texture and especially it presents a different pathology from the query. In extension of this study, we had completed the aspect of precision by query (ie. image content and/or semantic attributes) in the following paragraph.

Figure 8. Search results by content: mammography-query in the MIAS databases

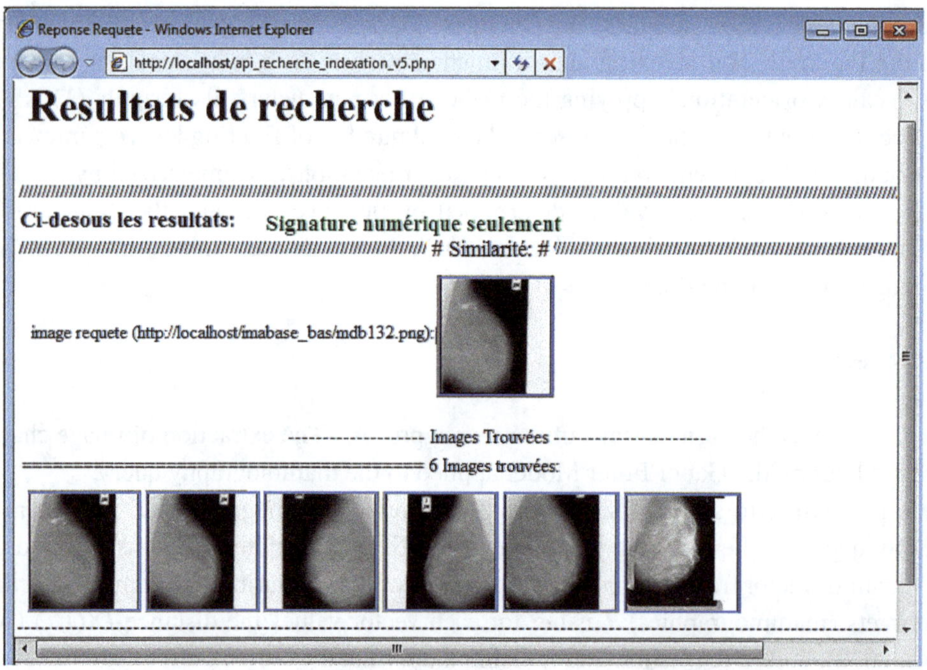

Intermodal Analysis, Indexing, and Searching

The proposed intermodal system combines the two indexing approaches proposed previously. At this level, they are considered as two communicating subsystems in the same environment (Lin, Wu, & Chaovalitwongse, 2015),(Eschler, O'Leary, Kendall, Ralston, & Pratt, 2015),(Thomas & Sael, 2015). In synthesis, our final system, as illustrated in the Figure 9, is a hybrid model that exploits the functionalities of each subsystem (ie. content based image and semantic description) to enhance the hybrid system's responses and limit the impact of weaknesses for each approach.

In addition, we show as illustrated in the Figure 10, the twelve response results combining in the same query a set of semantic attributes (ie. Background = 'F', Type = 'CIRC') and the numeric signature of the image- query (ie. Query = 'mdb005.png').

The intermodal system responses had shown relevant images. In addition, it had shown some non-relevant selected images. In synthesis, we can observe that the hybrid system has been enhanced with the combination of the two approaches. For a better system evaluation (Schreier, Schwarz, Modre-Osprian, Kastner, Scherr, & Fruhwald, 2013),(Maybury, 2011), we will complete the performance study as follows.

Material and Methods for Performance Study

The number of new cases of breast cancer in the world was estimated into 2012 at 1.7 million cases with 0.522 million cases of deaths. Breast cancer is the most frequent cause of death per cancer among women in the world (International Agency for Research on Cancer [IARC], 2015). Thus the critical need

Figure 9. Intermodal system of indexing and search applying content and/or semantic attributes

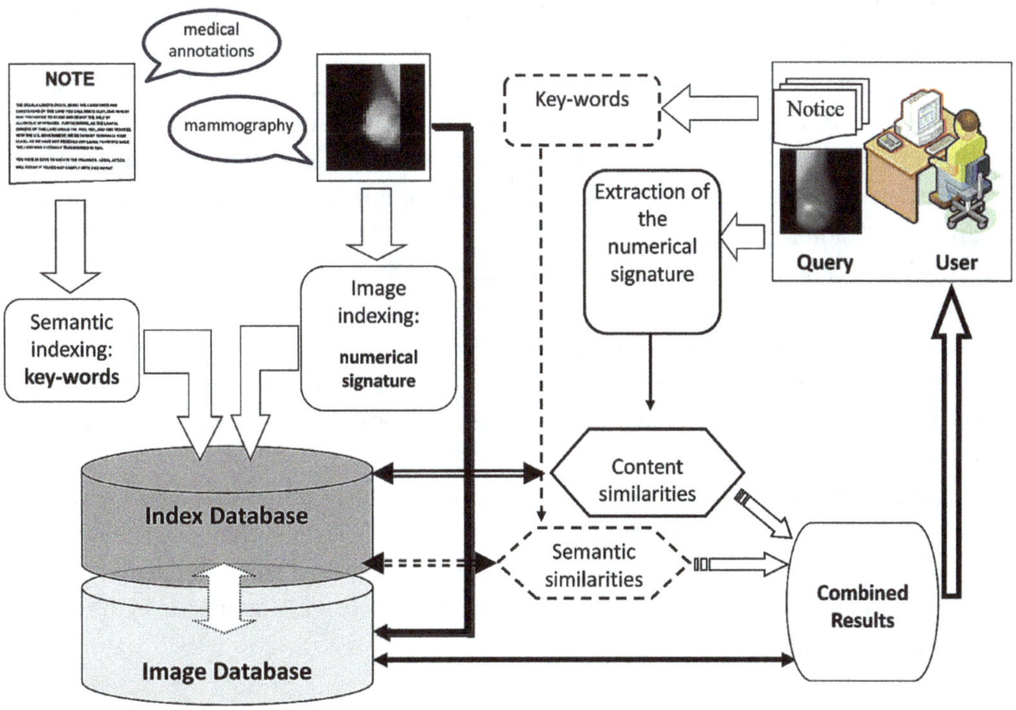

Figure 10. Results of the intermodal system

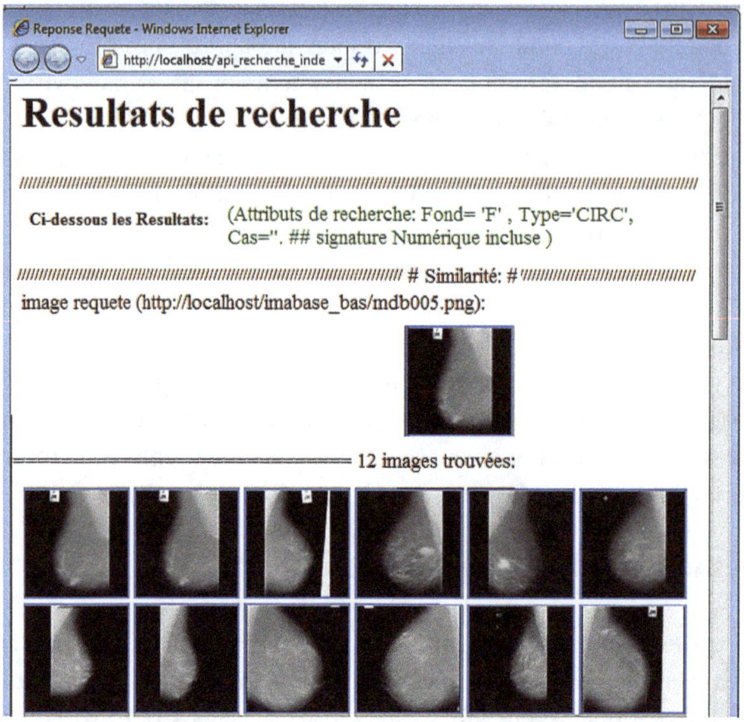

for diagnosis on medical image analysis allowing assistance and decision-making by the professional in medicine. It is found that the learning curve for professional radiologists in Europe and particularly in France reached 13 years of training. That is why a learning tool in this context is with major interest for the tutored training.

Our experiment tests are based on training databases of medical images (from MIAS databases: *Mammographic Image Analysis Society*) containing 320 mammography diagnosed by medical specialists. To evaluate the performance of our system, we are interested in the computing of precision and recall ratios. The relevance in this case study is based on three mammography characteristics: "tissue type", "tumor shape" and "pathology case".

In a practical application when user formulates a query, the system processing according to this formulation is based on: (i) the semantic attributes (from professional descriptions), (ii) the digital signature (from Gabor Filter Model), (iii) or the both approaches (Conti, Ucelli, & De Amicis, 2005),(Sebestyenova & Kurdel, 2014). The system relevance is based primarily on the "pathology case". Considering that our system is dedicated to diagnosis assistance and to decision-making when the breast cancer diagnosis is confirmed.

The performance in information retrieval (IR) is simultaneously proportional to the response time and the precision of the system. Generally, in the information retrieval system (IRS) based on images, the user is much more interested in the relevant output (or similar images to the image-query) than in the time-response system. To evaluate our system effectiveness, we were interested in the computing of two standard ratios: "recall" and "precision".

The precision *(P)* also called 'positive predictive value', is the fraction of retrieved images that are relevant, and formulated like:

$$P = \frac{NIP}{NIT}$$

where

NIP: Is the number of relevant founded images, and
NIT: Is the total number of founded images by the system.

The recall (*R*) also known as 'sensitivity' is the fraction of relevant images that are retrieved, and formulated like:

$$R = \frac{NIP}{NIPDB}$$

where

NIPDB: Is the number of relevant images in the databases.

In practice, in order to assess the system, we use several queries and thus to compute the "average in precision" (PM) corresponding to each level of recall according to the following formula:

$$PM = \overline{P(R)} = \sum_{i=1}^{N_{req}} \frac{P_i(R)}{N_{req}}$$

where

$\overline{P(R)}$**:** Average precision with recall R,
N_{req}**:** Number of queries,
$P_i(R)$**:** Precision of query (i) with recall R.

In statistics, the Table 1 summarizes the average values obtained by the indexing system using the content based approach and the intermodal approach.

However, the relevance in our case study is defined on the three mammography characteristics (ie."tissue type", "tumor shape" and "pathology case"). But, we underlined another characteristic (case: benign/malignant) which is not known by the doctor and it is required. Therefore, in the first system based on semantic descriptors, it will be judicious to specify only the first characteristics in the query.

The curves (1) and (2) of the Figure 11 illustrate the various values of the average precision according to the recalls obtained respectively by the systems (A) and (B).

Table 1. Precisions obtained according to three values of the recall: 0.25, 0.5, and 0.75

Approach	Average Values	
Content based: *System A.*	**Recall (R)**	**Precision (PM)**
	0.25	0.73
	0.50	0.45
	0.75	0.21
Intermodal: *System B.*	**Recall (R)**	**Precision (PM)**
	0.25	0.87
	0.50	0.66
	0.75	0.33

Figure 11. Average of precision according to the recalls in the two systems (A) and (B)

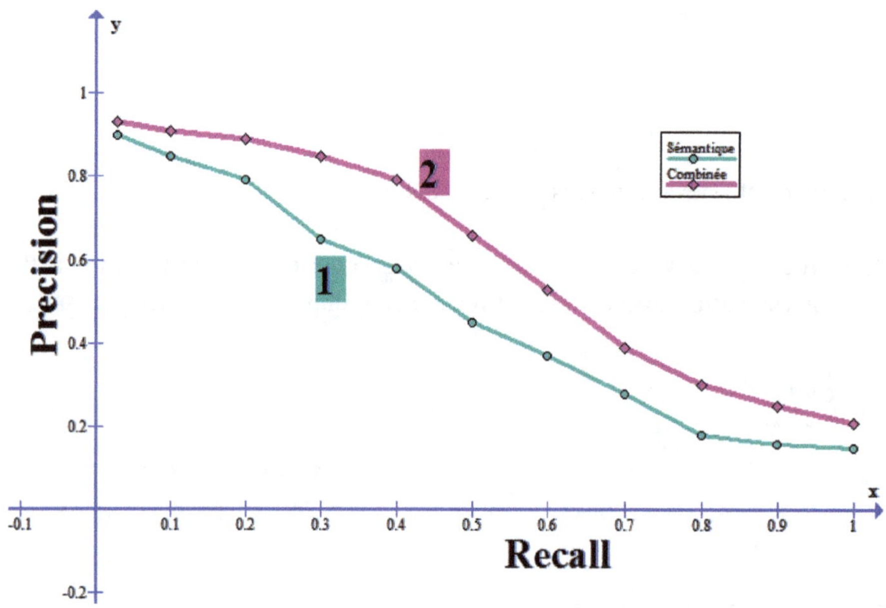

An improvement of the performance is remarkable by using the system (B) (or intermodal approach). However, another statistics report was made: it is acted on the computing time that each query requires, a significant decrease in accuracy for higher rates recall than 0.45.

OPTIMIZATION OF SOLUTIONS AND RECOMMENDATIONS

The Gabor filter application requires processing an image pixel by pixel. As a consequence, the indexing time is directly proportional to the image dimension (image *I(x, y)* having dimensions *MxN pixels*). Thus, it is more suitable to use reduced image or a significant image zone (Nagashree, Aswini, Dyana,

Figure 12. Extraction of the tumoral zone interest in mammography of 128x128 pixels

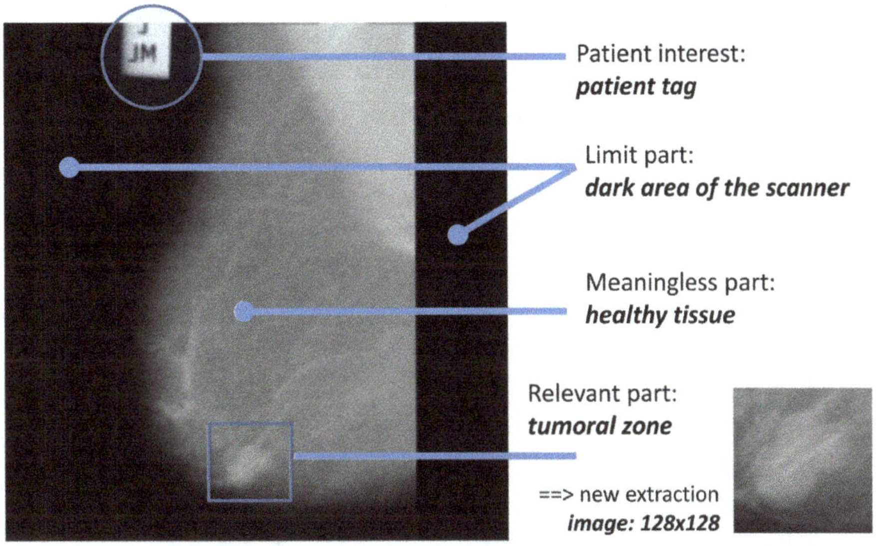

& Srinivas Rao, 2014), (Mitrea, Nedevschi, & Badea, 2014) instead of all the pixels in image. To adapt this "sensible idea" to our case studies, we extracted all the significant zones from the mammography database in MIAS: what was significant in the extraction was the tumoral zone according to the semantic description of the medical professionals. This part is spread out, almost in all the cases of this particular study, over a radius which does not exceed 70 pixels. Then, the mammography images of 128x128 pixels centred with the tumoral zones are localized. The Figure 12 illustrates this procedure processing the pertinent part in image based on tumoral zone located.

In the Figure 12, we can distinguish four different parts (or zones):

1. **The White Zone in the Surrounding Black Content:** It is generally information about the patient;
2. **The Black Zone of the Image:** It is the black bottom of the negative scanner;
3. **The Healthy Tissue:** It concerns all the mammography without the tumor;
4. **The Tumoral Zone:** It concerns the desciption by professional locating the tumor, its pathology, xy-coordination (that gives the projection for the new optimized solution), etc.

The first two zones of the mammography are interesting from the point of view of an informational purpose. The third one is significant but less informative than the zone four (or the tumoral zone). Moreover, this last zone is the most relevant one in the case of breast cancer.

For this specific report, we created a new database containing the reduced images and incorporating only the relevant zone of the mammography: results illustrated in the Figure 13.

Keeping *URLs* of the original mammographies, the system can restore the full image by clicking on the reduced image treated: it is not enough to treat a significant part in the tumoral zone if the professional can locate the tumor in the full mammography to observe similarities.

In this new application method, we brought to the system an average-time gain equal to 69.24% in statistical terms with a significant contribution to recall and precision ratios of the system.

Figure 13. New intermodal system using the tumoral zones in image sources 128x128 pixels

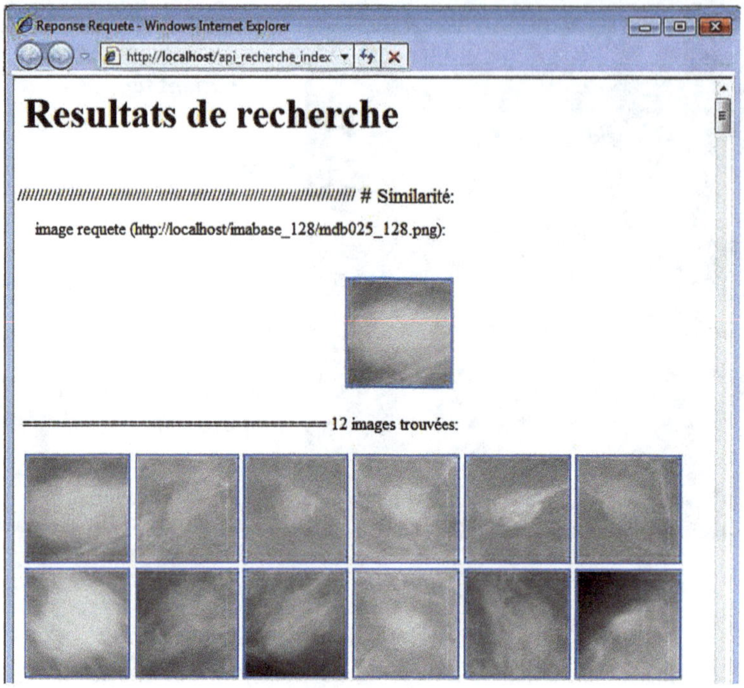

The Figure 14 illustrates the optimized results on reduced tumoral zone in images with high levels in recall and precision of the system compared to its treatments on image sources.

Figure 14. High levels in recall and precision using the tumoral zone in mammographies

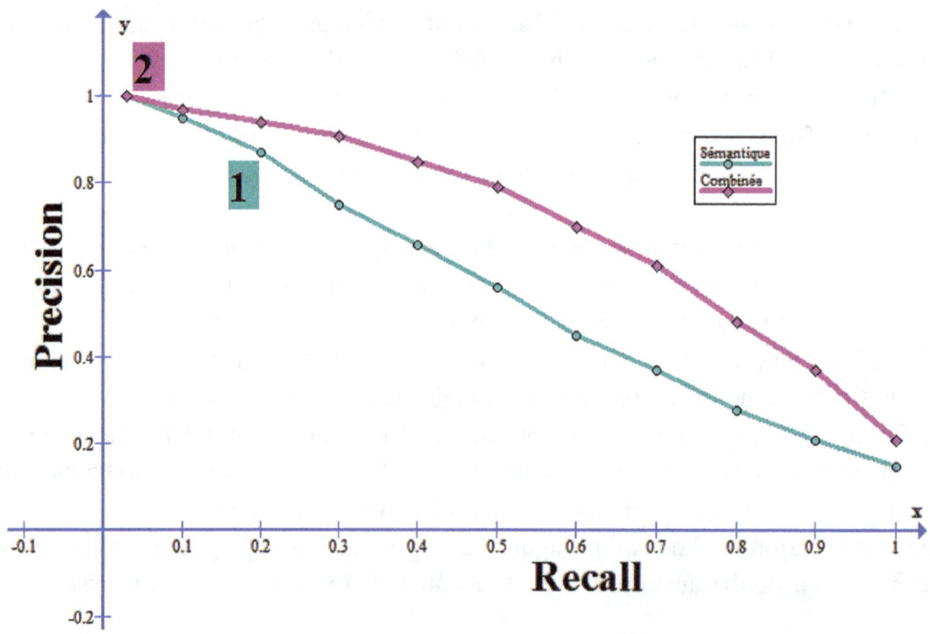

Table 2. Precisions obtained according to three principal values of the recall: 0.25, 0.5, and 0.75

Approach	Numerical Signature	Intermodal	Optimized
Recall	**Precision**	**Precision**	**Precision**
0.25	0.73	0.87	0.92
0.50	0.45	0.66	0.79
0.75	0.21	0.33	0.56

In Table 2, we recapitulate the principal average values of precisions obtained after each set of experimented approaches applying: numerical signature (based on image content), intermodal (semantic attributes and image content) and optimized zone processing (only tumoral zone in the mammography).

The use of the reduced images (or the interest zone in mammography image) enabled us to optimize our system. An average gain in the time equal to *69.24%* was carried out. In addition to the improvement of the precision according to the recall: *79%* for a recall of 0.5.

FUTURE RESEARCH PERSPECTIVES

The application of Gabor Filters requires the time-processing of the image pixel by pixel. As a new result, the indexing time-processing is directly proportional to the image dimensions. The idea in our case study and the experimental contribution is to process the significant zone (or tumoral zone) from the mammography image. Consequently, the image processing is only applied to the selected zone to obtain significant results with high level results in the indexing time-processing and in recall and precision ratios for the system.

CONCLUSION

In this research work we start presenting the tests of two linked subsystems: the indexing by the semantic attributes and the indexing by the digital signature on image. In the first subsystem we tested our application based on mammography images. In digital training, each image was enriched by professional medical notes describing its pathology case. We exploited these professional notes for better semantic indexing. However this approach shows its limits. Thus, we have extended treatments with the level of image content.

The proposed system characterized the image by its numerical signature that represents its morphological aspects (texture, shape and grayscale). An accuracy of 0.45 for a recall of 0.5 was obtained. In order to improve this result we worked out the intermodal system by combining the two subsystems. For a Recall of 0.5 we could have, with this new system, an accuracy of *66%*. This precision is being improved but is not sufficient. More especially as the computing time is considerable and proportional to the dimension of the image. The use of the reduced images or the significant zone of interest from the image source enabled us to optimize our system. An average gain in the time equal to *69.24%* was achieved. In addition to the improvement of the precision according to the recall: *79%* for a recall of 0.5.

Considering that our system can be used in diagnosis assistance and decision-making when the breast cancer diagnosis is confirmed: in the future, professionals in medicine can take advantage of this tool that has not stopped progress in its objectives.

REFERENCES

Agarwal, M., & Maheshwari, R. P. (2012). *Content Based Image Retrieval Based on Log Gabor Wavelet Transform. Advanced Materials Research*. Switzerland: Trans Tech Publications.

Akgül, C. B., Rubin, D. L., Napel, S., Beaulieu, C. F., Greenspan, H., & Acar, B. (2011). Content-Based Image Retrieval in Radiology: Current Status and Future Directions. *Journal of Digital Imaging*, *24*(2), 208–222. doi:10.1007/s10278-010-9290-9 PMID:20376525

Al-Marzouqi, H., & Al Regib, G. (2014). Texture similarity using periodically extended and adaptive curvelets. In *Signal and Information Processing (GlobalSIP), 2014 IEEE Global Conference*. doi:10.1109/GlobalSIP.2014.7032261

Alzu'bi, A., Jaber, T., & Amira, A. (2014). The effectiveness of LSI-based CBIR with image noise using wavelet-based texture. In *Image Processing Theory, Tools and Applications (IPTA), 2014 4th International Conference*. DOI: doi:10.1109/IPTA.2014.7001969

Anju, T. A., & Chandy, D. A. (2014). Brain image retrieval using Local Ternary Co-Occurrence Pattern and CDF 9/7 wavelet. In *Electronics and Communication Systems (ICECS), 2014 International Conference*. DOI: doi:10.1109/ECS.2014.6892540

Bhatt, P., Rusiya, P., & Birchha, V. (2014). WAGBIR: Wavelet and Gabor Based Image Retrieval Technique for the Spatial-Color and Texture Feature Extraction Using BPN in Multimedia Database. In *Computational Intelligence and Communication Networks (CICN), 2014 International Conference*. DOI: doi:10.1109/CICN.2014.71

Bhatt, P., Rusiya, P., & Birchha, V. (2014). WAGBIR: Wavelet and Gabor Based Image Retrieval Technique for the Spatial-Color and Texture Feature Extraction Using BPN in Multimedia Database. In *Computational Intelligence and Communication Networks (CICN), 2014 International Conference*. DOI: doi:10.1109/CICN.2014.71

Bloch, I., Gousseau, Y., Maître, H., Matignon, D., Schmitt, F., Sigelle, M., & Tupin, F. (2005). *Le traitement des images*. Département TSI – Télécom-Paris.

Camargo, J. E., Caicedo, J. C., & Gonzalez, F. A. (2013). A kernel-based framework for image collection exploration. *Journal of Visual Languages and Computing*, *24*(1), 53–57. doi:10.1016/j.jvlc.2012.10.008

Candemir, S., Jaeger, S., Palaniappan, K., Musco, J. P., Singh, R. K. Xue, Z., … McDonald, C.J. (2014). Lung Segmentation in Chest Radiographs Using Anatomical Atlases With Nonrigid Registration. IEEE Transactions on Medical Imaging, 33(2), 577-590. DOI: doi:10.1109/TMI.2013.2290491

Chen, C.-M., Lu, H. Y. H.-S., & Han, K.-C. (2000). A textuel approch based on gabor fonctions for texture edge detection in ultrasound images. Institute of Biomedical Engineering, National Taiwan University and Institute of Statistics, National Chiao-Tung University.

Cheng, G., Han, J., Guo, L., Liu, Z., Bu, S., & Ren, J. (2015). Effective and Efficient Midlevel Visual Elements-Oriented Land-Use Classification Using VHR Remote Sensing Images. IEEE Transactions on Geoscience and Remote Sensing, 53(8). DOI: doi:10.1109/TGRS.2015.2393857

Choi, C., Choi, Y. K., & Park, C. C. (2004). The color retrieval system with color component analysis. *Imaging Systems and Techniques, 2004. (IST). 2004 IEEE International Workshop*. doi:10.1109/IST.2004.1397277

Clausi, D.A., & Jernigan, M.E. (1999). *Designing Gabor Filters for optimal texture separability*. Department of Systems Design Engineering, University of Waterloo.

Conti, G., Ucelli, G., & De Amicis, R. (2005). Automatic extraction of semantic information for a context sensitive multimodal framework for VR. In *Cyberworlds, 2005. International Conference*. doi:10.1109/CW.2005.25

Costa Oliveira, M., & Raniery Ferreira, J. (2013). A Bag-of-Tasks approach to speed up the lung nodules retrieval in the BigData age. In *e-Health Networkg, Applications & Services (Healthcom), 2013 IEEE 15th International Conference*. DOI: doi:10.1109/HealthCom.2013.6720753

Costianes, P. J., & Plock, J. B. (2010). Gray-level co-occurrence matrices as features in edge enhanced images. In *Applied Imagery Pattern Recognition Workshop (AIPR), 2010 IEEE 39th*. doi:10.1109/AIPR.2010.5759705

Costianes, P. J., & Plock, J. B. (2010). Gray-level co-occurrence matrices as features in edge enhanced images. In *Applied Imagery Pattern Recognition Workshop (AIPR), 2010 IEEE 39th*. doi:10.1109/AIPR.2010.5759705

Das, S., & Kundu, M. K. (2012). *Effective Management of Medical Information Through A Novel Blind Watermarking Technique*. Springer Science & Business Media, LLC.

Datta, R., Joshi, D., Li, J., & Wang, J. Z. (2008). Image Retrieval: Ideas, Influences, and Trends of the New Age. *ACM Computing Surveys*, *40*(2), 1–60. doi:10.1145/1348246.1348248

De Oliveiraa, J., Machadob, A., & Chaveza, G. (2010). MammoSys: A content-based image retrieval system using breast density patterns. *Computer Methods and Programs in Biomedicine*.

Eakins, J. P., Boardman, J. M., & Graham, M. E. (1998). Similarity retrieval of trade mark images. *IEEE Multimedia*, *5*(2), 53-63.

Eschler, J., O'Leary, K., Kendall, L., Ralston, J. D., & Pratt, W. (2015). Systematic Inquiry for Design of Health Care Information Systems: An Example of Elicitation of the Patient Stakeholder Perspective. In *System Sciences (HICSS), 2015 48th Hawaii International Conference*. DOI: doi:10.1109/HICSS.2015.339

Eschler, J., O'Leary, K., Kendall, L., Ralston, J. D., & Pratt, W. (2015). Systematic Inquiry for Design of Health Care Information Systems: An Example of Elicitation of the Patient Stakeholder Perspective. In *System Sciences (HICSS), 2015 48th Hawaii International Conference*. DOI: doi:10.1109/HICSS.2015.339

Florea, F., Rogozan, A., Bensrhair, A., Dacher, J.-N., & Darmoni, S. (2005). *Recherche des images médicales par contenu et type de ressource dans un catalogue de santé en ligne. Laboratoire Perception, Systèmes et Information, CNRS FRE-2645*. France: INSA & Université de Rouen.

Giro-i-Nieto, X., Ventura, C., Jordi Pont-Tuset, C., & Marques, F. (2010). *Content-Based Image Retrieval as a Web Service. Technical University of Catalonia*. UPC.

Haralick, R. M., Shanmugam, K., & Dinstein, I. (1973). Textural features for image classification. *IEEE Transactions on Systems, Man, and Cybernetics*, 3.

Harbaoui, A., Ghenima, M., & Sidhom, S. (2009). Enrichissement des contenus par la réindexation des usagers: un état de l'art sur la problématique. *SIIE'2009 International conference. HAL Id: inria-00426376*. Retrieved from https://hal.inria.fr/inria-00426376

He, C., Zhuo, T., Zhao, S., Yin, S., & Chen, D. (2015). Particle Filter Sample Texton Feature for SAR Image Classification. Geoscience and Remote Sensing Letters, 12(5). DOI: doi:10.1109/LGRS.2014.2386351

Hunter, J. (2008). Tracking the Progress of Multimedia Semantics – from MPEG-7 to Web 3.0. (Keynote Talk). In SAMT 2008 (LNCS), (vol. 5392). Springer-Verlag Berlin Heidelberg.

Ingole, P. V., & Kulat, K. D. (2012). A Chain Code Based Fuzzy Features for Brain MRI Retrieval. In *Emerging Trends in Engineering and Technology (ICETET), 2012 Fifth International Conference*. DOI: doi:10.1109/ICETET.2012.50

International Agency for Research on Cancer (IARC). (2015). *OMS organization: statistics of dec. 2012*. Retrieved from http://www-dep.iarc.fr/

Jai-Andaloussi, S., Lamard, M., Cazuguel, G., Tairi, H., Meknassi, M., Cochener, B., & Roux, C. (2010). Content Based medical Image Retrieval based on BEMD: Optimization of a similarity metric. In *Engineering in Medicine and Biology Society (EMBC), 2010 Annual International Conference of the IEEE*. DOI: doi:10.1109/IEMBS.2010.5626134

Kekre, H. B., & Mishra, D. (2010). CBIR using Upper Six FFT Sectors of Color Images for Feature Vector Generation. *IACSIT International Journal of Engineering and Technology*.

Khan, A., Deep, S., Li, J.-P., Kumar, K., Shaikh, R. A., & Hasan, F. (2014). Vision prehension with CBIR for cloud robo. In *Wavelet Active Media Technology and Information Processing (ICCWAMTIP), 2014 11th International Computer Conference*. doi:10.1109/ICCWAMTIP.2014.7073411

Kim & Park. (1999). Statistical textural features for detection of microcalcifications in digitized mammograms. IEEE Transactions Medical Imaging, 18(3), 231-238. DOI: doi:10.1109/42.764896

Lanata, A., Valenza, G., Nardelli, M., Gentili, C., & Scilingo, E. P. (2015). Complexity Index From a Personalized Wearable Monitoring System for Assessing Remission in Mental Health. Biomedical and Health Informatics, 19(1). DOI: . Publication Year: 2015, pp: 132 - 139 doi:10.1109/JBHI.2014.2360711

Li, C., Duan, G., & Zhong, F. (2015). Rotation Invariant Texture Retrieval Considering the Scale Dependence of Gabor Wavelet. IEEE Transactions on Image Processing, (99). DOI: doi:10.1109/TIP.2015.2422575

Lin, Wu, & Chaovalitwongse. (2015). Integrating Human Behavior Modeling and Data Mining Techniques to Predict Human Errors in Numerical Typing. IEEE Transactions Human-Machine Systems, 45(1). DOI: doi:10.1109/THMS.2014.2357178

Lu, K., He, N., & Li, L. (2012). Nonlocal Means-Based Denoising for Medical Images. Computational and Mathematical Methods in Medicine. doi:10.1155/2012/438617

Mammographic Image Analysis Society (MIAS). (2015). Retrieved from http://skye.icr.ac.uk/miasdb/miasdb.html

Marino, G., & Tarchi, D. (2014). MIMO radar imaging and geometrical target properties: A perspective from a classification point of view. In *EUSAR 2014; 10th European Conference on Synthetic Aperture Radar Proceedings*.

Maybury, M. (2011). Information Graphics in Multimodal Documents. In Multimedia Information Extraction: Advances in Video, Audio, and Imagery Analysis for Search, Data Mining, Surveillance and Authoring. DOI: doi:10.1002/9781118219546.ch15

Mitrea, D., Nedevschi, S., & Badea, R. (2014). The role of the Textural Microstructure Cooccurrence Matrices in the classification of the abdominal tumors, based on ultrasound images. In *Intelligent Computer Communication and Processing (ICCP), 2014 IEEE International Conference*. doi:10.1109/ICCP.2014.6936972

Mohammed, N., & Squire, D. M. (2013). Efficient and accurate independent component filter-based features for texure similarity. In *Image Processing (ICIP), 2013 20th IEEE International Conference*. doi:10.1109/ICIP.2013.6738594

Mundy, J., Binford, T., Boult, T., Hanson, A., Beveridge, R., Haralick, R., . . . Strat, T. (1992). The image understanding environment program. *Computer Vision and Pattern Recognition, 1992. Proceedings CVPR '92., 1992 IEEE Computer Society Conference*. DOI: doi:10.1109/CVPR.1992.223157

Nagashree, R. N., Aswini, N., Dyana, A., & Srinivas Rao, C. H. (2014). Detection and classification of ground penetrating radar image using textrual features. In *Advances in Electronics, Computers and Communications (ICAECC), 2014 International Conference*. doi:10.1109/ICAECC.2014.7002403

Oussalah, M. (2008). Content Based Image Retrieval: Review of State of Art and Future Directions. In Image Processing Theory, Tools and Applications, 2008. IPTA 2008. First Workshops. DOI: doi:10.1109/IPTA.2008.4743799

Pham, M., Mercier, G., & Michel, J. (2015). Pointwise Graph-Based Local Texture Characterization for Very High Resolution Multispectral Image Classification. Selected Topics in Applied Earth Observations and Remote Sensing, (99). DOI: doi:10.1109/JSTARS.2014.2386902

Prasad, B. E., Gupta, A., Toong, H.-M., & Madnick, S. E. (1987). A microcomputer-based image database management system. *IEEE Transactions on Industrial Electronics*, *IE-34*(1), 83–88. doi:10.1109/TIE.1987.350929

Raina, N., Roshi, N., Chauhan, R., & Goudar, R. H. (2014). A fused features approach on Content-Based Image Retrieval based on Fuzzy rule-set. In *Advances in Computing, Communications and Informatics (ICACCI), 2014 International Conference*. doi:10.1109/ICACCI.2014.6968407

Rajalakshmi, T., & Minu, R. I. (2014). Improving relevance feedback for content based medical image retrieval. In *Information Communication and Embedded Systems (ICICES), 2014 International Conference Proceedings*. DOI: doi:10.1109/ICICES.2014.7033863

Ramos, J., Kockelkorn, T., Ramos, I., Ramos, R., Ginneken, B., Viergever, M., … Grutters, J. (2015). Content Based Image Retrieval by Metric Learning from Radiology Reports: Application to Interstitial Lung Diseases. *IEEE Journal of Biomedical and Health Informatics*, (99). DOI: .10.1109/JBHI.2014.2375491

Rangayyan, R. M., Ayres, F. J., & Desautels, J. E. L. (2007). A Review of Computer-Aided Diagnosis of Breast Cancer: Toward the Detection of Subtle Signs. *Journal of the Franklin Institute*, *344*(3-4), 312–348. doi:10.1016/j.jfranklin.2006.09.003

Rangayyan, R. M., Mudigonda, N. R., & Desautels, J. E. L. (2000). Boundary modelling and shape analysis methods for classification of mammographic masses. Revue: Medical and Biological Engineering and Computing, Collection: Engineering, 38(5), 487-496.

Rao, P. S., & Raju, G. S. (2010). An approach for CBIR system through multilayer neural network. International Journal of Engineering Science and Technology, 2(4), 559-563.

Ravani, R., Mirali, M. R., & Baniasadi, M. (2010). *Parallel CBIR System Based on Color Coherence Vector*. In *17th International Conference on Systems, Signals and Image Processing*.

Regniers, O., Bombrun, L., Guyon, D., Samalens, J.-C., & Germain, C. (2015). Wavelet-Based Texture Features for the Classification of Age Classes in a Maritime Pine Forest. Geoscience and Remote Sensing Letters, 12(3). DOI: doi:10.1109/LGRS.2014.2353656

Sampat, M. P., Markey, M. K., & Bovik, A. C. (2005). Computer-Aided Detection and Diagnosis in Mammography. In *Handbook of Image and Video Processing*. Amsterdam: Elsevier Academic Press. doi:10.1016/B978-012119792-6/50130-3

Schreier, G., Schwarz, M., Modre-Osprian, R., Kastner, P., Scherr, D., & Fruhwald, F. (2013). Design and evaluation of a multimodal mHealth based medication management system for patient self administration. In *Engineering in Medicine and Biology Society (EMBC), 2013 35th Annual International Conference of the IEEE*. doi:10.1109/EMBC.2013.6611236

Sebestyenova, J., & Kurdel, P. (2014). Multimodal aspects of communication and data storage and managing systems. In *Intelligent Engineering Systems (INES), 2014 18th International Conference*. doi:10.1109/INES.2014.6909370

Sidhom, S., & David, A. (2007). Automatic indexing of multimedia documents as a starting point to annotation process. *ISKO: 9th International Conference*. Vienna, Austria: Ergon Verlag.

Singh, B. K., & Mazumdar, B. (2010). Content Retrieval From X-RAY Images Using Color & Texture Features. Department of Biomedical Engg. National Institute of Technology, Raipur (C.G).

Sinha, D., Ahmed, M. T., & Greenspan, M. (2014). Image Retrieval Using Landmark Indexing for Indoor Navigation. *Computer and Robot Vision (CRV), 2014 Canadian Conference*. doi:10.1109/CRV.2014.17

Sivakamasundari, J., Kavitha, G., Natarajan, V., & Ramakrishnan, S. (2014). Proposal of a Content Based retinal Image Retrieval system using Kirsch template based edge detection. In *Informatics, Electronics & Vision (ICIEV), 2014 International Conference*. DOI: doi:10.1109/ICIEV.2014.6850744

Suapang, P., Puttanakit, V., & Yimman, S. (2013). Mammography Archiving and Web Viewer. In *SICE Annual Conference (SICE), 2013 Proceedings*.

Thomas, J., & Sael, L. (2015). Overview of integrative analysis methods for heterogeneous data. In *Big Data and Smart Computing (BigComp), 2015 International Conference*. doi:10.1109/35021BIGCOMP.2015.7072811

Tong, X., Xie, H., & Weng, Q. (2014). Urban Land Cover Classification With Airborne Hyperspectral Data: What Features to Use? Selected Topics in Applied Earth Observations and Remote Sensing, 7(10). DOI: doi:10.1109/JSTARS.2013.2272212

Wang, D., Wang, Li, Liu, Li, & Zhang. (2007). Mapping Query to Semantic Concepts: Leveraging Semantic Indices for Automatic and Interactive Video Retrieval. In *Semantic Computing, 2007. ICSC 2007. International Conference*. DOI: doi:10.1109/ICSC.2007.105

Yuan, Y., Li, B., & Meng, M. Q.-H. (2015). Improved Bag of Feature for Automatic Polyp Detection in Wireless Capsule Endoscopy Images. IEEE Transactions Automation Science and Engineering, (99). DOI: doi:10.1109/TASE.2015.2395429

Zhang, Z., Zhang, R., Yao, J., Pu, G., Knudson, P.E., Weinstock, R.S., & Krol, A. (2005). Medical data on demand with WebMIA. Engineering in Medicine and Biology Magazine, 24(3). DOI: doi:10.1109/MEMB.2005.1436469

Zheng, J., Kuai, D., Liu, Z., Teng, Y., & Zhang, T. (2011). *Salient Feature Volume and Its Application in Brain MRI Image Registration. 4th International Conference on Biomedical Engineering and Informatics (BMEI).*

Zhuang, X., Yu, & Haralick. (1984). A new approach to the solution of the maximum entropy image reconstruction problem. In *Acoustics, Speech, and Signal Processing, IEEE International Conference on ICASSP '84*. DOI: doi:10.1109/ICASSP.1984.1172340

Chapter 9
Effect of Slow and Fast Music on the Autonomic Nervous System and Cardiac Health:
A Preliminary Investigation

Suraj Kumar Nayak
National Institute of Technology, Rourkela, India

Rudra Dutt Shukla
National Institute of Technology, Rourkela, India

Ipsita Panda
National Institute of Technology, Rourkela, India

Biswajeet Champaty
National Institute of Technology, Rourkela, India

Goutam Thakur
Manipal Institute of Technology, India

Biswajit Mohapatra
Vesaj Patel Hospital, India

D. N. Tibarewala
Jadavpur University, India

Kunal Pal
National Institute of Technology, Rourkela, India

ABSTRACT

In this study, the effect of slow and fast music on the heart rate variability and conduction pathway of the heart was studied. The results indicated an increase in the parasympathetic dominance as the volunteers were made to listen to music. The magnitude of the parasympathetic activity was higher when the volunteers were made to listen to fast music. This indicates that slow and fast music affected the sympatho-vagal balance in different proportions. The analysis of the ECG signal and wavelet transformed ECG signal suggested an alteration in the conduction pathway of the heart.

DOI: 10.4018/978-1-5225-0140-4.ch009

INTRODUCTION

Music has been reported to alter the physiological and the psychological states of humans (Kemp & Quintana, 2013).This results in the alteration of the cardiovascular activity (Levenson, 2014). The main reason for the alteration in the physiological activity of the heart has been described due to the intervention of the autonomic nervous system. In the last decade, there has been an immense increase in the stress and the anxiety of the persons. This, in turn, has resulted in the increase in the number of the diseases associated with the psychosomatic disorder (Dey, Banerjee, Bhattacharya, & Tibarewala, 2015). To alleviate such conditions, music therapy has been proposed due to its ability to alter the activity of the autonomic nervous system. Even though the music therapy has been found to change the emotional states of the patients, the mechanism of music therapy is still a gray area for the researchers (Z. Yang, Su, Ji, Zhu, & Bai, 2014). Music has been found to evoke a particular type of emotional state.

Many researchers have studied the effect of different types of music on the emotional states of the volunteers. In most of the studies, the response of the volunteers regarding their emotional states was recorded. Unfortunately, no other physiological responses were taken into account. Due to this reason, conflicting results were obtained. In some of the recent literature, it was found that listening to music decreases the sympathetic activity with the corresponding increase in the parasympathetic activity (Lee et al., 2012). The sympathetic and the parasympathetic activities, which form an integrated part of the autonomic nervous system, can be analyzed non-invasively by studying the heart rate variability (HRV) (Thoma et al., 2013). The analysis of the HRV helps in understanding the dynamic interactions among the sympathetic and parasympathetic systems, which constantly changes due to the internal and the external stimuli. Till date, very few reports were found which analyzes the effect of music on the conduction pathway of the heart. It is important to study this parameter because the autonomic nervous system innervates the sino-atrial (SA) node, which is regarded as the pacemaker of the heart. It is quite possible that the physiological changes in the conduction pathway may also alter the cardiac physiology.

In the present study, we have tried to understand the effect of slow and fast music on the activity of the autonomic nervous system and the conduction pathway of the heart. The activity of the autonomic nervous system was analyzed by studying the heart rate variability. The physiological changes in the conduction pathway of the heart were studied by analyzing the ECG signal. The ECG signal was analyzed either as acquired or after processing in the joint time-frequency domain using wavelet decomposition. The features of HRV, ECG signals and wavelet transformed ECG signals were used to predict the important parameters using linear (Analysis of Variance (ANOVA)) or non-linear (Classification and Analysis Regression Tree (CART), Boosted Tree (BT), Random Forest (RF)) classifiers. The important parameters were used as input predictors for the classification using Automated Neural Network (ANN).

BACKGROUND

Music has been instrumental in reducing the anxiety and mental-stress of people since the ancient days (Skånland, 2013). However, understanding the influences of music on the physiological parameters of the human body received a major thrust just more than a century ago (Davis, Gfeller, & Thaut, 2008). Extensive research has been done to analyze the effect of music on human health. A number of studies have suggested that listening to the music not only influences the emotional and mood states of a person but also modulates the physiological parameters like galvanic skin response, pulse rate, blood pressure, functionalities of the immune system and respiration rate to name a few (Altschuler, 2001; Bernardi, Porta, & Sleight, 2006; McCraty, Barrios-Choplin, Atkinson, & Tomasino, 1998; Siedliecki & Good, 2006). As an outcome, music therapy has received considerable attention of the healthcare professionals in recent years. It has been found that musical interventions are beneficial in reducing pain, anxiety and stress of patients in healthcare settings, even though the exact governing mechanism is still not well-known (Ising & Kruppa, 2004).

It has been reported by various researchers that listening to the music alters the functioning of the autonomic nervous system (Ellis & Thayer, 2010). This, in turn, results in the modulation of the cardiac physiology through the activation of either the sympathetic or the parasympathetic nervous system (White, 1999; Yamashita, Iwai, Akimoto, Sugawara, & Kono, 2006). The alteration in the autonomic nervous system activity can be understood non-invasively by analyzing the variation in the duration of the electrocardiogram (ECG) signal during consecutive heart-beats. The measurement of this variation is termed as heart rate variability (HRV) (Bilchick & Berger, 2006). The analysis of HRV can be done using various linear and non-linear methods to divulge valuable information regarding the autonomic nervous system activity and the cardiac health (Cardiology, 1996; Carvalho et al., 2011; Voss, Kurths, Kleiner, Witt, & Wessel, 1995). Latha *et al.* (2014) reported that classical music has beneficial effect on heart rate variability and also reduces the stress level of a person due to the parasympathetic dominance (Latha, Srikanth, Sairaman, & NR, 2014). However, different types of music have been found to influence the physiological parameters of the human body in different ways (Labbé, Schmidt, Babin, & Pharr, 2007). A number of studies have revealed that listening to a fast and dynamic piece of music has an excitative effect. On the other hand, listening to a slow and melodious music induces a sedative effect (Iwanaga & Tsukamoto, 1997). Also, an increase in the heart rate has been observed while listening to a fast music, whereas, a reduced heart rate is noted in response to a slow music, even though the change in heart rate may not be statistically significant (Iwanaga & Tsukamoto, 1997).

MAIN FOCUS OF THE CHAPTER

The main focus of this study is to analyze the effect of slow and fast music on the autonomic nervous system activity and the electrophysiology of the heart of healthy individuals. This study was encouraged by the keen interest to understand the physiological alterations prompted by listening to the different types of music (of a specific language to which a person is acquainted with) so that a suitable type of music with better salutary effect can be recommended.

Electrocardiogram (ECG)

The graphical representation of the electrical potential associated with the functioning of the heart is regarded as the Electrocardiogram (abbreviated as ECG or sometimes EKG). It was first detected by Waller in the year 1889 using a capillary electrometer (Zywietz, 2003), which was later modified in 1903 by Einthoven using a string galvanometer as the recording device. Einthoven introduced some concepts (e.g. labeling of the various ECG waves, electrode placement sites at the arms and legs etc.), which are still used today. The acronym EKG originates from Einthoven's native language (Dutch), where the word cardio is spelt using a *k* (Bronzino, 1999). An ECG waveform can be obtained by taking a differential recording between two points on the body surface using surface electrodes. Each differential recording is called as a lead (Figure 1). The three basic leads, numbered with roman characters I, II and III, are defined as given in Equations 1, 2 and 3.

$$I = V_{LA} - V_{RA} \tag{1}$$

$$II = V_{LL} - V_{RA} \tag{2}$$

$$III = V_{LL} - V_{LA} \tag{3}$$

where V_{LA}= left arm, V_{RA}= right arm and V_{LL}= left leg and $II = I + III$.

For the identification of basic arrhythmias, a single-lead ECG is adequate. Mostly, the lead II is preferred as it provides the largest waves. However, the continuous research carried out during the twentieth century has revealed additional arrangements which results in the generation of the 12-lead ECG (Lewell & Davis, 2011). The cardiologists use a 12-lead ECG for the diagnosis of complex arrhythmias, infarctions and hypertrophy (Fesmire, Percy, Bardoner, Wharton, & Calhoun, 1998).

The normal ECG signal itself consists of various waves, namely the P wave, the QRS complex and the T wave (Hurst, 1998). The P wave corresponds to the depolarization of the atrial muscle cells (Dilaveris & Gialafos, 2001). The contraction of the ventricular muscle cells is represented by the QRS complex (Wellens, Bär, & Lie, 2000). Hence, the P wave and the QRS complex are also known as depolarization waves. Often, the Q portion of the QRS complex is not perceptible and the RS complex represents the contraction of the ventricular muscle cells. The T wave indicates the repolarization of the ventricular muscle cells and is also known as repolarization wave (Opthof et al., 2007).

Figure 1.The standard limb leads I, II, and III

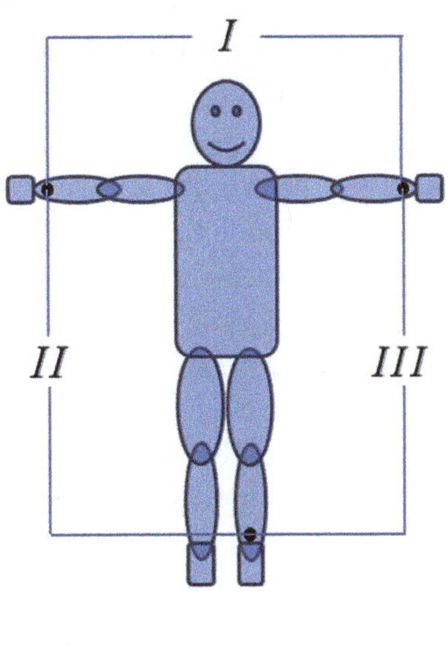

Discrete Wavelet Transform

The discrete wavelet transform (DWT) is a realization of the wavelet transform by a discrete set of the wavelet scales and translations following some defined rules. In other words, it decomposes the signal into mutually orthogonal set of wavelets. DWT presents adequate information both for analysis and synthesis of the original signal with a considerable decrease in the computation time. According to DWT, a discrete signal $f[n]$ can be approximated as given in Equation 4 (Liu, 2010).

$$f[n] = \frac{1}{\sqrt{M}} \sum_{k} W_{\phi}[j_0, k] \phi_{j_0,k}[n] + \frac{1}{\sqrt{M}} \sum_{j=j_0}^{\infty} \sum_{k} W_{\psi}[j, k] \psi_{j,k}[n] \tag{4}$$

where

$f[n], \phi_{j_0,n}[n], \psi_{j,k}[n]$ are discrete functions defined in [0, M-1]

The wavelet coefficients (approximation and detailed coefficients) are given by Equations 5 and 6 respectively.

$$W_{\phi}[j_0, k] = \frac{1}{\sqrt{M}} \sum_{n} f[n] \phi_{j_0,k}[n] \tag{5}$$

$$W_{\psi}[j, k] = \frac{1}{\sqrt{M}} \sum_{n} f[n] \psi_{j,k}[n] \tag{6}$$

Heart Rate Variability (HRV)

Heart rate variability (HRV) can be regarded as a measure of the temporal variation of the consecutive heart beats (Karim, Hasan, & Ali, 2011). It is also defined as the amount of the heart rate variation from the average heart rate (van Ravenswaaij-Arts, Kollee, Hopman, Stoelinga, & van Geijn, 1993). HRV is a useful tool to understand the effect of the parasympathetic and the sympathetic nervous systems (branches of autonomic nervous system) on the activity of the heart. The sympathetic nervous system increases the rate of contraction of the heart through the release of the hormones epinephrine and norepinephrine, which act on the sino-atrial and atrio-ventricular nodes. These hormones take a longer duration to exert their effect and form the low frequency power (LFP) component of the HRV spectrum (between 0.04 Hz and 0.15 Hz) (Karim et al., 2011). On the other hand, the parasympathetic nerves release acetylcholine that acts quickly on the above-mentioned nodes to decrease the rate of contraction of the heart and forms the high frequency power (HFP) component of the HRV spectrum that extends from 0.15 Hz to 4 Hz (Karim et al., 2011). As a consequence, the ratio of LFP to HFP gives a measure of the sympatho-vagal balance.

Many commercial devices are available now-a-days, which facilitate the automated measurement of HRV features. However, the analysis of the significance and meaning of various HRV features are much difficult. As a result, there is a high chance for getting incorrect conclusions. To mitigate the occurrence of such problems and for developing suitable standards, a task force was established jointly by the European Society of Cardiology and the North American Society of Electrophysiology in the year 1996. The main objectives of this establishment were to define the terms associated with HRV, protocol of its measurement and establish relation between physiological and pathophysiological conditions (Cardiology & Cardiology, 1996). According to the recommendations of the task force, both the time domain and the frequency domain measurements of HRV are feasible. The time domain methods are considered as the simplest and can be further classified as either statistical or classical. These methods may involve the determination of the heart rate at any given time interval or the measurement of the variations in time interval between successive QRS complexes. The time duration between successive QRS complexes is termed as NN interval and is useful for obtaining the various statistical and geometrical parameters of HRV. However, the frequency domain methods of HRV analysis utilize the very low frequency components (VLF) (less than 0.04 Hz), low frequency components (LF) (between 0.04 Hz and 0.15 Hz) and high frequency components (HF) (between 0.15 Hz to 4 Hz) of the HRV spectrum, while using short-term ECG signal (Parati, Saul, Di Rienzo, & Mancia, 1995). During the frequency domain analysis of HRV using long-term ECG, use of ultra-low frequency components has also been proposed (Kleiger, Stein, & Bigger, 2005).

HRV has evolved as a popular non-invasive research means for autonomic nervous system and cardiac health. A distressed HRV has been reported to be a predictor of risk after acute myocardial infarction (MI) and as an early indicator of diabetic neuropathy. Diabetic neuropathy (also known as diabetic automatic neuropathy (DAN)) is a complication associated with diabetes mellitus. It causes postural hypotension, persistent tachycardia, gustatory sweating, gastroparesis, bladder atony and nocturnal diarrhea (Cardiology, 1996). Other probable uses of HRV in clinical assessment include estimation of the integrity and physiological status of cardiac autonomic innervations and the susceptibility to different cardiac arrhythmias occurring due to autonomic disparity (Kautzner & John Camm, 1997).

METHODS

Volunteers

Fifteen male volunteers in the age group of 22.2 ± 1.46 years were selected for the study. A conscious effort was made for not including the smokers and athletes into the study. This was done to eliminate any autonomic nervous system interventions due to smoking or regular exercise. Also, ECG signals were recorded at least one week after mid-semester examination and two weeks before the start of the end-semester examination. This was done to avoid any anxiety and/or altered emotional state of the volunteers. The volunteers were informed about the study and the procedure was verbally explained to them in details. If the volunteers agreed to participate in the study, they were asked to fill up an informed consent form. Necessary approval for the acquisition of the ECG signal was obtained from the Institute ethical committee vide office order #NITRKL/IEC/FORM/2/25/4/11/001, dated 13/12/2013.

Acquisition of ECG Signals

The ECG signals were acquired in a laptop using portable ECG machine (EKG sensor, Vernier Software and Technology, USA). The output of the sensor was connected to the data acquisition system (USB-4704, Advantech Co. Ltd, USA). A suitable program was made using LabVIEW-2010 Software (National Instruments, USA). The program was capable of acquiring the ECG signals and save the data in a text file for further analysis. The volunteers were advised to report to the recording station consecutively for three days. On the first day, the ECG signal of the volunteers was recorded without any stimulus. This signal was used as the control. On the second day, the volunteers were made to listen to a slow music for 5 min. The ECG was recorded immediately after the stimulus was stopped. On the third day, the volunteers were made to listen to a fast music for 5 min and subsequently the ECG was recorded.

HRV Analysis

The recorded ECG was loaded in Biomedical Workbench Software (National Instruments, USA). The R-peaks of the ECG signal were extracted using a band-pass filter having lower and higher cutoff frequencies of 10Hz and 25Hz, respectively. The R-R intervals were calculated using the software and the file was saved in the computer. The saved file was used for the calculation of the HRV features. The important features were obtained from linear (ANOVA) and non-linear (CART, BT, RF) statistical methods. The important features, so obtained, were used as the predictors for probable classification using ANN method.

- **Time Domain Analysis:** Five second of ECG signal was extracted from the recorded ECG signals. Statistical features were calculated using a LabVIEW program. Similar to the method used for the classification of the ECG signal using HRV features, the classification of the signals using ANN was carried out.
- **Analysis using Wavelet Transformed ECG Signals:** The five second of ECG signal was decomposed and subsequently reconstituted using discrete wavelet transform (DWT). The reconstituted signal was used for the calculation of the statistical features and subsequent classification using ANN.
- **ANN Classification:** Predictor importance of > 95% was considered for classification using ANN method. MLP and RBF algorithms were used for the classifications. The ANN classification was carried using the trial version of Statistica software (version 12.0).

RESULTS AND DISCUSSIONS

HRV Analysis

Heart Rate Variability (HRV) has been defined as the physiological phenomenon, which is often used as a marker of the Autonomic Nervous System (ANS) activity (Dey, Palit, Bhattacharya, & Tibarewala, 2014). This is because the ANS is responsible for the activity of the SA node (present in the heart). Since SA node is regarded as the pacemaker of the heart and is responsible for the physiological activity of the cardiac muscles, any alteration in the ANS activity results in the change in the heart beat-to-beat variations. The heart beat-to-beat variations may be studied by monitoring the duration of the RR intervals. The ANS can be subdivided into sympathetic and parasympathetic (vagal) systems. The sympathetic system has been reported to increase the heart rate, whereas, the parasympathetic system decreases the heart rate (Mukherjee, Palit, Banerjee, & Bhattacharya, 2015). In our study, we have found that there was a reduction in the mean heart rate of the volunteers when they were subjected to the stimulus (music). The reduction in the heart rate was marginal when slow song stimulus was given. But when the volunteers were stimulated with the fast song, there was a drastic reduction in the heart rate. As discussed above, this indicated that listening to music increases parasympathetic activities. Parasympathetic activity is more pronounced when fast music was used as the stimulus. Similar observations have been reported by M. Iwanaga *et al.* (2013), where the authors have studied the effects of sedative and stimulative music on ANS (Jiang, Zhou, Rickson, & Jiang, 2013). Alike the variation in the heart rate (HR), the RR mean, RR standard deviation (RR-SD) and RMSSD also showed a similar trend.

Apart from the mean heart rate, the RR mean, the RR-SD, the RMSSD and some of the spectral components of HRV have been considered as the markers of ANS. The major components include high frequency HRV spectral components (HF), low frequency HRV spectral components (LF) and LF/HF ratio. HF component has been associated with the vagal activities. The LF/HF ratio provides information about the sympatho-vagal activity. In general, if the LF/HF ratio is greater than 4.8 then the sympathetic activity is considered to be predominant. On the contrary, the vagal activity is found to be dominant if the LF/HF ratio is lower than 1.3. From the results, it was observed that there was an increase in the HF component in the presence of stimulus. The increase was much higher in case of fast music. The LF component was also higher in the volunteers during post-stimulus period. But the increase was marginal as compared to the HF component increase. Hence, it can be predicted that listening to music stimulates mainly the parasympathetic system and has either no or marginal effect on the sympathetic system. In contradiction to the above results, the LF/HF ratio was found to be lower in the post-stimulus period after making the volunteers listening to the slow music, whereas, the ratio was higher in the volunteers who were made to listen to the fast music. Literature suggests that in many cases, the LF/HF ratio fails to predict the sympatho-vagal activity in a proper manner (Billman, 2013).

In total 29 HRV parameters were calculated. To determine the significant parameters, the obtained parameters were subjected to analysis of variance (ANOVA). The differences were considered to be significant if p-value was <0.05. ANOVA is a statistical model that helps analyzing the mean values among the different groups and is used in comparing the data for more than two groups. The ANOVA analysis of the HRV parameters suggested that only NN50 & pNN50 were significantly different. These (NN50 & pNN50) are the time domain parameters of the HRV analysis. The parameter NN50 is defined as the number of the RR interval differences of successive RR intervals, which are greater than 50ms. pNN50 is obtained by dividing NN50 by the total number of RR intervals (Equation 7). Both NN50 & pNN50 are inversely related with the HF (parasympathetic activity). Both the parameters were found to be lower under post-stimulus conditions. The activity was more pronounced when fast music was used as the stimuli. These values also suggested a parasympathetic dominance during post-stimulus measurements. Though Mean HR, LF component, HF component, LF/HF ratio, RR-SD and RMSSD were statistically insignificant, the results indicated the parasympathetic dominance during the post-stimulus period.

$$pNN50 = \frac{NN50}{Total\ number\ of\ RR\ intervals} \tag{7}$$

Decision tree-based analysis was done to determine the important features that might play important role in accurately classifying the different stimulus conditions. The decision trees may be broadly classified either as CART (Classification and Regression Tree), BT (Boosted Tree) or RF (Random Forest) analyses. In statistics, the combined analyses of both classification and regression using decision tree analysis are known as CART analysis. BT analysis is similar to CART analysis but shows better classification efficiency. This is due to the fact that CART analysis uses binary classification trees. The BT analysis uses a combination of binary classification trees. But the residual values from each tree is used for improved classification (Holden, Finch, & Kelley, 2011). RF classifier is also a decision tree based analysis method. It uses more number of decision trees as compared to CART and BT classifiers. Due to this reason, the classification achieved by RF classifier is far superior than the other above mentioned decision tree classifiers (Gokgoz & Subasi, 2015). The classification using CART classifier indicated that NN50 and LF Power (FFT) were the major predictors during the classification. Previously, it has been mentioned that NN50 is a predictor of parasympathetic dominance. LF Power (FFT) was found to be higher under post-stimulus conditions. It has been previously reported that an increase in the LF Power (FFT) is a marker of the parasympathetic dominance. From the boosted tree classification, it was found that RR-SD, LF Power (FFT), VLF Power (AR), HF Power (AR), LF % (AR) and LF n.u. (AR) were the important parameters during classification. The values of these predictors also indicated a parasympathetic dominance. The random forest classifier also showed that NN50 was the important predictor (Table 1). In gist, from the analysis of the HRV parameters, it may be concluded that the parasympathetic activity was increased during the post-stimulus (music) period. An increase in the parasympathetic activity is associated with the reduction in the heart rate and cardiac protection (Olshansky, Sabbah, Hauptman, & Colucci, 2008). To have an understanding whether the important predictors obtained from ANOVA and decision tree classifiers may be used for classifying the control group from the post-stimuli groups, the predictors were used as inputs for ANN classifiers. MLP (multi-layered perceptron) and RBF (radial basis function) algorithms were used. It was found that the RBF algorithms provided better results as compared to the MLP algorithms. This difference can be explained by comparing the inherent architecture of the networks. Firstly, the RBF network uses only one hidden layer and the inputs are weighted only after connecting to the hidden layer, whereas, the MLP algorithm has multiple hidden layers in which one layer is connected to other layers through a linear mathematical function (Nayak et al., 2015). Secondly, the RBF networks operate as local approximation networks as the formation of their outputs depends only on specific hidden units present in certain local receptive fields. On the other hand, MLP networks behave as global networks because their outputs are determined by all the neurons (Xie, Yu, & Wilamowski, 2011). RBF and MLP networks also differ in their classification mechanisms. The RBF networks use hyper-spheres to separate the data space, whereas, the MLP networks generate hyper-planes to achieve the same goal (Wang & Fu, 2006). Additionally, the RBF ANN networks are more resilient to bad training set than the MLP ANN networks due to higher values of d' sensitivity index (difference between the means of the two groups, normalized by the geometric means of their standard deviations) (Finan, Sapeluk, & Damper, 1996). Due to the above mentioned facts, RBF networks have been reported to provide a better efficiency than the MLP networks. A classification efficiency of 97.78% was obtained when HF Power (AR), LF% & LF n.u. were used as input for the classification. The RBF algorithm used 34 hidden nodes for the classification purpose. The details of the algorithm have been tabulated in Table 2 and the confusion matrix has been provided in Table 3. This indicated that though the above-mentioned features are not statistically significant (as per ANOVA), there is a non-linear function that can actually classify the features. It may be concluded from the above that ANN may be used to classify the emotional changes induced by listening to slow and fast music.

Table 1. Important predictors from HRV features

Classifiers	HRV Features	Control Group Mean±SD	Slow Music Mean±SD	Fast Music Mean±SD	p- Value	Predictor Importance
ANOVA	NN50	314.67±32.62	306.87±28.33	281.67±39.21	0.027207	--
	pNN50	80.40±3.69	78.33±4.04	71.40±4.67	0.000001	--
CART	NN50	314.67±32.62	306.87±28.34	281.67±39.21		0.98
	LF Power (FFT)	6086.67±1927.94	6300.00±2753.18	6820.22±3761.49		1.00
BT	RR SD(ms)	234.00±8.39	233.33±11.13	225.33±11.01		0.95
	LF Power (FFT)	6086.67±1927.94	6300.00±2753.18	6820.22±3761.49		0.95
	VLF Power AR	2126.00±901.38	2330.67±1886.37	2084.67±989.99		1.00
	HF Power AR	9846.67±4494.43	10246.67±4701.65	10206.00±6073.99		0.95
	LF % AR	34.67±1740.88	34.20±2200.58	35.60±2641.61		0.96
	LF n.u. AR	27.38±4.90	26.99±4.52	29.30±6.59		0.96
RF	NN50	314.67±32.62	306.87±28.33	281.67±39.21		1.00

Table 2. Parameters of the RBF (2-32-3) network

Networks	Features	Classification Efficiency	Algorithm	Error Function	Hidden Act.	Output Act.
RBF 2-32-3	HF,Power AR, LF%, LF n.u.	97.78	BFGS 35	SOS	Exponential	Exponential

Table 3.Confusion matrix of RBF (2-32-3) network

	Category-FM	Category-SM	Category-WM	Result
Total	15.00	15.00	15.00	45.00
Correct	14.00	15.00	15.00	44.00
Incorrect	1.00	0.00	0.00	1.00
Correct (%)	93.00	100.00	100.00	97.78
Incorrect (%)	6.00	0.00	0.00	2.22

Time Domain Analysis

The statistical parameters (e.g. arithmetic mean (AM), median, mode, kurtosis, skewness, root mean square (RMS), standard deviation, variance and summation) of the extracted 5 sec ECG signal were calculated. Analysis of the data using ANOVA suggested that no features were statistically different. CART analysis indicated that the important features were AM, median, mode, kurtosis and summation. Summation and median were found as the relevant parameters using boosted tree classifier. Random

Table 4. Important predictors from time domain features

Classifiers	Time Domain Features	Control Group Mean±SD	Slow Music Mean±SD	Fast Music Mean±SD	Predictor Importance
CART	AM	-0.0023±0.0053	-0.0016±0.0046	-0.0014±0.0041	1.0000
	kurtosis	16.8191±5.6433	17.0229±4.5284	16.1546±4.1924	0.9759
	Median	-0.0101±0.0077	-0.0119±0.0099	-0.0105±0.0086	0.9772
	Mode	0.0033±0.0135	0.0070±0.0091	0.0053±0.0174	0.9514
	Summation	-11.5877±26.5039	-8.1666±23.3935	-7.3880±20.8084	1.0000
BT	Median	-0.0101±0.0077	-0.0119±0.0099	-0.0105±0.0086	1.0000
RF	Skewness	2.7380±0.9149	2.8358±0.8005	2.6700±0.8098	1.0000

forest classifier suggested skewness as the only important parameter (Table 4). An analysis of the above-mentioned features as predictors for ANN showed that AM, median, mode, kurtosis and summation were able to classify the signals with an efficiency of 86.86%. The details of the algorithm have been tabulated in Table 5 and the confusion matrix has been provided in Table 6. As per the literature, classification efficiency of more than 80% is acceptable (S. Yang & Naiman, 2014).

Figure 2. Wavelet decomposition and reconstruction of ECG signal

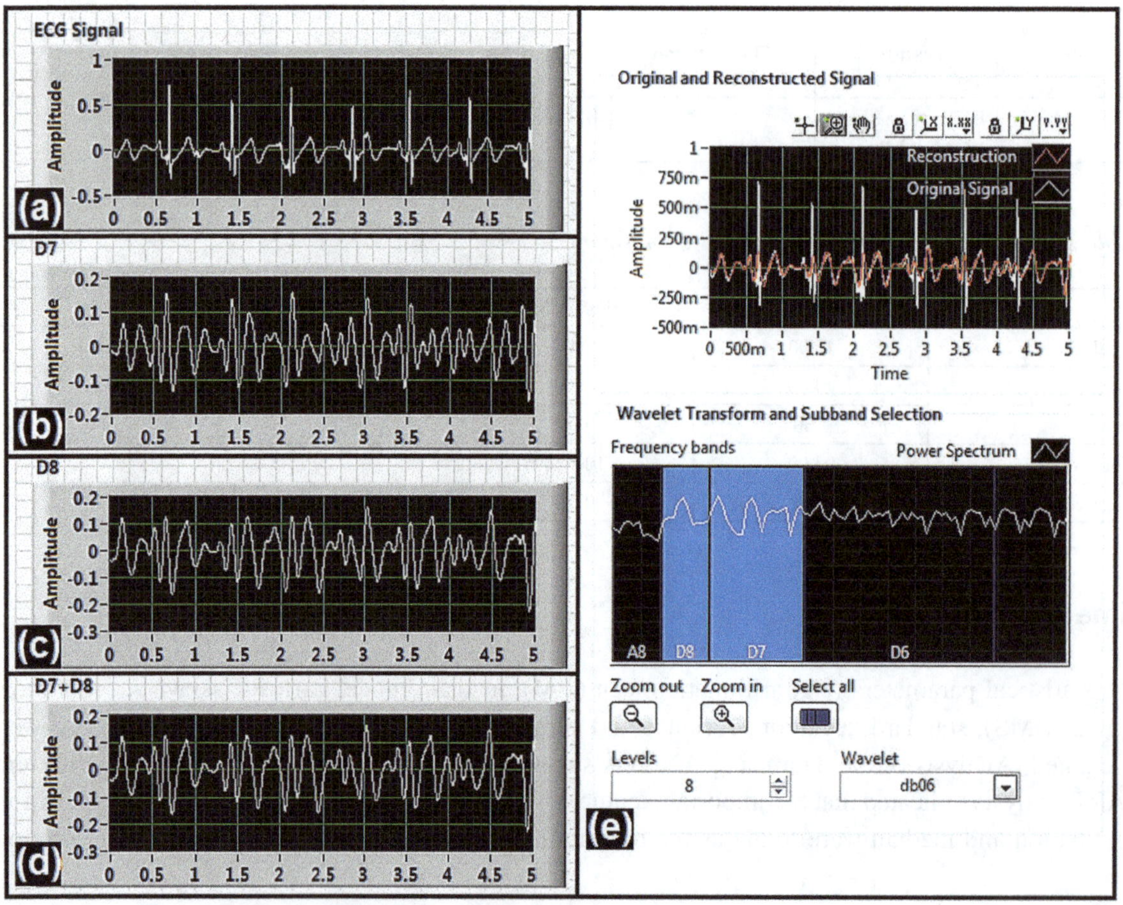

Table 5. Parameters of the RBF (5-32-3) network

Networks	Features	Classification Efficiency	Algorithm	Error Function	Hidden Act.	Output Act.
RBF 5-32-3	AM, Kurtosis, Median, Mode, Summation	86.87	RBFT	Entropy	Gaussian	Softmax

Table 6. Confusion matrix of RBF (5-32-3) network

	Category-FM	Category-SM	Category-WM	Result
Total	15.00	15.00	15.00	45.00
Correct	15.00	12.00	12.00	39.00
Incorrect	0.00	3.00	3.00	6.00
Correct (%)	100.00	80.00	80.00	86.87
Incorrect (%)	0.00	20.00	20.00	13.13

Table 7. Important predictors from time domain wavelet features

Classifiers	Wavelet Features	Control Group Mean±SD	Slow Music Mean±SD	Fast Music Mean±SD	Predictor Importance
CART	Median	-0.0096±0.0060	-0.0106±0.0105	-0.0112±0.0095	1.0000
BT	Median	-0.0097±0.0060	-0.0106±0.0105	-0.0112±0.0095	1.0000
	Mode	0.0027±0.0146	0.0047±0.0118	0.0084±0.0132	0.9646
RF	SD	0.1543±0.0500	0.1543±0.0923	0.1556±0.0609	1.0000

Table 8. Parameters of the RBF (2-18-3) network

Networks	Features	Classification Efficiency	Algorithm	Error Function	Hidden Act.	Output Act
RBF 2-18-3	Median & Mode	80.00	RBFT	CE	Gaussian	Softmax

Analysis using Wavelet Processed ECG Signals

The extracted ECG signal (5 sec) was decomposed using 8 levels of the db06 wavelet. The db06 wavelet was used because it has been reported to have good correlation with the ECG signal (Desai & Sankhe, 2012). The D7 & D8 components were used for the reconstruction of the ECG signal (Figure 2). The statistical parameters of the wavelet transformed ECG signal were determined. In this case also, no significantly different features were obtained from ANOVA. CART classifier indicated that median was the most important predictor. BT classifier showed that Median and Mode were the important predictors, whereas, RF showed that standard deviation (SD) was an important predictor (Table 7). ANN classification using median and mode features suggested that the signals may be classified with an efficiency of 80%. The details of the algorithm have been tabulated in Table 8 and the confusion matrix has been provided

Table 9. Confusion matrix of RBF (2-18-3) network

	Category-FM	Category-SM	Category-WM	Result
Total	15.00	15.00	15.00	45.00
Correct	14.00	12.00	10.00	36.00
Incorrect	1.00	3.00	5.00	9.00
Correct (%)	93.00	80.00	66.00	80.00
Incorrect (%)	6.00	20.00	33.00	20.00

in Table 9. Like the time domain ANN classification, ANN classification using wavelet processed signal also indicated the possibility of existence of a non-linear relationship that may be exploited to identify the emotional state of volunteers.

FUTURE RESEARCH DIRECTIONS

Though the results found in this study are encouraging, future studies can be conducted on a larger group of volunteers for the validation of the results. The exact alteration in the physiological parameters of the conduction pathway of the heart can be studied in-depth in the future course of time. The present study was dedicated to the analysis of the effect of different types of music (slow and fast) on the autonomic nervous system and the physiology of the heart. However, future research can be carried out to investigate the effect of music on other physiological parameters such as galvanic skin response, blood pressure and respiration rate.

CONCLUSION

The use of music in altering the emotional state of patients is being studied by many researchers (Latha, Tamilselvan, Susiganeshkumar, & Sairaman, 2015). Many scientists have reported that listening of music results in the increase in parasympathetic dominance due to the increased vagal activity. In our study, we have tried to determine the alteration in the ANS activity by making the volunteers listen to slow and fast music. A marginal increase in the parasympathetic dominance was observed when the volunteers listened to the slow music. But when the volunteers listened to the fast music, there was a dramatic increase in the parasympathetic activity. The mean heart rate values were found to be statistically insignificant. NN50 & pNN50 were found to be statistically significant. NN50 & pNN50 are associated with the variation in the RR intervals. This means that they might provide information about the conduction pathway of the heart. Hence, it can be assumed that the listening of music not only alters the ANS activity but is also capable of altering the physiology of the conduction pathway of the heart. To confirm this, statistical features of the time domain ECG signals and wavelet transformed ECG signals were calculated and were used for classification using ANN. Using features of both the time domain and the wavelet transformed ECG signals, a classification efficiency of $\geq$ 80% was achieved. This confirmed that listening to music also affects the conduction pathway of the heart.

REFERENCES

Altschuler, I. (2001). A psychiatrist's experience with music as a therapeutic agent. *Nordic Journal of Music Therapy*, *10*(1), 69–76. doi:10.1080/08098130109478019

Bernardi, L., Porta, C., & Sleight, P. (2006). Cardiovascular, cerebrovascular, and respiratory changes induced by different types of music in musicians and non-musicians: The importance of silence. *Heart (British Cardiac Society)*, *92*(4), 445–452. doi:10.1136/hrt.2005.064600 PMID:16199412

Bilchick, K. C., & Berger, R. D. (2006). Heart rate variability. *Journal of Cardiovascular Electrophysiology*, *17*(6), 691–694. doi:10.1111/j.1540-8167.2006.00501.x PMID:16836727

Billman, G. E. (2013). The LF/HF ratio does not accurately measure cardiac sympatho-vagal balance. *Frontiers in Physiology, 4*.

Bronzino, J. D. (1999). *Biomedical engineering handbook* (Vol. 2). CRC Press.

Cardiology, T. F. E. S. (1996). Heart rate variability standards of measurement, physiological interpretation, and clinical use. *European Heart Journal*, *17*(3), 354–381. doi:10.1093/oxfordjournals.eurheartj.a014868 PMID:8737210

Cardiology, T. F. E. S., & Cardiology, T. F. E. S. (1996). the North American Society of Pacing and Electrophysiology. Heart rate variability: Standards of measurement, physiological interpretation and clinical use. *Circulation*, *93*(5), 1043–1065. doi:10.1161/01.CIR.93.5.1043 PMID:8598068

Carvalho, T. D., Pastre, C. M., de Godoy, M. F., Fereira, C., Pitta, F. O., & de Abreu, L. C. (2011). Fractal correlation property of heart rate variability in chronic obstructive pulmonary disease. *International Journal of Chronic Obstructive Pulmonary Disease*, *6*, 23. doi:10.2147/COPD.S15099 PMID:21311690

Davis, W. B., Gfeller, K. E., & Thaut, M. H. (2008). *An introduction to music therapy: Theory and practice*. ERIC.

Desai, K., & Sankhe, M. S. (2012). *A real-time fetal ECG feature extraction using multiscale discrete wavelet transform.* Paper presented at the Biomedical Engineering and Informatics (BMEI), 2012 5th International Conference on. doi:10.1109/BMEI.2012.6512966

Dey, A., Banerjee, A., Bhattacharya, D., & Tibarewala, D. (2015). *Does Music Affect HRV Impulse? A Time Domain Study. In Computational Advancement in Communication Circuits and Systems* (pp. 453–461). Springer.

Dey, A., Palit, S. K., Bhattacharya, D., & Tibarewala, D. (2014). Significance Analysis of Different Time Domain Measures Of HRV to Differentiate Normal and On-Music States. *Significance*, *3*(3).

Dilaveris, P. E., & Gialafos, J. E. (2001). P-wave dispersion: A novel predictor of paroxysmal atrial fibrillation. *Annals of Noninvasive Electrocardiology*, *6*(2), 159–165. doi:10.1111/j.1542-474X.2001.tb00101.x PMID:11333174

Ellis, R. J., & Thayer, J. F. (2010). Music and autonomic nervous system (dys) function. *Music Perception*, *27*(4), 317–326. doi:10.1525/mp.2010.27.4.317 PMID:21197136

Fesmire, F. M., Percy, R. F., Bardoner, J. B., Wharton, D. R., & Calhoun, F. B. (1998). Usefulness of automated serial 12-lead ECG monitoring during the initial emergency department evaluation of patients with chest pain. *Annals of Emergency Medicine*, *31*(1), 3–11. doi:10.1016/S0196-0644(98)70274-4 PMID:9437335

Finan, R., Sapeluk, A., & Damper, R. (1996). *Comparison of multilayer and radial basis function neural networks for text-dependent speaker recognition.* Paper presented at the Neural Networks, 1996, IEEE International Conference on. doi:10.1109/ICNN.1996.549207

Gokgoz, E., & Subasi, A. (2015). Comparison of decision tree algorithms for EMG signal classification using DWT. *Biomedical Signal Processing and Control*, *18*, 138–144. doi:10.1016/j.bspc.2014.12.005

Holden, J. E., Finch, W. H., & Kelley, K. (2011). A comparison of two-group classification methods. *Educational and Psychological Measurement*, *71*(5), 870–901. doi:10.1177/0013164411398357

Hurst, J. W. (1998). Naming of the waves in the ECG, with a brief account of their genesis. *Circulation*, *98*(18), 1937–1942. doi:10.1161/01.CIR.98.18.1937 PMID:9799216

Ising, H., & Kruppa, B. (2004). Health effects caused by noise: Evidence in the literature from the past 25 years. *Noise & Health*, *6*(22), 5. PMID:15070524

Iwanaga, M., & Tsukamoto, M. (1997). Effects of excitative and sedative music on subjective and physiological relaxation. *Perceptual and Motor Skills*, *85*(1), 287–296. doi:10.2466/pms.1997.85.1.287 PMID:9293589

Jiang, J., Zhou, L., Rickson, D., & Jiang, C. (2013). The effects of sedative and stimulative music on stress reduction depend on music preference. *The Arts in Psychotherapy*, *40*(2), 201–205. doi:10.1016/j.aip.2013.02.002

Karim, N., Hasan, J. A., & Ali, S. S. (2011). Heart rate variability–a review. *Journal of Basic and Applied Sciences*, *7*(1), 71–77.

Kautzner, J., & John Camm, A. (1997). Clinical relevance of heart rate variability. *Clinical Cardiology*, *20*(2), 162–168. doi:10.1002/clc.4960200214 PMID:9034646

Kemp, A. H., & Quintana, D. S. (2013). The relationship between mental and physical health: Insights from the study of heart rate variability. *International Journal of Psychophysiology*, *89*(3), 288–296. doi:10.1016/j.ijpsycho.2013.06.018 PMID:23797149

Kleiger, R. E., Stein, P. K., & Bigger, J. T. (2005). Heart rate variability: Measurement and clinical utility. *Annals of Noninvasive Electrocardiology*, *10*(1), 88–101. doi:10.1111/j.1542-474X.2005.10101.x PMID:15649244

Labbé, E., Schmidt, N., Babin, J., & Pharr, M. (2007). Coping with stress: The effectiveness of different types of music. *Applied Psychophysiology and Biofeedback*, *32*(3-4), 163–168. doi:10.1007/s10484-007-9043-9 PMID:17965934

Latha, R., Srikanth, S., & Sairaman, H. (2014). Effect of music on heart rate variability and stress in medical students. *International Journal of Clinical and Experimental Physiology*, *1*(2), 131. doi:10.4103/2348-8093.137409

Latha, R., Tamilselvan, K., Susiganeshkumar, E., & Sairaman, H. (2015). Effect of Classical music on heart rate variability between genders. *International Journal of Biomedical Research*, *6*(3), 192–195. doi:10.7439/ijbr.v6i3.1841

Lee, K.-C., Chao, Y.-H., Yiin, J.-J., Hsieh, H.-Y., Dai, W.-J., & Chao, Y.-F. (2012). Evidence that music listening reduces preoperative patients' anxiety. *Biological Research for Nursing*, *14*(1), 78–84. doi:10.1177/1099800410396704 PMID:21278165

Levenson, R. W. (2014). The autonomic nervous system and emotion. *Emotion Review*, *6*(2), 100–112. doi:10.1177/1754073913512003

Lewell, M., & Davis, M. (2011). *12 Lead ECG*. Academic Press.

Liu, C.-L. (2010). *A tutorial of the wavelet transform*. Taiwan: NTUEE.

McCraty, R., Barrios-Choplin, B., Atkinson, M., & Tomasino, D. (1998). The effects of different types of music on mood, tension, and mental clarity. *Alternative Therapies in Health and Medicine*, *4*(1), 75–85. PMID:9439023

Mukherjee, S., Palit, S. K., Banerjee, S., & Bhattacharya, D. (2015). A Comparative Study on Three Different Types of Music Based on Same Indian Raga and Their Effects on Human Autonomic Nervous Systems *Chaos* [Springer.]. *Complexity and Leadership*, *2013*, 243–254.

Nayak, S. K., Panda, I., Champaty, B., Bagh, N., Pal, K., & Tibarewala, D. (2015). *Automated Neural Network Based Classification of HRV and ECG Signals of Smokers: A Preliminary Study. In Advancements of Medical Electronics* (pp. 271–279). Springer.

Olshansky, B., Sabbah, H. N., Hauptman, P. J., & Colucci, W. S. (2008). Parasympathetic nervous system and heart failure pathophysiology and potential implications for therapy. *Circulation*, *118*(8), 863–871. doi:10.1161/CIRCULATIONAHA.107.760405 PMID:18711023

Opthof, T., Coronel, R., Wilms-Schopman, F. J., Plotnikov, A. N., Shlapakova, I. N., Danilo, P. Jr, & Janse, M. J. et al. (2007). Dispersion of repolarization in canine ventricle and the electrocardiographic T wave: T pe interval does not reflect transmural dispersion. *Heart Rhythm*, *4*(3), 341–348. doi:10.1016/j.hrthm.2006.11.022 PMID:17341400

Parati, G., Saul, J. P., Di Rienzo, M., & Mancia, G. (1995). Spectral analysis of blood pressure and heart rate variability in evaluating cardiovascular regulation a critical appraisal. *Hypertension*, *25*(6), 1276–1286. doi:10.1161/01.HYP.25.6.1276 PMID:7768574

Siedliecki, S. L., & Good, M. (2006). Effect of music on power, pain, depression and disability. *Journal of Advanced Nursing*, *54*(5), 553–562. doi:10.1111/j.1365-2648.2006.03860.x PMID:16722953

Skånland, M. S. (2013). Music, health, and well-being. *International Journal of Qualitative Studies on Health and Well-being*, 8. PMID:23930993

Thoma, M. V., La Marca, R., Brönnimann, R., Finkel, L., Ehlert, U., & Nater, U. M. (2013). The effect of music on the human stress response. *PLoS ONE*, *8*(8), e70156. PMID:23940541 van Ravenswaaij-Arts, C. M., Kollee, L. A., Hopman, J. C., Stoelinga, G. B., & van Geijn, H. P. (1993). Heart rate variability. *Annals of Internal Medicine*, *118*(6), 436–447. doi:10.7326/0003-4819-118-6-199303150-00008 PMID:8439119

Voss, A., Kurths, J., Kleiner, H., Witt, A., & Wessel, N. (1995). Improved analysis of heart rate variability by methods of nonlinear dynamics. *Journal of Electrocardiology*, *28*, 81–88. doi:10.1016/S0022-0736(95)80021-2 PMID:8656135

Wang, L., & Fu, X. (2006). *Data mining with computational intelligence*. Springer Science & Business Media.

Wellens, H. J., Bär, F. W., & Lie, K. (2000). *The value of the electrocardiogram in the differential diagnosis of a tachycardia with a widened QRS complex*. Springer.

White, J. M. (1999). Effects of relaxing music on cardiac autonomic balance and anxiety after acute myocardial infarction. *American Journal of Critical Care*, *8*(4), 220. PMID:10392221

Xie, T., Yu, H., & Wilamowski, B. (2011). *Comparison between traditional neural networks and radial basis function networks*. Paper presented at the IEEE International Symposium on Industrial Electronics. doi:10.1109/ISIE.2011.5984328

Yamashita, S., Iwai, K., Akimoto, T., Sugawara, J., & Kono, I. (2006). Effects of music during exercise on RPE, heart rate and the autonomic nervous system. *The Journal of Sports Medicine and Physical Fitness*, *46*(3), 425. PMID:16998447

Yang, S., & Naiman, D. Q. (2014). Multiclass cancer classification based on gene expression comparison. *Statistical Applications in Genetics and Molecular Biology*, *13*(4), 477–496. PMID:24918456

Yang, Z., Su, Z., Ji, F., Zhu, M., & Bai, B. (2014). Mechanisms of behavior modification in clinical behavioral medicine in China. *International Journal of Behavioral Medicine*, *21*(4), 580–583. doi:10.1007/s12529-014-9405-7 PMID:24842543

Zywietz, C. (2003). *A brief history of electrocardiography-progress through technology*. Hannover: Biosigna Institute for Biosignal Processing and Systems Research.

ADDITIONAL READING

Ahearn, G. S., Tapson, V. F., Rebeiz, A., & Greenfield, J. C. Jr. (2002). Electrocardiography to define clinical status in primary pulmonary hypertension and pulmonary arterial hypertension secondary to collagen vascular disease. *CHEST Journal*, *122*(2), 524–527. doi:10.1378/chest.122.2.524 PMID:12171826

Burns, N. (2013). *Cardiovascular physiology*: Retrieved from School of Medicine, Trinity College, Dublin. http://www. medicine. tcd. ie/physiology/assets/docs12_13/lecturenotes/NBurns/Trinity% 20CVS% 20lecture.

Chou, T.-C., & Knilans, T. K. (1996). *Electrocardiography in clinical practice: adult and pediatric*. WB Saunders Company.

Connes, P. (2010). Heart rate variability. *Exercise Physiology: From a Cellular to an Integrative Approach, 75*, 162.

Ellis, R. J., Koenig, J., & Thayer, J. F. (2012). Getting to the heart autonomic nervous system function in the context of evidence-based music therapy. *Music and Medicine, 4*(2), 90–99. doi:10.1177/1943862112437766

Ellis, R. J., & Thayer, J. F. (2010). Music and autonomic nervous system (dys) function. *Music Perception, 27*(4), 317–326. doi:10.1525/mp.2010.27.4.317 PMID:21197136

Gillen, E., Biley, F., & Allen, D. (2008). Effects of music listening on adult patients' pre-procedural state anxiety in hospital. *International Journal of Evidence-Based Healthcare, 6*(1), 24–49. PMID:21631813

Haun, M., Mainous, R. O., & Looney, S. W. (2001). Effect of music on anxiety of women awaiting breast biopsy. *Behavioral Medicine (Washington, D.C.), 27*(3), 127–132. doi:10.1080/08964280109595779 PMID:11985186

Iwanaga, M., Kobayashi, A., & Kawasaki, C. (2005). Heart rate variability with repetitive exposure to music. *Biological Psychology, 70*(1), 61–66. doi:10.1016/j.biopsycho.2004.11.015 PMID:16038775

Juslin, P. N., & Västfjäll, D. (2008). Emotional responses to music: The need to consider underlying mechanisms. *Behavioral and Brain Sciences, 31*(05), 559–575. doi:10.1017/S0140525X08005293 PMID:18826699

Katz, A. M. (2010). *Physiology of the Heart*. Lippincott Williams & Wilkins.

Kim, J., & André, E. (2008). Emotion recognition based on physiological changes in music listening. *Pattern Analysis and Machine Intelligence. IEEE Transactions on, 30*(12), 2067–2083.

Krout, R. E. (2007). Music listening to facilitate relaxation and promote wellness: Integrated aspects of our neurophysiological responses to music. *The Arts in Psychotherapy, 34*(2), 134–141. doi:10.1016/j.aip.2006.11.001

Lacourse, E., Claes, M., & Villeneuve, M. (2001). Heavy metal music and adolescent suicidal risk. *Journal of Youth and Adolescence, 30*(3), 321–332. doi:10.1023/A:1010492128537

Lee, K.-C., Chao, Y.-H., Yiin, J.-J., Hsieh, H.-Y., Dai, W.-J., & Chao, Y.-F. (2012). Evidence that music listening reduces preoperative patients' anxiety. *Biological Research for Nursing, 14*(1), 78–84. doi:10.1177/1099800410396704 PMID:21278165

Liu, Y. H., Chang, M. Y., & Chen, C. H. (2010). Effects of music therapy on labour pain and anxiety in Taiwanese first-time mothers. *Journal of Clinical Nursing, 19*(7-8), 1065–1072. doi:10.1111/j.1365-2702.2009.03028.x PMID:20492051

Lundqvist, L.-O., Carlsson, F., Hilmersson, P., & Juslin, P. (2008). Emotional responses to music: Experience, expression, and physiology. *Psychology of Music, 37*(1), 61–90. doi:10.1177/0305735607086048

Malik, M. (1998). Heart rate variability. *Current Opinion in Cardiology, 13*(1), 36–44. doi:10.1097/00001573-199801000-00006 PMID:9559255

McCraty, R., Atkinson, M., Rein, G., & Watkins, A. D.WATKINS. (1996). Music enhances the effect of positive emotional states on salivary IgA. *Stress Medicine*, *12*(3), 167–175. doi:10.1002/(SICI)1099-1700(199607)12:3<167::AID-SMI697>3.0.CO;2-2

McCraty, R., Barrios-Choplin, B., Atkinson, M., & Tomasino, D. (1998). The effects of different types of music on mood, tension, and mental clarity. *Alternative Therapies in Health and Medicine*, *4*(1), 75–85. PMID:9439023

Rauscher, F. H., Spychiger, M., Lamont, A., Mills, J., Waters, A. J., & Gruhn, W. (1998). Responses to Katie Overy's Paper," Can Music Really'Improve'the Mind?" Psychology of Music, 26, 97-99. *Psychology of Music*, *26*(2), 197–210. doi:10.1177/0305735698262007

Rautaharju, P. M., Surawicz, B., & Gettes, L. S. (2009). AHA/ACCF/HRS recommendations for the standardization and interpretation of the electrocardiogram: part IV: the ST segment, T and U waves, and the QT interval a scientific statement from the American Heart Association Electrocardiography and Arrhythmias Committee, Council on Clinical Cardiology; the American College of Cardiology Foundation; and the Heart Rhythm Society Endorsed by the International Society for Computerized Electrocardiology. *Journal of the American College of Cardiology*, *53*(11), 982–991. doi:10.1016/j.jacc.2008.12.014 PMID:19281931

Roque, A. L., Valenti, V. E., Guida, H. L., Campos, M. F., Knap, A., Vanderlei, L., & de Abreu, L. C. et al. (2013). The effects of different styles of musical auditory stimulation on cardiac autonomic regulation in healthy women. *Noise & Health*, *15*(65), 281. doi:10.4103/1463-1741.113527 PMID:23771427

Scherer, K. R., & Zentner, M. R. (2001). Emotional effects of music: Production rules. *Music and emotion: Theory and research*, 361-392.

Schorr, J. A. (1993). Music and pattern change in chronic pain. *ANS. Advances in Nursing Science*, *15*(4), 27–36. doi:10.1097/00012272-199306000-00004 PMID:8512302

Sokhadze, E. M. (2007). Effects of music on the recovery of autonomic and electrocortical activity after stress induced by aversive visual stimuli. *Applied Psychophysiology and Biofeedback*, *32*(1), 31–50. doi:10.1007/s10484-007-9033-y PMID:17333313

Stauss, H. M. (2003). Heart rate variability. *American Journal of Physiology. Regulatory, Integrative and Comparative Physiology*, *285*(5), R927–R931. doi:10.1152/ajpregu.00452.2003 PMID:14557228

Tabloski, P. A., Mckinnon-Howe, L., & Remington, R. (1995). Effects of calming music on the level of agitation in cognitively impaired nursing home residents. *American Journal of Alzheimer's Disease and Other Dementias*, *10*(1), 10–15. doi:10.1177/153331759501000105

Thoma, M. V., La Marca, R., Brönnimann, R., Finkel, L., Ehlert, U., & Nater, U. M. (2013). The effect of music on the human stress response. *PLoS ONE*, *8*(8), e70156. doi:10.1371/journal.pone.0070156 PMID:23940541

Valenti, V. E., Guida, H. L., Frizzo, A. C., Cardoso, A. C., Vanderlei, L. C. M., & Abreu, L. C. (2012). Auditory stimulation and cardiac autonomic regulation. *Clinics (Sao Paulo)*, *67*(8), 955–958. doi:10.6061/clinics/2012(08)16 PMID:22948465

Vuust, P., & Frith, C. D. (2008). Anticipation is the key to understanding music and the effects of music on emotion. *Behavioral and Brain Sciences*, *31*(05), 599–600. doi:10.1017/S0140525X08005542

Weeks, B. P., & Nilsson, U. (2011). Music interventions in patients during coronary angiographic procedures: A randomized controlled study of the effect on patients' anxiety and well-being. *European Journal of Cardiovascular Nursing*, *10*(2), 88–93. doi:10.1016/j.ejcnurse.2010.07.002 PMID:20685168

Yamasaki, A., Booker, A., Kapur, V., Tilt, A., Niess, H., Lillemoe, K. D., & Conrad, C. et al. (2012). The impact of music on metabolism. *Nutrition (Burbank, Los Angeles County, Calif.)*, *28*(11), 1075–1080. doi:10.1016/j.nut.2012.01.020 PMID:22858194

KEY TERMS AND DEFINITIONS

Autonomic Nervous System: Autonomic nervous system is a part of the peripheral nervous system, responsible for the control of the involuntary functions of the body. It helps in maintaining homeostasis through the regulation of heart rate, blood pressure, respiration rate and breathing.

Classification and Regression Tree (CART): The supervised learning method that performs the analyses of both classification and regression using decision trees.

Decision Tree: Decision tree is a way of displaying an algorithm in a tree-like structure. It is mainly used the field of operations research.

Electrocardiogram (ECG): Electrocardiogram is the representation of the electrical activity of the heart measured from the skin surface. It comprises of various waves such as P-wave, QRS-complex and T-wave.

Heart Rate Variability (HRV): Heart rate variability can be considered as a measure of the temporal variation of the consecutive heart beats. It is an indispensable tool for the non-invasive measurement of the effect of autonomic nervous system on the cardiac health.

Parasympathetic Nervous System: The parasympathetic nervous system is that part of the autonomic nervous system which promotes the normal functioning of a number of organ systems. Its dominance results in efficient digestion, normal heart rate, etc.

Sympathetic Nervous System: The sympathetic nervous system is that branch of the autonomic nervous system which acts in stressful situations and exerts opposite effects to that of the parasympathetic nervous systems (e.g. increase in the heart rate, decrease in the efficiency of digestion etc.).

APPENDIX: ABBREVIATIONS

ANN: Artificial Neural Network
ANS: Autonomic Nervous System
BT: Boosted Tree
CART: Classification And Regression Tree
ECG: Electrocardiogram
HRV: Heart Rate Variability
HF: High Frequency
LF: Low Frequency
MLP: Multi Layer Perceptron
p.u.: per unit
RBF: Radial Basis Function
RF: Random Forest
RMSSD: Root Mean Square Standard Deviation
SD: Standard Deviation
VLF: Very Low Frequency.

Section 5

Assortment of Medical Imaging Applications–Based Classification

Chapter 10
Development of Ultrasound Imaging CAD Tool for Assessment of Pathologies in Supraspinatus Tendon

Rishu Gupta
Universiti Teknologi Petronas, Malaysia

Irraivan Elamvazuthi
Universiti Teknologi Petronas, Malaysia

John George
University of Malaya Research Imaging Centre, Malaysia

ABSTRACT

Non-invasive diagnostic imaging methods for diagnosis of pathological conditions is increasingly gaining popularity resulting from speedy and effective recovery during follow up in several clinical trials. The accuracy of the diagnosis depends on the experience and knowledge of physicians conducting the trial. In such scenario, the need for quantitative measures for details such as shape and size of tissue can assist physicians for better intuitive understanding of tissue and its pathologies. Computer aided diagnosis (CAD) tool incorporating methods for segmentation, texture analysis and area computation can increase the accuracy of diagnosis by providing quantitative analysis of the image. This chapter briefly describes issues and challenges for building the CAD tool followed by brief description about the methods involved. The methods are validation are also discussed briefly. To summarize the work, brief discussion about a new software or CAD tool for diagnosis of pathologies supraspinatus tendon with the help of ultrasound images is provided. The new software has an intuitive user interface which is easy, quick and suitable for medical work.

DOI: 10.4018/978-1-5225-0140-4.ch010

INTRODUCTION

In recent times, non-invasive medical imaging modalities such as ultrasound, magnetic resonance imaging (MRI), computed tomography (CT), X-ray are increasingly helpful for the preliminary diagnosis of the patients. The modalities assist medical practitioners by non-invasively providing the details of anatomical parts suffering from pathological conditions. The visual analysis of the tissue under examination gives qualitative understanding on the pathological state of tissue based on experience and expertise. However, since the visual analysis gives the qualitative assessment, the quantitative details regarding the shape, size of the tissues and pathological condition can provide better and intuitive understanding during follow up for physicians to better diagnose and treat the patients. Computer aided diagnosis (CAD) tools are becoming useful and effective for assistive diagnosis since last decade. The quantitative details helpful for physicians can be thickness, area of the tissue or the type and area of pathological condition within the tissue. The CAD tool incorporating the methods for assessment and measurements of pathological conditions in tissue structure can be developed using advanced imaging concepts.

Non-invasive imaging modalities such as X-ray, CT/PET, MRI and ultrasound offers several advantages and disadvantages. X-ray, CT/PET uses ionizing radiations which is harmful for human body, at the same time also provides very good contrast images for diagnosis. In MRI, the contrast of the images is very good and modality does not use ionizing radiations but MRI is not recommended for the patients with pacemakers, certain implants and intraocular metallic foreign bodies. Other challenge with MRI is its use with patients suffering from claustrophobia. Ultrasound imaging modality poses several benefits such as it is safe, as it uses non-ionizing sound pulses for scanning; it provides real time image or continuous frames for examination; it is compact and portable making it available for easy transportation; it is highly economical compared to other modalities and also the patients acceptability for ultrasound equipment is higher. Despite several advantages, ultrasound images has major drawback of low contrast and resolution which makes the modality highly operator dependent and also the diagnosis results are not easily reproducible.

Due to its benefits and capability to image the pathological condition in real time with motion it is being rigorously used for MSK applications. The ultrasound imaging allows physicians to have the real time and more flexible view of pathological tissues under examination. This chapter provides understanding about the development of CAD tool for Supraspinatus tendon. The possible reasons for development of pathological condition in the muscle are tendon rupture or inactivity. The types of tendon pathologies are:

1. Tendinosis;
2. Tear.

Tendinosis occurs due to overuse of the shoulder. In athletes participating in sports involving repetitive arm motion, such as swimming, throwing, racquet, whereas, in non-athletes it occurs due to the probable existing history of heavy weight lifting or sudden pull. Continuous or permanent rubbing also tends to weaken tendon. Tear is when tendon is no longer fully attached to the humerus, in young generation it occurs due to fall or accident, whereas for adults tear occurs due to redundant overhead movement.

CAD tool can be incorporated in diagnosis for assisting medical practitioners in two different ways. First method involves modification of existing equipment with request to original equipment manufacturer. Second method involves providing a standalone tool for assessment of tissues which should be installed along with imaging equipment. However, it should be considered that research on CAD is done not to eliminate the need for an expert, rather to help or provide radiologist with the second rational opinion to make diagnosis confident and accurate thereby saving time and effort.

Therefore, development of CAD tool should be carried out based on the application and modality. The algorithms can be generated in many ways that can help radiologist to identify the pathological conditions better compared to original image such as

1. To implement a method for enhancing the quality of an image thereby providing medical practitioners with an image better than original image for diagnosis.
2. To propose a method for extraction of region of interest or tissue having pathological condition that will allow physicians for focused analysis of tissue.
3. The method can also be devised to calculate the area of pathological condition to monitor the healing of tissues or calculate the topological information from tissue such thickness or area.

In the work on Supraspinatus tendon, three different methods were proposed. Firstly, enhancement method for the image is proposed which performs the enhancement based on the understanding of the underlying gray level distribution in the image. Secondly, segmentation method is proposed which takes into account the invariant features from the image and extracts the region of interest which helps in focused assessment of pathological conditions. As an outcome for segmentation region of interest i.e., SSP tendon is extracted from the ultrasound image which helps radiologist for focused assessment of pathologies. Thirdly, for objective assessment of pathological conditions clustering method is developed. The clustering method incorporates information from edges, and neighborhood pixels in the form of spatial distance and gray level intensities. The information is incorporated using the edge adaptive directional kernel which is computed using the singular value decomposition of the gradient image and calculating the orientation, scaling, and elongation parameter for particular pixel based on neighborhood information. The developed clustering algorithm clusters the region of interest into pathological and non-pathological region.

In this chapter the development of CAD tool for Supraspinatus (SSP) tendon in shoulder is described in detail. The chapter also briefly discusses about the challenges and issues faced in the development of CAD tool followed by brief discussion on the techniques evolved and validation methods adopted. To summarize the work brief introduction about the new developed CAD tool which can be used for image assessment of supraspinatus ultrasound image is provided.

BACKGROUND

In literature, researchers have used ultrasound imaging modalities to quantify the details of anatomical body parts; nearly three decades ago, studies were proposed on how to use ultrasound signals to obtain quantitative estimates explaining the soft tissue properties extensively. The earliest literature providing encouraging experimental results and theoretical framework for usage of quantitative ultrasound for characterization of tissues and microstructure can be found in (Insana & Hall, 1990; F. L. Lizzi, Greenebaum, Feleppa, Elbaum, & Coleman, 1983). Following these studies, other applications of ultrasound imaging also introduced quantitative measures such as cyst size measurement (Tomonaga, Filipi, Lowham, & Martinez, 1999), foetal measurements during pregnancy (Carneiro, Georgescu, Good, &

Comaniciu, 2007, 2008), detection and quantification of prostate cancer (Feleppa, Mamou, Porter, & Machi, 2011), cardiac function by tissue characterization (Frederic L. Lizzi et al., 1997; Perez et al., 1992), characterization of breast tissue (Liao et al., 2012; Mohana Shankar et al., 2001), characterization of diffused liver diseases (Kadah, Farag, Zurada, Badawi, & Youssef, 1996), and characterization of cancerous lymph nodes (Ahuja et al., 2008; Mamou et al., 2011). Some other application of ultrasound imaging which includes comparative analysis of four different methods for quantitative assessment of coronary artery calcium lesions using intravascular ultrasound (Araki et al., 2015), improved correlation between carotid and coronary atherosclerosis SYNTAX score using automated ultrasound carotid bulb plaque IMT measurement.(Ikeda et al., 2015) In MSK ultrasound researchers have ventured to obtain quantitative information regarding cross sectional area and thickness (Eranki, Cortes, Feren, ek, & Sikdar, 2013; Habermeyer, Krieter, Tang, Lichtenberg, & Magosch, 2008; Horng, 2013; Katayose & Magee, 2001; Leung & Griffith, 2008; Ming-Huwi Horng & Chen, 2009; P. K. Nielsen, Jensen, Darvann, Jorgensen, & Bakke, 2006; Scholten, Pillen, Verrips, & Zwarts, 2003) of tendon. In another application, ultrasound was used to calculate muscle kinematics during vibrant activities such as drop landing in healthy subjects (Eranki, et al., 2013). Tissue classification in tendon was attempted in (P. K. Nielsen, et al., 2006; Pernille Kofoed Nielsen, Jensen, Darvann, Jørgensen, & Bakke, 2000) to characterize the tissues based on the gray level information provided by ultrasound images. In recent research (Harris-Love, Monfaredi, Ismail, Blackman, & Cleary, 2014), measurement of muscle dystrophy and sacropenia is studied based on changes in muscle quality via echogenicity measurements using gray scale images. Present state of art equipment for diagnosis of ultrasound images failed to analyze accurate tendon pathology and is subjective to operator assessments. And also available techniques for improved, focused and objective assessment of pathologies are very scarce. To overcome the existing problems a CAD tool using advanced image processing techniques is developed which can assist radiologists for reliable diagnosis. To develop CAD tool that fulfills the needs of medical practitioners is a tedious task due to the existing variabilities such as

1. Different soft tissues under imaging offers different acoustic impedance and hence different response to sound waves.
2. The physical properties of tissue under imaging such as on shape, size, and number of scatterers varies with anatomical position.
3. Physics of the equipment.
4. Variability in patients based on height, body weight, BMI.

The challenges and issues faced in the development of CAD tools are discussed in subsequent section.

CHALLENGES AND ISSUES

Challenges being faced in the development of CAD tool for different anatomical body parts are as follows:

1. The major impediment for the development of CAD tool using advanced imaging methods for ultrasound images is the contrast and resolution of images. Different anatomical body part shows different properties towards the ultrasound pulses being fired based on its acoustic impedance. Therefore none of the developed methods for imaging in ultrasound can be globally used for all

anatomical parts. The developed methods are mostly application specific such as cardiac, fetal, liver, kidney etc. Therefore a fresh analysis of the anatomical body part in consideration has to be performed.

2. Present state of art equipment for diagnosis of ultrasound images specifically in supraspinatus tendon failed to analyze accurate tendon pathology and are subjective to operator assessments.
3. The other major issue for development of CAD tool is credibility and validation of the system due to inter and intra-observer variability within and between radiologist's assessments at different time intervals.

The development of CAD tool that can be effectively used for diagnostic purposes in medical setting is a challenging task and requires special attention. Some more issues that were faced and investigated in the development of methods incorporated in tool for assessment of Supraspinatus tendon were

1. Will the enhancement of ultrasound image of SSP tendon assist radiologist for improved diagnosis of pathologies in SSP tendon?
2. How will the region of interest segmentation impact the diagnosis of pathologies in SSP Tendon?
3. The diagnosis of pathological conditions in ultrasound image depends on the deviation of gray level in the image from healthy tissues; can clustering of segmented SSP tendon be used for quantified analysis of pathological conditions?
4. Identification of the method of validation on different avenues in research.

The development of the CAD tool requires rigorous testing and validation both qualitative and quantitative with the help of experienced medical practitioners. The brief discussion about the details of methods is summarized in subsequent section.

BRIEF OVERVIEW OF METHODS

To develop a method which is robust and invariant to variations in ultrasound images, the task was subdivided into separate sections. For enhancement, the statistical properties of SSP tendon ultrasound images were studied based on the gray level intensity pattern in normal tissues and pathological tissues. From the observed details provided by the preliminary analysis, four statistical models namely Rayleigh, Weibull, normal and log-normal were considered. Further, goodness of fit test and significance value of fit for pathological tissue and normal tissues using different statistical models was calculated. The enhancement of ultrasound images was performed based on chosen statistical models providing improved diagnosis of SSP tendon.

For segmentation, analysis of feature extraction methods from images was done. Different methods such as statistical, scale space decomposition, texture based methods were studied. Curvelet decomposition method was chosen due to its properties of directionality and anisotropy. The image was reconstructed using the curvelet coefficients and to obtain the mask for SSP tendon morphological and logical operators along with connected component analysis was used. The ground truth for SSP tendon was procured with the help of radiologist's delineation of SSP tendon from set of ultrasound images.

For clustering, methods for choosing number of clusters were studied. Basic concept of Fuzzy C means algorithm and its recent developments in the domain of image processing were clearly understood. Further, kernel regression method for image enhancement and modifications were detailed.

The validation of the algorithm and methods developed was performed quantitatively and qualitatively. For qualitative assessment, two experienced radiologist assessment were considered and statistical analysis of their visual assessment was performed. For quantitative assessment, several parameter metrics such as universal quality index, signal to noise ratio, structure similarity index mean square error, and structural content were considered for enhancement, true positive rate, false positive rate and accuracy was included for segmentation and segmentation accuracy and entropy computation methods were used for clustering algorithm. The methods used for qualitative and quantitative assessment of developed imaging algorithms are summarized in section to follow.

VALIDATION METHOD

Validation of research in medical imaging is of utmost importance. For validation purposes, phantoms, animal model, clinical studies based on the manual delineation performed by radiologists are generally preferred. In ultrasound imaging, very little work is performed using phantoms or simulated images which clearly explain the difficulty faced to procure realistic phantoms and simulations for tissues. Another impediment for validation of research on ultrasound images is non-availability of standard database for images for comparison of results. Field II ultrasound simulation package is used in limited cases in some of the applications (Hassenpflug, Prager, Treece, & Gee, 2005; Ledesma-Carbayo et al., 2005) for validation purposes.

Lack of standardized measures for quantitative assessment of ultrasound images makes it difficult to compare results obtained from using different methods. By far, most extensively used technique for validation of results in ultrasound imaging is manual delineation of clinical data with the help of radiologist (Noble & Boukerroui, 2006). In most of the recent literature (Ghose et al., 2012; Massich et al., 2010; Noble, 2010; Noble & Boukerroui, 2006; Prevost et al., 2014; Rueda et al., 2014), for validation of segmentation in ultrasound images, models manually delineated images by radiologist are used as ground truth. Numerous literature, suggests use of manual delineation being used as a reference for research validation in applications on different anatomical part such as cardiac, prostate, IVUS, kidney and many others (Ghose, et al., 2012; Ledesma-Carbayo, et al., 2005; Massich et al., 2012; Rueda, et al., 2014). Inter- and intra- variability is a concern because manual segmentation is not the task radiologist intends to do often. Therefore, the comparisons for the results are performed by statistical methods generally using the clinical assessment of images with delineation performed by different radiologists. Inter and intra variability for diagnosis is calculated based on radiologist's assessment of several images at different time intervals. After the procurement of assessment results obtained by different radiologist statistical methods are used to validate the results of the algorithm. In the proposed work on Supraspinatus tendon three different methods for improvement in the diagnosis were proposed. In the first method, enhancement of images was performed which should provide better visualization of abnormalities or pathological conditions. In second method, automated segmentation of region of interest i.e. Supraspinatus tendon was provided for focused assessment of pathologies. In the third method, a clustering method was provided which can effectively cluster noisy images of ultrasound to provide delineated region which can successfully be diagnosed for quantitative pathological region. In the section to follow, brief discussion about the method of validation is provided for enhancement, segmentation and clustering subsequently.

Assessment of Enhancement

For medical ultrasound images, to be able to design the reliable and accurate algorithm for assessment of ultrasound images, it is necessary that images are relevant as per radiologist satisfaction. When observing an image, the quality depends on many factors such as sharpness, contrast, viewing angle, resolution and other factors (A. J. Ahumada & Null, 1993). For ultrasound images, unfortunately subjective quality of an image cannot be explained figuratively, and hence final opinion depends on expert's evaluation of the image. The evaluation of image by radiologist also depends on expertise. Although, ultrasound imaging modality contains artifacts and is subjected to the radiologist assessment; on several occasions it has been verified that ultrasound tend to provide comparable accuracy with that of MRI or arthroscopy (Lenza et al., 2013; Teefey, Middleton, Bauer, Hildebolt, & Yamaguchi, 2000; Teefey et al., 2004). The validation methods espoused in the literature (Harold L. Kundel, 2003; Naredo et al., 2006; Zhong, Tagare, & Beaty, 2006) have been used in this research work. This observation regarding the nature of ultrasound images motivates use of different image quality assessment and expert's assessment for outcome of different algorithms to quantify the quality of algorithm. Assessment for enhancement of SSP tendon ultrasound image is performed using qualitative and quantitative methods.

Qualitative Assessment

The performance of the proposed techniques was evaluated based on the radiologist's assessment of the enhanced images. The algorithms were tested for ensuring:

1. Consistence performance of method;
2. Reliability of the method;
3. Overall estimate to check the significance of enhancement.

Three rounds of assessments were performed by two radiologists on enhanced images using different methods (Drakonaki, Allen, & Wilson, 2009; Ottenheijm et al., 2014). The blind evaluation was conducted for each image; the assessment was performed using three enhanced and one original image. The resultant images were provided to radiologist with no prior information given regarding clinical history of patient. All four images were shown to radiologist at the same time for evaluation with no mention about the technique used for enhancement. For intra-observer variability, readings from the same radiologist were taken again after the period of three weeks. The total of three evaluations for each image was performed and images were shown in random manner to radiologist at every evaluation. The assessment sheet for evaluation of the established techniques is shown in Table 1. The sheets were provided for every enhanced technique and image. Therefore, for each image four assessment sheets were given to radiologists one for each technique. The assessment sheets obtained with the help of radiologist was then further evaluated using statistical method to report the accuracy of the method.

The sheet contains information regarding three different pathological conditions i.e. tear and tendinosis and the pathological conditions were classified as

Table 1. Assessment sheets for radiologists

Tissue Classification	TP	FP	TN	FN
Tendinosis				
Tear in normal SSP				
Rank				

1. **True Positives (TP):** Ailment present and diagnosed correctly.
2. **True Negatives (TN):** Ailment not present and not diagnosed.
3. **False Positives (FP):** Disease not present but diagnosed.
4. **False Negatives (FN):** Disease present but cannot be diagnosed.

The final row for rank assessment is over-all assessment of the enhancement of image on the scale of 1-4 where 1 was given to worst performer and 4 was given to best performer.

Inter-observer and intra-observer variability was calculated to estimate the enhancement in the images and its relevance to the diagnosis. The analysis was performed based on the overall assessment of the images. The Cohen (κ) value is calculated to determine the inter-observer agreement (Harold L. Kundel, 2003). Cohen(κ) values (Landis JR, 1977) greater than .80 shows almost complete agreement and less than 20 shows no agreement, whereas 21-40 gives fair, 41-60 indicates moderate and 61-80 specifies considerable level of agreement among radiologists The formula for computing κ value is given below,

$$\kappa = \frac{p_0 - p_e}{1 - p_e} \tag{1}$$

where, p_0 overall agreement between two observer, p_e is agreement expected to occur by chance, $p_{0,}$ p_e can be calculated as follows,

$$p_0 = \frac{P_{pos} + P_{neg}}{T} \tag{2}$$

where, P_{pos} is the positives in agreement, P_{neg} is the negatives in agreement, T is the total number of images and p_e is calculated as the joint positive and joint negative responses from both radiologists, the calculation for p_e is done using formula

$$p_e = \frac{P_{pos1}}{T} * \frac{P_{pos2}}{T} + \frac{P_{neg1}}{T} * \frac{P_{neg2}}{T} \tag{3}$$

where, P_{pos1} and P_{pos2} is the total number of positives for radiologist 1 and radiologist 2 respectively, P_{neg1} and P_{neg2} are the total number of negatives for radiologist 1 and radiologist 2 respectively. For intra-observer variability, separate assessment for tear and tendinosis was performed. Percentage agreement between the readings taken from radiologist was computed, the computation was performed by taking the average of percentage agreement found in first round-second round (FR-SR), second round-third round (SR-TR) and third round-first round (TR-FR) agreement for both the radiologists.

Quantitative Assessment

The quantitative assessment was further performed using various image metrics to correlate the results obtained qualitatively. For synthetic or optical image, where original image $X_{i,j}$ are available, various quantitative parameters are used to validate the outcome of the resultant image $Y'_{i,j}$ which we have introduced to quantify the performance of enhancment. In the below equations from (4.59) – (4.63), μ and σ are respectively the mean and variance within the images. The different quantitative measurement indices investigated are:

1. **Universal Quality Index (UQI):** This performance measure models distortion in image as factor of three components (Zhou & Bovik, 2002), contrast distortion, luminance distortion, and loss of correlation. The numerical formula for the metric is given by

$$UQI = \frac{\sigma_{XY}}{\sigma_x \sigma_Y} * \frac{2\mu_X \mu_Y}{\mu_X^2 + \mu_Y^2} * \frac{2\sigma_X \sigma_Y}{\sigma_X^2 + \sigma_Y^2} \tag{4}$$

Metric provides information about extent of structure preservation, luminance variance and contrast dependence of two images.

2. **Mean Square Error (MSE):** Estimates the overall change in the quality of the image in original and enhanced image. The computation is performed using

$$MSE = \frac{1}{NM} \sum_{i,j=1}^{N,M} \left(X_{i,j} - Y_{i,j} \right)^2 \tag{5}$$

Although mean square error is often used to judge image quality, it does not sufficiently correlate to the perceptual quality of image. Therefore, it is advised to use it in combination with other parameter metrics.

3. **Signal to Noise Ratio (SNR):** Although sensitivity to signal and noise are important for algorithms by themselves, what really matters is the ratio of signal to noise which is calculated as

$$SNR = 10 \log \left(\frac{\sum_{i,j=1}^{N,M} X_{i,j}^2}{\sum_{i,j=1}^{N,M} \left(X_{i,j} - Y_{i,j} \right)^2} \right) \tag{6}$$

4. **Structural Similarity Index (SSI):** Measures any distortion in the image into three factors: luminance, contrast distortion and loss of correlation. The formula for computation of SSI is given by

$$SSI = \frac{\left(2\mu_X\mu_Y + c_1\right)\left(2\sigma_X\sigma_Y + c_2\right)}{\left(\mu_X^2 + \mu_Y^2 + c_1\right)\left(\sigma_X^2 + \sigma_Y^2 + c_2\right)} \quad (7)$$

where, $c_1 = 01(DR)$ and $c_2 = 03(DR)$ are that depends on the dynamic range (DR=255) of the image and used to stabilize the division with weak denominator. The range of output values from SSI is from -1 to 1 where -1 stands for poor similarity and 1 stands for good similarity between the original image and enhanced image.

5. **Structural Content (SC):** Explains the similarity between enhanced and the original image; higher value suggests that algorithm employing image enhancement have lenient effect on structures.

$$SC = \frac{\sum_{i=1}^{N}\sum_{j=1}^{M} X_{i,j}^2}{\sum_{i=1}^{N}\sum_{j=1}^{M} Y_{i,j}^2} \quad (8)$$

Assessment of Segmentation

For the assessment of segmentation, qualitative measures were adopted both for performance of the algorithm and improvement in diagnostic capabilities.

Performance of Segmentation Algorithm: Qualitative Assessment

The quantitative method uses three parameter metrics: 1) False positive rate (FPR); 2) True positive rate (TPR) (Madabhushi & Metaxas, 2003); 3) Accuracy (ACC). The measurement metrics were calculated based on the area of segmentation. The regions were classified as true positives, false positives, and false negatives. Pictorial representation for corresponding area is shown in Figure 1.

Figure 1. Corresponding areas for false positive, false negative and true positives

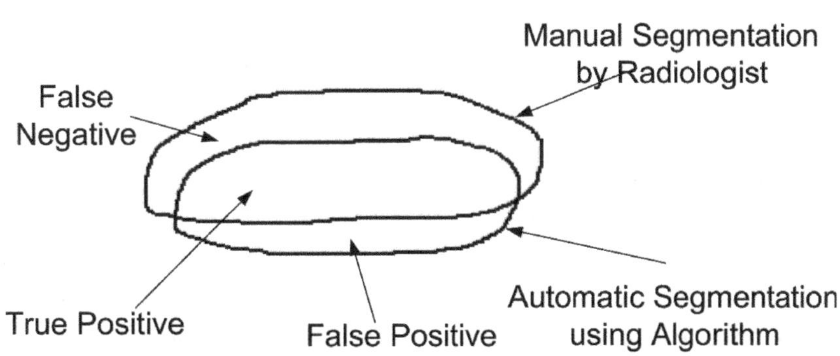

The performance metrics can be calculated using the formula below,

$$TPR = \frac{TP}{TP + FN} \tag{9}$$

$$FPR = \frac{FP}{FP + TN} \tag{10}$$

$$ACC = \frac{TP + TN}{TP + FP + TN + FN} \tag{11}$$

where, *TP* is region of SSP tendon accurately segmented by algorithm, *FP* is the region segmented by proposed method but does not exist in radiologist delineation, *FN* is the region delineated by radiologist and not existent in region segmented by proposed method, *TN* do not exist for assessment of segmentation. The images for visualization were also provided.

Performance on Diagnostics: Qualitative Assessment

The SSP tendon segmentation from ultrasound image results in the focused assessment of the tendon for pathological condition. The results were validated by providing the segmented image to radiologist and performing the assessment based on the radiologist interpretation of pathologies from focused images. The pathological conditions considered for evaluation in this case were tears, which could be partial thickness tears (PTTs) or full thickness tears (FTTs). The specificity and sensitivity values were calculated from radiologist assessment of the segmented image using the formula,

$$\begin{aligned} Sensitivity &= \frac{TP}{TP + FN}, \\ Sensitivity &= \frac{TN}{FP + TN} \end{aligned} \tag{12}$$

Also, the results of evaluation performed by radiologist were compared to that of existing results for the evaluation of PTTs and FTTS using ultrasound image.

Assessment of Clustering

The proposed clustering algorithm for sub-gray level segmentation of gray scale images has been validated using both qualitative and quantitative assessment methods. For qualitative assessment, algorithm is tested on synthetic, real as well as medical images (MRI, Ultrasound) by Gaussian noise, salt and pepper noise and speckle noise by varying the percentage of noise levels by 10%, 30% and 50%.

Figure 2. Synthetic images for testing clustering algorithms

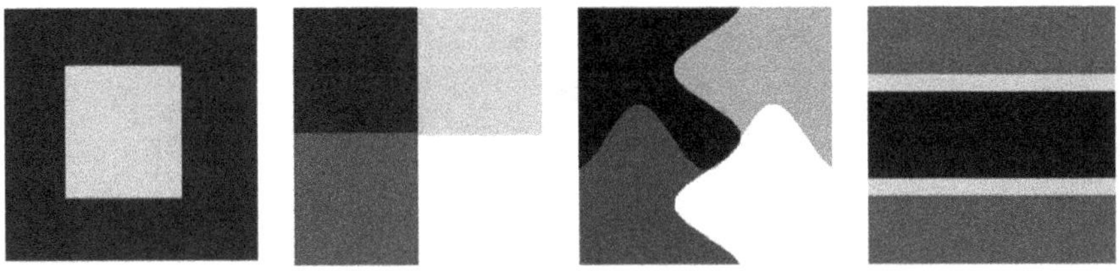

For qualitative assessment, the results of algorithm were compared with the radiologist delineation of pathologies in ultrasound images. The details regarding the quantitative and qualitative assessment are detailed in subsequent sections.

Quantitative Assessment: Validation

The visual results and the quantitative comparison of the proposed algorithm is provided with existing state of art clustering methods such as N-cut (Fowlkes, Belongie, Fan, & Malik, 2004), FLICM (Krinidis & Chatzis, 2010), RFLICM (Maoguo, Zhiqiang, & Jingjing, 2012), and KWFLICM (Maoguo, Yan, Jiao, Wenping, & Jingjing, 2013). The synthetic images used for validating the proposed algorithm are shown in Figure 2. For all the synthetic images, the noise level and type of noise was varied. The results of proposed algorithm over images with 50% Gaussian noise, 50% salt and pepper noise and 50% speckle noise are provided for visual analysis and to quantitatively estimate the performance of algorithm measurement metric was used.

The clustering accuracy of the different algorithms was compared with respect to the segmentation accuracy (SA) (Chunming et al., 2011). The formula for the computation of segmentation accuracy is calculated as the ratio of sum number of pixel correctly identified to that of the total sum of number of pixels in the image.

$$SA = \sum_{i=1}^{c} \frac{R_i \cap I_i}{\sum_{j=1}^{c} I_i} \tag{13}$$

where, c denotes the number of clusters, R_i are the set of pixels belonging to the i_{th} cluster found by the algorithm and I_i are the set of pixels belonging to the i_{th} cluster in the referenced image taken for segmentation.

The optical images used for validation of the proposed algorithms were cameraman image and coins image with four and ten coins shown in Figure 3. And, since the algorithm was developed for medical images with the objective to delineate the tissues underneath for better visualization and diagnosis, therefore algorithm was also tested on MRI brain medical images shown in Figure 4.

Due to unavailability of ground truth images in the medical domain segmentation accuracy (SA) cannot be calculated. Therefore, the accuracy of the algorithm was objectively evaluated using entropy based information (H Zhang, J. Fritts, & Goldman, Jan. 2004), which often is used for evaluating the clustering accuracy for images with no ground truth. The entropy for region j can be written as,

Figure 3. Real image for assessment of clustering algorithm

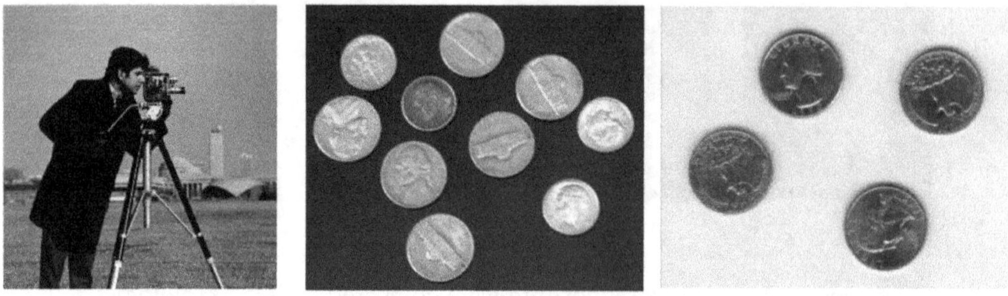

Figure 4. MRI medical images of brain

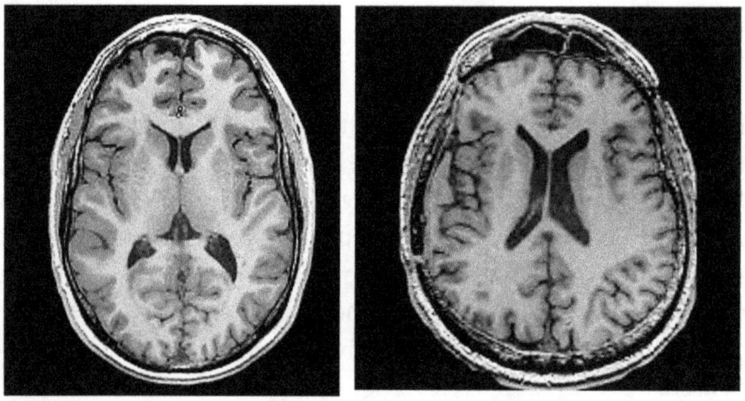

$$H(R_j) = -\sum_{m \in V_j} \frac{L_j(m)}{S_j} \log \frac{L_j(m)}{S_j} \tag{14}$$

The expected region entropy $H_r(I)$ of the segmented image is,

$$H_r(I) = \sum_{j=1}^{c} \frac{S_j}{S_I} H(R_j) \tag{15}$$

The layout entropy, $H_l(I)$, is defined as,

$$H_l(I) = -\sum_{j=1}^{c} \frac{S_j}{S_i} \log \frac{S_j}{S_I} \tag{16}$$

The entropy based assessment parameter, E combining both layout entropy and expected region entropy can be calculated as,

$$E = H_r(I) + H_l(I) \tag{17}$$

where, C is the number of clusters, R_j is the region of original image, $L_j(m)$ denotes the number of pixels in the cluster j having gray intensity value equal to m, V_j contains all the available gray levels in the region R_j, S_j is the number of pixels in region R_j. The concept behind this measurement index is that clustering should maximize the pixel uniformity in segmented region and minimize uniformity across regions. Therefore, good clustering is achieved when calculated entropy, E is least. The method was compared by the latest state of art algorithms such as N-cut, FLICM, RFLICM, and KWFLICM. The algorithm with minimum difference from the original ground truth image is the best clustering performer. The similar values were computed, after performing segmentation based on other clustering methods. Finally the algorithm is tested on ultrasound images and the results are provided to radiologist for assessment of the pathological regions extracted using proposed algorithms.

Qualitative Assessment: Pathology Identification

After the step of sub-gray level clustering, pathologies are clearly visible to the radiologists. The area of pathological condition is computed using region growing technique, wherein the seed point is selected by radiologist intervention using the clustered image. The segmented region identified as pathological condition is compared with the region of pathology identified by radiologist on the ultrasound image. The visual image showing the comparison of the extracted area by radiologist and area delineated by proposed algorithm is shown for assessment. For qualitative assessment of the proposed algorithm area based metric (Ladak et al., 2000) is proposed which is summarized as follows.

1. Compute the area of true positive (*TP*) which is defined as the common area between the radiologist delineation and area extracted by proposed algorithm.
2. Compute the region of false positives (FP), which is area in proposed algorithm but not included in the region extracted by radiologist.
3. Calculate the false negative (*FN*) which is the region belonging to the radiologist delineation but outside the region extracted by proposed method.

The corresponding region of *TP*, *FP*, and *FN* are shown in Figure 1. To estimate the performance of the algorithm two parameter metrics were calculated

$$\begin{aligned} Sensitivity &= \frac{TP}{TP + FN}, \\ Accuracy &= 1 - \left(\frac{FP + FN}{TP + FN}\right) \end{aligned} \tag{18}$$

Higher accuracy and sensitivity of the segmentation assures better result understanding and visualization regarding the pathological conditions resulting in improved diagnostic and faster recovery of patients. The next section briefly gives the details of results obtained for enhancement, segmentation and clustering along with assessment by medical practitioners.

DEVELOPMENT OF CAD TOOL

CAD tool development involves pre-processing of images, region of interest segmentation, identification of pathologies and report generation after the examination of the patient. The stages of CAD development are shown in Figure 5.

In this research ultrasound image is acquired with the help of experienced radiologist and further pre-processing involves enhancement of image which provides improved diagnosis and also proves as input for feature extraction which is next step for automatic segmentation. The segmentation is performed so as to provide focused assessment of the pathological conditions to radiologist and is carried out using morphological, logical and connected component analysis. The objective assessment of pathological

Figure 5. Steps for CAD tool

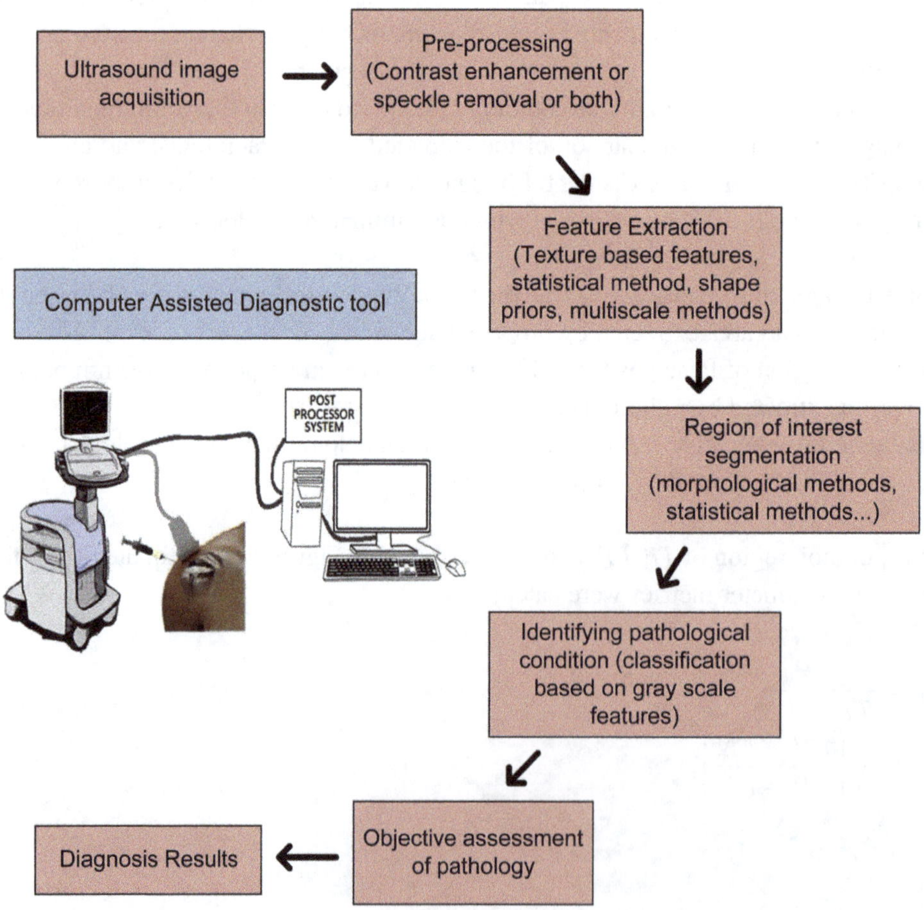

conditions involves sub-gray level segmentation of segmented tendon image and identification of pathology by radiologist intervention. The CAD tool for this particular application was divided to provide four ways for assisting radiologist for diagnosis of SSP tendon

1. Improved diagnosis of SSP tendon for pathologies by implementation of adaptive contrast enhancement produced by Rayleigh distribution.
2. Focused assessment of pathologies by provide automatic segmentation of SSP tendon.
3. Objective assessment of the identified pathological conditions.
4. Report generation for the performed examination by the radiologist.

The detailed description about the steps followed is described in the following sections.

SOFTWARE DEVELOPMENT PLATFORM

The CAD tool was developed using MATLAB software. The developed software was divided into two panels. On the left panel affiliation is shown at the top followed by the two axes for display of original image and output image after performing the set of operations. The right panel contains the tabs for radiologist to perform algorithmic operations for improved, focused and objective assessment. The detail of each section is provided as follows.

Execution of Graphical User Interface (GUI)

Figure 6 shows graphical user interface for the CAD tool developed. The software is executed by scribing MENSAA (given name) on command prompt.

The left panel shows two axes, the top axis is for original image and the bottom axis is for processed image. The right panel shows the different function available for radiologist to perform the diagnosis of the patient. The right panel is further subdivided into three subsections from top to bottom; the first section encapsulates function regarding the image input and image enhancement, followed by second section of automatic segmentation and third section of problem identification and area computation.

Load Input Image

Click on 'load Image' tab shown in Figure 7 in color box.

The window will appear as shown in Figure 7. User can select one image from set of images for further processing. The square shows the tab for load image. Figure 8, shows the image of MENSAA with original image to be diagnosed.

The image file location and size can be seen in the tab next to load image button and made bold with color. The original input image can be seen in the top left corner of the GUI.

Figure 6. MENSAA layout for diagnosis

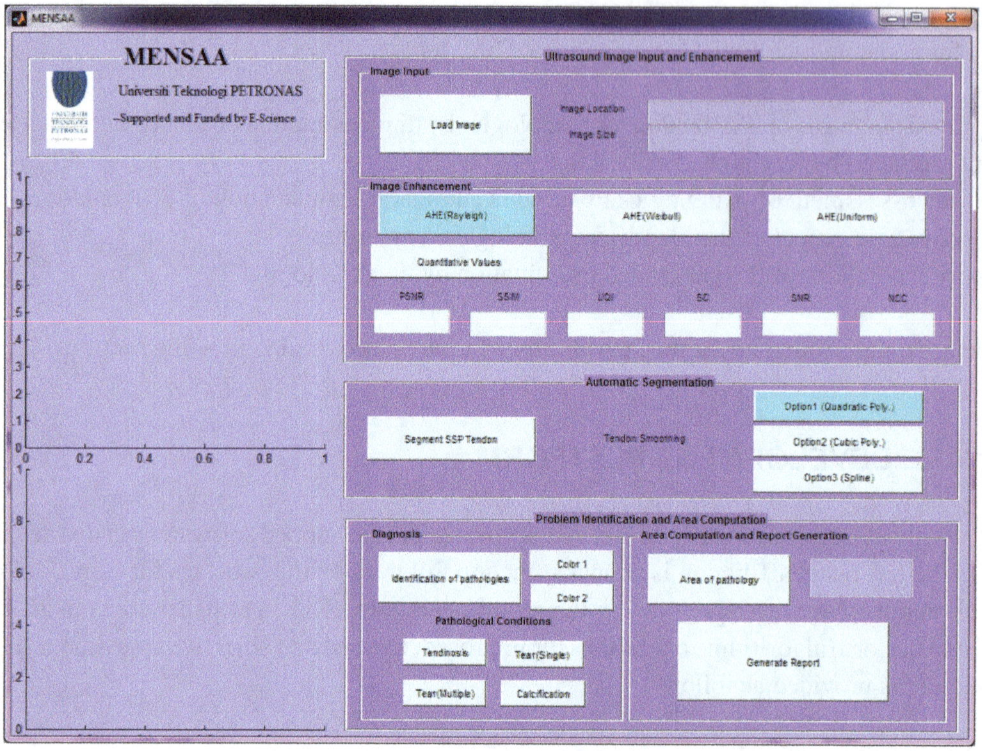

Figure 7. Upload image for analysis

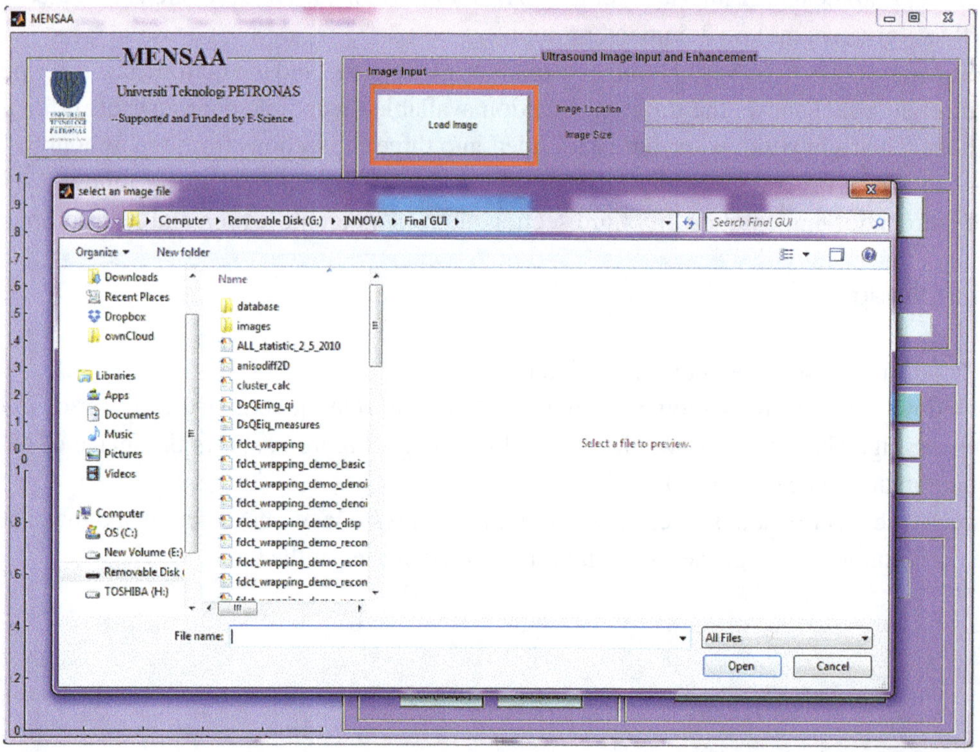

Figure 8. Original image shown for analysis

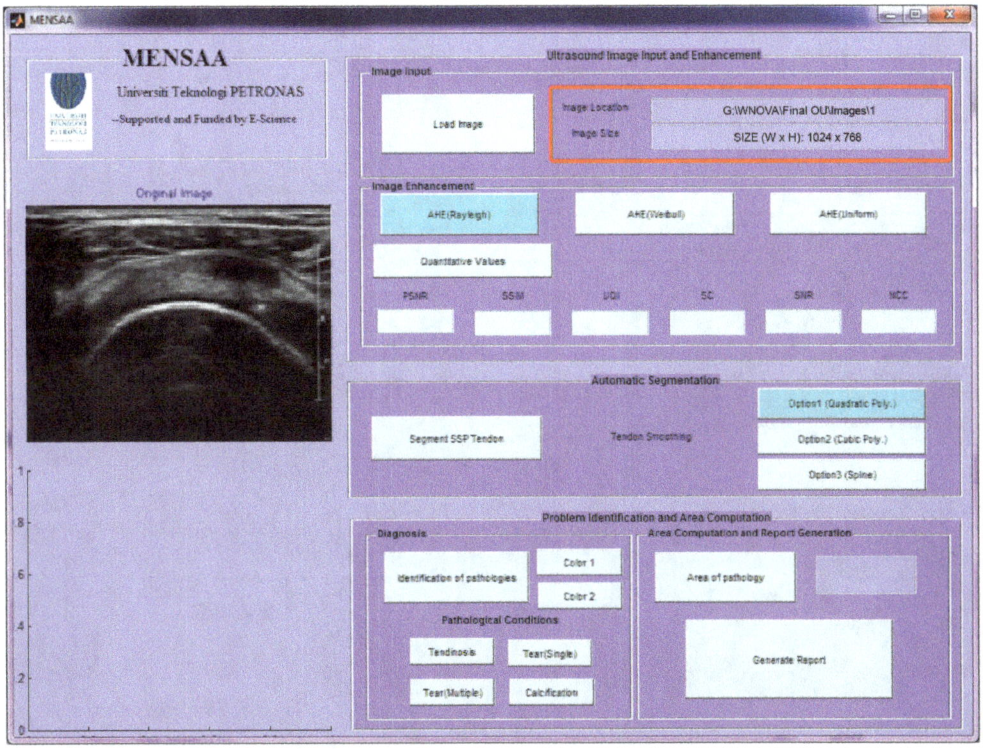

Enhancement: Improved Diagnosis

The image enhancement is performed with the help of tabs provided namely Rayleigh enhancement, Weibull enhancement and normal enhancement. All the three tabs are encapsulated in the box and shown in Figure 9.

By clicking on the tab respective enhanced image can be seen on axis 2. The tabs for quantitative assessment of images are also provided under the image enhancement tabs and shown in box in Figure 10.

The quantitative image assessment is provided to assist inexperienced radiologist to choose the best image for analysis of the SSP tendon. The quantitative assessment tabs made available are peak signal to noise ratio (PSNR), structural similarity index measurement (SSIM), universal quality index (UQI), structural content (SC), signal to noise ratio (SNR), and normalized cross correlation (NCC). The inexperienced operator can use the quantitative information to perform effective evaluation. The metrics are calculated by clicking the button 'Quantitative values' shown in color box Figure 10, shows the image with enhanced image and parameter values for the enhancement performed using the algorithm.

Segmentation: Focused Assessment

Automatic segmentation of SSP tendon ultrasound image can be performed by clicking the "Segment SSP tendon" tab shown in color box in Figure 11.

Figure 9. Image enhancement

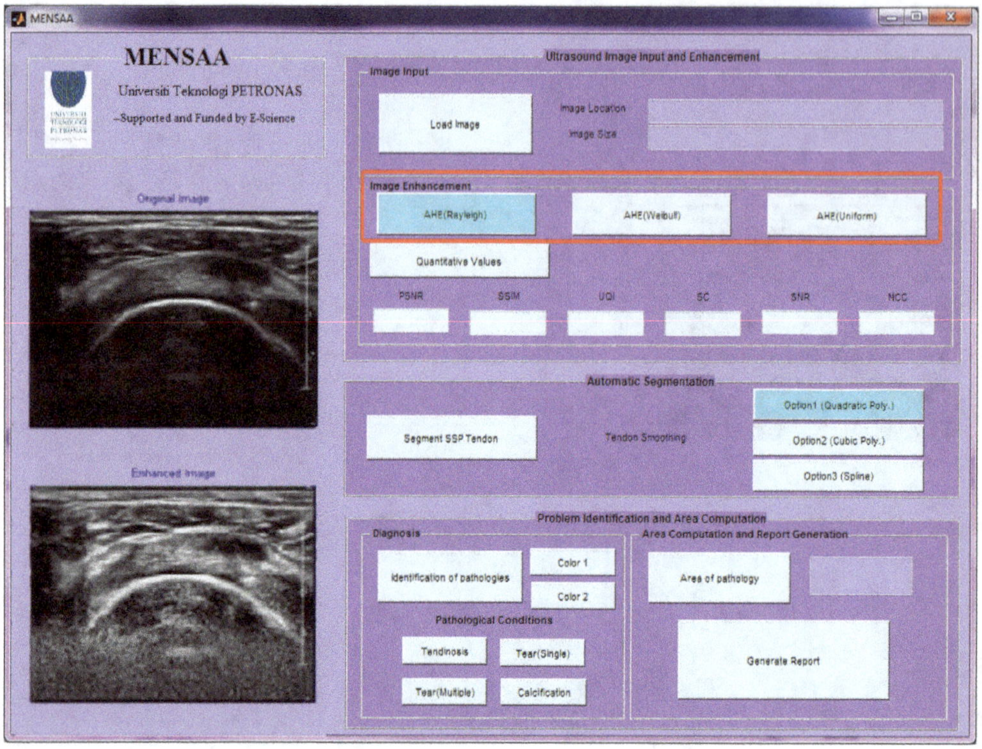

Figure 10. Quantitative information for enhancement

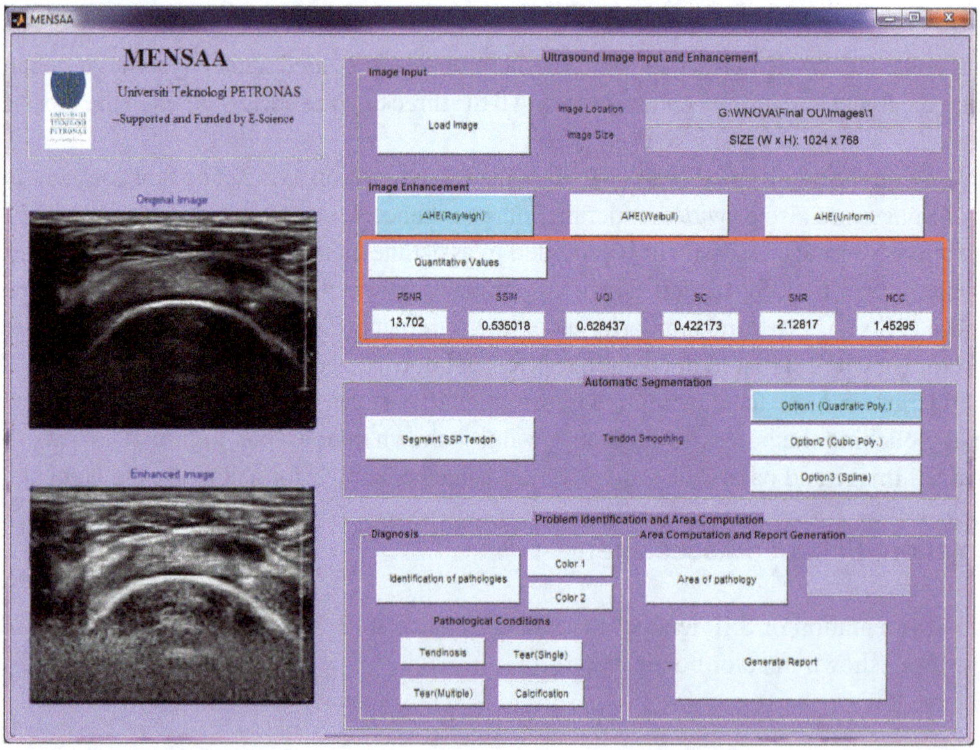

Figure 11. SSP tendon segmentation

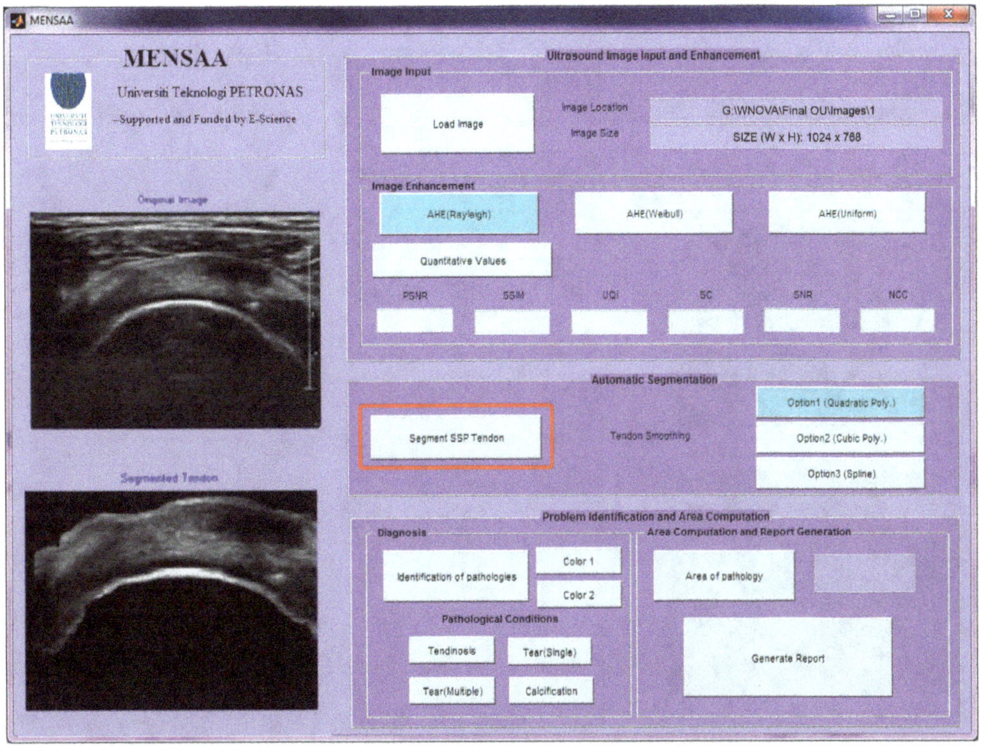

Figure 12. Smoothed SSP tendon

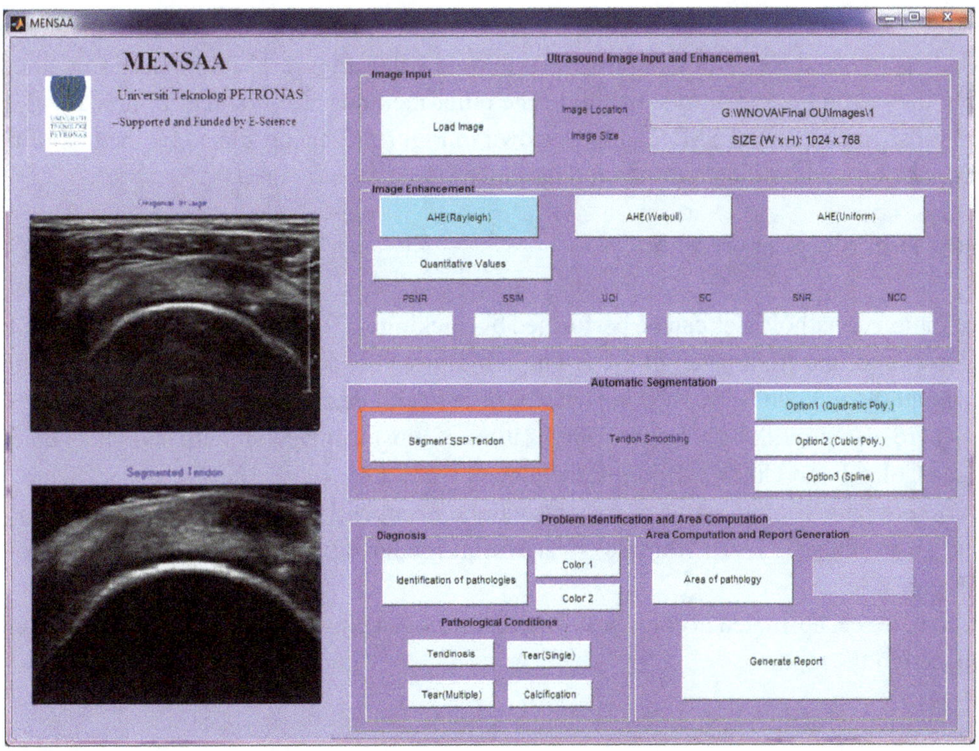

Figure 13. Identification of pathologies

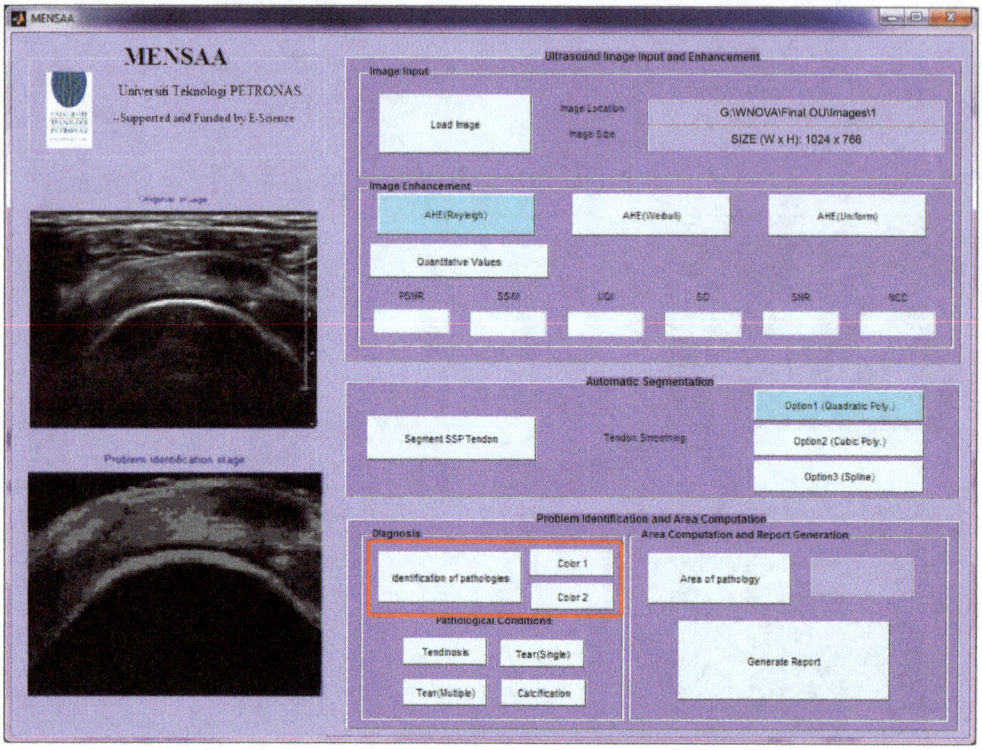

The tendon extracted is irregular in shape as shown in Figure 11. In the next step, the tendon structure is smoothed for better visualization and diagnosis. There are three options available for smoothing of tendon. The best method for smoothing is shown in bold color. Figure 12, shows the smoothed tendon image using the quadratic polynomial method. The other methods are shown as option 2 and option 3.

The tab for segmentation of SSP tendon is shown in Figure 12 encapsulated by the box of red color. The other options for smoothing are shown adjacently.

Clustering: Pathology Identification

The identification of pathologies can be performed by clicking on the tab “identification of pathologies” in the last section of the right panel of GUI. The sub-cluster image is shown in Figure 13 wherein the detection of pathologies can be easily done by experienced and inexperienced radiologist. Two different color spaces are also provided for better visualization of cluster image and are shown as color tabs in Figure 13, as Color 1 and Color 2. Buttons are shown in color.

Four different pathological states of patients can be examined using MENSAA. Four tabs namely Tendinosis, Tear (Single), Tear (Multiple), tear within tendinosis can be seen in the diagnosis panel shown in Figure 14.

The buttons are encapsulated in color box. When radiologist clicks on the tab the response is recorded to be published in the report.

Figure 14. Pathological conditions

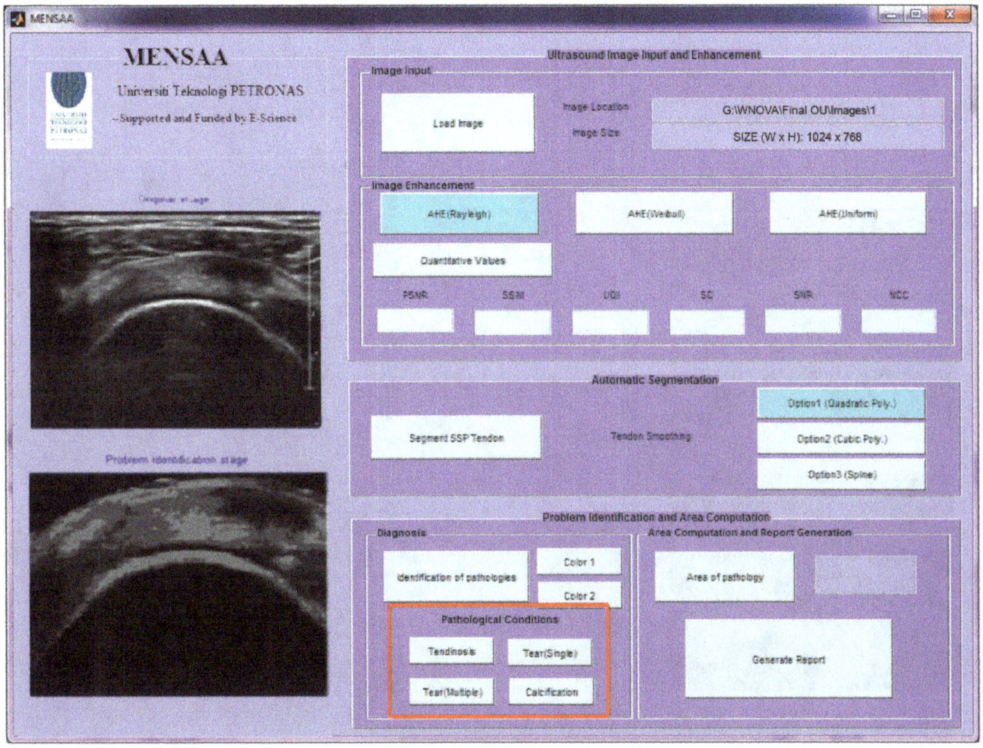

Area Computation and Report Generation

The user input is needed to compute the area of diagnosed pathological condition, radiologist after the identification of the pathological regions has to provide a seed point or chose a pixel from the pathological region and algorithm will automatically provide the region of pathology with the area in the tab next to "area of pathology". Figure 15 shows the "area of pathology" tab encapsulated in the color box along with the unit of area of pathology.

After the complete examination of the pathologies and region of pathology computation report can be generated. The final report for diagnosis with quantitative information regarding the pathology can be made available by clicking on the button "Generate Report" shown in Figure 16.

The CAD tool developed is highly intuitive and user friendly with the capability to transform predictable pathology in SSP tendon to objective detection of the pathological conditions. The system developed is highly reliable because of qualitative and quantitative assessment performed with the help of radiologist on the developed algorithms. The provided system gives increased accuracy in the diagnosis by providing improved, focused and objective assessment of pathological conditions in SSP tendon. The results for assessment are provided in the subsequent section for every stage in the CAD tool.

Figure 15. Area of pathology

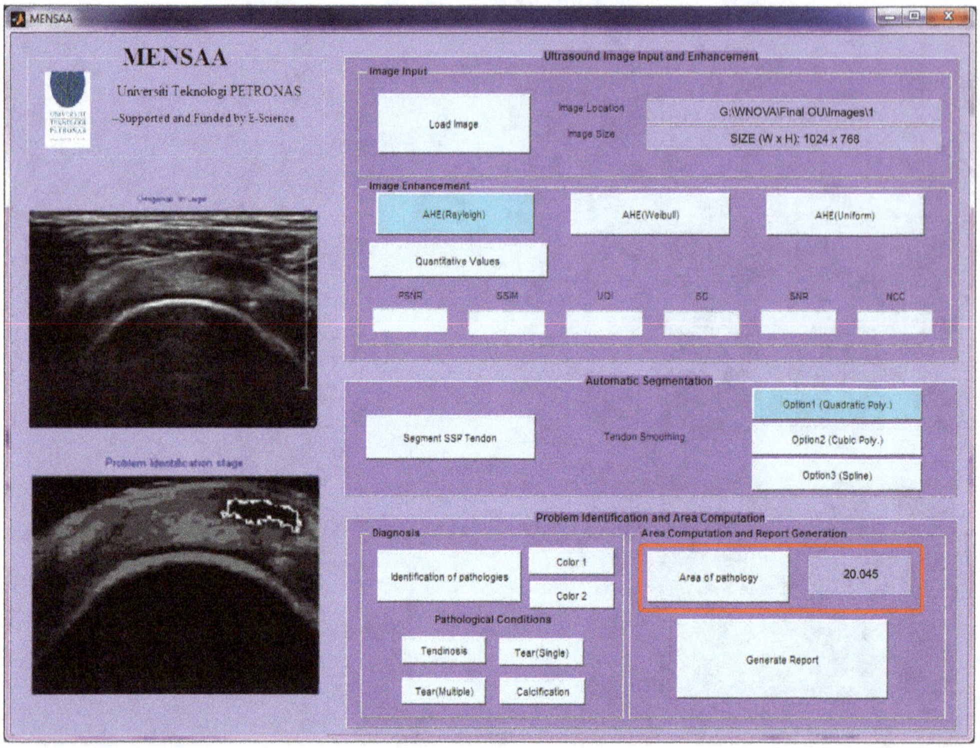

Figure 16. Generate report

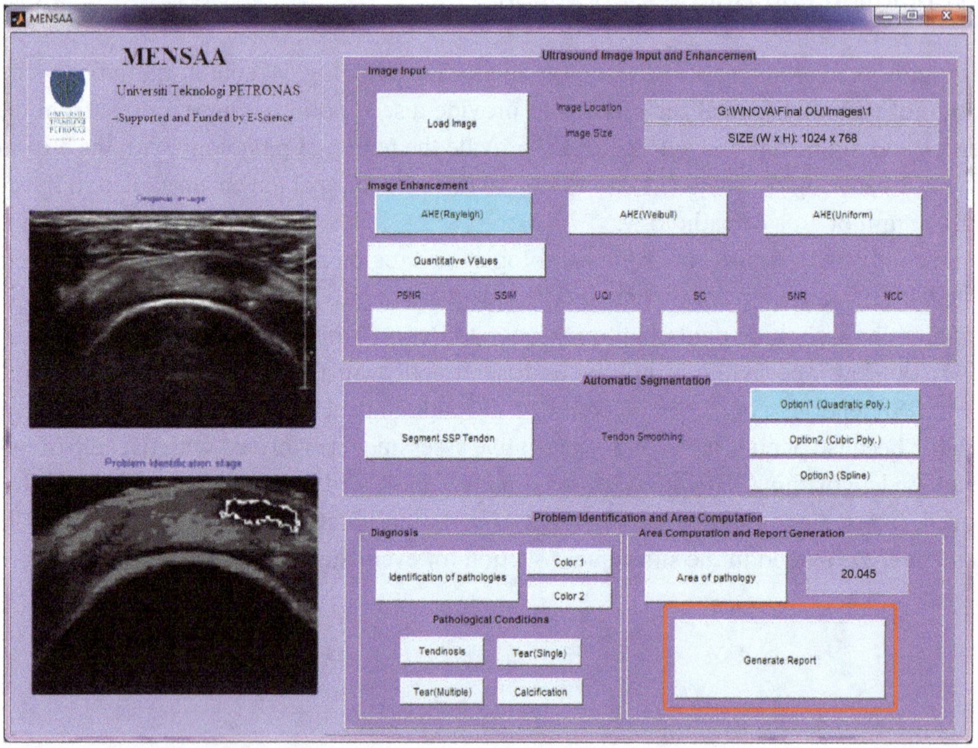

Figure 17. Universal quality index

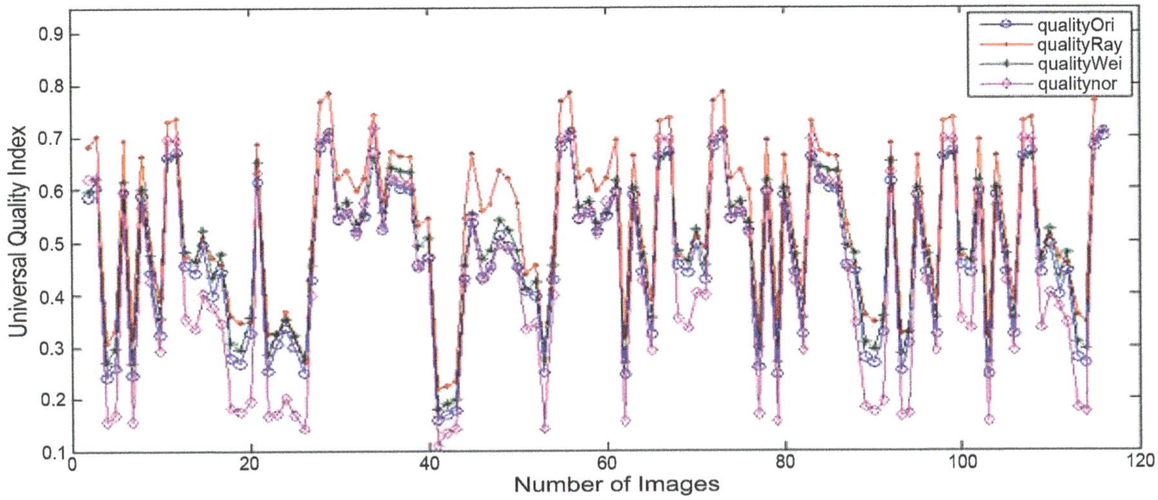

QUANTITATIVE ASSESSMENT RESULTS AT DIFFERENT STAGES

The quantitative results obtained for enhancement, segmentation and clustering are provided. The values for quantitative assessment for enhancement is provided first followed by results for segmentation and clustering.

Quantitative Assessment for Enhancement

The plot for evaluation metrics are shown in Figure 17, Figure 18, Figure 19, Figure 20, and Figure 21 for universal quality index, signal to noise ratio, structure similarity index, structural content and mean square error respectively.

Figure 18. Signal to noise ratio

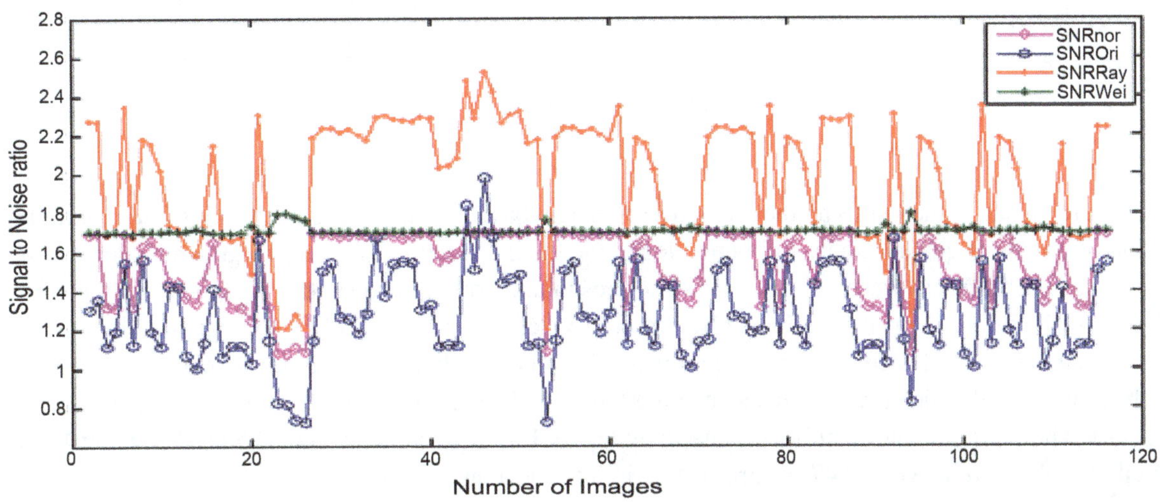

Figure 19. Structural similarity index

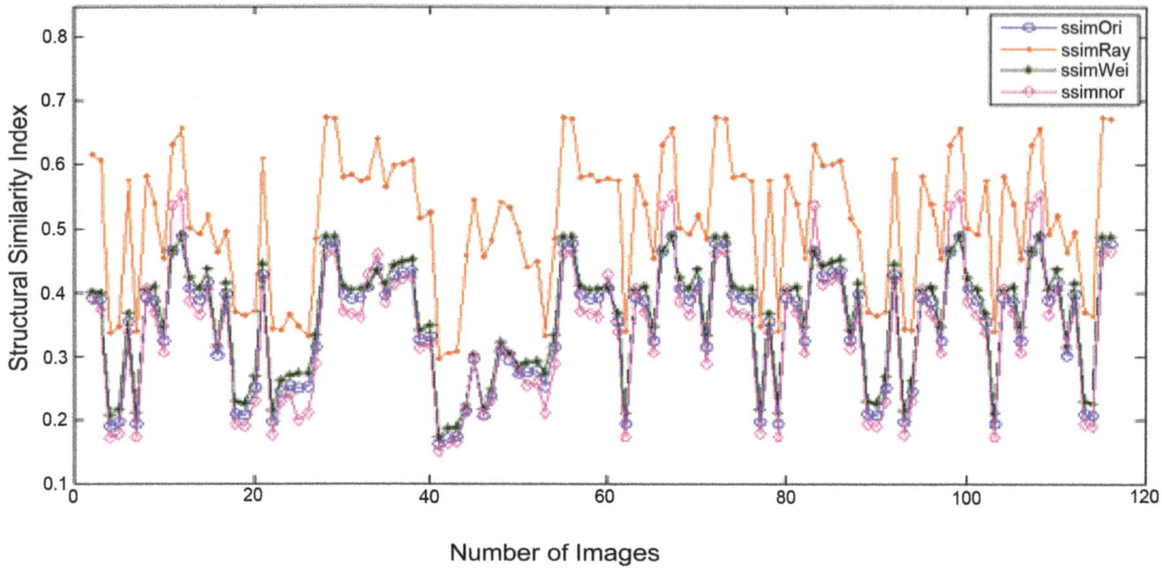

Figure 20. Structural content

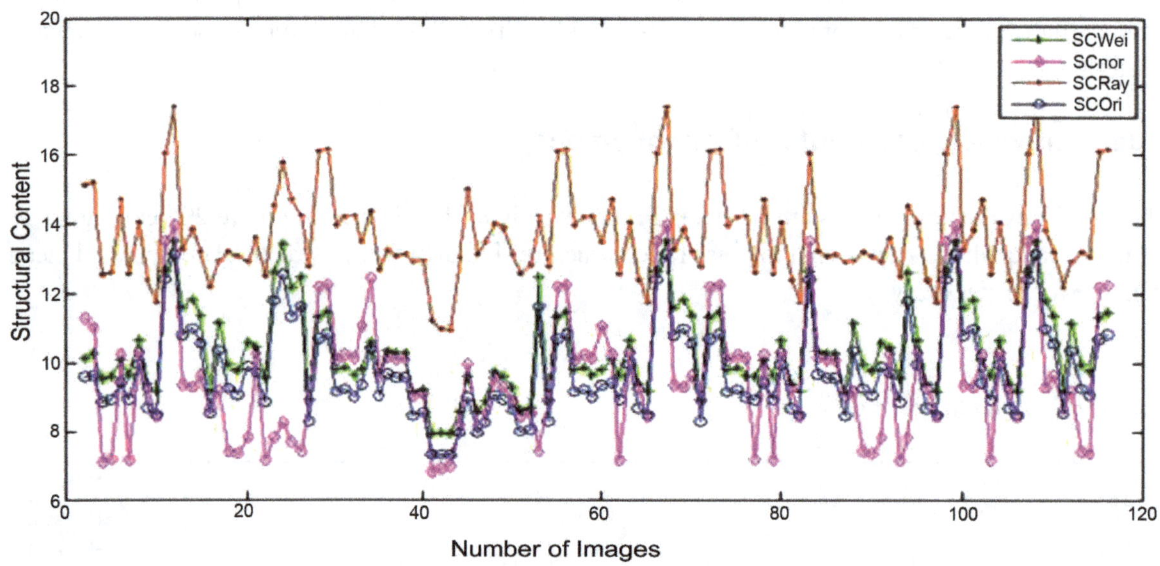

Figure 17, shows the results for the evaluation of images based on universal quality index. The maximum value of universal quality index is obtained for Rayleigh enhanced ultrasound image which depicts the methods capabilities to preserve the tissue structures in ultrasound image better than the other methods. The Rayleigh enhancement is followed by Weibull which was qualitatively also suggested by experts as the second best enhancement method after the Rayleigh method. Original ultrasound image results to be at number 3 which again justifies the qualitative analysis followed by the normal enhancement at the last. The average value of universal quality index for Rayleigh enhancement is 54 followed by 49 for Weibull enhanced image and 47 for original and 43 for normal enhanced image.

Figure 21. Mean square error

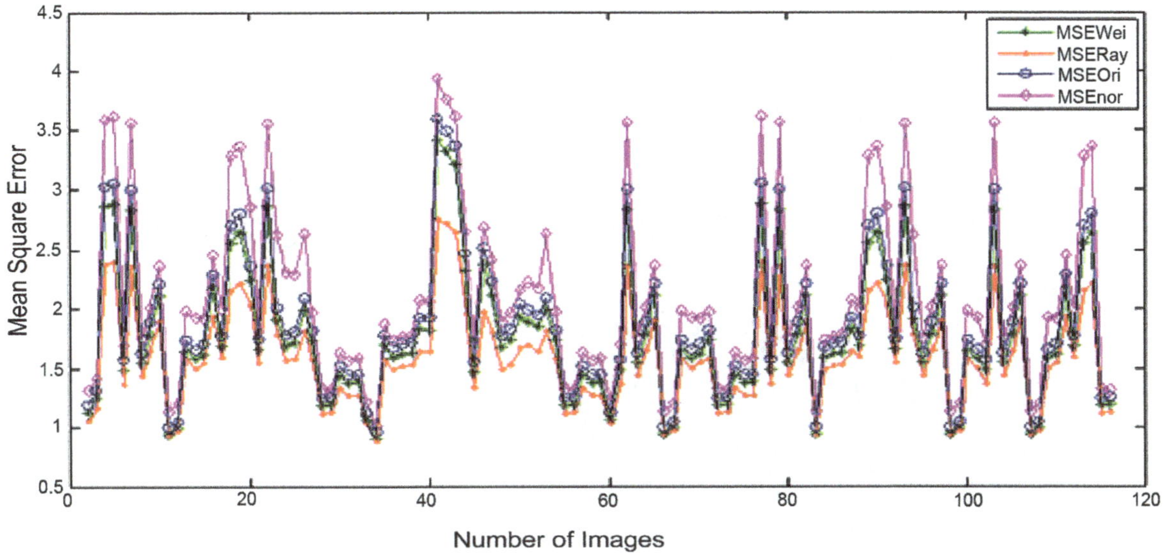

Figure 18, shows the result obtained by signal to noise ratio measurement index with maximum average SNR value of 1.98 for Rayleigh enhancement SSP tendon image followed by original image at number 2 with the average SNR value of 1.71 and Weibull enhanced image with very slight difference of 03 in the values of SNR with original image at number 3 and finally the performance of normal enhanced image is last with the average SNR value of 1.27. The results from SNR values rates Rayleigh enhanced ultrasound image to contain more signal to noise ratio compared to other methods for enhancement.

Figure 19, shows the result of four considered algorithms with respect to the structure similarity index parameter metric. The average value of Rayleigh enhanced image is 512 followed by 49 for Weibull, 43 for normal enhanced image and 35 for original image. The results obtained from the SSIM index shows the best preservation of the structure details in Rayleigh enhanced image which is similar to the results obtained from qualitative analysis performed with the help of experienced radiologists.

Figure 20 gives the quantitative result of the algorithm based on the structural content parameter with average value of 13.76 for Rayleigh enhancement followed by 14 for Weibull enhancement, 9.74 for original image and 9.61 for normal enhanced ultrasound image. The results are consistent for Rayleigh enhanced ultrasound image showing maximum diagnostic capabilities for detection of pathological region in SSP tendon. The results are also consistent with the radiologist assessment of the ultrasound images.

Figure 21 shows the results from last quantitative parameter introduced based on the error introduced in the images after the enhancement. Mean square error for all the enhanced images was calculated and average value of MSE for Rayleigh is 1.601 followed by 1.78 by Weibull enhanced image, 1.87 from original image and 2.10 from norm enhanced ultrasound image. The MSE for Rayleigh enhancement is lowest suggesting the maximum enhancement and minimum introduction of the unnecessary details to ultrasound images after enhancement.

Figure 22. Results from manual segmentation of radiologist and automatic segmentation using proposed algorithm

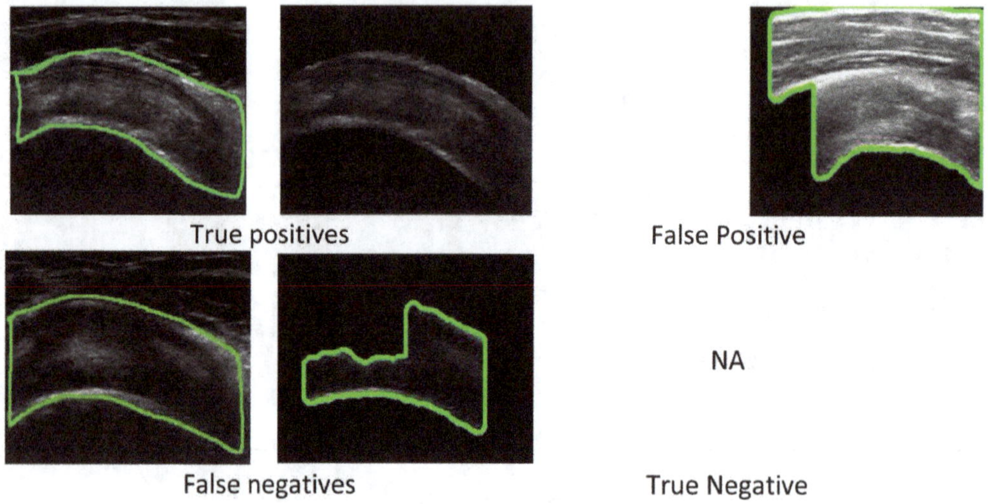

Quantitative Assessment for Segmentation

Out of the total 116 images, 109 images were correctly classified. In 3 images algorithm failed to extract SSP tendon and outliers were more prominent. In 4 images, the complete tendon was segmented but with outliers accompanied with it. Figure 22, shows the visualization of the results using manual segmentation by radiologist and result obtained using proposed algorithm.

Figure 22(a) shows the true positive results wherein accurate segmentation as per radiologist requirement was attained followed by Figure 22(b) it can be seen that the region segmented by radiologist is present in the result with an outlier region shown. The false positives arise because of the inaccurate detection of muscle fat outlier which plays important role in segmentation. In Figure 22(c), result shows inaccuracy of the algorithm in the form of detection of false negatives, wherein the reason for inaccuracy is poor visibility of bursae. No cases of true negatives were found (true negatives are cases when the segmentation area completely lies outside the region manually segmented by radiologists). The qualitative assessment of results obtained using proposed algorithm was performed using true positive rate, false positive rate and accuracy of segmentation. Table 2 shows the measurement values of the algorithm for true positive rate, false positive rate and accuracy. The accuracy of the algorithm obtained for the provided data set was 94.82% i.e. out of 116 images taken, the proposed algorithm was able to segment

Table 2. Performance result of the algorithm

Performance Metric	Evaluation Result
True positive rate (TPR)	9137
False positive rate (FPR)	0862
Accuracy (ACC)	9482

SSP tendon from 103 images successfully. And the true positive rate of 91.37% which is number correct segmentation over total correct segments and false negatives and false positive rate of 8.62% which is total number of false positive over conditional negatives.

The performance of the algorithm was also tested based on the improvement in the diagnostic capabilities due to focused SSP tendon image generated by algorithm. The assessment was performed with the help of radiologist and discussed in next section.

Quantitative Assessment for Segmentation

For precise evaluation of the region of pathologies identified using proposed algorithm all images must be taken into account. The region of pathologies is evaluated in comparison to the assessment performed by radiologist on real ultrasound image. The area of pathological condition is marked by radiologist in the original ultrasound image and later that area is compared to the region extracted using the proposed algorithm. The area extracted using the proposed algorithm is classified as either true positive (TP), false positive (FP), false negative (FN). For instance, the original ultrasound image for SSP tendon is shown in Figure 23(a) which shows the pathological region in the right top corner of tendon, which by radiologist was classified as region of tendinosis. In the clustered image shown in Figure 23(b), the region of tendinosis is clearly segmented out along with possible regions of tear which in the initial diagnosis performed by radiologist were not very visible. The area of region is computed based on the pixel values.

In Figure 23, the white line is the region segmented by radiologist whereas the green line is the region segmented with the help of proposed algorithm. The true positive is the number of pixels that are correctly identified by the proposed algorithm. False positive are area extracted by radiologist but excluded by proposed algorithm and false negatives are the areas delineated by radiologist but excluded by proposed method. The accuracy and sensitivity for the results in Figure 23 is calculated as follows:

The area is computed based on the analysis of number of pixels enclosing the manual segmented region and radiologist segmented region.

- **TP:** Number of pixels correctly identified by proposed algorithm.
- **FN:** Total number of pixels extracted by radiologist – TP.
- **FP:** Total number of pixels extracted by proposed algorithm – TP.

For Figure 23:

TP = 4489 pixels;
Region segmented by radiologist = 4757 pixels;
Region segmented by proposed algorithm = 5167 pixels;
FP = 5167-4489 = 678
FN = 4757-4489 = 268

$$Accuracy = 1 - \left(\frac{FP + FN}{TP + FN}\right) = 1 - 1989 = 8011$$

Figure 23. Assessment of segmentation for SSP tendon ultrasound image with pathological condition tear within tendinosis

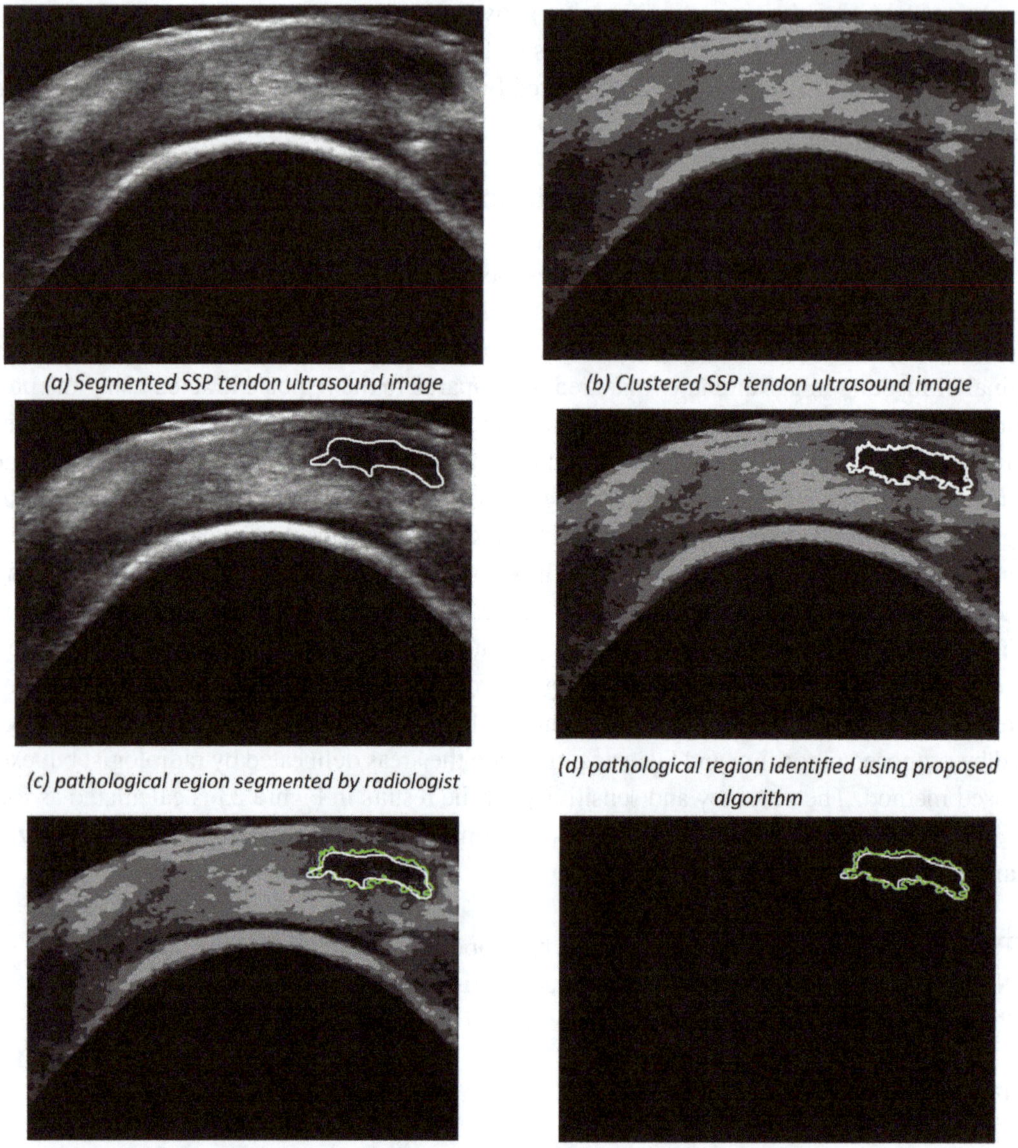

(a) Segmented SSP tendon ultrasound image

(b) Clustered SSP tendon ultrasound image

(c) pathological region segmented by radiologist

(d) pathological region identified using proposed algorithm

(e) Overlay of region segmented by radiologist and proposed algorithm over clustered image

(f) Overlay of region segmented by radiologist and proposed algorithm over dark background.

$$Sensitivity = \frac{TP}{TP + FN} = \frac{4489}{4489 + 268} = 9437$$

In the second image shown in Figure 24 the primary or initial diagnosis of radiologist suggested patient to be suffering from tendinosis and tear in the tendon. The clustered segmented image confirms diagnosis. The region for pathological condition is clearly segmented in clustered image. The analysis

Figure 24. Assessment of segmentation of SSP tendon ultrasound image with tear as pathological condition

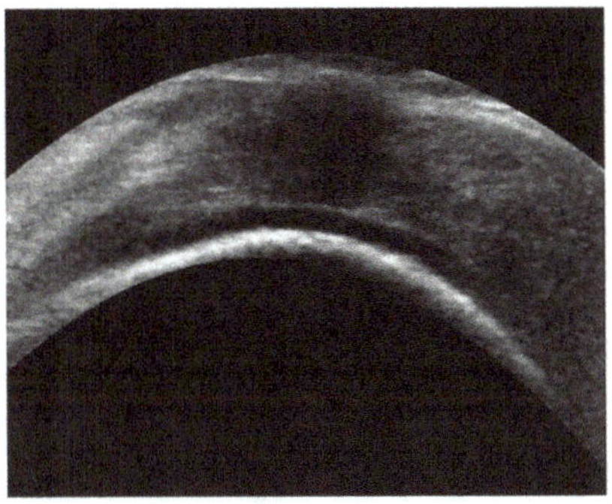

(a) Segmented SSP tendon ultrasound image

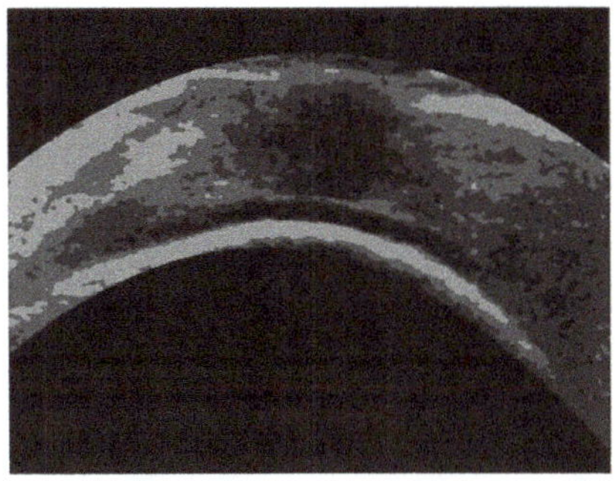

(b) Clustered SSP tendon ultrasound image

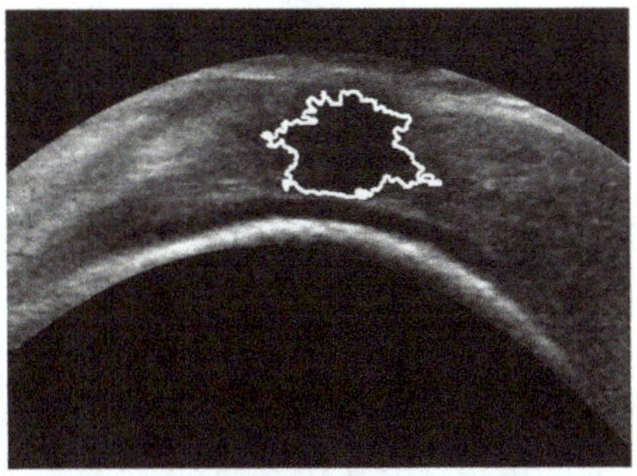

(c) patholgoical region segmented by radiologist

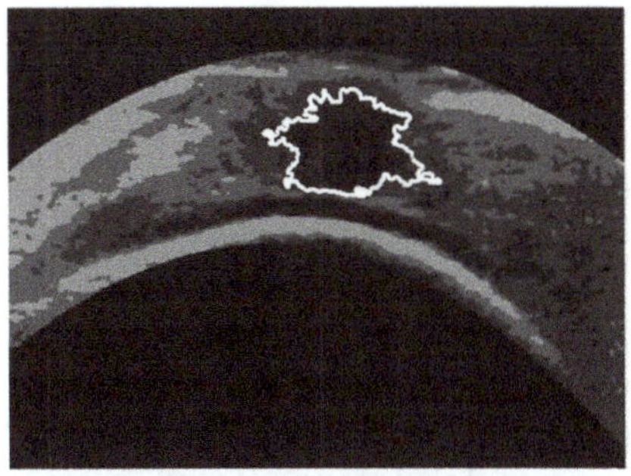

(d) pathological region identified using proposed algorithm

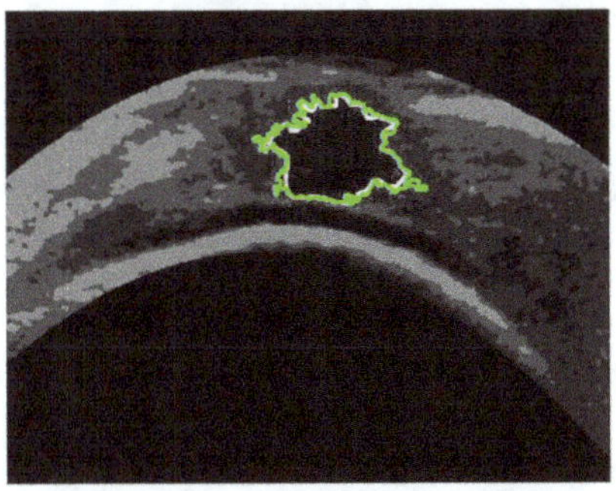

(e) Overlay of region segmented by radiologist and proposed algorithm over clustered image

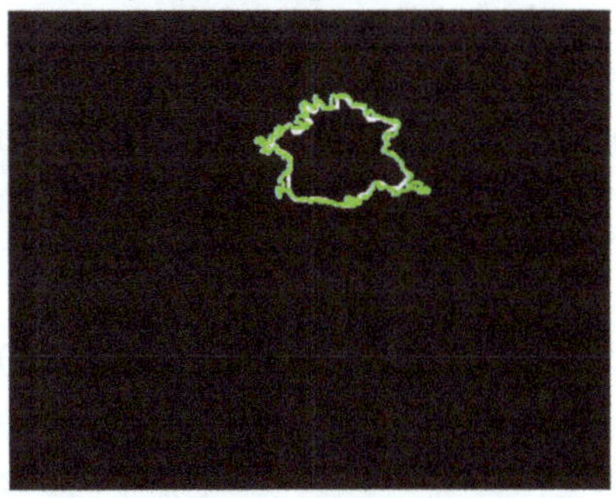

(f) Overlay of region segmented by radiologist and proposed algorithm over dark background

for the results was performed based on the comparison with the radiologist delineation of the pathological region. The quantitative values regarding the performance are calculated in the form of accuracy and sensitivity.

The area is computed based on the analysis of number of pixels enclosing the manual segmented region and radiologist segmented region.

- **TP:** Number of pixels correctly identified.
- **FN:** Number of pixels extracted by radiologist – TP.
- **FP:** Number of pixels extracted by proposed algorithm – TP.

For Figure 24:

TP = 7887 pixels;
Region segmented by radiologist = 8024 pixels;
Region segmented by proposed algorithm = 8542 pixels;
FP = 8942-7887 = 1055
FN = 8024 – 7887 = 137

$$Accuracy = 1 - \left(\frac{FP + FN}{TP + FN} \right) = 1 - 1486 = 8514$$

$$Sensitivity = \frac{TP}{TP + FN} = \frac{7887}{7887 + 137} = 9842$$

The accuracy of the algorithm for this image is calculated to be 85.14% and sensitivity is calculated as 98.42%. The quantitative analysis of the 30 images is provided in Table 3.

Table 4 details the summary of the proposed algorithm using sensitivity and accuracy based on 30 images.

The standard deviation in the results obtained for sensitivity and accuracy is also tabulated with sensitivity as 9195±0789 and accuracy as 8071±0724.

SUMMARY OF PROPOSED CAD TOOL

The developed CAD tool successfully implemented three algorithms for assessment of Supraspinatus tendon. The brief summary about enhancement, segmentation and clustering is provided in subsequent section.

Enhancement: Improved Visualization of SSP Tendon

This work studies the statistical nature of SSP tendon ultrasound image for normal and pathological tissue and based on the analysis of gray levels in tissues, four possible statistical distributions were considered for further investigation. The goodness of fit test was conducted and significance values were calculated to evaluate the fitness of different models for SSP tendon image. The analysis suggested Rayleigh as the best fit for SSP tendon data followed by Weibull, normal and log-normal distributions. Since the significance value for log-normal enhanced image was very low, therefore, the enhancement was performed using Rayleigh, Weibull and normal distributions.

Table 3. Accuracy and sensitivity analysis for proposed method of pathologies assessment

Image Number	Sensitivity	Accuracy
1	9614	8441
2	9086	7965
3	8857	7936
4	9723	8365
5	9124	8234
6	9352	8125
7	9154	8025
8	9312	8153
9	9736	8412
10	9152	8025
11	9456	8324
12	9125	8061
13	8763	7825
14	9245	8125
15	9786	8352
16	9824	8456
17	9752	8497
18	8516	7632
19	8612	7756
20	9763	8564
21	9154	8065
22	9438	8152
23	9515	8291
24	9671	8451
25	9327	8215
26	9457	8312
27	8632	7842
28	5516	4478
29	9736	8672
30	9458	8406
Average	**9195**	**8071**

Table 4. Summary of pathology assessment

Total Images	Sensitivity ± Std. Dev.	Accuracy ± Std. Dev.
30	9195±0789	8071±0724

The resultant images obtained were compared with original image generated by ultrasound equipment. The comparison was performed based on qualitative and quantitative assessment of resultant images. For qualitative assessment, two experienced radiologist were involved for the validation of obtained enhanced images in three different rounds of assessment. The statistical analysis of the assessment obtained by radiologist was performed for inter and intra variability test. For quantitative assessment, several parameter metrics such as universal quality index, signal to noise ratio, structural similarity index, structural content and mean square error were considered.

It was concluded both quantitatively and qualitatively that assessment of SSP tendon ultrasound image using Rayleigh distribution has improved results for diagnosis of tear, and tendinosis as pathological conditions in SSP tendon.

Segmentation: Focused Assessment

For focused assessment of SSP tendon, algorithm was developed that extracts SSP tendon from ultrasound image. The shape and anatomical features of SSP tendon were taken into consideration. In all ultrasound images of SSP tendon taken by different radiologist and machines, convex shape of ultrasound image is common. The anatomical location of SSP tendon in ultrasound image suppressed between humeral cortex and bursae also gives a unique feature which was exploited for generating mask for SSP tendon. The feature extraction was performed using curvelet method due to its property of preserving edges along the curves and unique features of SSP tendon ultrasound image. The image reconstructed using extracted curvelet coefficients contain outliers which has to be removed for accurate extraction of tendon. Therefore, to accomplish the task of extraction of SSP tendon mask from reconstructed image, morphological and logical operators along with connected component analysis was performed. The method was successfully tested over available database of SSP tendon ultrasound image. To sum up, the method of segmentation of SSP tendon gives us two-fold purpose. First, it provides us new method for extraction of features from curvelet coefficients by computing the energy from image reconstructed using curvelet coefficients and image delineated by radiologist. Second, it solves the purpose for focused assessment of SSP tendon.

The method was tested qualitatively for performance of the algorithm by calculating the true positive rate, false positive and accuracy of the algorithm and qualitative assessment for enhanced diagnostic capabilities was performed with the help of radiologists by assessing the pathological conditions of PTTs and FTTs in SSP tendon. The obtained result shows increased sensitivity and specificity for diagnosis of PTTs and FTTs over existing methods.

Clustering: Pathologies Identification

For objective assessment, clustering algorithm is proposed which uses the concept of Fuzzy C-means clustering and edge adaptive directional kernel regression method. The determination of number of clusters was done by computing between to within variability among the structures in SSP tendon. The proposed method incorporates information from local neighborhood, information from spatial distance of local pixels and also gradient information from the neighborhood pixels within the window.

The proposed algorithm was tested with the synthetic, optical and medical images by varying noise type (Gaussian, salt and pepper, and speckle) and level (10%, 30%, and 50%). The accuracy for synthetic images was evaluated based on the segmentation accuracy of the algorithm; results obtained were compared with existing state of art methods for clustering. Later, the algorithm was tested with real optical images of cameraman, four coins image, eight coins image by varying noise type (Gaussian, salt and pepper, and speckle) and level (10%, 30%, and 50%). For real images, segmentation accuracy cannot be taken as the quantitative parameter due to the lack of ground truth image. Therefore, entropy based parameter has been used which calculates the layout entropy and expected region entropy to evaluate the performance of the clustering algorithm. The method was also tested for two medical brain MRI images, by varying noise type (Gaussian, salt and pepper, and speckle) and level (10%, 30%, and 50%). The obtained result for medical images indicates the performance of proposed algorithm better than previous compared algorithms in preserving details and insensitiveness to outliers.

The clustering algorithm was further used to objectively calculate the region of pathologies in SSP tendon. The assessment of the clustering results was performed based on the comparison of radiologist delineation of pathological region and region identified using proposed algorithm. The result obtained shows the improvement in the diagnosis of pathologies in SSP tendon and also confirms the reproducibility of the diagnostics.

FUTURE RECOMMENDATIONS

In each step of proposed algorithms, key issues have been discussed. Here are some points which appears throughout and raises perspectives worth investigating for future development of the methods.

In the first part of the CAD tool, results suggest increased accuracy of method for diagnosing the pathologies in SSP tendon. The results obtained were verified both qualitatively and quantitatively. The method used Rayleigh, Weibull, normal and log-normal distributions for enhancing the contrast of images for diagnosis of tear and tendinosis. However, it is of utmost importance to investigate the presence of other pathological conditions in SSP tendon, particularly, identification of calcification. To this purpose, it could be useful to consider other statistical models or mixture models such as Nakagami, K-, Gamma, Rician or even combination of such distributions to form a mixture model.

For the second part, i.e., segmentation of SSP tendon the accuracy of the algorithm is calculated to be 94.82%. To increase the accuracy, modifications in existing protocols for diagnosis of SSP tendon should be devised so as to get clear picture of tendon. The reason for false segmentation was lack of bursae structure or isotropic nature of ultrasound imaging, both of which are caused due to orientation and alignment of transducer towards the SSP tendon to be imaged.

In the objective assessment of pathological condition, the area of pathology is determined by the proposed method. The identification of pathology is performed by radiologist with the help of clustered image provided by proposed algorithm. To automate the identification and classification of pathologies and thereby assisting radiologist, the texture features of clustered image can be studied.

CONTROVERSIES

The major controversies for the development of CAD tool for medical assistance in ultrasound is the effectiveness and credibility of the tool. Since ultrasound medical imaging modality provides the tomographical view of tissue under imaging for which ground truth is mostly not available and radiologist delineation of tissue is considered as ground truth. Therefore, quantitative validation of the proposed method cannot be performed. The method of validation mostly depends on medical practitioners and is qualitative in nature.

DISCUSSION AND CONCLUSION

For enhancement of SSP tendon ultrasound images, average cohen (κ) value were calculated for three assessments performed by radiologists. For qualitative assessment, interobserver and intraobserver agreement between the radiologist was calculated using (Harold L. Kundel, 2003; Naredo, et al., 2006). For quantitative assessment, different image measurement metrics such as UQI, SNR, SSI, MSE, and SC were included (Zhou & Bovik, 2002). The results obtained shows the average interobserver agreement was 7394 for Rayleigh distribution followed by 7232 for Weibull, 6886 for original image and 6016 for normal enhanced image. The computed cohen (κ) values suggest considerable agreement between the radiologist for Rayleigh, Weibull and original image whereas for normal enhanced image moderate agreement has been observed based on the values of parameter metric in (Harold L. Kundel, 2003; Naredo, et al., 2006). For tear, intra-observer agreement using enhancement performed by Rayleigh is 76.33% for radiologist 1 and 833% for radiologist 2, which was followed by Weibull with percentage agreement of 76% by radiologist 1 and 77% by radiologist 2; original image shows the agreement of 72.66% by radiologist 1 and 76.33% by radiologist 2. The enhancement performed by normal enhanced image gives intra-observer agreement for radiologist 1 to be 69.33% and for radiologist 2 to be 68.66% which is lower than that for original image. For tendinosis, observation of results suggested Rayleigh to be having higher percentage agreement within radiologist with 80% for radiologist 1 and 83% for radiologist 2 followed by original with agreement of 73.33% by radiologist 1 and 79.33% from radiologist 2, Weibull with agreement of 72.33% and 76.33% for radiologist 1 and radiologist 2 respectively. Normal enhanced image gives the lowest percentage for intraobserver agreement between three rounds. The intraobserver agreement for Rayleigh was found to be higher for tear and tendinosis. Further for tendinosis, original image is at second position, Weibull at third position and normal enhanced image with least intraobserver agreement. The inter and intraobserver agreement are in accordance with the literature in (El Khouli et al., 2009). The pattern for pathological condition tear was bit different with Rayleigh at first position followed by Weibull at second and original at third, normal enhanced image gives least intraobserver agreement. The quantitative assessment of the results obtained was performed further using five different performance parameter metrics. The qualitative and quantitative results of the enhancement ensures Rayleigh to provide best results followed by Weibull at second position and original image at third followed by normal enhanced image giving least values.

The segmentation of the SSP tendon from ultrasound image is intended to provide a focused assessment of the tendon to the radiologist. The accuracy for extracting the tendon from the ultrasound image is computed to be 94.82% when considering a database of 116 images. Being a pioneer work the database for the segmentation comparison was not available. Therefore, a study was conducted based on the comparison of diagnosis of pathological conditions using normal images and focused SSP tendon images. The pathological conditions of partial thickness tear (PTT) and full thickness (FTT) was diagnosed and compared, results obtained shows increased performance in the detection of pathological conditions, PTT and FTT, compared to the previous work (Abd-ElGawad, Ibraheem, & Fouly, 2013; Rutten, Jager, & Kiemeney, 2010; Singh, 2012). The focused SSP tendon gives the sensitivity of 94% and specificity of 93.6% for PTT compared to sensitivity of 92.3% and specificity of 92.6% reported in the previous work. Similarly, for diagnosis of FTT the sensitivity and specificity is increased from 92.6% and 94% to respectively 95.6% and 95.6%.

Lastly, clustering method was proposed for objective assessment using basic concept of Fuzzy C means and edge adaptive kernel regression, the assessment performed yielded sensitivity and accuracy of 9195±0789 and 8071±0724 for assessment of pathological conditions. The proposed algorithm for clustering was tested with the synthetic images, real images, and medical images by varying noise type (Gaussian, salt and pepper, and speckle) and level (10%, 30%, and 50%). The accuracy of the proposed algorithm was compared with existing state of art clustering methods such as N-cut (Fowlkes, et al., 2004), FLICM (Krinidis & Chatzis, 2010), RFLICM (Maoguo, et al., 2012), and KWFLICM (Maoguo, et al., 2013). For quantitative validation, the accuracy for synthetic images was evaluated based on the segmentation accuracy of the algorithm; results obtained were compared with existing state of art methods for clustering. For real images, segmentation accuracy cannot be taken as the quantitative parameter due to the lack of ground truth image. Therefore, entropy based parameter has been used which calculates the layout entropy and expected region entropy to evaluate the performance of the clustering algorithm. The entropy index for the proposed method was found to be lowest compared to other methods. The method was also tested for medical images (MRI and ultrasound), the speckle noise of 50% was introduced to the images and entropy was calculated for resultant images for proposed algorithm and four other algorithms. The obtained result for medical images indicates higher performance of proposed algorithm over previous algorithms in preserving details and its insensitiveness to outliers. The visual results obtained from the algorithm on ultrasound images is also provided, the results yield increased accuracy for assessment of pathological condition in SSP tendon.

The developed CAD tool for diagnosis of SSP tendon has been developed, tested and proven to be efficient for diagnosis of pathological conditions by radiologists. The tool is tested successfully to tackle pathological conditions such as tear and tendinosis. Since its foundations are mathematical and depends on the invariant features of SSP tendon image, therefore, the method is applicable to all the images of SSP tendon taken from different source and radiologists. The developed tool incorporates the method for improved, focused and objective assessment of pathological condition: tear and tendinosis. The developed method can be applied for other applications of ultrasound imaging as well. It is envisaged that the developed methodology may fuel future research endeavors for improved and reliable diagnosis of medical images for other anatomical regions.

REFERENCES

Abd-ElGawad, E. A., Ibraheem, M. A., & Fouly, E. H. (2013). Evaluation of supraspinatus muscle tears by ultrasonography and magnetic resonance imaging in comparison with surgical findings. *The Egyptian Journal of Radiology and Nuclear Medicine*, *44*(4), 829–834. doi:10.1016/j.ejrnm.2013.08.001

Ahuja, A. T., Ying, M., Ho, S. Y., Antonio, G., Lee, Y. P., & King, A. D. (2008). Ultrasound of malignant cervical lymph nodes. *Cancer Imaging; the Official Publication of the International Cancer Imaging Society*, *8*, 48–56. PMID:18390388

Ahumada, A. J., & Null, C. H. (1993). *Digital images and human vision. chapter Image quality: a multidimensional problem*. Cambridge, MA: MIT Press.

Araki, T., Ikeda, N., Dey, N., Chakraborty, S., Saba, L., Kumar, D., & Suri, J. S. et al. (2015). A comparative approach of four different image registration techniques for quantitative assessment of coronary artery calcium lesions using intravascular ultrasound. *Computer Methods and Programs in Biomedicine*, *118*(2), 158–172. doi:10.1016/j.cmpb.2014.11.006 PMID:25523233

Carneiro, G., Georgescu, B., Good, S., & Comaniciu, D. (2007). Automatic fetal measurements in ultrasound using constrained probabilistic boosting tree. *Med Image Comput Comput Assist Interv*, *10*(Pt 2), 571–579. PMID:18044614

Carneiro, G., Georgescu, B., Good, S., & Comaniciu, D. (2008). Detection and Measurement of Fetal Anatomies from Ultrasound Images using a Constrained Probabilistic Boosting Tree. Medical Imaging. *IEEE Transactions on*, *27*(9), 1342–1355.

Chunming, L., Rui, H., Zhaohua, D., Gatenby, J. C., Metaxas, D. N., & Gore, J. C. (2011). A Level Set Method for Image Segmentation in the Presence of Intensity Inhomogeneities With Application to MRI. Image Processing. *IEEE Transactions on*, *20*(7), 2007–2016.

Drakonaki, E. E., Allen, G. M., & Wilson, D. J. (2009). Real-time ultrasound elastography of the normal Achilles tendon: Reproducibility and pattern description. *Clinical Radiology*, *64*(12), 1196–1202. doi:10.1016/j.crad.2009.08.006 PMID:19913130

El Khouli, R. H., Macura, K. J., Jacobs, M. A., Khalil, T. H., Kamel, I. R., Dwyer, A., & Bluemke, D. A. (2009). Dynamic contrast-enhanced MRI of the breast: Quantitative method for kinetic curve type assessment. *AJR. American Journal of Roentgenology*, *193*(4), W295-300. doi:10.2214/AJR.09.2483 PMID:19770298

Eranki, A., Cortes, N., Feren, Z. G., & Sikdar, S. (2013). *A Novel Application of Musculoskeletal Ultrasound Imaging*. Academic Press.

Feleppa, E. J., Mamou, J., Porter, C. R., & Machi, J. (2011). Quantitative ultrasound in cancer imaging. *Seminars in Oncology*, *38*(1), 136–150. doi:10.1053/j.seminoncol.2010.11.006 PMID:21362522

Fowlkes, C., Belongie, S., Fan, C., & Malik, J. (2004). Spectral grouping using the Nystrom method. *Pattern Analysis and Machine Intelligence. IEEE Transactions on*, *26*(2), 214–225.

Ghose, S., Oliver, A., Marti, R., Llado, X., Vilanova, J. C., Freixenet, J., & Meriaudeau, F. et al. (2012). A survey of prostate segmentation methodologies in ultrasound, magnetic resonance and computed tomography images. *Computer Methods and Programs in Biomedicine*, *108*(1), 262–287. doi:10.1016/j.cmpb.2012.04.006 PMID:22739209

Habermeyer, P., Krieter, C., Tang, K. L., Lichtenberg, S., & Magosch, P. (2008). A new arthroscopic classification of articular-sided supraspinatus footprint lesions: A prospective comparison with Snyder's and Ellman's classification. *Journal of Shoulder and Elbow Surgery*, *17*(6), 909–913. doi:10.1016/j.jse.2008.06.007 PMID:18818103

Harold, L., & Kundel, M. P. (2003). Measurement of Observer Agreement. *Radiology*, *228*(2), 303–308. doi:10.1148/radiol.2282011860 PMID:12819342

Harris-Love, M. O., Monfaredi, R., Ismail, C., Blackman, M. R., & Cleary, K. (2014). Quantitative ultrasound: Measurement considerations for the assessment of muscular dystrophy and sarcopenia. *Front Aging Neurosci*, *6*, 172. doi:10.3389/fnagi.2014.00172 PMID:25071570

Hassenpflug, P., Prager, R. W., Treece, G. M., & Gee, A. H. (2005). Speckle classification for sensorless freehand 3-D ultrasound. *Ultrasound in Medicine & Biology*, *31*(11), 1499–1508. doi:10.1016/j.ultrasmedbio.2005.07.007 PMID:16286028

Horng, & Chen, S.-M. (2009). Multi-class Classification of Ultrasonic Supraspinatus Images based on Radial Basis Function Neural Network. *Journal of Medical and Biological Engineering*, *29*(5), 242–250.

Horng, M.-H. (2013). The Glowworm Swarm Optimization for Training the Radial Basis Function Network in Ultrasonic Supraspinatus Image Classification. *Advanced Science Letters*, *19*(9), 2724–2727. doi:10.1166/asl.2013.4977

Ikeda, N., Gupta, A., Dey, N., Bose, S., Shafique, S., Arak, T., & Suri, J. S. et al. (2015). Improved correlation between carotid and coronary atherosclerosis SYNTAX score using automated ultrasound carotid bulb plaque IMT measurement. *Ultrasound in Medicine & Biology*, *41*(5), 1247–1262. doi:10.1016/j.ultrasmedbio.2014.12.024 PMID:25638311

Insana, M. F., & Hall, T. J. (1990). Characterising the microstructure of random media using ultrasound. *Physics in Medicine and Biology*, *35*(10), 1373–1386. doi:10.1088/0031-9155/35/10/003 PMID:2243842

Kadah, Y. M., Farag, A. A., Zurada, J. M., Badawi, A. M., & Youssef, A. M. (1996). Classification algorithms for quantitative tissue characterization of diffuse liver disease from ultrasound images. *IEEE Transactions on Medical Imaging*, *15*(4), 466–478. doi:10.1109/42.511750 PMID:18215928

Katayose, M., & Magee, D. J. (2001). The cross-sectional area of supraspinatus as measured by diagnostic ultrasound. *The Journal of Bone and Joint Surgery. British Volume*, *83*(4), 565–568. doi:10.1302/0301-620X.83B4.11153 PMID:11380133

Krinidis, S., & Chatzis, V. (2010). A Robust Fuzzy Local Information C-Means Clustering Algorithm. Image Processing. *IEEE Transactions on*, *19*(5), 1328–1337.

Ladak, H. M., Mao, F., Wang, Y., Downey, D. B., Steinman, D. A., & Fenster, A. (2000). Prostate boundary segmentation from 2D ultrasound images. *Medical Physics*, *27*(8), 1777–1788. doi:10.1118/1.1286722 PMID:10984224

Landis, K. G. Jr, & Koch, G. G. (1977). The measurement of observer agreement for categorical data. *Biometrics*, *33*(1), 159–174. doi:10.2307/2529310 PMID:843571

Ledesma-Carbayo, M. J., Kybic, J., Desco, M., Santos, A., Suhling, M., Hunziker, P., & Unser, M. (2005). Spatio-temporal nonrigid registration for ultrasound cardiac motion estimation. *IEEE Transactions on Medical Imaging*, *24*(9), 1113–1126. doi:10.1109/TMI.2005.852050 PMID:16156350

Lenza, M., Buchbinder, R., Takwoingi, Y., Johnston, R. V., Hanchard, N. C., & Faloppa, F. (2013). Magnetic resonance imaging, magnetic resonance arthrography and ultrasonography for assessing rotator cuff tears in people with shoulder pain for whom surgery is being considered. *Cochrane Database of Systematic Reviews*, *9*, CD009020. PMID:24065456

Leung, J. L., & Griffith, J. F. (2008). Sonography of chronic Achilles tendinopathy: A case-control study. *Journal of Clinical Ultrasound*, *36*(1), 27–32. doi:10.1002/jcu.20388 PMID:17721925

Liao, Y. Y., Li, C. H., Tsui, P. H., Chang, C. C., Kuo, W. H., Chang, K. J., & Yeh, C.-K. (2012). Strain-compounding technique with ultrasound Nakagami imaging for distinguishing between benign and malignant breast tumors. *Medical Physics*, *39*(5), 2325–2333. doi:10.1118/1.3700167 PMID:22559602

Lizzi, F. L., Astor, M., Liu, T., Deng, C., Coleman, D. J., & Silverman, R. H. (1997). Ultrasonic spectrum analysis for tissue assays and therapy evaluation. *International Journal of Imaging Systems and Technology*, *8*(1), 3–10. doi:10.1002/(SICI)1098-1098(1997)8:1<3::AID-IMA2>3.0.CO;2-E

Lizzi, F. L., Greenebaum, M., Feleppa, E. J., Elbaum, M., & Coleman, D. J. (1983). Theoretical framework for spectrum analysis in ultrasonic tissue characterization. *The Journal of the Acoustical Society of America*, *73*(4), 1366–1373. doi:10.1121/1.389241 PMID:6853848

Madabhushi, A., & Metaxas, D. N. (2003). Combining low-, high-level and empirical domain knowledge for automated segmentation of ultrasonic breast lesions. *IEEE Transactions on Medical Imaging*, *22*(2), 155–169. doi:10.1109/TMI.2002.808364 PMID:12715992

Mamou, J., Coron, A., Oelze, M. L., Saegusa-Beecroft, E., Hata, M., Lee, P., & Feleppa, E. J. et al. (2011). Three-dimensional high-frequency backscatter and envelope quantification of cancerous human lymph nodes. *Ultrasound in Medicine & Biology*, *37*(3), 345–357. doi:10.1016/j.ultrasmedbio.2010.11.020 PMID:21316559

Maoguo, G., Yan, L., Jiao, S., Wenping, M., & Jingjing, M. (2013). Fuzzy C-Means Clustering With Local Information and Kernel Metric for Image Segmentation. Image Processing. *IEEE Transactions on*, *22*(2), 573–584.

Maoguo, G., Zhiqiang, Z., & Jingjing, M. (2012). Change Detection in Synthetic Aperture Radar Images based on Image Fusion and Fuzzy Clustering. Image Processing. *IEEE Transactions on*, *21*(4), 2141–2151.

Massich, J., Meriaudeau, F., Pérez, E., Martí, R., Oliver, A., & Martí, J. (2010). Lesion Segmentation in Breast Sonography. In J. Martí, A. Oliver, J. Freixenet, & R. Martí (Eds.), *Digital Mammography* (Vol. 6136, pp. 39–45). Springer Berlin Heidelberg. doi:10.1007/978-3-642-13666-5_6

Massich, J., Meriaudeau, F., Sentís, M., Ganau, S., Pérez, E., & Martí, R. et al.. (2012). Automatic Seed Placement for Breast Lesion Segmentation on US Images. In A. A. Maidment, P. Bakic, & S. Gavenonis (Eds.), *Breast Imaging* (Vol. 7361, pp. 308–315). Springer Berlin Heidelberg. doi:10.1007/978-3-642-31271-7_40

Mohana Shankar, P., Dumane, V. A., Reid, J. M., Genis, V., Forsberg, F., & Piccoli, C. W. (2001). Classification of ultrasonic B-mode images of breast masses using Nakagami distribution. *Ultrasonics, Ferroelectrics and Frequency Control. IEEE Transactions on*, *48*(2), 569–580.

Naredo, E., Moller, I., Moragues, C., de Agustin, J. J., Scheel, A. K., & Grassi, W. (2006). Interobserver reliability in musculoskeletal ultrasonography: Results from a "Teach the Teachers" rheumatologist course. *Annals of the Rheumatic Diseases*, *65*(1), 14–19. doi:10.1136/ard.2005.037382 PMID:15941835

Nielsen, P. K., Jensen, B. R., Darvann, T., Jørgensen, K., & Bakke, M. (2000). Quantitative ultrasound image analysis of the supraspinatus muscle. Clinical Biomechanics, 15. *Supplement, 1*(0), S13–S16.

Nielsen, P. K., Jensen, B. R., Darvann, T., Jorgensen, K., & Bakke, M. (2006). Quantitative ultrasound tissue characterization in shoulder and thigh muscles--a new approach. *BMC Musculoskeletal Disorders, 7*(1), 2. doi:10.1186/1471-2474-7-2 PMID:16420695

Noble, J. A., & Boukerroui, D. (2006). Ultrasound image segmentation: A survey. Medical Imaging. *IEEE Transactions on, 25*(8), 987–1010.

Noble, J. A., & Wells, P. N. T. (2010). Ultrasound image segmentation and tissue characterization. *Proceedings of the Institution of Mechanical Engineers. Part H, Journal of Engineering in Medicine, 224*(2), 307–316. doi:10.1243/09544119JEIM604 PMID:20349821

Ottenheijm, R. P., van't Klooster, I. G., Starmans, L. M., Vanderdood, K., de Bie, R. A., Dinant, G. J., & Cals, J. W. L. (2014). Ultrasound-diagnosed disorders in shoulder patients in daily general practice: A retrospective observational study. *BMC Family Practice, 15*(1), 115. doi:10.1186/1471-2296-15-115 PMID:24916105

Perez, J. E., Miller, J. G., Wickline, S. A., Holland, M. R., Waggoner, A. D., Barzilai, B., & Sobel, B. E. (1992). Quantitative ultrasonic imaging: Tissue characterization and instantaneous quantification of cardiac function. *The American Journal of Cardiology, 69*(20), 104H–111H. doi:10.1016/0002-9149(92)90653-G PMID:1605115

Prevost, R., Mory, B., Cuingnet, R., Correas, J.-M., Cohen, L., & Ardon, R. (2014). Kidney Detection and Segmentation in Contrast-Enhanced Ultrasound 3D Images. In A. S. El-Baz, L. Saba, & J. Suri (Eds.), *Abdomen and Thoracic Imaging* (pp. 37–67). Springer. doi:10.1007/978-1-4614-8498-1_2

Rueda, S., Fathima, S., Knight, C. L., Yaqub, M., Papageorghiou, A. T., Rahmatullah, B., & Noble, J. A. et al. (2014). Evaluation and comparison of current fetal ultrasound image segmentation methods for biometric measurements: A grand challenge. *IEEE Transactions on Medical Imaging, 33*(4), 797–813. doi:10.1109/TMI.2013.2276943 PMID:23934664

Rutten, M. J., Jager, G. J., & Kiemeney, L. A. (2010). Ultrasound detection of rotator cuff tears: Observer agreement related to increasing experience. *AJR. American Journal of Roentgenology, 195*(6), W440-446. doi:10.2214/AJR.10.4526 PMID:21098177

Scholten, R. R., Pillen, S., Verrips, A., & Zwarts, M. J. (2003). Quantitative ultrasonography of skeletal muscles in children: Normal values. *Muscle & Nerve, 27*(6), 693–698. doi:10.1002/mus.10384 PMID:12766980

Singh, J. P. (2012). Shoulder ultrasound: What you need to know. *Indian J Radiol Imaging, 22*(4), 284–292. doi:10.4103/0971-3026.111481 PMID:23833420

Teefey, S. A., Middleton, W. D., Bauer, G. S., Hildebolt, C. F., & Yamaguchi, K. (2000). Sonographic differences in the appearance of acute and chronic full-thickness rotator cuff tears. *Journal of Ultrasound in Medicine, 19*(6), 377–378, quiz 383. PMID:10841058

Teefey, S. A., Rubin, D. A., Middleton, W. D., Hildebolt, C. F., Leibold, R. A., & Yamaguchi, K. (2004). Detection and quantification of rotator cuff tears. Comparison of ultrasonographic, magnetic resonance imaging, and arthroscopic findings in seventy-one consecutive cases. *The Journal of Bone and Joint Surgery. American Volume*, *86-A*(4), 708–716. PMID:15069134

Tomonaga, T., Filipi, C. J., Lowham, A., & Martinez, T. (1999). Laparoscopic intracorporeal ultrasound cystic duct length measurement: A new technique to prevent common bile duct injuries. *Surgical Endoscopy*, *13*(2), 183–185. doi:10.1007/s004649900935 PMID:9918627

Zhang, H., Fritts, J., & Goldman, S. (2004). An entropy-based objective evaluation method for image segmentation. *Proc. SPIE- Storage and Retrieval Methods and Applications for Multimedia, 5307*, 38–49.

Zhong, T., Tagare, H. D., & Beaty, J. D. (2006). Evaluation of Four Probability Distribution Models for Speckle in Clinical Cardiac Ultrasound Images. Medical Imaging. *IEEE Transactions on*, *25*(11), 1483–1491.

Zhou, W., & Bovik, A. C. (2002). A universal image quality index. *Signal Processing Letters, IEEE*, *9*(3), 81–84. doi:10.1109/97.995823

ADDITIONAL READING

Angelsen, B. (2000). *Ultrasound Imaging: Waves, Signals, and Signal Processing*. Emantec.

Bezdek, J. C., Ehrlich, R., & Full, W. (1984). FCM: The fuzzy c-means clustering algorithm. *Computers & Geosciences, 10*(2–3), 191-203. doi:

Candès, E., Demanet, L., Donoho, D., & Ying, L. (2006). Fast Discrete Curvelet Transforms. *Multiscale Modeling & Simulation, 5*(3), 861-899. doi: doi:11137/05064182X

Goodman, J. W. (1975). *Statistical properties of laser speckle patterns* (Vol. 9). Springer Berlin Heidelberg.

Maoguo, G., Yan, L., Jiao, S., Wenping, M., & Jingjing, M. (2013). Fuzzy C-Means Clustering With Local Information and Kernel Metric for Image Segmentation. *Image Processing, IEEE Transactions on, 22*(2), 573-584. doi: 11109/tip.2012.2219547

Nazarian, L. N., Jacobson, J. A., Benson, C. B., Bancroft, L. W., Bedi, A., McShane, J. M., . . . Yamaguchi, K. (2013). Imaging algorithms for evaluating suspected rotator cuff disease: Society of Radiologists in Ultrasound consensus conference statement. *Radiology, 267*(2), 589-595. doi: 11148/radiol.13121947

Roy, J. S., Braen, C., Leblond, J., Desmeules, F., Dionne, C. E., MacDermid, J. C., . . . Fremont, P. (2015). Diagnostic accuracy of ultrasonography, MRI and MR arthrography in the characterisation of rotator cuff disorders: a meta-analysis. *Br J Sports Med*. doi: 11136/bjsports-2014-094148

Sanches, J. M., Laine, A. F., & Suri, J. S. (2011). *Ultrasound Imaging: Advances and Applications*. Springer.

KEY TERMS AND DEFINITIONS

Body Mass Index (BMI): The measure of body fat based on height and weight.

CAD Tool: Computer aided diagnosis tool designed to assist radiologist for second rational opinion regarding diagnosis and also to make the diagnostic results reproducible.

Clustering: Method of separating gray level image into different clusters or regions based on homogeneous properties such as intensity, gradient, texture, etc.

Musculoskeletal (MSK): Musculoskeletal system comprises of bones, muscles, ligaments, joints and other connective tissues which maintains strength and stability in a body.

Supraspinatus Tendon: One of the four muscles in rotator cuff in shoulder responsible outward motion away from the body. Of all the four muscles supraspinatus tendon is affected earliest for any pathological changes.

Ultrasound: A medical imaging modality providing details regarding the anatomical structure under examination using the ultra-high frequency sound waves and helps in the identification of pathological conditions.

Chapter 11
New Imaging and Computational Technology as a Guide for Catheter Ablation of Incessant Tachyarrhythmias

Carlo Pappone
University of Milan, Italy

Vincenzo Santinelli
University of Milan, Italy

Carmine Garzillo
University of Naples, Federico II, Italy

Simonetta Crisà
University of Milan, Italy

ABSTRACT

Computational technology in the era of catheter ablation (RFA) has made it possible to experience relief from incessant atrial tachyarrhythmias (AT) by 3D electroanatomical mapping (EAM) systems. The Authors report the results of such technology in > 500 consecutive patients (57% males, mean age 56.9 years) with incessant refractory post-ablation left AT (mean cycle length 256 ms). Patients underwent electroanatomical-mapping systems, which combine electrophysiological and spatial information allowing accurate reconstruction of the whole atria with real-time activation sequence guiding RFA for continuous transmural linear lesions. Color-coded voltage and/or activation maps were successfully performed in all patients. Mapping distinguished clearly and rapidly between micro-macro-reentrant (>80%) and focal mechanisms. Acute success was obtained without major complications, with repeated procedures in about 5% of patients. EAM technology allows determining both mechanism and location of arrhythmia, ensuring successful elimination of complex arrhythmogenic substrates.

INTRODUCTION

An Epochal Change in the Management of Complex Tachyarrhythmias: Background

In the last two decades the rapid expansion of indications for catheter ablation from common supraventricular tachycardias to very complex tachyarrhythmias including atrial fibrillation, incessant atrial tachycardia and ventricular tachycardia led electrophysiologists to face more prolonged procedure times

DOI: 10.4018/978-1-5225-0140-4.ch011

with excessive fluoroscopy exposure and, then the need for stable and reproducible catheter movement, all of which require a substantial improvement in the existing traditional 2D mapping technology, and new developments (Silka, Gillette, et al., 1985; Van Hare, Velvis, & Langberg, 1990; Kay, Chong, et al., 1993; Chen, Chiang, et al., 1994; Lesh, Van Hare, et al., 1994; Poty, 1996; Chen, Tai, et al., 1998; Haissaguerre, Jais, et al., 1998; Schilling, Peters, Davies, 1998; Gornick, Adler, et al., 1999; Jais, Shah, et al., 2000; Kottkamp, Hugl, et al., 2000; Willems, Weiss, et al., 2000; Saoudi, Cosío, et al., 2001). As a result, in the last years different electroanatomical mapping systems using different ablation catheters have been increasingly developed to definitively eliminate complex refractory tachyarrhythmias in many patients with or without structural heart diseases, (Nakagawa, Shah, et al., 2001; Dixit, & Callans, 2002; Friedman, 2002; Friedman, Asirvatham, et al., 2002; Kirchhof, Loh, et al., 2002; de Groot, Schalij, et al., 2003; Kopelman, Prater, et al., 2003; Macle, Jais, et al., 2003; Marrouche, Martin, et al., 2003; Oral, Scharf, et al., 2003; Pappone, Rosanio, et al., 2003; Schenider, Ndrepepa, et al., 2003; Pappone, Manguso, et al., 2004; Pappone, Santinelli, et al., 2004; Sporton, Earley, 2004; Ventura, Rostock, et al., 2004; Corrado, Basso, et al., 2005; Gurevitz, Glikson, et al., 2005; Packer, 2005; Rotter, Takahashi, et al., 2005; Earley, Showkathali, et al., 2006; Estner, Deisenhofer, et al., 2006; Kistler, Rajappan, et al., 2006; Oral, Pappone, et al., 2006; Pappone, Augello, et al., 2006; Pappone, & Santinelli, 2006; Roberts-Thomson, Kistler, et al., 2006; Chae, Oral, et al., 2007; Jais, Matsuo, et al., 2009; Martinek, Nesser, et al., 2007; Matsuo, Lim, et al., 2007; Medi, Kalman, et al., 2009; Del Carpio Munoz, Buescher, et al., 2010; Wilber, Pappone, et al., 2010; Khaykin, Oosthuizen, et al., 2011; Barbhaiya, Kumar, et al., 2014; Kang, Etheridge et al., 2014; Kapa, & Asirvatham, 2014; Sun, & Piccini, 2014 Anter, Tschabrunn, & Josephson, 2015; Buch, & Shivkumar, 2015; Ceresnak, Nappo, & Janson, 2015; Scherr, Derval, et al., 2015; N Wang, Ouyang, et al., 2015; Winterfield, Jensen, et al., 2015; Zipes, Calkins, et al., 2015). Since 1990s catheter ablation has been commonly used to treat supraventricular tachyarrhythmias with a success rate of over 90 percent, a low risk of complications while the patient can resume the normal activities in a few days (Silka, Gillette, et al., 1985; Van Hare, Velvis, Langberg, 1990; Kay, Chong, et al., 1993; Kopelman, Prater, et al., 2003; Chen, Chiang, et al., 1994; Lesh, Van Hare, et al., 1994; Poty, 1996; Kopelman, Prater, et al., 2003). It causes little or no discomfort and is done under mild sedation with local anesthesia. In structural heart diseases, catheter ablation is usually performed for drug inefficacy or intolerance or as adjunctive therapy in patients with an implantable cardioverter-defibrillator, who are experiencing frequent DC schock discharges. Consensus groups from the European Society of Cardiology and the North American Society of Pacing and Electrophysiology have defined regular atrial tachycardia (AT) as either focal or macro-reentrant, classified according to electrophysiological mechanisms and anatomical structures (Saoudi, Cosío, et al., 2001). Focal ATs are characterised by a focal origin with subsequent centrifugal spread, with a mech- anism based in abnormal automaticity, triggered activity or micro re-entry (Chen, Tai, et al., 1998; Roberts-Thomson, Kistler, et al., 2006). Macro-reentrant ATs, by contrast, involve a larger re-entry circuit, conventionally defined by a diameter in excess of 2 cm. The most common form of macro-reentrant AT involves the cavo-tricuspid isth- mus (CTI) as a critical region and has traditionally been referred to as 'typical atrial flutter'. Since this classifi- cation, a third category of atrial tachycardia has been defined. This is termed small circuit re-entry and is "some- where between micro and macro". These circuits most commonly occur after atrial fibrillation (AF) ablation pro- cedures involving extensive left atrial ablation. Radiofrequency catheter ablation was first described in pediatric patients in the early 1990s (van Hare, Velvis, & Langberg, 1990). Since then, multiple advances in the technology and understanding of this procedure have allowed this technique to blossom into one of the most powerful therapeutic tools available particularly to the pediatric electrophysiologists for children with complex tachyarrhythmias. This treatment has, in the majority of cases, replaced arrhythmia surgery as the definitive cure for most arrhythmias. Newer advances now permit therapeutic ablations using a transcatheter approach. In this technique, an electrode catheter inserted through a blood vessel during electrophysiologic studies is used to perform targeted radiofrequency applications in the heart. A patient can be cured through ablative therapy, so antiarrhythmic medication is no longer needed. There are several advantages to this therapy when used in the common indications: no exercise restrictions, no need for chronic drug therapy, and the avoidance of hospital visits for breakthrough episodes.

From Conventional Two Dimensional Fluoroscopy to Recent Three Dimensional Electroanatomic Mapping Systems

Before an ablation procedure can be performed, the electrophysiologists must first identify the area where abnormal rhythm is coming from (arrhythmogenic substrate). Then, they should record the surrounding local electrical activity during abnormal rhythm or arrhythmia inducibility to create a detailed "map" of the precise area of heart muscle responsible, which require a complete understanding of current mapping techniques to exactly identify the arrhythmia substrate for successful ablation/elimination (Silka, Gillette, et al., 1985; Van Hare, Velvis, Langberg, 1990; Kay, Chong, et al., 1993; Chen, Chiang, et al., 1994; Lesh, Van Hare, et al., 1994; Poty, 1996; Kopelman, Prater, et al., 2003). Fluoroscopy alone has been always used to locate and direct catheters to potential areas that cause arrhythmias. However, fluoroscopy has several risks. Indeed, fluoroscopic mapping has low 2 D spatial resolution interfering with ablation procedures that require substrate modification in which it is imperative to locate scar tissue and maintain an electrically active isthmus in the atrial or ventricular myocardium (Kottkamp, Hugl, et al., 2000; Willems, Weiss, et al., 2000). In addition, X-ray exposure may negatively affect the patient and medical staff increasing the incidence of diseases, such as dermatitis, cataracts, birth defects and cancer. Pediatric patients are also at risk, especially from gonad and thyroid irradiation. Complex electrophysiological procedures may involve a significant duration for the fluoroscopy Kottkamp, Hugl, et al., 2000; Willems, Weiss, et al., 2000; Kirchhof, Loh, et al., 2002; Rotter, Takahashi, et al., 2005). Therefore, lead aprons are worn by the medical team as well as placed over patient thyroid and gonads, and acrylic plates as well as special glasses are used to block radiation and reduce such risks. In the last two decades, the rapid expansion of indications from common supraventricular tachyarrhythmias to more complex supraventricular and/or ventricular tachyarrhythmias led electrophysiologists to face more prolonged procedure times with excessive fluoroscopy exposure and the need for stable and reproducible catheter movement, all of which require a substantial improvement in the existing traditional 2D fluoroscopic mapping technology. The recent advent of electroanatomic mapping (EAM) systems has facilitated three-dimensional imaging without X-rays, thus reducing the risks associated with fluoroscopy. Therefore, non-fluoroscopic mapping, including electroanatomic mapping (EAM), has altered percutaneous treatment of complex tachyarrhythmias, such as atrial tachycardia and atrial fibrillation (Kottkamp, Hugl, et al., 2000; Willems, Weiss, et al., 2000; Pappone, Rosanio, et al., 2003; Pappone, Manguso, et al., 2004; Pappone, Santinelli, et al., 2004). This technology is based on a simple principle by measuring the difference between the electrical potential detected on the patient surface and from the catheter in the patient's vascular structure. Therefore, the three-dimensional shape of the cavity where the catheter is located can be reconstructed with pinpoint accuracy (Pappone, Rosanio, et al., 2003;

Pappone, Manguso, et al., 2004; ; Pappone, Santinelli, et al., 2004). Thus, structures, such as veins, arteries and heart chambers, can be visualized in real-time and manipulated to discern localization of arrhythmogenic points, which can be successfully treated using ablation.

Why Use an Electroanatomical Mapping System?

While having an electroanatomic mapping system available for every ablation procedure may seem like an advantage, their expense and the additional preparatory time must be justified. This may be relatively easy to do when complex incessant tachyarrhythmias or cardiac anatomy are anticipated (Nakagawa, Shah, et al., 2001; Dixit, & Callans, 2002; Friedman, 2002; Friedman, Asirvatham, et al., 2002; Kirchhof, Loh, et al., 2002; de Groot, Schalij, et al., 2003; Pappone, Rosanio, et al., 2003; Pappone, Manguso, et al., 2004; Pappone, Santinelli, et al., 2004). When available information suggests an arrhythmia mechanism located near important structures such as a manifest bypass tract originating near the AV node, electroanatomic mapping may allow for marking of such structures so that they may be avoided. Similarly, when complex anatomy and areas of scar contributing to macroreentry are anticipated, electroanatomic mapping may allow demarcation of such regions so that they may be isolated. Non-sustained tachycardias or rapid rhythm disturbances resulting in hemodynamic compromise lend themselves well to certain electroanatomic mapping systems, as suspected sites of tachycardia origin may be more accurately recorded and targeted for ablation than with fluoroscopy alone. Chief among these, however, is electroanatomic mapping's ability to reliably allow catheter positioning without the use of fluoroscopy, a distinct advantage for both patient and operator (Pappone, Rosanio, et al., 2003; Pappone, Manguso, et al., 2004; Pappone, Santinelli, et al., 2004). Several studies have confirmed these advantages, with comparable success rates to conventional, non- electroanatomic mapping-guided approaches. Fluoroscopy time and radiation dose are indeed reduced with electroanatomic mapping when compared to conventional mapping strategies (Kottkamp, Hugl, et al., 2000; Willems, Weiss, et al., 2000; Pappone, Manguso, et al., 2004). This is true for a variety of rhythm disturbances including AV node reentry and bypass tract-mediated arrhythmias (Kirchhof, Loh, et al., 2002; Kopelman, Prater, et al., 2003) . The greatest impact of electroanatomic mapping is its application to facilitate elimination of incessant atrial tachyarrhythmias or pulmonary vein isolation for treatment for atrial fibrillation (Marrouche, Martin, et al., 2003; Oral, Scharf, et al., 2003; Pappone, Rosanio, et al., 2003; Pappone, Manguso, et al., 2004; Pappone, Santinelli, et al., 2004), but these benefits must be weighed against their added expense (Friedman, 2002).

Current Electroanatomic Mapping Systems

The currently available models include the Carto®, EnSite (NAVx)®, and Localiza® systems (Pappone, Rosanio, et al., 2003; Pappone, Manguso, et al., 2004; Pappone, Santinelli, et al., 2004; Packer, 2005; Oral, Pappone, et al., 2006; Pappone, Augello, et al., 2006; Pappone, & Santinelli, 2006; Del Carpio Munoz, Buescher, et al., 2010; Wilber, Pappone, et al., 2010; Khaykin, Oosthuizen, et al., 2011). Three-dimensional electroanatomical mapping systems have evolved as curative strategies for several refractory complex rhythm disturbances. The general principles, rationale, and working of the various mapping systems have been explained well in the existing literature (Pappone, Rosanio, et al., 2003; Pappone, Manguso, et al., 2004; ; Pappone, Santinelli, et al., 2004; Packer, 2005; Winterfield, Jensen, et al., 2015). Briefly, these systems use an electromagnetic (CARTO) or impedance-based (NAVx) catheter location method, which permits reconstruction of a color-coded three-dimensional anatomic shell of any cardiac chamber of interest. During mapping, the electrogram obtained at a given site is stored and the local activation time catalogued as compared with some selected electric signal preference. The accrued points in the map are assigned to an isochronal color-scale based on their respective local activation times. In addition to the local activation map, maps that display the voltage of the recorded electrograms can be created. For accurate interpretation of these color-coded electroanatomical maps (EAM), there are many considerations to do. Optimal catheter wall contact, appropriate interpretation of the colors on the color-coded map, appropriate choice of the reference electrogram, sufficient number of collected points for a complete and anatomical correct mapping of the chamber of interest, and strategies to address catheter tip migration with respiration or change in cardiac rhythm and annotation of complex intracardiac signals are all examples of such requisites for successful reconstruction and ablation. Among the data provided by electroanatomic mapping are local activation mapping. Several electroanatomic mapping systems have specific features, including enhanced ability to map non-sustained or hemodynamically unstable tachyarrhythmias, ability to display diagnostic as well as mapping catheter positions, and wide compatibility with a variety of catheters. Very recently, the 3D electroanatomical mapping systems with multipolar catheters have been created to provide faster data collection to efficiently deal with complex tachyarrhythmias by rapidly evaluating additional regions safer and more precisely (Barbhaiya, Kumar, et al., 2014; Sun, & Piccini, 2014). Each electroanatomic mapping system has its strengths and weaknesses, and the system chosen is essentially based on what data are required for procedural success (local activation mapping, substrate mapping, cardiac geometry), the anticipated arrhythmia, the compatibility of the system with adjunctive tools (i.e. diagnostic and ablation catheters), and, most importantly, the operator's experience with the selected system (Buch, & Shivkumar, 2015). Incorrect or inappropriate application of electroanatomic color-coded mapping can hamper mapping and procedural success, and should not replace careful interpretation of data with adherence to electrophysiological principles (Del Carpio Munoz, Buescher, et al., 2010).

Noncontact Mapping

The noncontact mapping system utilizes a multi-electrode array (MEA) catheter to simultaneously record multiple areas of endocardial activation (Dixit, & Callans, 2002; Beukema, Elvan et al., 2012; Ceresnak, Nappo, & Janson, 2015; Scherr, Derval, et al., 2015; Wang, Ouyang, et al., 2015). Hence, relatively high-density mapping can be performed from even a single beat of tachycardia. Three-dimensional (3D) localization of the MEA surface electrodes is achieved by applying a low-level 5.6 kHz current between an electrode on the distal end of the MEA catheter and two ring electrodes along its shaft, proximal and distal to the MEA itself. (Beukema, Elvan et al., 2012) Similarly, a separate mapping catheter's position can be determined by delivering current between its electrode and these two ring electrodes. Chamber geometry can be reconstructed by manipulating this mapping catheter within the chamber of interest and the corresponding electrical isopotentials can be "plotted" on this geometric representation of the endocardial surface. Advantages of the EnSite mapping system include acquisition of multiple endocardial electrograms from a single beat, rendering it quite useful in mapping atrial and ventricular ectopic beats, non-sustained arrhythmias, and rhythm disturbances that are poorly tolerated hemodynamically. Any mapping/ablation catheter is also compatible with this system. Disadvantages include inaccuracy of electrogram timing and morphology at greater distances from the MEA, difficulty in positioning the MEA balloon, and inaccuracy in reconstructing certain features of chamber geometry (Beukema, Elvan et al., 2012).

Ablation Catheters: From Single-Tip Point-by-Point to Multipoint Catheters

Traditionally, radiofrequency (RF) catheter ablation is performed using rigid single-tip, point-by-point technique, which is often time consuming and requires a high degree of operator skill. A significant number of complications may be associated with rigid irrigated-tip catheters, including but not limited to thromboembolism, pulmonary vein stenosis and atrio-oesophageal fistulae. Consequently, innovative technologies are being developed to make the catheter ablation of atrial fibrillation safer and easier (Wilber, Pappone, et al., 2010; Anter, Tschabrunn, & Josephson, 2015; Buch, & Shivkumar, 2015; Winterfield, Jensen, et al., 2015). Multipoint catheters have been recently developed representing a big advancement for successful ablation of tachyarrhythmias (Anter, Tschabrunn, & Josephson, 2015), and, currently are commonly used in our laboratory. If multipoint catheter technology is not available in electrophysiology laboratories, the Authors suggest to take at least 100 points for automatic tachycardias and 200 points for reentrant arrhythmias in a given chamber for successful ablation (Pappone, & Santinelli, 2006). More important than this arbitrary number is the need to be certain of the completeness of the map in terms of chamber geometry. Expected anatomic boundaries such as the vena cava, great arteries, and atrioventricular annuli should be included in the map. Causes for incomplete chamber mapping include an inappropriately placed reference patch (such that some points, for example, taken in a very large ventricle, will not appear in the map), diverticula, aneurysms, or pouches that have not been entered and yet may house the arrhythmogenic substrate and the need for specific epicardial mapping. Even with an automatic tachycardia, a complete map is desirable to accurately establish targeted areas for ablation (Willems, Weiss, et al., 2000; de Groot, Schalij, et al., 2003; Pappone, Manguso, et al., 2004; Packer, 2005; Pappone, & Santinelli, 2006). Flexible catheter technology may offer a promising approach, since it is relatively easy to use. It is well-known that conventional tip-irrigated catheters, being rigid, cannot always adapt to anatomical targets due to the limited contact area (Winterfield, Jensen, et al., 2015). This makes RF applications challenging, time consuming or even ineffective. The Cool Flex (St Jude Medical, St Paul, MN) is a novel, flexible and fully-irrigated tip catheter with an innovative design. It can be used in a parallel, perpendicular or angular orientation to better adapt the ablation catheter tip with the surrounding tissue (Winterfield, Jensen, et al., 2015). In addition to flexibility, the laser-cut design permits fluid to be infused around the whole catheter tip ablation electrode. The catheter deflects up to 20° with 20g of pressure. Compared with conventional rigid-tip catheters, the Cool Flex catheter is able to better adapt to a greater range of cardiac tissue anatomy using different angles of approach. This ultimately makes RF application more effective and safer (Winterfield, Jensen, et al., 2015). The unique, laser-cut electrode tip of the Therapy Cool Flex catheter has been designed to provide optimal irrigation flow over the entire tip for improved cooling compared to conventional irrigated catheter designs. The catheter electrode features irrigation slits arranged in a zigzag pattern. Four ports at the distal end of the tip to allow irrigation to flow around the surface area. In addition to this, the effect of the catheter tip bending and conforming to the tissue opens the irrigation slits on the side of the catheter tip facing the tissue. Therefore, saline flows directly to the area where it is most required. Preliminary experience with this new ablation catheter is reported in the treatment of different tachyarrhythmias, including slow and accessory pathway ablation, cavotricuspid isthmus-dependent atrial flutter and atrial fibrillation (Winterfield, Jensen, et al., 2015). One or two radiofreqency applications may be sufficient to eliminate the arrhythmogenic substrate in most patients without complications.

MAIN FOCUS OF THE CHAPTER

The purpose of this chapter was to report, describe and discuss the large experience of the Authors on the features and management of highly symptomatic patients returning with refractory incessant atrial tachycardias after atrial fibrillation ablation. The Authors also illustrate and discuss current three-dimensional electroanatomic mapping systems for successful catheter ablation examining how to create and evaluate electroanatomic maps focusing on key issues related to the latest mapping systems and ablation catheters with success rates and complications.

Methodology: Proposed Systems and Recommendations

For correct interpretation of any electroanatomical 3D maps, a variety of considerations must be understood, discussed, meticulously managed and anticipated. The good catheter contact, the appropriate choice of both the reference point and window of interest, the exit site (focal or reentrant), the complete mapping of the correct chamber of interest, the correct interpretation of the colors in the map, and the strategies to address catheter tip migration with respiration or change in cardiac rhythm with annotation of complex intracardiac signals, are all examples of such methodological pre-requisites for success of catheter ablation among patients with complex atrial tachyarrhythmias (Del Carpio Munoz, Buescher, et al., 2010; Wang, Ouyang, et al., 2015; Winterfield, Jensen, et al., 2015; Zipes, Calkins, et al., 2015). In addition, interpreting color activation maps is facilitated by knowledge of the likely arrhythmia mechanism: focal or reentrant (Del Carpio Munoz, Buescher, et al., 2010). Finally, regardless of the mechanism and when using traditional common point-by-point catheters the operator should also consider whether a sufficient number of points have been taken to adequately define both activation and anatomy, and then, whether the reference electrogram and window of interest have been appropriately selected to exactly evaluate arrhythmia mechanism (Del Carpio Munoz, Buescher, et al., 2010). The required number of points needed to construct a reliable map is dependent not only on the tachycardia mechanism, but also on the size/geometry of the chamber being mapped and on the potential involvement of other chambers that may need to be mapped (Del Carpio Munoz, Buescher, et al., 2010). It should also be emphasized that the number of points that can reasonably be obtained may be limited by the hemodynamic stability of the patient and stability of the arrhythmia (Del Carpio Munoz, Buescher, et al., 2010).

The Reference Point

During the activation sequence mapping, many data points are usually acquired as the catheter navigates across the endocardial wall of the chamber of interest and the timing of these electrograms are compared with a predetermined reference point, usually the coronary sinus for its stability (Del Carpio Munoz, Buescher, et al., 2010). As this acquisition process continues, a color-coded scheme begins to emerge on the map. With current systems, areas of red color indicate sites of "early activation" and the activation becomes progressive later proceeding through the colors of the rainbow to yellow-green, and finally the blue and purple hues defining areas of late activation relative to the reference electrogram. These colors are displayed as an isochronal time bar adjacent to the 3D map. The color-coded map is useful to accurately identify ablation targets as well as to guide as to where radiofrequency energy should be delivered

(Del Carpio Munoz, Buescher, et al., 2010). If a focal tachycardia is the arrhythmia being mapped, the earliest activation time, usually indicated on the color-coded map as "red region" represents the ablation target and then should be the optimal site for successful ablation. At successful sites of focal tachycardia, the earliest bipolar electrogram in the "red region" will precede the QRS or P wave by at least 20 to 30 ms and have a QS complex in the unipolar electrogram (Del Carpio Munoz, Buescher, et al., 2010). If the arrhythmia is due to a reentry circuit, the correct interpretation of color-coded activation maps may be more difficult. Indeed, there is no unique "early or late" area, as in focal tachycardias, because any given activation area may have other sites, which can be activated before or after that location. However, if the complete reentry circuit is extensively and accurately mapped, the red area of earliest activation should be adjacent to a purple area of latest activation, because the circulating wave front moves from the purple region back into the red region to complete the circuit. If one changes the selected reference time, as a consequence this will change the location of the red region and the same tachycardia mapped by 2 different operators, both of whom chose 2 different but appropriate reference electrograms for the map, may have a very different color-coded map sequence. If the annotation is correct, however, the sequence of activation from region to region will be the same. The proximal/mid CS electrodes are often selected as a timing reference as the atrial EGM in these poles are often of greater amplitude and fidelity than their ventricular counterparts, preventing inappropriate timing using the ventricular electrograms. Such inaccurate results can be observed if the distal CS electrodes are selected as the timing reference, for example, where the ventricular EGM amplitude is equivalent to, or even larger than the atrial EGM. The ventricular EGM may then be inappropriately taken as the timing reference yielding an incorrect and confusing activation map. When mapping ventricular tachycardias or premature ventricular complexes, a right ventricular apical recording may be chosen as a stable timing reference for ventricular activation. The timing window refers to the range of activation times surrounding reference EGM activation. Proper timing window definition requires accurate determination of the underlying tachycardia mechanism (focal versus macroreentrant tachycardia); erroneously diagnosed tachycardia mechanism will result in vastly incorrect timing window definition and consequently, creation of an invalid activation map. Once the correct tachycardia mechanism has been diagnosed, the timing window may be defined to include the extremes of cardiac activation preceding and following reference EGM activation.

The Window of Interest

In addition to selecting a reference point, electroanatomic mapping systems also select a window of interest for mapping by specifying an interval "before and after" the reference point determining the position of the reference point in the window (Del Carpio Munoz, Buescher, et al., 2010). The signals of local activation map are calculated to a reference point and the surface ECG is choosen as the electrical reference. The window of interest defines the time interval to a reference during which the local electrogram is acquired and its local acquisation time is determined and completeness is composed of two intervals, one before and one after the reference. The multipoint technology with a velocity software (Afocus for Ensite and Pentarray for CARTO) allows multiple points to be simultaneously collected, a more dense collection of map points, and greater detail on the chamber of interest. Voltage and activation contact or noncontact maps of the endocardium can be rapidly deployed using both unipolar and bipolar signals. For macroreentrant tachycardias, this window is typically specified such that the sum of the intervals approximates the tachycardia cycle length, but the window settings specifying how much of the cycle length being mapped should be shown as being before or after a particular reference electrogram is arbitrary. Two different operators may correctly choose 2 different windows of reference, again giving rise to 2 different locations for "red areas" for the same tachycardia. As a result, the red or "early" site is an entirely arbitrary area for macroreentrant arrhythmias and should not be considered as a target site for successful ablation. For focal tachycardias, the window of reference does not have to be precisely chosen. Anticipating that the true early site of activation is rarely earlier than 50 ms from the start of the surface ECG (P wave or QRS) and appreciating which component of the ECG or specific electrogram is being chosen, one can quite easily choose how much earlier than the reference the window should start. For example, if a focal ventricular tachycardia has a total QRS duration of 180 ms, a window that begins 300 ms before the peak QRS should be more than sufficient to identify the earliest site. With a focal left atrial tachycardia in a normal heart, activation beginning 160 ms earlier than a coronary sinus activation site probably would be sufficient. On the other hand, with a focal atrial tachycardia arising from the right atrium in a patient with a diseased heart and slow intra-atrial conduction, the earliest site of activation could be close to 300 ms earlier than a lateral coronary sinus reference site, and the beginning of the mapping window should exceed this time interval. Significantly more consideration is required when choosing the window of interest for reentrant tachycardias. Generally, the window of interest is chosen to be 10 or 20 ms less than the tachycardia cycle length. If the window is too short, the entire cycle length cannot be mapped, and 2 different points in the circuit may be catalogued with similar timing (for example, a tachycardia cycle length 300 ms, total window of interest 200 ms starting 100 ms before and ending 100 ms after the reference point, points that 210 to 250 ms ahead of the earliest site could all appear with the same red color annotation). On the other hand, if too large a window of interest is chosen, 2 electrograms representing activation of the same site may appear within the window of interest. If the operator does not consistently take either the earliest or later electrogram, an entirely meaningless map will be created.

The Exit Site

The exit site probably determines the surface ECG morphology (P wave or QRS complex), and activation of this region precedes the onset of the QRS or P wave in the surface ECG (Del Carpio Munoz, Buescher, et al., 2010). Whether the "red area" on color-coded electroanatomic maps is able to identify the exit site of a reentrant tachycardia requires to be clarified. Indeed, as previously discussed, the site of the red "early" region depends on both the reference point and mapping window of interest, and then it does not necessarily is able to identify the true exit of the reentry circuit. However, if the onset of the QRS or P-wave is clearly defined, we can appropriately identify the window of interest, and then the red region on the map represents the local endocardial activation immediately preceding the QRS or P-wave onset, which reasonably is the exit region. Sometimes, the complete reentry circuit (with activation spanning the entire tachycardia cycle length) cannot be identified because some areas of the circuit may be intramural/epicardial or can be associated with low-amplitude electrograms, which are not detectable by the recording system. In such circumstances, the 3D color-coded map essentially identifies the "focal" exit site of the tachycardia circuit in that chamber. If this is the circuit exit, pace mapping at that site typically resembles the tachycardia. Understanding this possibility, however, it should be remembered, as emphasized above, that when dealing with a reentrant tachycardia, the color scheme alone is not a sufficient guide to choose appropriate ablation sites.

Conduction Velocity

Commonly, reentrant tachycardias are supported by areas of slow conduction. Valuable information about conduction velocity may be gleaned from the color local activation map (Del Carpio Munoz, Buescher, et al., 2010). Each color shift represents a temporal fraction of the entire tachycardia cycle length. Thus, multiple colors evident over a small distance in the heart suggest a region of slow conduction. Interpreting color maps to ascertain conduction velocity assumes, however, that the wave front of activation is propagating roughly linearly through the region from the earlier side to the later side. That is, along the vector of the color changes. This is, however, not always the case. For example, in bystander areas of slow conduction or when adjacent areas are separated by conduction block, the wave front may reach adjacent locations from different paths. This creates a "pseudointerval" between each of these isochrones that may give the false appearance of slow conduction or the appearance of conduction when there is block between regions. This potential pitfall is influenced by the "fill threshold." Mapping systems assign an activation time over the area around an acquired point. The size of this area is determined by setting the "fill threshold." If inadequate numbers of points are taken and the fill threshold allows interpolation over a large area, the colors will not represent a true picture of either conduction velocity or activation sequence and the anatomy may also be distorted.

Characterization, Definition, and Mechanisms of Atrial Tachycardia

Atrial tachycardias are defined as either:

1. **Macro–Re-Entrant:** Continuous propagation sequence with earliest and latest activation adjacent to each other and range of activation times encompassing most of the tachycardia cycle length (Willems, Weiss, et al., 2000; Pappone, Manguso, et al., 2004), or
2. **Focal:** Radial spread of activation not covering most of the tachycardia cycle length, with ablation of the focus interrupting the tachycardia (Jais, Shah, et al., 2000; Willems, Weiss, et al., 2000; Saoudi, Cosío, et al., 2001; Pappone, Manguso, et al., 2004; Wang, Ouyang, et al., 2015; Winterfield, Jensen, et al., 2015; Zipes, Calkins, et al., 2015).

The re-entrant circuit is characterized as single or dual loop, rotating around natural anatomic barriers or previously ablated areas, which are demonstrated by activation mapping and characterized by the presence of double potential along the lines. Gaps are usually defined as breakthroughs in a previously ablated area, evidenced by activation mapping and by the absence of double potentials. A critical isthmus is commonly defined as a narrow passage between fixed obstacles, demonstrated to be a crucial component of the circuit by activation mapping. Termination of the tachycardia with ablation across the isthmus confirmed its critical role. Anatomic positions were arbitrarily defined as lateral, septal, or posterior wall. Septal and lateral LAs were subdivided in inferior, middle, and superior (roof) segments.

Macro–Reentrant Tachycardia

Catheter ablation of macro–re-entrant tachycardias is initially attempted across the critical isthmus, using an 8-mm or 3.5 mm tip irrigated ablation catheter with pulses at a target temperature of 60°C and 40°, respectively and a maximum power output of 100 W or 30 W, respectively (Willems, Weiss, et al., 2000;

Pappone, Manguso, et al., 2004). The catheter is dragged after 15 to 30 s, after causing an effective lesion, demonstrated by a reduction of the local electrogram amplitude by ≥80% or a splitting into double potentials. If the tachycardia is not interrupted, ablation is directed to close identifiable gaps involved in the circuit, or an outer loop between fixed obstacles, such as the posterior wall or the mitral isthmus. Electroanatomic-guided ablation of macro–re-entrant AT has proven to be feasible and effective (Pappone, Manguso, et al., 2004). The arrhythmia circuit can be rapidly and accurately characterized in the majority of patients, particularly using multipoint catheters. As expected, most of the tachycardias are related to discontinuities on previous ablation lines (Figures 2, 3, 4, 5, 6, 7, 8, 9, 10). In many patients, the arrhythmias are entirely related to gaps on lines at the mitral isthmus and posterior wall, and less frequently patients have lines deployed at the posterior wall during circumferential pulmonary vein ablation. Incomplete lines or recovery of conduction at these areas can create the slow conduction necessary to sustain re-entry. Although ablation at these sites are designed to avoid macro–re-entry, it is still not clear whether they actually prevent or contribute to it, and further studies are needed to define their role in circumferential pulmonary vein ablation (Pappone, Manguso, et al., 2004). The Authors observed a tendency of gaps and foci to occur at the septal aspect of the right PVs (Figures 6-10), and at the superior segment of the lateral LA, anterior to the LSPV. Many macro–reentrant tachycardias have critical components at these areas (Willems, Weiss, et al., 2000; Pappone, Manguso, et al., 2004). Continuous linear lesions are difficult to achieve, even under direct visualization during intraoperative ablation. Creating transmural, permanent lines of block with a percutaneous approach can be even more challenging at these sites (Pappone, Manguso, et al., 2004). Technical factors can be used to explain the propensity to discontinuities at specific areas. Frequently, only a narrow rim of atrial tissue between the LSPV and the LA appendage is present, which makes stable catheter positioning difficult to attain. In addition, the presence of dense pectinate muscle in the LA appendage, contiguous to the normal atrial wall, can make transmural lesion more difficult to achieve in this area. Good access to the postero-septal area is essential to perform the encircling lines of the right PVs. A very high or posterior transeptal puncture may make stable catheter positioning over the septum difficult, with the distal electrode in poor contact or inadequate orientation with the endocardial surface. Another possible explanation is the presence of muscle bundles deeply located in the epicardial fat of the posterior interatrial and atrioventricular groove.

RESULTS

Study Population

From January 1999 to January 2015 the Authors have extensively used both the CARTO and NavX systems in five hundred thirteen patients (mean age 56.9 ±3.4 years, 57% males). All patients underwent mapping and ablation of 645 left ATs (mean cycle length 256 ±110 ms), after a mean follow-up of 4.3 ± 1.2 months from the previous index ablation procedure for atrial fibrillation (Figures 1-10). Three-dimensional reconstruction of the LA was performed with an average of 95 ± 23 points. In 28 patients, the number of mapping points was limited by the nonsustained nature of the arrhythmia. Mean fluoroscopy exposure was 9.7 ± 3.6 min and procedural duration, from transseptal puncture to the end of LA ablation, was 27.5 ± 7 min. Conventional, multipoint or deflectable mapping/ablation catheters were used. Using point-by-point conventional mapping catheters with at least 100 points and coverage of at least 90% of the tachycardia cycle length the Authors have been able to accurately reconstruct

Figure 1. Panel A, top: Isochronal electroanatomical activation map of focal left atrial tachycardia using contact technique and Ensite Velocity System in left lateral projection showing centrifugal activation of the left atrium (LA) from the left atrial appendage (LAA). Bottom. The activation wavefront spreads from the LAA apex (white color) to the rest of the LA. Electrograms recorded on distal ablation catheter during atrial tachycardia show conduction delay with fractionated, double atrial electrograms, which constituted the ablation target. Panel B, bottom: Left lateral tilted electroanatomic activation map as in Panel A. The lower half of the panel shows intracardiac distal ablation electrograms during RF application at the time of AT termination with restoration of sinus rhythm.

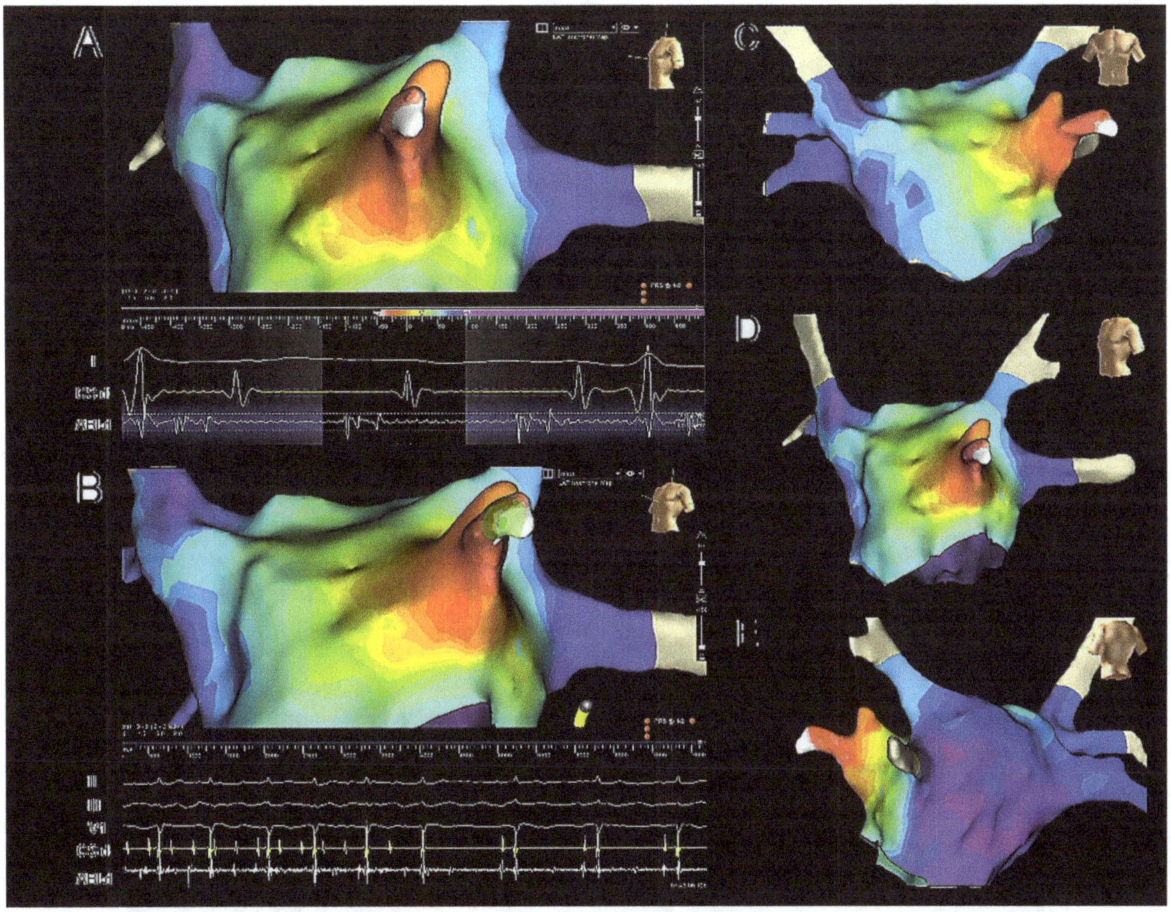

complete electroanatomical anatomical or color-coded maps in all patients in a relatively short time (mean, 25±7.3 minutes). Using multipoint technology (CARTO and Ensite systems) accurate mapping was performed with shorter (5.4±3.2 minutes) procedure times (Figures 2-10). Atrial size and geometry were automatically performed, measured and displayed by a dedicated software. During tachycardia appropriate location/timing reference and window of inerest was accurately defined and selected for each patient, as required. In all patients during tachyarrhythmias the coronary sinus was the optimal choice as a timing reference, due to its stable positioning and lower likelihood of being dislodged and disrupting activation mapping (compared to a high right atrial catheter, for example, that may be dislodged by a roving mapping catheter). Propagation maps were easily reconstructed in all patients and played back from data obtained through activation mapping, demonstrating spread of activation throughout a cardiac

Figure 2. Left lateral view of a macro-reentrant left atrial tachycardia with critical isthmus involving the mitral valve annulus showing a close spatial relationship between the earliest and latest activation "head meets tail". The color-coded maps were performed by using the focus multipoint 20 poles catheter of the Ensite system. LL: left lateral

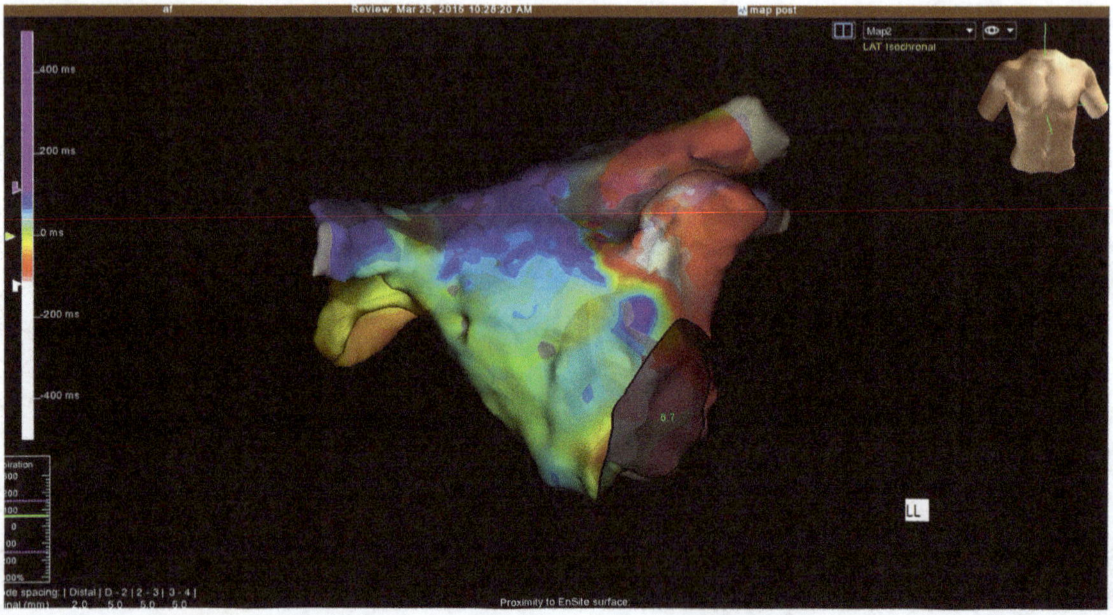

Figure 3. Antero-Posterior view of a macro-reentrant left atrial tachycardia with critical isthmus involving the mitral valve annulus showing a close spatial relationship between the earliest and latest activation "head meets tail". The color-coded maps were performed by using the focus multipoint 20 poles catheter of the Ensite system. AP: Antero-posterior

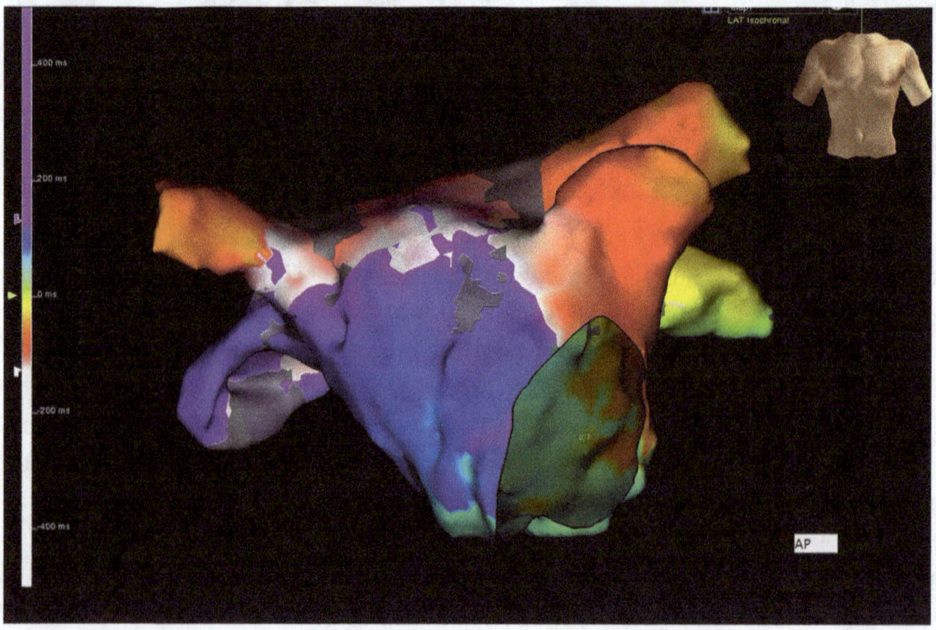

Figure 4. Left Anterior Oblique view of a macro-reentrant left atrial tachycardia with critical isthmus involving the mitral valve annulus showing a close spatial relationship between the earliest and latest activation "head meets tail". The color-coded maps were performed by using the focus multipoint 20 poles catheter of the Ensite system. LAO: Left anterior oblique

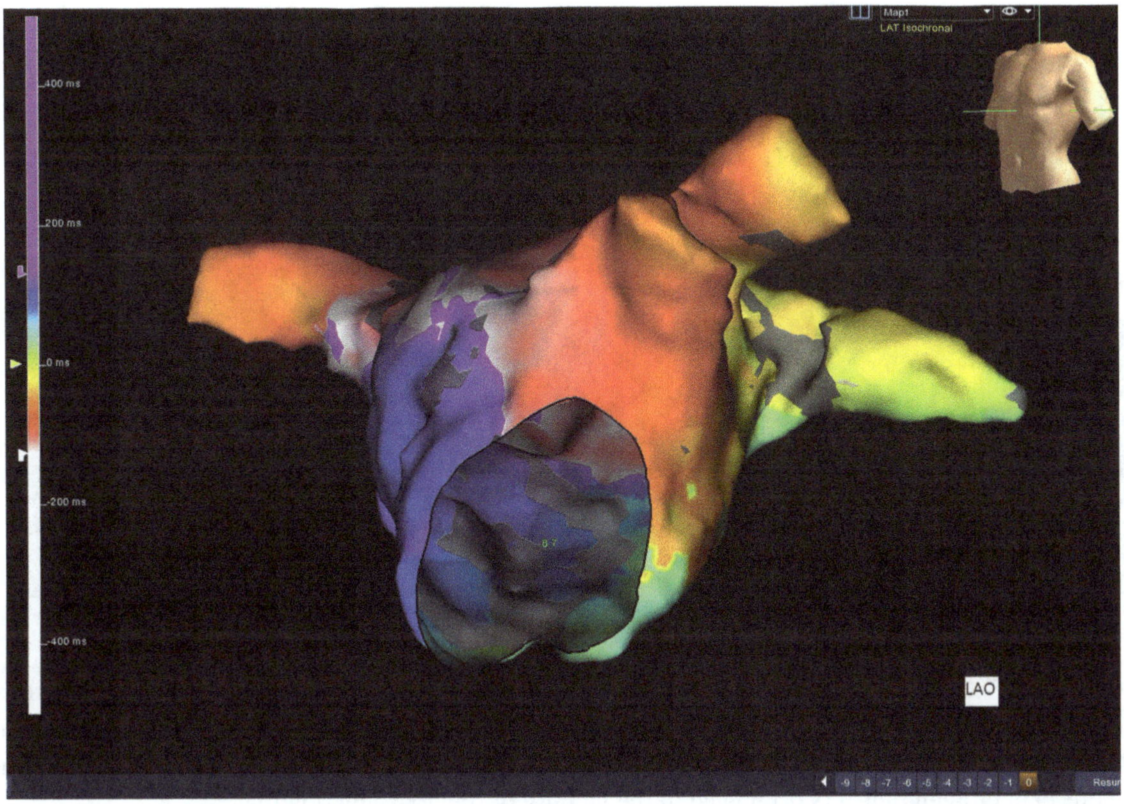

chamber during arrhythmia. Figures 1-10 are examples of local activation maps from both focal and macroreentrant mechanisms. Early and late activation sites during tachycardia were easily and rapidly displayed in all patients, commonly appearing as colored red and purple, respectively. Also, because the tachycardia was known to be in the left atrium, initially a left atrial map alone was rapidly reconstructed by such electroanatomical systems. If the chamber of origin was uncertain, as it was in 35 patients, sequential activation maps of the right and left atrium, or of coronary sinus were separately created.

Arrhythmia Characterization

Among 645 incessant left ATs, 554 (86%) were due to macro-reentrant circuits with earliest atrial activation on prior circumferential ablation lesions and 91 were due to a focal/micro-reentrant pattern (Figures 1-10). The commonest macroreentrant AT was the macroreentrant mitral annular tachycardia (Figures 2-5). Among the 91 focal/microreentrant left ATs, 55 patients were truly focal AT (mean cycle length: 266 ± 35.9 ms; Figure 1) while 36 micro-reentrant left ATs (mean cycle length: 277 ± 24 ms). The tachycardia was induced by programmed stimulation in 25 patients and was incessant in all but one. Among focal ATs, arrhythmia foci were frequently located close to the septal aspect of the right PVs

Figure 5. Postero-Anterior view of a macro-reentrant left atrial tachycardia with critical isthmus involving the mitral valve annulus showing a close spatial relationship between the earliest and latest activation "head meets tail". The color-coded maps were performed by using the focus multipoint 20 poles catheter of the Ensite system. PA: Postero-anterior

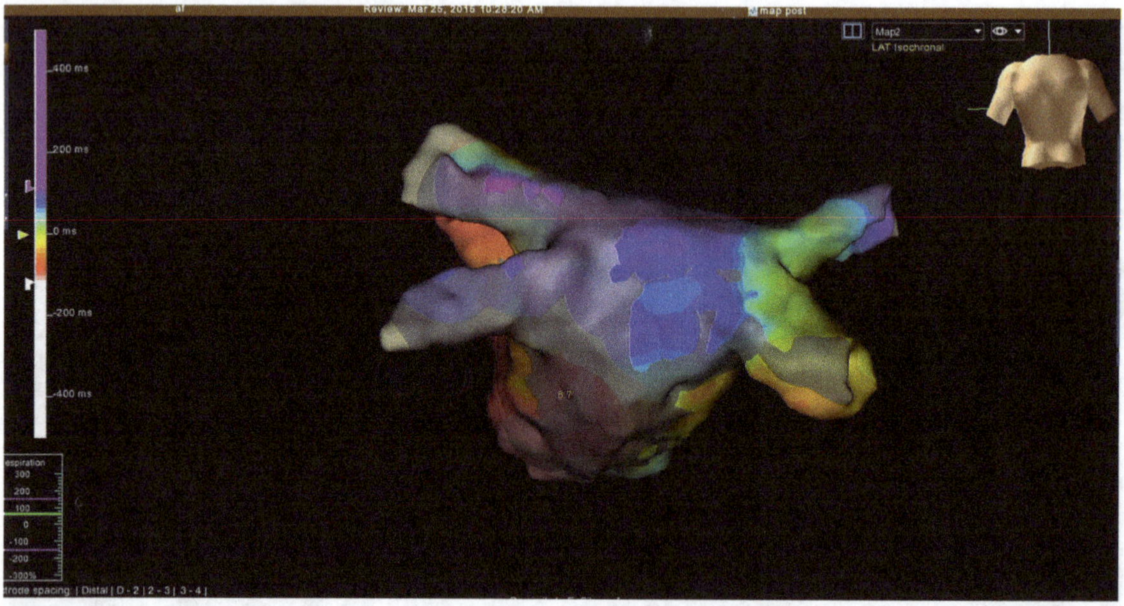

ostia (37 cases), and rarely on the left atrial appendage (Figure 1). In microreentrant ATs, the earliest activation was frequently mapped at the superior segment of the lateral LA (26 cases), anterior to the left superior pulmonary vein (LSPV) or in the posterior wall of the left atrium (10 cases). All but one (Figure 1) microreentrant ATs originated in the vicinity of previous ablation lines.

Of the 554 tachycardias characterized as macro–re-entrant (mean cycle length: 295 ± 25 ms), 315 showed single loop circuits involving the mitral isthmus (315 ATs, 57%; mean cycle length 390 ms), the remaining 239 ATs had earliest activation using gaps on the previous encircling lines at the septal aspect of the right PVs (121 ATs), at the superior segment of the lateral LA, anterior to the LSPV (91 ATs) or on the posterior wall of the LA (27 ATs). Single, fragmented electrograms were recorded at these propagating sites, with continuous areas of double potentials interposed, representing obstacles to activation. Color-coded electroanatomical maps showed single –loop reentrant circuit tachycardia in the majority of cases (525 ATs) or less frequently (29 ATs) dual-loop circuit tachycardias, frequently involving the mitral isthmus and the LA posterior wall.

RF Ablation

Catheter ablation resulted in arrhythmia termination (both focal and reentrant ATs) in all patients without major complications.

In truly focal ATs RF applications were done at earliest site of endocardial activation as guided by electroanatomical maps (Figure 1) by 8 mm or 3.5 mm tip-irrigated catheters with pulses of up to 30 s. Unipolar recordings showing negative (QS) pattern with sharp initial deflection also were considered

Figure 6. CARTO map with a Left Lateral view of the left atrium during incessant atrial tachycardia. The activation color-coded electroanatomical maps using the Pentarray multipoint catheter show a macro-reentrant septal atrial tachycardia. During application of RF energy it is possible to tag each application directly in the map to visualize the ablation line (white dots superimposed on the septal region of the map). LL: Left Lateral

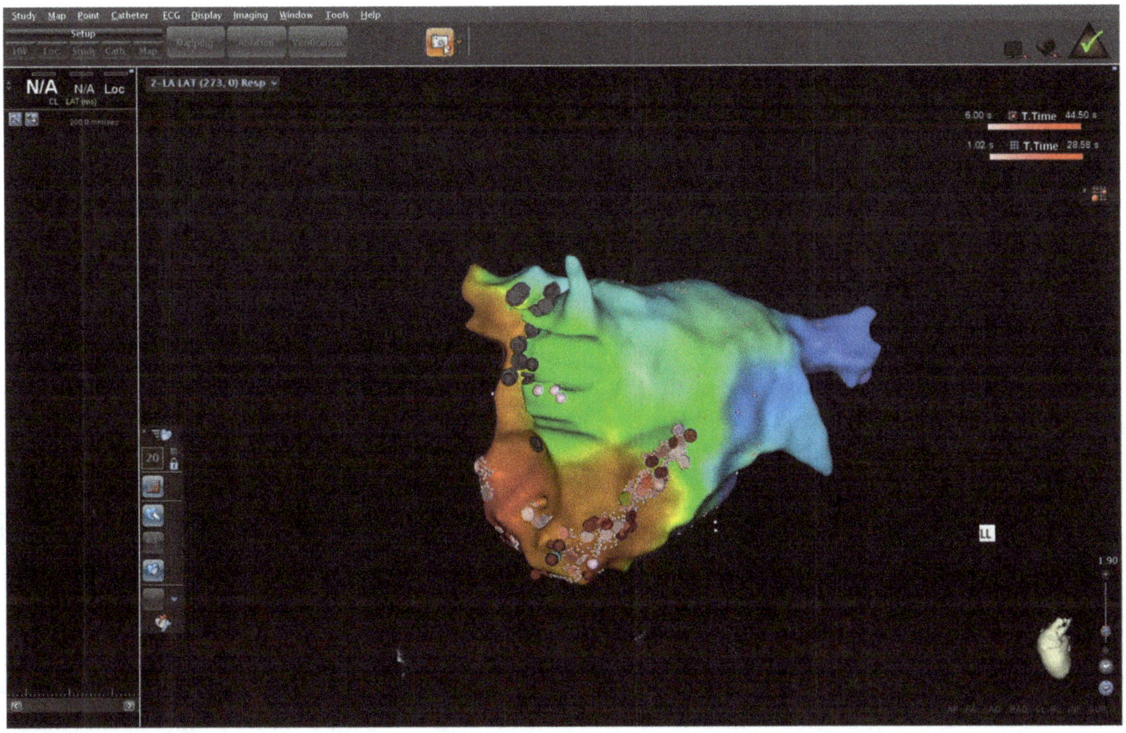

indicative of the focus. In focal micro-reentrant ATs related to gaps in prior ablation lines, gaps were eliminated by a single RF application and the ablation effect was consolidated by extending ablation to a short line (Figure 6-10). In micro-reentrant ATs local atrial electrograms at the site of earliest atrial activation appeared of low amplitude and/or fragmented or rarely, with double potentials. Despite restoration of sinus rhythm and non-inducibility of AT after successful ablation, 3D mapping revealed residual conduction gaps in many (30%) patients, all of which were definitively eliminated by further RF applications.

Ablation of macro–reentrant ATs was initially attempted across critical isthmuses, using 8-mm ablation catheter with pulses at a target temperature of 60°C and a maximum power output of 100 W or using 3.5 mm tip-irrigated catheter with temperature setting of 35°C and maximum power of 30 W. The ablation catheter was dragged after 15 to 30 s, after causing an effective lesion, demonstrated by a reduction of the local electrogram amplitude by ≥80% and/or a splitting into double potentials. If the tachycardia was not interrupted, ablation was directed to close identifiable gaps involved in the circuit, or an outer loop between fixed obstacles, such as the posterior wall or the mitral isthmus. Mitral annulus macroreentrant ATs were treated by long linear lesions connecting two adjacent non-conductive structures as guided by color-coded electroanatomical maps (Figures 6-10).

Figure 7. CARTO map with an Antero-Posterior view of the left atrium during incessant atrial tachycardia. The activation color-coded electroanatomical maps using the Pentarray multipoint catheter show a macro-reentrant septal atrial tachycardia. During application of RF energy it is possible to tag each application directly in the map to visualize the ablation line (white dots superimposed on the septal region of the map). AP: Antero-posterior

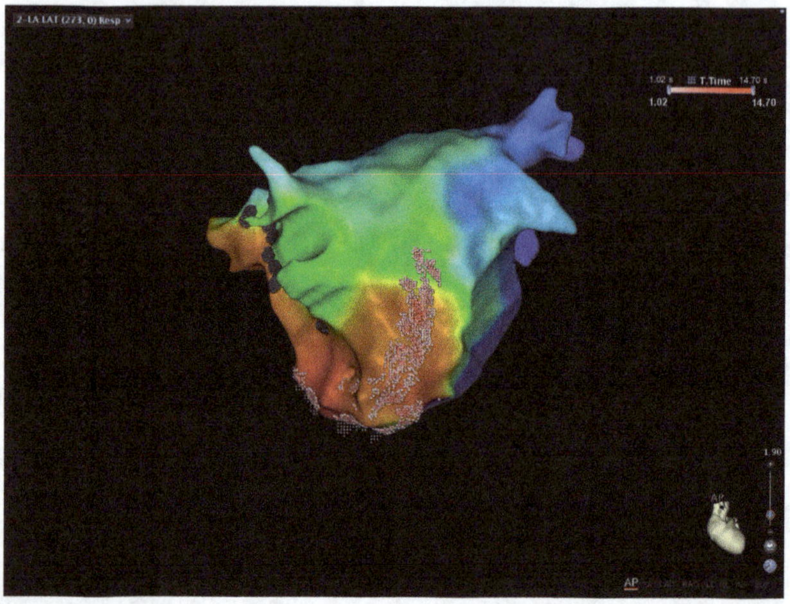

Figure 8. CARTO map with a Left Anterior Oblique view of the left atrium during incessant atrial tachycardia. The activation color-coded electroanatomical maps using the Pentarray multipoint catheter show a macro-reentrant septal atrial tachycardia. During application of RF energy it is possible to tag each application directly in the map to visualize the ablation line (white dots superimposed on the septal region of the map). LAO: Left Anterior Oblique

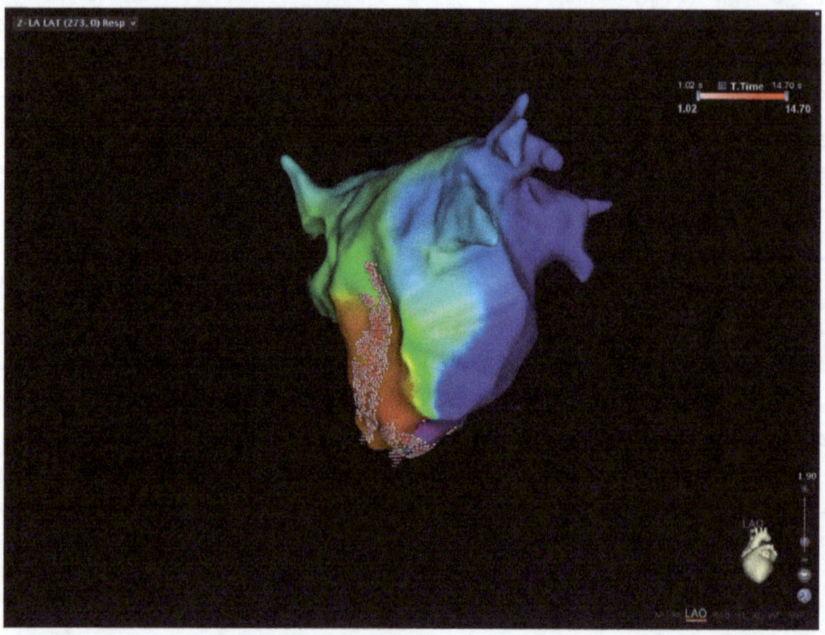

Figure 9. CARTO map with a Postero-Anterior view of the left atrium during incessant atrial tachycardia. The activation color-coded electroanatomical maps using the Pentarray multipoint catheter show a macro-reentrant septal atrial tachycardia. During application of RF energy it is possible to tag each application directly in the map to visualize the ablation line (white dots superimposed on the septal region of the map). PA: Postero-Anterior

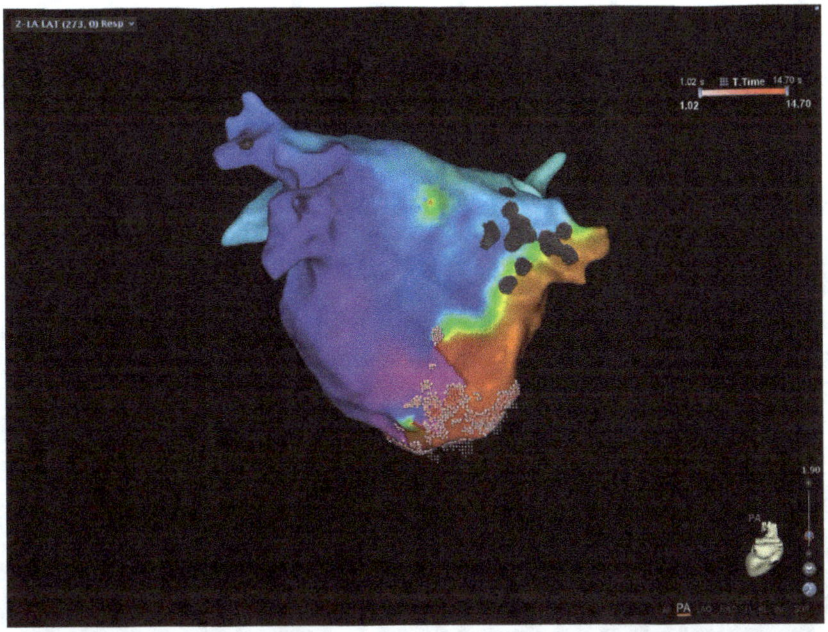

After a mean follow-up of 35 ± 12 months, no AT recurrences were reported in all but 10 patients (8 patients developed persistent AF after a mean of 2.3 months of the left AT ablation and 2 patients had a new incessant arrhythmia after 1 and 3 months of the left AT ablation, which proved to be a different focal LA tachycardia. This arrhythmia was successfully mapped and ablated at the anterior aspect of the left superior PV ostium.

FUTURE RESEARCH DIRECTIONS

Discussion

This study reports the largest number of post-ablation incessant left atrial tachycardias successfully treated by radiofrequency catheter ablation exclusively using current electroanatomical mapping systems and ablation catheters including the more recent multipoint mapping and ablation catheters. The results demonstrate this strategy can be performed without fluoroscopy with satisfactory results for short procedure times, high success with low complication rates.

It is well known that in patients who undergo catheter ablation for atrial fibrillation the highest incidence of post-ablation incessant atrial tachyarrhythmias occurs after an ablation strategy involving multiple and extensive lesions in the left atrium (pulmonary vein isolation, additional linear ablation associated with targeting of complex fractionated electrograms) (Jais, Shah, et al., 2000; Pappone, Rosanio et al.,

Figure 10. CARTO map with a Right Anterior Oblique view of the left atrium during incessant atrial tachycardia. The activation color-coded electroanatomical maps using the Pentarray multipoint catheter show a macro-reentrant septal atrial tachycardia. During application of RF energy it is possible to tag each application directly in the map to visualize the ablation line (white dots superimposed on the septal region of the map). RAO: Right anterior oblique

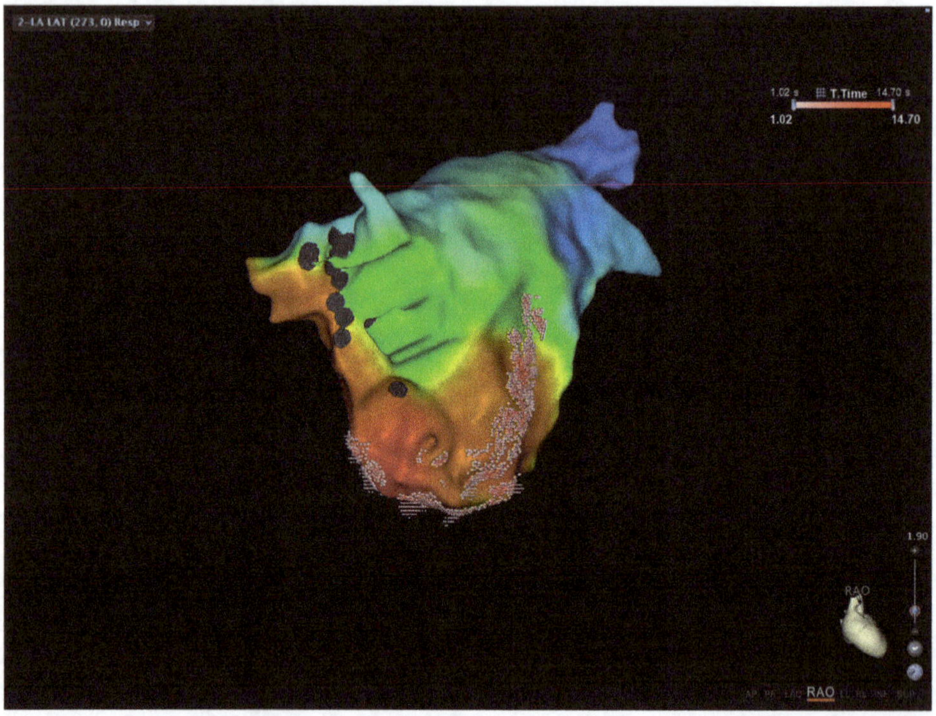

2003; Pappone, Manguso, et al., 2004; Packer, 2005; Oral, Pappone, et al., 2006; Pappone, Augello, et al., 2006; Pappone, & Santinelli, 2006; Chae, Oral, et al., 2007; Jais, Matsuo, et al., 2009; Zipes, Calkins, et al., 2015). The Authors report in this study all consecutive patients who experienced incessant left ATs after catheter ablation for atrial fibrillation including PV isolation with substrate ablation in the left atrium. It is conceivable that after prior extensive substrate elimination due to the index procedure, reentrant (both macro and micro-reentrant) left ATs originating on ablation lines were more common than focal ATs, representing about 90% of all cases. In agreement with these results, several studies reported reentrant circuits to be a major mechanism of incessant ATs following left AF ablation involving a large substrate modification (Jais, Shah, et al., 2000; Pappone, Manguso, et al., 2004; Chae, Oral, et al., 2007; Jaïs, Matsuo, et al., 2009; Scherr, Derval, et al., 2015). Jais, Shah, et al., (2000) performed a detailed study of 22 left atrial macro-reentrant ATs. Seventy-seven percent of the study cohort had significant structural heart disease, including significant mitral valve dysfunction, previous mitral valve surgery or left ventricular systolic dysfunction with marked left atrial dilatation. Most patients had single circuits, with a smaller group having multiple or highly complex circuits. Ablation of a critical isthmus of slow conduction resulted in 91% acute procedural success rate, with sinus rhythm maintained in 73% at 15 months. Jais, Matsuo, et al., (2009) have recently reported a cohort of 128 consecutive patients with 246 left ATs in the context of prior extensive AF ablation. Forty-six percent were demonstrated to be macro-reentrant ATs while 54% were confirmed to be micro-reentrant or less frequently truly focal ATs. Indeed, of non macroreentrant ATs, 26% were demonstrated to arise from a discrete point source as "truly focal" AT but 74% were found to arise from a small reentrant circuit 1–2 cm in diameter, with activation recordable throughout ≥75% of the tachycardia cycle in this small region and subsequent centrifugal spread to the remainder of the left atrium. Of interest, such circuits were preferentially found at the sites of previous ablation, where zones of slow conduction were demonstrable. The results reported in our study confirm and extend such data remaining a debate as to whether these circuits represent the underlying primary drivers of AF uncovered by ablation and substrate modification or, more likely, are simply secondary to prior ablation with reentry around scar due to previous ablation lesions.

Electroanatomic Mapping as a Guide for Post-Ablation Atrial Tachycardia

The results of the present study demonstrate that when using the methodology proposed in this chapter, electroanatomic-guided ablation of incessant post-ablation ATs is safe, feasible and effective. Indeed, the arrhythmia mechanism (reentrant circuits or foci) was easily and rapidly identified in all patients without or with minimal use of fluoroscopy and, as expected, most of reentrant arrhythmias related to discontinuities on previous ablation lines can be definitively eliminated by targeted RF applications. In many patients, the LA posterior wall and the mitral isthmus are involved in the reentrant circuits. In our series, accurate electroanatomical maps by multipoint mapping catheters allowed to demonstrate that the shortest cycle lengths usually occur with circuits rotating around closely positioned gaps, rather than with large circuits, such as in mitral isthmus dependent re-entry. This observation emphasizes the importance of deploying continuous lesion at the encircling lines during the index procedure to avoid post-ablation rapid ATs. The results of this study further indicate that although acute electrical remodeling is achieved in all patients after the index ablation procedure without apparently identifiable gaps, the recovery of conduction in such critical points on the ablation lines can occur later, representing the basic mechanism of macro-reentrant or micro-reentrant focal activity. Incomplete lines or recovery of conduction at these areas can create the slow conduction necessary to sustain re-entry (Jais, Shah, et al., 2000; Pappone, Manguso, et al., 2004; Jais, Matsuo, et al., 2009). Although during the index procedure ablation lines at these critical sites are designed to avoid post-ablation macro–re-entry, it is still not clear whether they actually prevent or contribute to it, and further studies are needed to define their role. There are relatively few reports describing re-entrant circuits in detail (Nakagawa, Shah, et al., 2001; Pappone, Manguso, et al., 2004). This study is indeed original providing additional data on the electrophysiologic findings in a large consecutive series of patients with left AT after ablation for atrial fibrillation using different electroanatomic mapping systems. In fact, this series demonstrates that focal activity may be a potential alternative mechanism in a minority of patients after ablation (10%). "Truly " post-ablation focal atrial tachycardias, as demonstrated by color-coded electroanatomical activation and propagation maps, are less common than reentrant tachycardias, representing less than 10% of cases and electroanatomical-map guided catheter ablation is highly effective in eliminating such tachyarrhythmias, as with reentrant arrhythmias. Several studies have reported success rates between 69% and 100% with most reporting success rates between 85% and 95% with low complication rates, as it was in our series (Chen, Chiang, et al., 1994; Lesh, Van Hare, et al., 1994; Poty, 1996; Chen, Tai, et al., 1998; Roberts-Thomson, Kistler, et al., 2006; Chae, Oral, et al., 2007; Jais, Matsuo, et al., 2009; Kang, Etheridge et al., 2014; Anter, Tschabrunn, & Josephson, 2015). Chen, Tai, et al., (1998) have analyzed clinical and electrophysiologic characteristics that predicted success from catheter ablation of focal AT in reports published between 1969 and 1997. They reported an overall recurrence rate of 7% after successful catheter ablation. Older age, background structural heart disease and multiple foci of AT were risk factors for arrhythmia recurrence. Creating transmural, permanent lines of block with a percutaneous approach can be even more challenging, but the results of this study indicate that electroanatomical-guided catheter ablation is very useful to definitively eliminate such tachyarrhythmias. Frequently, only a narrow rim of atrial tissue between the LSPV and the LA appendage is present, which makes stable catheter positioning difficult to attain in the absence of accurate anatomical maps. In addition, the presence of dense pectinate muscle in the LA appendage, contiguous to the normal atrial wall, can make transmural lesion more difficult to achieve in this area as it was in one patient in this series (Figure 1). Good access to the postero-septal area is essential to perform the encircling lines of the right PVs. A very high or posterior transseptal puncture may make stable catheter positioning over the septum difficult, with the distal electrode in poor contact or inadequate orientation with the endocardial surface.

Clinical Implications

Our experience suggests that the septal aspect of ablation lines encircling the right PVs and the area anterior to the left superior PV are particularly vulnerable to recovery of conduction after the index ablation procedure, predisposing patients to the development of left AT. Particular attention should be paid at these sites to ensure continuous, transmural lesions by accurate and detailed electroanatomical mapping systems. Meticulous mapping to define the LA anatomy, particularly between the LSPV and the LA appendage, is necessary to guide linear ablation. Further research is needed to define the role of lines in the mitral isthmus and the posterior wall. The recognition of focal tachycardia as a possible mechanism can further assist the treatment because detailed mapping with high density of points is necessary only at the sites of early activation, shortening the procedure time and fluoroscopy exposure. The impact of other image methods or new catheter designs on the occurrence and characteristic of these arrhythmias is unclear.

Limitations

The Authors used conventional 8 mm, tip-irrigated 3.5 mm mapping/ablation catheters or multipoint mapping/ablation catheters. These tools and settings may not be appropriate in centers with less experience or lower volumes of cases.

CONCLUSION

Atrial tachycardia is a generic term for a range of differing circuits. These can be broadly divided by mechanism into macro-reentrant, focal and small circuit re-entry. The advent of sophisticated mapping solutions has rendered the vast majority of these atrial circuits curable with catheter ablation, with high success rates and very low incidence of complications. Electroanatomic mapping systems are effective in characterizing incessant refractory atrial tachycardias, which currently are increasingly referred worldwide to electrophysiology laboratories representing an important midterm complication following catheter ablation of atrial fibrillation. This sustained tachyarrhythmia can be due to either re-entrant or focal mechanisms. Re-entry occurs most commonly using gaps on previously continuous ablation lines. Such gaps have shown a tendency to occur at critical sites such as the septal aspect of the right PVs, between the LSPV and the LA appendage, the mitral isthmus and/or the posterior wall of the LA. Electroanatomical mapping systems are useful to ensure accurate anatomical and electrical identification of targeted areas and that linear lesions are continuous and transmural for successful ablation.

REFERENCES

Anter, E., Tschabrunn, C. M., & Josephson, M. E. (2015). High-resolution mapping of scar-related atrial arrhythmias using smaller electrodes with closer interelectrode spacing. *Circulation: Arrhythmia and Electrophysiology*, *8*(3), 537–545. doi:10.1161/CIRCEP.114.002737 PMID:25792508

Barbhaiyam, C. R., Kumar, S., Ng, J., Tedrow, U., Koplan, B., John, R., & Michaud, G. F. et al. (2014). Overdrive pacing from downstream sites on multielectrode catheters to rapidly detect fusion and to diagnose macroreentrant atrial arrhythmias. *Circulation*, *129*(24), 2503–2510. doi:10.1161/CIRCULATIONAHA.113.008494 PMID:24812357

Beukema, R. J., Elvan, A., Smit, J. J., Delnoy, P. P., Misier, A. R., & Reddy, V. (2012). Pulmonary vein isolation to treat paroxysmal atrial fibrillation: Conventional versus multi-electrode radiofrequency ablation. *Journal of Interventional Cardiac Electrophysiology*, *34*(2), 143–152. doi:10.1007/s10840-011-9653-2 PMID:22354772

Buch, E., & Shivkumar, K. (2015). Catheter Ablation of Atrial Fibrillation: Advent of Second-Generation Technologies. *Journal of the American College of Cardiology*, *66*(12), 1361–1363. doi:10.1016/j.jacc.2015.07.056 PMID:26383723

Ceresnak, S. R., Nappo, L., Janson, C. M., & Pass, R. H. (2015). Tricking CARTO: Cryoablation of Supraventricular Tachycardia in Children with Minimal Radiation Exposure Using the CARTO3 System. *Pacing and Clinical Electrophysiology*, *28*(Sep). doi: doi:10.1111/pace.12754 PMID:26412504

Chae, S., Oral, H., Good, E., Dey, S., Wimmer, A., Crawford, T., & Chugh, A. et al. (2007). Atrial tachycardia after circumferential pulmonary vein ablation of atrial fibrillation: Mechanistic insights, results of catheter ablation, and risk factors for recurrence. *Journal of the American College of Cardiology*, *50*(18), 1781–1787. doi:10.1016/j.jacc.2007.07.044 PMID:17964043

Chen, S., Chiang, C., Yang, C., Cheng, C., Wu, T., Wang, S., & Chang, M. S. et al. (1994). Sustained atrial tachycardia in adult patients. Electrophysi- ological characteristics, pharmacological response, possible mechanisms, and effects of radiofrequency ablation. *Circulation*, *90*(3), 1262–1278. doi:10.1161/01.CIR.90.3.1262 PMID:8087935

Chen, S. A., Tai, C. T., Chiang, C. E., Ding, Y. A., & Chang, M. S. (1998). Focal atrial tachycardia: Reanalysis of the clinical and electrophysiologic characteristics and prediction of successful radiofrequency ablation. *Journal of Cardiovascular Electrophysiology*, *9*(4), 355–365. doi:10.1111/j.1540-8167.1998.tb00924.x PMID:9581952

Corrado, D., Basso, C., Leoni, L., Tokajuk, B., Bauce, B., Frigo, G., & Thiene, G. et al. (2005). Three-dimensional electroanatomic voltage mapping increases accuracy of diagnosing arrhythmogenic right ventricular cardiomyopathy/dysplasia. *Circulation*, *111*(23), 3042–3050. doi:10.1161/CIRCULATIONAHA.104.486977 PMID:15939822

de Groot, N. M., Schalij, M. J., Zeppenfeld, K., Blom, N. A., Van der Velde, E. T., & Van der Wall, E. E. (2003). Voltage and activation mapping: How the recording technique affects the outcome of catheter ablation procedures in patients with congenital heart disease. *Circulation*, *108*(17), 2099–2106. doi:10.1161/01.CIR.0000092893.11893.38 PMID:14517169

Del Carpio Munoz, F., Buescher, T. L., & Asirvatham, S. J. (2010). Three-dimensional mapping of cardiac arrhythmias: What do the colors really mean? *Circulation: Arrhythmia and Electrophysiology*, *6*(6), 6–11. doi:10.1161/CIRCEP.110.960161 PMID:21156773

Dixit, S., & Callans, D. J. (2002). Role of contact and noncontact mapping in the curative ablation of tachyarrhythmias. *Current Opinion in Cardiology*, *17*(1), 65–72. doi:10.1097/00001573-200201000-00010 PMID:11790936

Earley, M., Showkathali, R., Alzetani, M., Kistler, P. M., Gupta, D., Abrams, D. J., & Schilling, R. J. et al. (2006). Radiofrequency ablation of arrhythmias guided by non-fluoroscopic catheter location: A prospective randomized trial. *European Heart Journal*, *27*(10), 1223–1229. doi:10.1093/eurheartj/ehi834 PMID:16613932

Estner, H. L., Deisenhofer, I., Luik, A., Ndrepepa, G., von Bary, C., Zrenner, B., & Schmitt, C. (2006). Electrical isolation of pulmonary veins in patients with atrial fibrillation: Reduction of fluoroscopy exposure and procedure duration by the use of a non-fluoroscopic navigation system (navx). *Europace*, *8*(8), 583–587. doi:10.1093/europace/eul079 PMID:16831837

Friedman, P. A. (2002). Novel mapping techniques for cardiac electrophysiology. *Heart (British Cardiac Society)*, *87*(6), 575–582. doi:10.1136/heart.87.6.575 PMID:12010949

Friedman, P. A., Asirvatham, S. J., Grice, S., Glikson, M., Munger, T. M., Rea, R. F., & Hammill, S. C. et al. (2002). Noncontact mapping to guide ablation of right ventricular outflow tract tachycardia. *Journal of the American College of Cardiology*, *39*(11), 1808–1812. doi:10.1016/S0735-1097(02)01864-8 PMID:12039496

Gornick, C., Adler, S., Pederson, B., Hauck, J., Budd, J., & Schweitzer, J. (1999). Validation of a new noncontact catheter system for electroanatomic mapping of left ventricular endocardium. *Circulation*, *99*(6), 829–835. doi:10.1161/01.CIR.99.6.829 PMID:9989971

Gurevitz, O. T., Glikson, M., Asirvatham, S., Kester, T. A., Grice, S. K., Munger, T. M., & Friedman, P. A. et al. (2005). Use of advanced mapping systems to guide ablation in complex cases: Experience with noncontact mapping and electroanatomic mapping systems. *Pacing and Clinical Electrophysiology*, *28*(4), 316–323. doi:10.1111/j.1540-8159.2005.09477.x PMID:15826266

Haissaguerre, M., Jais, P., Shah, D. C., Takahashi, A., Hocini, M., Quiniou, G., & Clémenty, J. et al. (1998). Spontaneous initiation of atrial fibrillation by ectopic beats originating in the pulmonary veins. *The New England Journal of Medicine*, *339*(10), 659–666. doi:10.1056/NEJM199809033391003 PMID:9725923

Jais, P., Matsuo, S., Knecht, S., Weerasooriya, R., Hocini, M., Sacher, F., & Haïssaguerre, M. et al. (2009). A deductive mapping strategy for atrial tachycardia following atrial fibrillation ablation: Importance of localized reentry. *Journal of Cardiovascular Electrophysiology*, *20*(5), 480–491. doi:10.1111/j.1540-8167.2008.01373.x PMID:19207747

Jais, P., Shah, D. C., Haissaguerre, M., Hocini, M., Peng, J. T., Takahashi, A., & Clémenty, J. et al. (2000). Mapping and ablation of left atrial flutters. *Circulation*, *101*(25), 2928–2934. doi:10.1161/01.CIR.101.25.2928 PMID:10869265

Kang, K. T., Etheridge, S. P., Kantoch, M. J., Tisma-Dupanovic, S., Bradley, D. J., Balaji, S., & Sanatani, S. et al. (2014). Current management of focal atrial tachycardia in children: A multicenter experience. *Circulation: Arrhythmia and Electrophysiology*, *3*(4), 664–670. doi:10.1161/CIRCEP.113.001423 PMID:25015944

Kapa, S., & Asirvatham, S. J. (2014). You can't know where you're going until you know where you've been: The clinical relevance of differences in accurate assessment of catheter location with mapping technologies. *Journal of Cardiovascular Electrophysiology*, *25*(1), 84–86. doi:10.1111/jce.12287 PMID:24118496

Kay, G. N., Chong, F., Epstein, A. E., Dailey, S. M., & Plumb, V. J. (1993). Radiofrequency ablation for treatment of primary atrial tachycardias. *Journal of the American College of Cardiology*, *21*(4), 901–909. doi:10.1016/0735-1097(93)90345-2 PMID:8450158

Khaykin, Y., Oosthuizen, R., Zarnett, L., Wulffhart, Z. A., Whaley, B., Hill, C., & Verma, A. et al. (2011). Carto-guided vs. Navx-guided pulmonary vein antrum isolation and pulmonary vein antrum isolation performed without 3-d mapping: Effect of the 3-d mapping system on procedure duration and fluoroscopy time. *Journal of Interventional Cardiac Electrophysiology*, *30*(3), 233–240. doi:10.1007/s10840-010-9538-9 PMID:21253840

Kirchhof, P., Loh, P., Eckardt, L., Ribbing, M., Rolf, S., Eick, O., & Haverkamp, W. et al. (2002). A novel nonfluoroscopic catheter visualization system (LocaLisa) to reduce radiation exposure during catheter ablation of supraventricular tachycardias. *The American Journal of Cardiology*, *90*(3), 340–343. doi:10.1016/S0002-9149(02)02481-5 PMID:12127630

Kistler, P. M., Rajappan, K., Jahngir, M., Earley, M. J., Harris, S., Abrams, D., & Schilling, R. J. et al. (2006). The impact of ct image integration into an electroanatomic mapping system on clinical outcomes of catheter ablation of atrial fibrillation. *Journal of Cardiovascular Electrophysiology*, *17*(10), 1093–1101. doi:10.1111/j.1540-8167.2006.00594.x PMID:16989651

Kopelman, H., Prater, S., Tondato, F., Chronos, N. A., & Peters, N. S. (2003). Slow pathway catheter ablation of atrioventricular nodal re-entrant tachycardia guided by electroanatomical mapping: A randomized comparison to the conventional approach. *Europace*, *5*(2), 171–174. doi:10.1053/eupc.2002.0296 PMID:12633642

Kottkamp, H., Hugl, B., Krauss, B., Wetzel, U., Fleck, A., Schuler, G., & Hindricks, G. (2000). Electromagnetic versus fluoroscopic mapping of the inferior isthmus for ablation of typical atrial flutter. A prospective randomized study. *Circulation*, *102*(17), 2082–2086. doi:10.1161/01.CIR.102.17.2082 PMID:11044424

Lesh, M., Van Hare, G., Epstein, L., Fitzpatrick, A., Scheinman, M., Lee, R., & Griffin, J. C. et al. (1994). Radiofrequency catheter ablation of atrial arrhythmias. Results and mechanisms. *Circulation*, *89*(3), 1074–1089. doi:10.1161/01.CIR.89.3.1074 PMID:8124793

Macle, L., Jais, P., Scavee, C., Weerasooriya, R., Hocini, M., Shah, D. C., & Haïssaguerre, M. et al. (2003). Pulmonary vein disconnection using the LocaLisa three-dimensional nonfluoroscopic catheter imaging system. *Journal of Cardiovascular Electrophysiology*, *14*(7), 693–697. doi:10.1046/j.1540-8167.2003.03012.x PMID:12930247

Marrouche, N. F., Martin, D. O., Wazni, O., Gillinov, A. M., Klein, A., Bhargava, M., & Natale, A. et al. (2003). Phased-array intracardiac echocardiography monitoring during pulmonary vein isolation in patients with atrial fibrillation: Impact on outcome and complications. *Circulation*, *107*(>21), 2710–2716. doi:10.1161/01.CIR.0000070541.83326.15 PMID:12756153

Martinek, M., Nesser, H. J., Aichinger, J., Boehm, G., & Purerfellner, H. (2007). Impact of integration of multislice computed tomography imaging into three-dimensional electroanatomic mapping on clinical outcomes, safety, and efficacy using radiofrequency ablation for atrial fibrillation. *Pacing and Clinical Electrophysiology*, *30*(10), 1215–1223. doi:10.1111/j.1540-8159.2007.00843.x PMID:17897124

Matsuo, S., Lim, K. T., & Haissaguerre, M. (2007). Ablation of chronic atrial fibrillation. *Heart Rhythm*, *4*(11), 1461–1463. doi:10.1016/j.hrthm.2007.07.016 PMID:17954407

Medi, C., Kalman, J. M., Haqqani, H., Vohra, J. K., Morton, J. B., Sparks, P. B., & Kistler, P. M. (2009). Tachycardia-mediated cardiomyopathy secondary to focal atrial tachycardia: Long-term outcome after catheter ablation. *Journal of the American College of Cardiology*, *53*(19), 1791–1797. doi:10.1016/j.jacc.2009.02.014 PMID:19422986

Nakagawa, H., Shah, N., Matsudaira, K., Overholt, E., Chandrasekaran, K., Beckman, K. J., & Jackman, W. M. et al. (2001). Characterization of reentrant circuit in macroreentrant right atrial tachycardia after surgical repair of congenital heart disease: Isolated channels between scars allow "focal" ablation. *Circulation*, *103*(5), 699–709. doi:10.1161/01.CIR.103.5.699 PMID:11156882

Oral, H., Pappone, C., Chugh, A., Good, E., Bogun, F., Pelosi, F. Jr, & Morady, F. et al. (2006). Circumferential pulmonary vein ablation for chronic atrial fibrillation: A randomized, controlled study. *The New England Journal of Medicine*, *354*(9), 934–941. doi:10.1056/NEJMoa050955 PMID:16510747

Oral, H., Scharf, C., Chugh, A., Hall, B., Cheung, P., Good, E., & Morady, F. et al. (2003). Catheter ablation for paroxysmal atrial fibrillation: Segmental pulmonary vein ostial ablation versus left atrial ablation. *Circulation*, *108*(19), 2355–2360. doi:10.1161/01.CIR.0000095796.45180.88 PMID:14557355

Packer, D. (2005). Three-dimensional mapping in interventional electrophysiology: Techniques and technology. *Journal of Cardiovascular Electrophysiology*, *16*(10), 1110–1116. doi:10.1111/j.1540-8167.2005.50161.x PMID:16191123

Pappone, C., Augello, G., Sala, S., Gugliotta, F., Vicedomini, G., Gulletta, S., & Santinelli, V. et al. (2006). A Randomized Trial of Circumferential Pulmonary Vein Ablation versus Antiarrhythmic Drug Therapy in Paroxysmal Atrial Fibrillation. The Ablation for Paroxysmal Atrial Fibrillation (APAF) Study. *Journal of the American College of Cardiology*, *48*(11), 2340–2347. doi:10.1016/j.jacc.2006.08.037 PMID:17161267

Pappone, C., Manguso, F., Vicedomini, G., Gugliotta, F., Santinelli, O., Ferro, A., & Santinelli, V. et al. (2004). Prevention of Iatrogenic Atrial Tachycardia following ablation of Atrial Fibrillation. A prospective randomized study comparing circumferential pulmonary vein ablation with a modified approach. *Circulation*, *110*(19), 3036–3042. doi:10.1161/01.CIR.0000147186.83715.95 PMID:15520310

Pappone, C., Rosanio, S., Augello, G., Gallus, G., Vicedomini, G., Mazzone, P., & Alfieri, O. et al. (2003). Mortality, Morbidity and Quality of Life after Circumferential Pulmonary Vein Ablation for Atrial Fibrillation. Outcomes from a Controlled not Randomized Long-Term Study. *Journal of the American College of Cardiology*, *42*(2), 185–197. doi:10.1016/S0735-1097(03)00577-1 PMID:12875749

Pappone, C., & Santinelli, V. (2006). How to perform encircling ablation of the left atrium. *Heart Rhythm*, *3*(9), 1105–1109. doi:10.1016/j.hrthm.2006.03.003 PMID:16945812

Pappone, C., Santinelli, V., Manguso, F., Vicedomini, G., Gugliotta, F., Augello, G., & Alfieri, O. et al. (2004). Pulmonary vein denervation enhances long-term benefit after circumferential ablation for paroxysmal atrial fibrillation. *Circulation*, *109*(3), 327–334. doi:10.1161/01.CIR.0000112641.16340.C7 PMID:14707026

Poty, H., Saoudi, N., Haïssaguerre, M., Daou, A., Clémenty, J., & Letac, B. (1996). Radiofrequency catheter ablation of atrial tachycardias. *American Heart Journal*, *131*(3), 481–489. doi:10.1016/S0002-8703(96)90526-8 PMID:8604627

Roberts-Thomson, K. C., Kistler, P. M., & Kalman, J. M. (2006). Focal atrial tachycardia II: Management. *Pacing and Clinical Electrophysiology*, *29*(7), 769–778. doi:10.1111/j.1540-8159.2006.00433.x PMID:16884515

Rotter, M., Takahashi, Y., Sanders, P., Haissaguerre, M., Hsu, L. F., Sacher, F., & Hocini, M. et al. (2005). Reduction of fluoroscopy exposure and procedure duration during ablation of atrial fibrillation using a novel anatomical navigation system. *European Heart Journal*, *26*(14), 1415–1421. doi:10.1093/eurheartj/ehi172 PMID:15741228

Saoudi, N., Cosío, F., Waldo, A., Chen, S. A., Iesaka, Y., Lesh, M., & Schoels, W. et al. (2001). A classification of atrial flutter and regular atrial tachycardia according to electrophysiological mechanisms and anatomical bases; a Statement from a Joint Expert Group from The Working Group of Arrhythmias of the European Society of Cardiology and the North American Society of Pacing and Electrophysiology. *European Heart Journal*, *22*(14), 1162–1182. doi:10.1053/euhj.2001.2658 PMID:11440490

Schenider, M., Ndrepepa, G., Dobran, I., Schreieck, J., Weber, S., Plewan, A., & Schmitt, C. et al. (2003). LocaLisa catheter navigation reduces fluoroscopy time and dosage in ablation of atrial flutter: A prospective randomized study. *Journal of Cardiovascular Electrophysiology*, *14*(6), 587–590. doi:10.1046/j.1540-8167.2003.03017.x PMID:12875418

Scherr, D., Derval, N., Sohal, M., Pascale, P., Wright, M., Jadidi, A., & Knecht, S. et al. (2015). Length of the Mitral Isthmus But Not Anatomical Location of Ablation Line Predicts Bidirectional Mitral Isthmus Block in Patients Undergoing Catheter Ablation of Persistent Atrial Fibrillation: A Randomized Controlled Trial. *Journal of Cardiovascular Electrophysiology*, *26*(6), 629–634. doi:10.1111/jce.12667 PMID:25786517

Schilling, R., Peters, N., & Davies, D. (1998). Simultaneous endocardial mapping in the human left ventricle using a noncontact catheter. Comparison of contact and reconstructed electrograms during sinus rhythm. *Circulation*, *98*(9), 887–898. doi:10.1161/01.CIR.98.9.887 PMID:9738644

Silka, M. J., Gillette, P. C., Garson, A. Jr, & Zinner, A. (1985). Transvenous catheter ablation of a right atrial automatic ectopic tachycardia. *Journal of the American College of Cardiology*, *5*(4), 999–1001. doi:10.1016/S0735-1097(85)80448-4 PMID:3973306

Sporton, S., Earley, M., Nathan, A., & Schilling, R. J. (2004). Electroanatomic versus fluoroscopic mapping for catheter ablation procedures: A prospective randomized study. *Journal of Cardiovascular Electrophysiology*, *15*(3), 310–315. doi:10.1111/j.1540-8167.2004.03356.x PMID:15030422

Sun, A. Y., & Piccini, J. P. (2014). Validation of non-contact and point-to-point mapping in a single electroanatomic map. *Europace*, *16*, 371–375. PMID:24158252

Van Hare, G. F., Velvis, H., & Langberg, J. J. (1990). Successful transcatheter ablation of congenital junctional ectopic tachycardia in a ten-month-old infant using radiofrequency energy. *Pacing and Clinical Electrophysiology*, *13*(6), 730–735. doi:10.1111/j.1540-8159.1990.tb02099.x PMID:1695353

Ventura, R., Rostock, T., Klemm, H., Lutomsky, B., Demir, C., Weiss, C., & Willems, S. et al. (2004). Catheter ablation of common-type atrial flutter guided by three-dimensional right atrial geometry reconstruction and catheter tracking using cutaneous patches: A randomized prospective study. *Journal of Cardiovascular Electrophysiology*, *15*(10), 1157–1161. doi:10.1046/j.1540-8167.2004.04064.x PMID:15485440

Wang, Z., Ouyang, J., Liang, Y., Jin, Z., Yang, G., Liang, M., & Han, Y. et al. (2015). Focal atrial tachycardia surrounding the anterior septum: Strategy for mapping and catheter ablation. *Circulation: Arrhythmia and Electrophysiology*, *8*(3), 575–582. doi:10.1161/CIRCEP.114.002281 PMID:25908691

Wilber, D. J., Pappone, C., Neuzil, P., De Paola, A., Marchlinski, F., Natale, A., & Berry, D. A. et al. (2010). ThermoCool AF Trial Investigators. *Journal of the American Medical Association*, *303*, 333–340. doi:10.1001/jama.2009.2029 PMID:20103757

Willems, S., Weiss, C., Ventura, R., Rüppel, R., Risius, T., Hoffmann, M., & Meinertz, T. (2000). Catheter ablation of atrial flutter guided by electroanatomic mapping (CARTO): A randomized comparison to the conventional approach. *Journal of Cardiovascular Electrophysiology*, *12*(11), 1223–1230. doi:10.1046/j.1540-8167.2000.01223.x PMID:11083243

Winterfield, J. R., Jensen, J., Gilbert, T., Marchlinski, F., Natale, A., Packer, D., & Wilber, D. J. et al. (2015). Lesion Size and Safety Comparison between the Novel Flex Tip on the FlexAbility Ablation Catheter and the Solid Tips on the ThermoCool and ThermoCool SF Ablation Catheters. *Journal of Cardiovascular Electrophysiology*, *11*(Sep). doi: doi:10.1111/jce.12835 PMID:26359632

Zipes, D.P., Calkins, H., Williams, E.S., & Halperin, J.L. (2015, September 16). ACC/AHA/HRS Advanced Training Statement on Clinical Cardiac Electrophysiology (A Revision of the ACC/AHA 2006 Update of the Clinical Competence Statement on Invasive Electrophysiology Studies, Catheter Ablation, and Cardioversion). *Heart Rhythm*.

Chapter 12
An Optimized Graph-Based Metagenomic Gene Classification Approach:
Metagenomic Gene Analysis

Md Sarwar Kamal
East West University, Bangladesh

Mohammad Ibrahim Khan
Chittagong University of Engineering and Technology, Bangladesh

Kaushik Dev
Chittagong University of Engineering and Technology, Bangladesh

Linkon Chowdhury
Chittagong University of Engineering and Technology, Bangladesh

Nilanjan Dey
Techno India College of Technology, India

ABSTRACT

Biological interaction mainly depends on the interactions of various genes and genomes. To identify actual meaning of interactions we have to find out the facts and reasons for these interactions. Gene analysis allows to verify such environment. Gene annotation means to identify the exon regions in metagenomic samples. The de Bruijn graph plays significant role in gene prediction and next generation sequencing (NGS). Apart from that, Eular Path of de Bruijn graph introduced generalized gene annotation for translational and splicing signals, exon introns separation and coding regions. set of graph reduction rules have used to build a de Bruijn graph. Accurate solution for large scale sequencing, trims space complexity and generates optimal gene annotation have tested.

INTRODUCTION

The approach that specifies or categorized the genetic substance from environmental collections is called metagenomics. This process is important due to its uniqueness on data clustering facilities. I.e. the system permits to organize huge molecular data into a small area. By imposing metagenomics concept, various vital and unique molecules with pivotal activities and applications have been determined. The

DOI: 10.4018/978-1-5225-0140-4.ch012

populations and demand of foods and daily necessary goods are increasing day by day. To fulfill the demand of daily commodities as well as medical support, metagenomics will play very important role. Lot of companies are willing and investing in this sector to clear the unknown genetic information. So metagenomics gene analyses will dominant in enzymes processes, medicines, agriculture, ecology and new generic products. Metagenomics ensure to supply new molecules and novel enzymes with dynamic activities and provide factors from set of enzymes from the cultivable microorganisms. Apart from that, the uses of metagenomics are used to uncovering novel biocatalysts from nature, bioremediation and xenobiotic metabolism.

DNA sequence consists of four nucleotides A, G, C and T. These sequencing efforts generate a large amount of raw data as the DNA sequence of a eukaryote is often longer than a hundred million base pairs. The genome of human has 3.2 billion (appx) base pairs. The annotation of these sequences of biological data is needed as a computation tool for gene finding. Locating the genes is not only helpful but also a prerequisite for further analysis, such as the characterization of the function of the gene product, determining the phylogeny of different species or understanding gene regulation. But the problem of finding genes in a genomic DNA sequence is difficult and high space complexity.

Metagenomics, the investigation of crude bacterium under the study of genomic substances gathered precisely from natural data sets, has been applied to analyze the shape, activities, and mechanical interactions of small communities. Various analysis permit us to know about different microbes in multiple areas (Ley et al., 2008; Rusch et al., 2007; Wu et al., 2011), their composite architectures of the communities they built (Huttenhower et al., 2012), and the pivotal encounter they maintain on the associated environment (Tyson et al., 2004). It important to analyze the various bacterium interactions however, human metagenomics interactions are very essential to utilize the meaningful result due to its impact on mankind need as drugs, foods and diseases identifications (Qin et al., 2012; Behre C.J, et al., 2013; Greenblum et al., 2011).

In the age of information superhighway, numerous metagenomic analyses are based on gene-centric processes and as well as new aim to cluster the complete genomic shape of the association by virtue of shotgun metagenomics. Mathematical analysis based on shotgun sequencing impact helped to mapped database to a orthologous gene groups such as KEGG (Kanehisa et al., 2012), COG (Tatusov et al., 2003), EggNOG (Powell et al., 2012), M5NR (wike et al., 2012) to investigate similarities to genes or proteins with real and annotated activities. It is important to know that the biological activities among similar genes are work together in contrast, with taxonomic identify resulted in the experimental analysis. BLAST is frequently used to mapped to obtain greater score values on sequence alignment and annotations (Dalevi et al., 2008). This annotation mechanism and the measurements of the data set alignment that mapped individual activity is a an important part in computational metagenomic research and it helps to identify the functional shifts related with disease, as it is the basis of general genomic of analyses.

An important hypothesis afterwards, this annotation process and the key to properly saving the absolute structures of the metagenome alignment where small genome sequencing input holds abundant information to precise map to the exact activity. By considering different annotation rules and assumptions that each input will be directed to either its gene of or to an orthologous gene from an efficient distant genome annotated with the same function. These rules for future assumption that input initiating from intergenic regions or from orthology collection with unknown activity will not be properly mapped to any of the active annotated genes in our database. These considerations are vital for both estimation as well as identifying the presence or absence of gene groups. Now-a-days, but, no details and systematic studies has not checked this analysis on a broad scale, nor have rules for this annotation system been regulated.

The shortage of such systematic analysis produce the results sketched for different metagenomics studies are very difficult to quantify and compile and challenges any steps to compare research outcomes.

Microarray data set is a collection of chemically coated glass, nylon membrane or silicon. A microarray is a small chip (made of chemically coated glass, nylon membrane, or silicon. It comprises of millions of information for metagenomics genome or DNA sequence analysis. Metagenomics based research or microarray engineering organized an environment to measures automated process to check up the expressions and interactions of genes in all respects as drug design, disease investigations, protein-protein interactions and sequence analysis. But, very large data set in genes and biological network creates computational complexities in efficient data handling. To overcome the overcome the difficulties, classification and clustering techniques help optimize data processing. Subgroups help to organize the data set separately and consecutive ways. This clustering process is important for better data processing. Various clustering algorithms have been contributing the better data processing. A microarray based computational algorithm (Jiang et al., 2004) leveled data set into three distinct parts that helps to maintain group based data separation. But unsupervised data management produces some pitfall of this algorithm. Total number of groups and subgroups were unknown it becomes problematic for very large data processing. Microarray DNA sequence and gene analysis plays an important role towards the generations of drugs and diseases investigations. This system allows thousand of small DNA molecules in a small storage area. In current time, microarray data processing is very important in the field of Computational Biology. Consequently, microarray image processing enables proper information generation in gene annotations (Karim et al., 2011). Moreover, complete or global metagenomics processing opens verification techniques for gene expressions interactions. Formal and basic approaches of measuring gene study focused on a specific factor that led a limited area of biological data processing as well as information generation. Due to limitations, lots of vital biological changes were lost or misjudged. In this regards global data processing are very much efficient to cover all the facts related to the overall data set (Fryer et al., 2002).

In addition, de bruijn graph runs much faster and requires less memory space than most of compared methods, and exhibits competitive CPU time. The performance of optimized de bruijn graph is even comparable with the other gene assembler in both sensitivity and accuracy. Reduced de bruijn graph also runs much faster for gene annotation.

BACKGROUND

De-Bruijn graph is a directed graph that crates edges among all existing nodes in such a way that $P = (p1, p2, p3, \ldots, an)$ to $Q = (q1, q2, q3, \ldots, bn)$ with Q being a left sided part of P, or $q1 = p2$, $q2 = q3$. The critical benefit of this graph is that it mathematical tools that helps to remove assembly faults and get optimal solutions. Transcription assembler iterative De Bruijn graph approach (T-IDBA) (Peng et al., 2011) is an modified approach of iterative de Bruijn graph that rearrange positive genome segments from large sets of irregular data set of genes. Velvet (Zerbino at el., 2008) is a complete tool that quickly manage de Bruijn graph to curtail false reads and cut the redundant input sequences in genome segments. Velvet is a strong and efficient and simple dBG-oriented assembler. ABySS (Simpson et al., 2009) is a parallel and cluster based a measurement which is used to employ storage space for large-scale data volumes using the de Bruijn based classification. This package support and indicate the K-mer graphs and strongly connected graph calculation for a certain amounts of nodes that requires large storage area. AllPaths (Butler et al., 2008) is another de Bruijn Graph based assembly tool which can manage large amounts of genome sequencing. It is expandable in both prototype and real data sets. Apart from that, this package holds an algorithm that is used to read corrected input genome sequences. An organized research paper (Sonia and Sarwar, 2015) on Next Generation Sequencing has narrated the graph based approaches for genome assembly. MIRA3 is an organized framework of overlap layout consensus (OLC) under greedy algorithms (Zang et al., 2000). It is a tedious assembler that can read and manage older errors by the support of OLC and greedy mechanisms. Mosaik (http://bioinformatics.bc.edu/marthlab/Mosaik) is a history oriented sequencing process that aligns parallel sequencing in an exact analysis using Smith–Waterman algorithm with the help of hash-based table for shorter sequence reads. Another OLC-based automated tool is Newbler (Margulies et al., 2005) which is massively re-arranged by the famous 454 Life Science in gene sequencing and analysis. The starting point of this tool is used to sequence the DNA or RNA without the support of pairwise alignments where the sequence lengths were near about 120 bp. This automated computational tool has been updated that can organize the pairwise alignments as well as distinct alignments. From 2005, OLC was introducing for two basic ways as, OLC could build unitigs from input data and second it constructs huge contigs from unitigs. The pivotal benefits of Newbler are uses of sequence reads coverage and reduced matching errors. Graphlet degree vectors (Sonia and Sohel, 2014) are tinny strongly connected level graph under a large graph network. It supports to verify the gene annotations as well as interactions.

The research area of finding the protein coding genes in a eukaryotic genomic sequence by computational methods has become competitive. Most of the estimated 30000-40000 human genes code for proteins. Cells make a protein molecule from a DNA sequence containing the gene (Figure 1). First, a copy of a contiguous region of DNA is larger than actually coding part. This process is called transcription. Out of this sequence the introns are spliced out and the result is the concatenation of the exons, so called messenger RNA (mRNA). The number of exons varies in per gene. Some genes consist of only one exon and therefore do not contain introns. The human muscle protein constitutes the other extreme. It consists of 178 exons. In human, it is estimated that there are on average nine exons in per gene (Brown, 2002). In metagenomic analysis is defined as the classification of microbial genomes via the direct isolation of genomic sequences from the environment without prior cultivation (Handelsman, 2007).

Figure 1. The central dogma is a framework for understanding the flow of genetic information. It states that DNA makes RNA, and RNA makes protein (amino acid.)In transcription process DNA convert into RNA specially mRNA(messenger RNA) and in translation RNA convert into protein(amino acid).

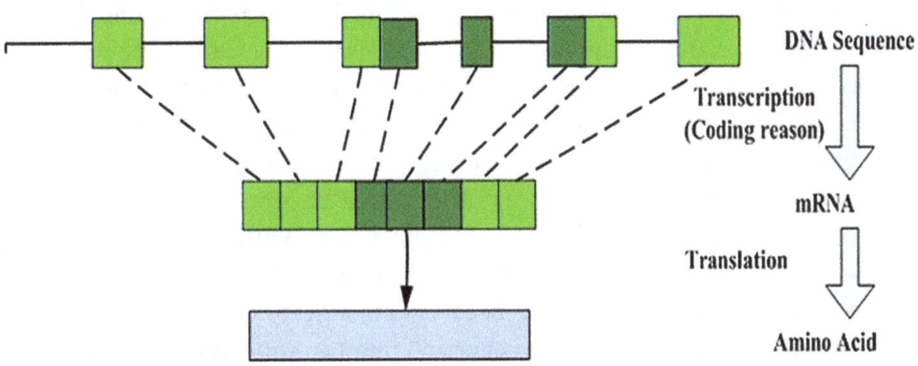

The whole genome of an organism sequence is assembled and then genes are predicted. In metagenomic, a single genome cannot be assembled and therefore, it is a challenge to predict genes within these short sequences (Hoff et al., 2009). Accurate gene annotation for environmental samples is needed so that genes can be classified to their correct functions, and it paves the way for functional studies in metagenomic. In the chromosomes the DNA sequence is found in a double stranded sequence, where each nucleotide in one strand is opposed by a complementary nucleotide in the other strand. A(Adenine) is the complement of T(Thiamine) and vice versa. In the same way C(Cytosine) and G(Guanine) are complementary bases. As the sequence of nucleotides of one strand is fully determined by the sequence of nucleotides on the opposite strand, we only need to know the sequence of one of the strands. Usually two neighboring genes (regardless whether they are on the same strand or on opposite strands) are separated by an inter-genomic region, but exceptions to this organization are known. In the human mitochondrial genome the coding regions (sic) of the genes ATP8 and ATP6, which are on the same strand, overlap by 46 nucleotides (the reading frames in the overlapping region are different). An example of a gene lying within another gene is the human neurofibromatosis type I gene on chromosome 17, which has three short genes on the opposite strand within one of its introns. Each of these internal genes has introns itself.

LITERATURE OVERVIEW

Bridger (Chang et al., 2015) is a software package that calculates the genome arrangements with the help of de novo transcriptome assembler where Cufflinks based methods are employed to decrease drawback of ongoing de novo assemblers. Justification of this tool are made with real data sets of human, and mouse RNA. It reduces the errors of false positive selections and operates substantially faster and holds much less storage areas than most existing assemblers. Consequently, Bridger restricted the sensitivity and accuracy with Cufflinks. However, this process is not fit for handling overlapped sequences. VirAmp (Yinan et al., 2015) is an integrated assembler that comprised with the techniques of existing assemblers as well as web-based interactive interfaces. This assembler supports multiple pipeline environments for data set classifications. This package also enables representations of large number of data set into a single platform. The interactive interface is the key advantages of this tool. However, this tool is also not free from overlapped genome sequencing and it takes more time to handle interconnected genome sets. ClusDCA (Wang et al., 2015) is ontology based automated environment that relocate information among all data set that has unique activity to mitigate the overfitting difficulties for sparsely annotated functions. To depict interconnected data, ontology based method takes more time due to absence of mapping. A mapping based analysis overcomes the difficulties where a reads mapping algorithm utilize short reads onto a de Bruijn graph of assemblies (Yuzhen et al., 2015). The prime consideration is a hash table that organizes the relationship of k-mers (mer: from Greek meaning "part") to enable faster mapping of reads to the graph. This is a reference-centric technique to metatranscriptome assembly that utilizes graphs of metagenome assembly as the reference. The experiments however notice that, this process has missed mapping of shorter fraction of multi-edge-spanning reads. While there is a sequencing defect in classification of k-mer, this algorithm is unable to detect the location of the error.

Accurate gene annotation for sample data is needed so that genes can be classified to their correct functions. Gene prediction programs can be categorized into two different groups. First, the ab initio programs that employ training set with known annotation for training the parameters of their models, are widely used in gene prediction (Mario et al., 2003). There are a large number of gene-finding programs of this kind, e.g. GENIE,(Martin et.al., 2000) GENSCAN, (Christopher, 1997) GENEID, (Gens et al., 2000) and GLIMMER (Arthur et al., 2007).Other gene prediction program known as similarity-based programs, use external information about the input sequence to predict genes. Some popular similarity based programs are GENEWISE,(Ewan et al., 2004) AGenDA (Leila, 2003) and the well known BLAST which searches the input. Open Reading Frame (ORF) is a conventional approach in gene prediction which began with a start codon and end with in-frame stop codon (Hoff et al., 2009). Generally, genes in prokaryotes are 1000-bp in length on average (Xu et al., 2006). Due to the short sequence length of metagenomic, they contain incomplete ORFs that lack start and/or stop codon, thus conventional ab-initio programs cannot be applied to metagenomic. Similarly, homology-based approaches for gene predictions rely on databases that only contain known, and thus a limited set of genes. Therefore, both of these categories do not work well for metagenomic fragments which are about 700 bp less than 400 bp when produced by Sanger and next generation sequencing, respectively (Mardis, 2008).Sequence similarity search has been proved useful in many cases, it is seen that only a fraction of newly discovered sequences have identifiable homolog in the current databases. Proteins might have already included representatives of most ancient conserved regions (ACRs, regions of protein sequences showing highly significant similarity across phyla) and that new sequences not similar to any database sequence are unlikely to contain ACRs (Green et al.,1993). The proportion of vertebrate genes with no detectable similarity in other phyla is estimated to be 50%.This is supported by a recent analysis of human chromosome 22 where only 50% of the proteins are found to be similar to previously known proteins. Therefore, recent tools have emerged to address these problems for metagenomic reads. Three programs are widely used for this purpose: Orphelia (Hoff, 2009), MetaGene (MG) (Noguchi et al., 2006), Meta Gene Annotator (MGA) (Noguchi et al., 2008), and Gene-Mark (Besemer et al., 1999). We demonstrate a memory efficient technique for metagenomic large scale data. We used bipartite graph and Euler path for finding gene from large DNA data set.

ARCHITECTURAL APPROACH

The structure of this work is built based on gene annotation (Figure 2).Our method works based on three phases: Data collection, Graph generation and Gene Annotation. The sample data are the data set of DNA nucleotides of human, plants or micro organ. Sample data are character of set of DNA nucleotide data stream. In graph generation phase divided into sub phases: generation of signed graph and graph reduction. In graph generation phase, we generate a undirected sign graph with multiple edges and loop. Graph reduction rules are used for graph rewriting. Basic reduction rule for graph rewriting technique is used for specification and generation of graph optimization.

After graph optimization we performed gene annotation. In next phase, gene annotation process is applied with euler path by using optimize de Brujin graph. We transform de Bruijn graph into series of equivalence sub graps. Euler path of every sub graphs represent the sub solution of the problem. Euler path is an efficient algorithm that is solved in a linear time. To combine the every solution of sub graphs represent the solution of gene annotation. In exon transcription, we marked initial and stopping sites in optimize de Brujin graph and find out euler path from intial site to stopping sites. Initial and stopping site indicates the exon annotation region.

Figure 2. Semantic view of the proposed methodology for genome assembly; our architecture has two phases: graph generation and genome assembly. In graph generation phase, an optimized de brujin graph is generated and genome assembly phase different type sequence are assembled (i.e. Exon separation or Genome fragmentation etc.).

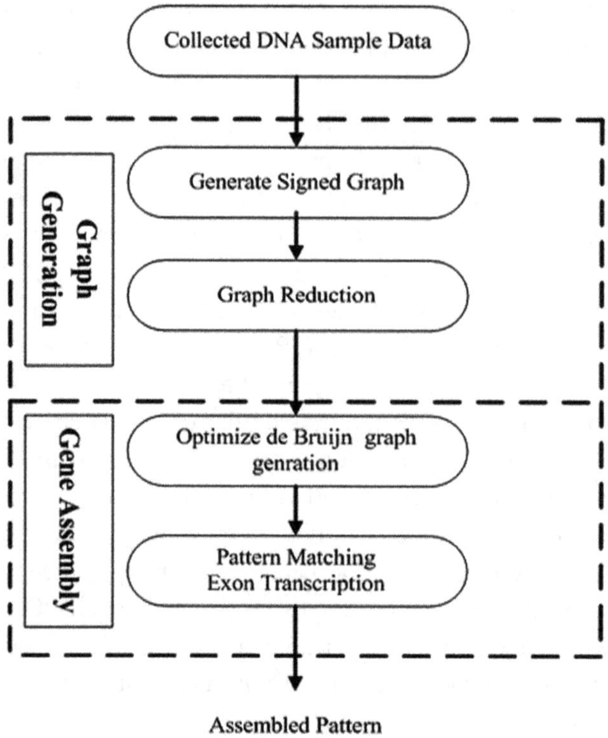

SIGNED GRAPH

In this section we have introduced basic notations for signed graph. Let G=(V,E) be a finite undirected graph with multiple edges and self loop. The number of $|\upsilon|$ the vertices, is called the order of G and the connected number of $|e|$ is called the degree of G. We write $\upsilon \in G$ if υ is vertex and $e \in G$ if e is edge of G. The neighborhood of a vertex υ is $N_G(\upsilon)=\{u|(\upsilon,u) \in G\}$.The vertex υ is isolated if $N_G(\upsilon)=0$.If a vertex has exactly one neighbor, it is denoted as a leap. We called G is discrete graph if all vertices are isolated. A subset $A \subseteq G$ is stable if there is no edges (υ,u) with $\upsilon,u \in A$. Graph A is complete if any two vertices of G are adjacent.

A signed graph $G=(V,E,\phi)$ consists of vertices and edges (V,E) together with a labeling function $\phi:V\rightarrow\{+,-\}$ of vertices V.A vertex $\upsilon \in G$ said to be positive and negative if $\varphi(v)=+$ and $\varphi(v)=-$ respectively. We let

$$G^{+}=\{v \mid \varphi(v)=+\} \text{ and } G^{-}=\{v \mid \varphi(v)=-\} \quad (1)$$

We say that a signed graph is negative if all its vertices are negative (Figure 3). Also, an edge $e=\{u,v\}$ is called negative, if $v,u \in G^{-}$.

Figure 3. A simple signed graph with positive or negative edges; an edge will negative if edges is connected with negative nodes and edges are positive if edges are connected with positive nodes.

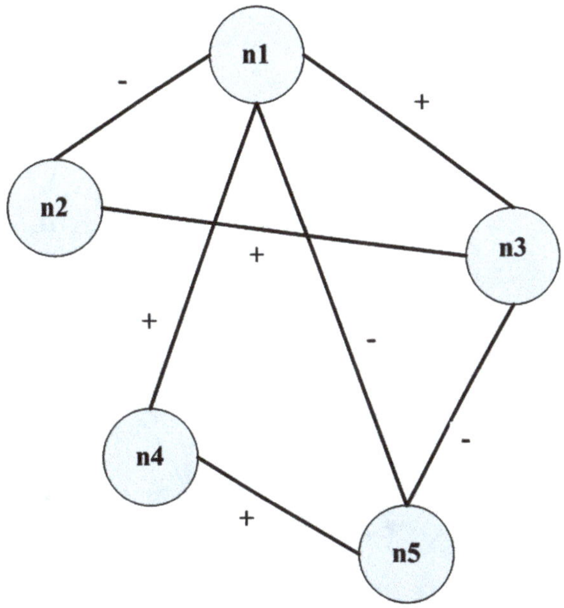

If G and H constitute a two signed graph and its two disjoint vertex sets are V(G) and V(H), let $G \oplus H$ be their disjoint union, the vertex set of $G \oplus H$ is $V(G) \cup V(H)$ (Figure 4a) and its edge forms,

$$E(G \oplus H) = E(G) \cup E(H) \tag{2}$$

The complete connection $G \otimes H$ has the vertices set and the edge set is (Figure 4b)

$$E(G \otimes H) = E(G) \cup E(H) \cup \{(v,u) \mid v \in G, u \in H\} \tag{3}$$

We used undirected sign graph for graph analysis and transformation which are performed in graph reduction technique. It is more compatible and easy in graph analysis in which enlarging graph by joining new edges with information and reduction by deleting edges or replacing sub graphs.

GRAPH REDUCTION RULE

There are three basic fundamental operations of reductions rule for signed graph. The molecular operations are translated into following operations:

Let u and v be two vertices:

1. The negative graph rule for v is applicable to G if $v \in G^{-}$ and it is isolated in G. The result is the signed graph $nr_{v}(v) = G - \{v\}$. The number of vertices is $\mid nr_{v} \mid = \{v\}$.

Figure 4. Two basic operations of signed graph: (a) And operation for two disjoint graph where two vertices convert into one vertex (b) complete operation for disjoint graph where two disjoint graph convert into one graph

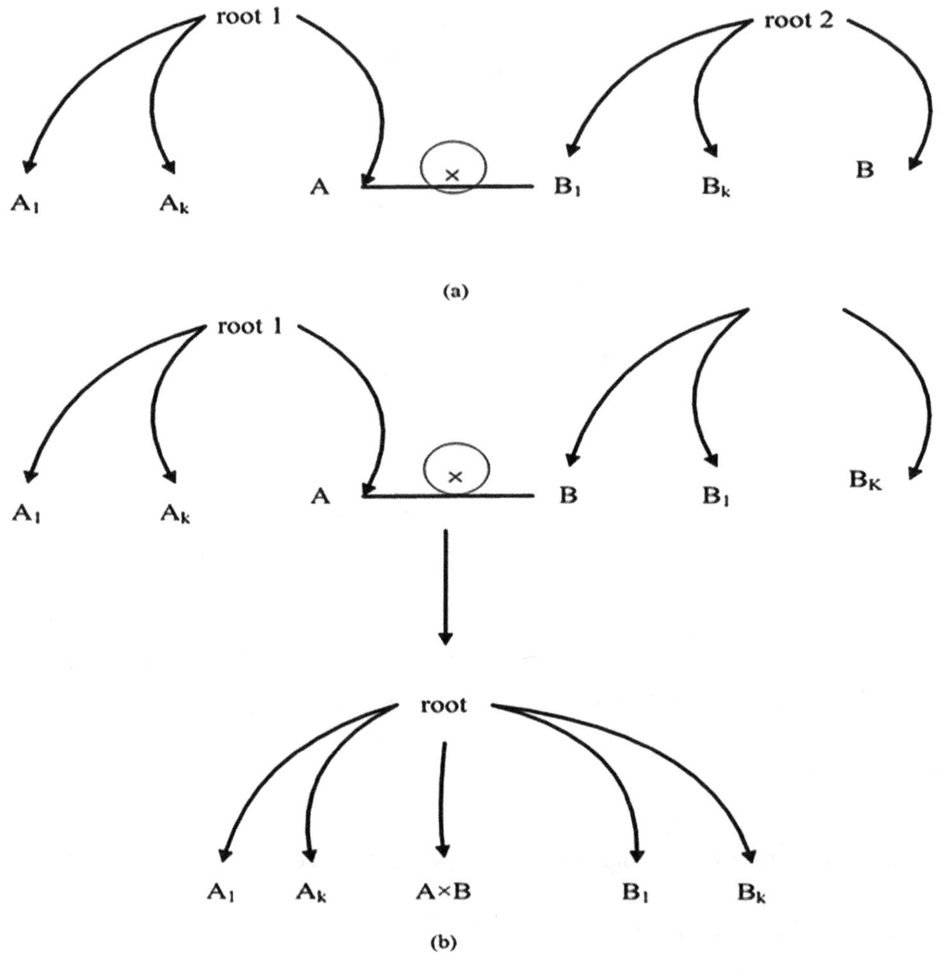

2. The positive graph rule for v is applicable to G if $v \in G^{+}$. The result is the signed graph $np_{v}(v) = G - \{v\}$. The number of vertices is $|\, nr_{v} \,| = \{v\}$.
3. The double rule for v≠u is applicable to G if $v, u \in G^{-}$ and $e = \{v, u\} \in E(G)$. The result for signed graph $dr(v) = G - \{(u, v), E', \varphi'\}$ where φ' is obtained to $G - \{u, v\}$ and E' obtained from complementary of E.

In basic reduction rule, graph rewriting technique is used for specification and generation of graph optimization. Graph analysis and transformation are performed by graph rewriting technique. Analyzing graph means enlarging graph by joining new edges with information and graph transformation means reduced into the graph rewriting by deleting and attaching sub graphs. In reduction rules we delete or replace two or more nodes by another node (Figure 5).

Figure 5. Graph reduction rule with termination point; in graph reduction rule it reduces the edges (paths) . A,B,C,D,E are nodes of the graph and Φ is termination point. D and E nodes are reduced by F or G.C,D and E nodes can also replaced by H. Here termination point indicates the ending point or pattern in transcription region. Replacement nodes reduce the graph complexity.

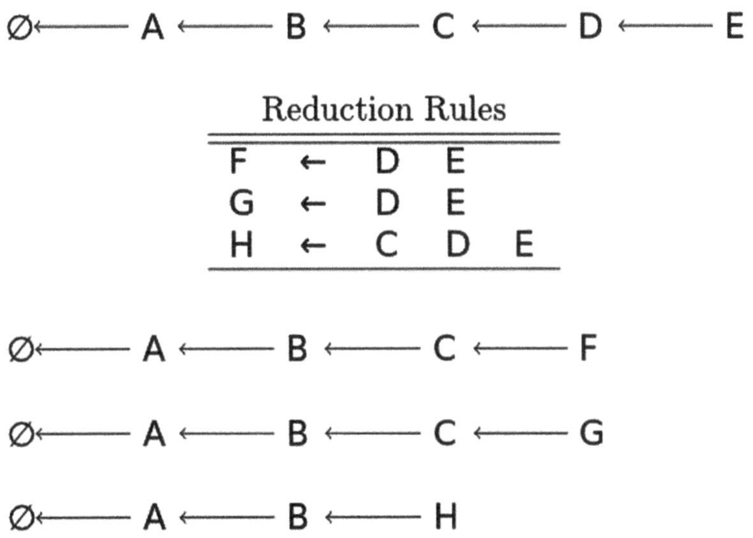

In graph reduction rules, node D and E are rewritten by F (Figure 5).Here D and E nodes can correlate with F, redundant nodes D and E are replaced by F. Node C,D and E are rewritten by new node H. Reduced edges are encrypted with new edge. Termination by edges accumulation and termination by edges subtraction is used for graph termination process. When, we reached to null point (Φ) that indicates the termination (Figure 5).

OPTIMIZE DE BRUJIN GRAPH

A sets of reads $S=\{s_1.......s_n\}$,define the de Bruijn graph $G(S_l)$ with (l-1) vertices.An (l- 1) tuple $v\epsilon S_{l-1}$ is joined by directed with l-edges. If S_l contains l-tuple for which the first (l-1) nucleotides coincide with v and last (l-1) nucleotides coincide with tuple w. Each l-tuple from S_l corresponds to an edge in G. If S contains the only sequence S_1, then this sequence corresponds to a path visiting each edge of the de Bruijn graph. A de Bruijn can substitute every edge by k parallel edges, where k is the number of times the edge is used. If S contains the only sequence S_1,this operation creates k parallel edges for every l-tuple repeating k times in S_1.Euler path is an efficient algorithm that is solved in a linear time.

In de Bruijn graph, a vertex v is called a source if indegree(v) =0,a sink if outdegree(v)=0 and branching vertex if indegree(v).outdegree(v)>1.A path $v_1......v_n$ in the de Bruijn graph is called a repeat pattern if indegree(v_1)>1,outdegree(v_n)>1 and indegree(v_i)=outdegree(v_i)=1,for $1\leq i\leq n-1$.Repeat pattern starts with v_i node and $v_{n,}$ are called exits from a repeat (Figure 6). An Eulerian path visits a repeat some times by visiting entrance and exit nodes. An Eulerian path covers a repeat if it contains an entrance into and exits from repeat by using end node. Every covering read-path reveals some information about the gene annotation between entrances and exit.

Figure 6. The overlapping pattern with repeated vertices and edges.v_1 ········ v_n are repeated vertices in an overlapping graph. It is difficult to find out the read -length and contigs. Euler path gives the optimal solution for overlapping pattern. This overlapped graph divided into two sub graphs.

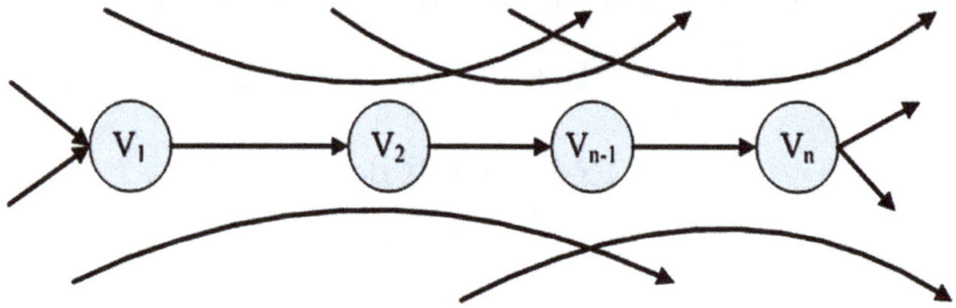

To solve the Euler path for gene annotation, we have transformed the both graph G and path P into new graph G_1 with path P_1. This is called equivalence if it exits one to one correspondence in (G, P) and (G_1, P_1).We transform de Bruijn graph into series of equivalence transformation:

$(G,P) \rightarrow (G_1,P_1) \rightarrow (G_2,P_2) \rightarrow \ldots\ldots\ldots \rightarrow (G_k,P_k)$

To combine the every solution of sub graphs represent the solution of gene annotation (exon/introns separation), Euler path solution is used. We describe a simple equivalence transformation that solves the Euler path problem where graph G has no multiple edges. We consider two cases of transformation; one is x-y detachment and another one is x-cut. Let $x=(v_{in},v_{mid})$ and $y=(v_{mid},v_{out})$ are two consecutive edges of graph G and $P_{x,y}$ be the collection of all paths of P that includes all sub paths. $P_{\rightarrow x}$ defines as a collection of paths from P that end with x and $P_{y\rightarrow}$ as a collection of paths from P that starts with y. Then x,y-detachment is a transformation that adds a new edge $z=(v_{in,}v_{out})$ and deletes the edges x and y from G (Figure 7a).This detachment transformation alters the systems of path P as follows:

1. Substitute z for x,y in all path from$P_{x,y}$.
2. Substitute z for x in all paths from $P_{\rightarrow x}$.
3. Substitute z for y in all paths from $P_{y\rightarrow}$.

Every detachment reduces the number of edges in G and reduces the complexity of Euler path problem. Consider a fragment of graph G with 5 edges or 4 paths y_3-x,y_4-x,x-y_1 and x-y_2 (fig-7b).For graph fragmentation n edges or paths, it will be y_n-x,y_{n-1}-x,....y_1-x. In symmetric situation, x is tangle (repeated pattern) and there is no available information to relate any of paths y_3-x and y_4-x to relate another paths x-y_1 and x-$y_{2.A}$n edge x=(v,w) is removable if

1. It is only incoming edge v and only one outgoing edge w.
2. x is either the initial or the terminal edge for every path P containing x.

An x-cut transformation P into a new system of paths by simply removing *x* from all paths in $P_{\rightarrow x}$ and $P_{x\rightarrow}$ without affected graph G itself (fig-7b).If x is a removable edge then x-cut is an equivalent transformation. Detachment and x cut proved to be powerful technique to build a simple de Bruijn graph and reduce fragments for all genome.

Figure 7. Equivalent transformation for Euler path; blue indicates the overlap paths and green line indicates equivalent paths.(a)X,Y –detachment which alters the systems of path for overlapped graph. In every detachment reduces the number of edges and reduces the complexity of Euler path. (b) X-cut which divide the overlapped graph into two or more sub graphs.

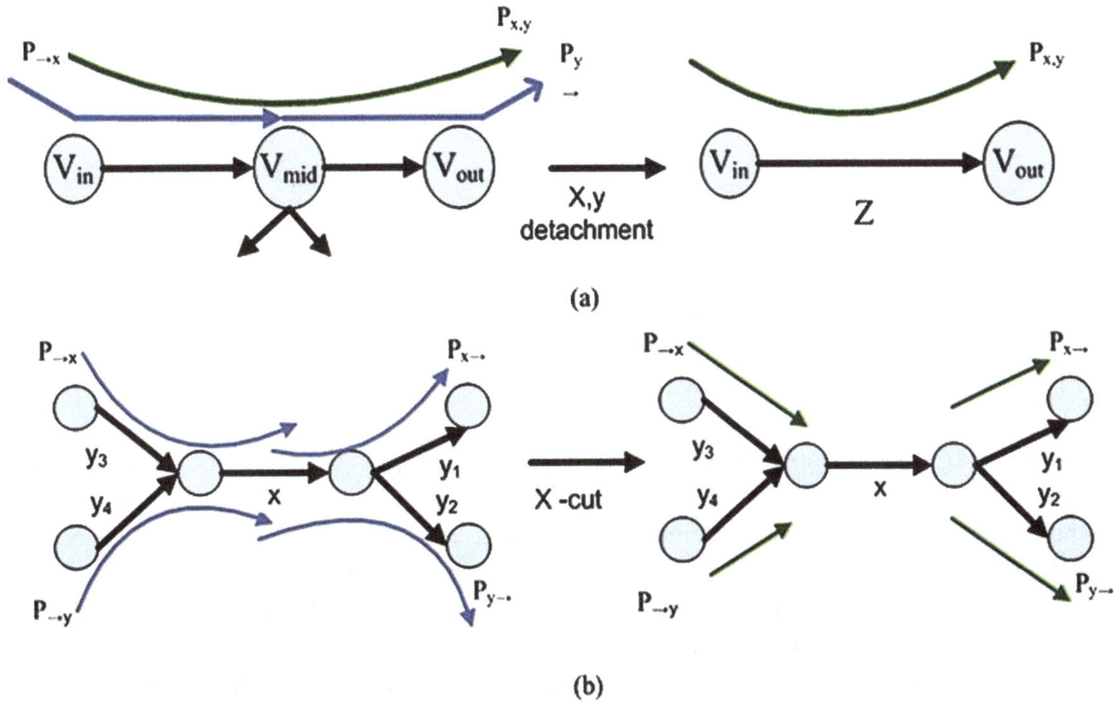

GENE ANNOTATION

De Bruijn graph is used for gene Annotation (Exon Intron separation) and next generation sequence assembler. It reduces computational effort by breaking read (sort sequence) into smallest part of DNA. Reads are called k-mer where the parameter k denotes the length of bases for these sequences. De Bruijn graph capture exon separation with considering exon initial and stop sites using k-mer (Figure 8).Construct a de Bruijn graph for exon introns where separation consists of the following steps:

1. **Structure of k-Spectrum:** Reads are divided into overlapping sequence of k. Every k-mer consists transcription and stopping site in exon chain.
2. **Node Generation:** Every (k-1) node generates for k-spectrum. In de Bruijn graph, exon initial site is marked as initial node (source), ending node (sink) represents stop site of exon chain and intermediate node serves donor and acceptor site for exon transcription.
3. **Edge Construction:** A directed edge is created from x node to y node if there exists k-mer such that its prefix is equal to x node to y node. Overlap path are reduced to euler path simplification which described in section 4.1.To traverse marked source node to sink node we had indentified the exon chain from whole DNA sequence.

By reducing whole data set into k-mer overlaps the de Bruijn graph reduces the high redundancy in short read data set. In exon annotation, imitation sites start with ATG and termination site with TAA or TAG or TGA. Another donor and acceptor site generates the internal node in de Bruijn graph. Initial and stopping site indicates the exon annotation region (Figure 8). By converting the set of reads into edges of the de Bruijn graphs, the annotation problem becomes equivalent to finding an Euler path graph. To reduce the exponential distinct Euler path, heuristics are usually applied to construct the graphs. The graphs are filtered of erroneous occurrences and nodes are unambiguously connected by edges which are merged together.

GENOME FRAGMENTATION

All sequencing platforms produce explanation of the target DNA molecule in the form of reads sequences of single-letter base pairs. (Miller et al., 2010). An example of a single-end read and a paired-end (Figure. 9a & Figure 9b). Genome assembly is two groups:

- **De Novo:** It is an assembly tools for DNA sequence. Contigs is A group of overlapping clones representing regions of the genome; the contiguous sequence of DNA created by assembling these overlapping chromosome fragments. In genome assembly scaffold is used to describe the first complete sequence assembly, to which new reads are aligned. Once have a scaffold you don't depend on de novo assembly anymore but can find a region to which any given new read is most similar and subsequently look for genetic variation.
- **Mapping/Reference:** In genomics complete genomes provide an outstanding resource for future sequencing projects. However, generating finished genomes is an exclusive and laborious endeavor. In some cases, the returns of finishing a genome are not worth the cost particularly when draft genomes can provide enough information for robust assembly process. Draft genomes contain a large number of unordered sequences of various lengths called contigs. Contigs can be joined into more contiguous sequences called scaffolds using paired-end reads. While a set of contigs/ scaffolds can be useful for a wide variety of projects (gene annotation, gene expression profiling,

Figure 8. The length of overlap k-1=2; green node indicates initial site and red node indicates termination site respectively. Black line indicates the order of k-mer. Two braches indicates the separate genome annotation and possible ways of exon chaining.

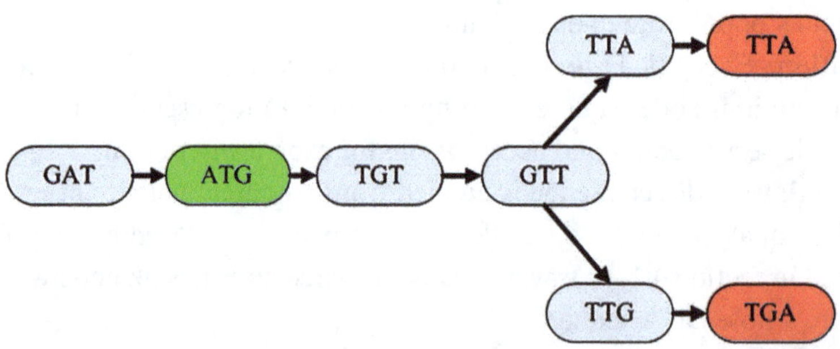

Figure 9. Example of DNA fragment read (a) single end (b) double end; single end read indicates the single DNA sequence fragmentation and double end read fragment the multiple sequences. Double end read reduces the time complexity than single end.

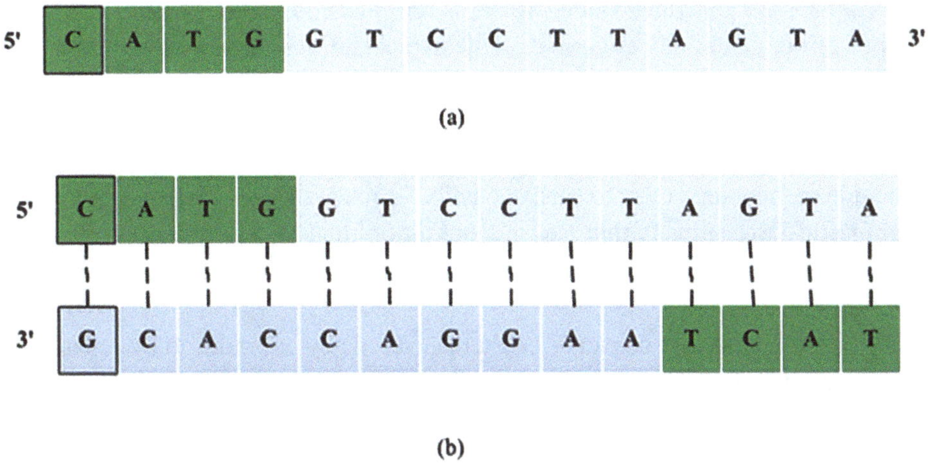

etc.), contig order provides vital information in comparative genomics and analyses of specific genomic regions. Typically, a rough ordering of contigs can be accomplished by mapping contigs to a closely related reference genome.

As a result of the de novo assembly stage, a set of scaffolded contigs is accessible. Besides ordered contigs, scaffolds also contain gaps of estimated length separating the contigs. Scaffolds are also often called supercontigs. Low risk assemblies consistent with almost all of the detectable pair-wise read overlaps are called unitigs.Sequence alignment is the procedure of comparing two or more sequences by searching for a series of individual base pairs or base pairs patterns that are in the same order in all sequences. In most cases, the sequences cannot be aligned perfectly due to their mismatch. In an optimal case, mismatch base pairs and gaps are placed, in order to match together as many identical or similar base pairs as possible.

Sanger's method is most popular sequence fragment assembly algorithms were focused on creating multiple overlapping alignments of the reads to produce a layout assembly of the data. The alignment is used to read the consensus sequence, from which the DNA sequence is incidental. The described method was called the overlap-layout-consensus approach (OLC). OLC approach is one of the two typical approaches of the de novo DNA assembly, and is effectively used during the assembly of long, high-quality reads. Another very important, and currently most utilized approach in combination with Next Generation Sequencing (NGS) data, is based on the de Bruijn graph. This approach was commonly known as short read assemblers. Unlike the computationally expensive step of determining overlap amongst reads, the de Bruijn graph is constructed from fixed-length subsequences. If the sequence length is m then that have a perfect (m-1) suffix to (m 1)-prefix overlap. In de Bruijn assembler include Euler, AllPaths and Velvet methods.

Both the OLC and the de Bruijn approaches are graph based. Another type approaches also do exist. They include greedy search methods i.e. dynamic approaches such as Taipan (Schmidt et al., 2009).Errors in assembly can occur for two main reasons: Firstly, incorrect or incomplete information provided to the assembler. The real-world WGS data that contains errors can induce the following problems in overlap and de Bruijn graphs (Miller et al., 2010):

- **Bubbles:** Bubbles are generated when two paths start and end nodes are same. Bubbles generated by causes of errors or biological variants. Dijksatra's and breath first algorithm is used the best path and remove such error.
- **Spurs:** Spurs are short, dead-end divergences from the main path. They are induced by sequencing error toward one end of a read. They can be induced by coverage dropping to zero. Possible causes include sequencing errors toward one end of a read, and low coverage.
- **Converging and Diverging Paths:** Reverse definition than for the bubbles, two paths converge into one, that later diverges again into two separate paths. Possible causes are repeats in the target or source genome.
- **Cycles:** Cycles are paths that converge on themselves. They are induced by repeats in the target. For instance, short tandem repeats induce small cycles.

Although sequencing technology has greatly enhanced, still no sequencing platform can produce sufficient data to assemble a complete genome from a single experiment. One of the key problems in shotgun sequencing is caused by repeats in genome sequences. Repeats, in cases when they are longer than fragment reads, persuade problems during the overlap phase of assembly. As a result, assemblies result in fragmented contigs, separated by gaps. Repeat caused fragmentation is more pronounced in the NGS technology. Assemblies containing gaps are called draft assemblies, while the process of filling the gaps is called finishing. Finishing involves obtaining missing sequences, improving low quality regions, resolving miss assemblies and ordering scaffolds. In order to fill gaps, further sequencing is usually required, either by amplifying and sequencing fragments spanning gaps, or by resequencing the entire DNA.

OVERLAP-LAYOUT-CONSENSUS APPROACHE

Let $N = \{n_1, n_{2,......} n_m\}$ be a set of non-empty strings over an alphabet. An overlap graph of G is a complete weighted directed graph where each string in N is a vertex and the length of an edge between vertices x and y. The construction of the overlap graph is the first step of the OLC approach. General process of this approach consists of three main phases from which it derives its name:

1. **Overlap:** An overlap graph is created by joining all the reads by their respective best overlapping reads. This step is similar to the greedy approach.
2. **Layout:** The overlap graph is analyzed and simplified with the application of graph algorithms to identify the appropriate paths traversing through the graph and produce an approximate layout of the reads along the genome. The ultimate goal is a single path that traverses each node in the overlap graph exactly once.
3. **Consensus:** Multiple sequence alignment of all reads covering the genome is performed, and the original sequence of the genome being assembled is contingent through the consensus of the aligned reads.

A very important observation is that the identification of a path that traverses every node in the graph only once is a computationally difficult Hamiltonian path problem. The problem is also known as the Travelling Salesman Problem and is NP-complete.

The evolution of assembly Overlap-Layout-Consensus (OLC) and de-bruijn graph (DBG) algorithms are widely used OLC generally works in three steps: first overlaps (O) among all the reads are found, then it carries out a layout (L) of all the reads and overlaps information on a graph and finally the consensus (C) sequence is inferred. It is an intuitionist assembly algorithm. In the OLC algorithm, the identification of overlap between each pair of reads is explicit; typically by doing all-against-all pair-wise reads aligning. As a result, the OLC algorithm constructs a reads graph, which places reads as nodes and assigns a link between two nodes when these two reads overlap larger than a cutoff length. The nodes number is equal to the reads number, increasing linearly with sequencing depth and the links number will increase by a logarithmic scale.

DBG is an anti-intuition algorithm, working by first chopping reads into much shorter k-mers and then using all the k-mers to form a DBG and finally inferring the genome sequence on the DBG. The DBG assemblers were initially successful on small genomes such as bacteria, and were then extended to large genomes. In the DBG algorithm, the overlap relationship between neighboring k-mers is established implicitly. This process is completed by chopping all the reads into k-mers and simultaneously recording their neighboring relations. DBG algorithm constructs a k-mer graph that places k-mer as nodes and assigns a link between two nodes when these two k-mers are neighbors on the genome.

EXON TRANSCRIPTION

As exons are not independent, by splicing exons together to assemble a gene one can further eliminate false exon predictions by imposing translatability (i.e. adjacent exons must maintain the open reading frame). The main difficulty in exon assembly is the combinatorial explosion problem: the number of ways N candidates' exons may be combined grows exponentially with N. The key idea of computational feasibility comes from dynamic programming (DP), which allows finding "optimal assembly" quickly without having to enumerate all possibilities. We can limit possible errors by assuming each entry with a correct annotation that should satisfy:

- The initiation site is ATG.
- The donor site is GT.
- The acceptor site is AG.
- The stopping site is either TAA or TAG or TGA.
- No stop codon interrupts the open reading frames.
- The length of coding regions is a multiple of three.

In pattern reorganization, the performance of a prediction system can be measured by the following statistics: true positive (TP), true negative (TN), false positive (FP) and false negative (FN). The internal exon prediction measurement on the nucleotide base pair in different level (Figure 10).

The accuracy of a prediction system is measured by sensitivity (SN), specificity (SP) and correlation co-efficiency (CC) as follows:

Figure 10. Measurement of Exon prediction comparing with predicted data set; True Positive (TP) indicates exon region consist both gene and predicted gene, True Negative (TN) indicates exon region not present both gene and predicted gene, in False Positive (FP) exon region is found in predicted pattern but not in real gene.

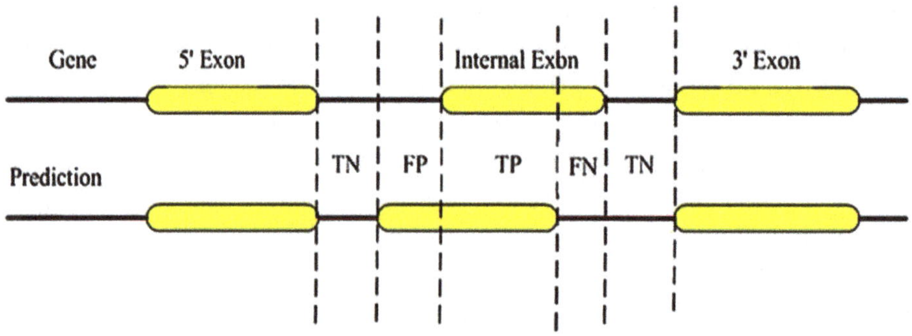

$$SN = \frac{TP}{TP + FN} \tag{4}$$

$$SP = \frac{TP}{TP + FP} \tag{5}$$

$$CC = \frac{TP \times TN - FP \times FN}{\sqrt{(TP + FN) \times (TN + FP) \times (TP + FP) \times (TF + FN)}} \tag{6}$$

RESULT

We experienced our gene analysis method on three data sets which are adh222, h178 and sag178 (Table 1). Adh22 is a single sequence of Drosophila melanogaster and 2.9Mb long. It is a well characterized sequence from the Adh22 region and has been used in the Genome Annotation Assessment Project(GASP). In the update version std1 contains 38 genes with a total of 111 exons and std3 contains 222 genes with a total of 909 exons. The genes lie on both strands. Both the authors of GENIE and of GENEID have used these two annotation sets for testing their programs. H178 is a set of 178 human genomic sequences with one complete gene each. Each contains one gene and a little neighboring DNA. The sequences are from EMBL, were compiled by[GAA+00] and have also been used by the author of GENSCAN for evaluation [YLB01]. The mean sequence length is 7169 bases. This set is known to contain three annotated genes which are very likely, if not known to be wrong. But we kept them for reasons of comparability. sag178 is a set of 43 sequences with 178 human genes. These sequences were also taken from [GAA+00]. The mean sequence length is 177 kilo bases (shortest 70, longest 282 kilo bases) and each sequence contains average 4.1 genes.

Table 1. Accuracy result on training data sets

Data Sets	Methods				
			Euler	GENESCAN	GENEID
adh22	Base	SP	97.3%	96%	96%
		SN	91%	92%	92%
	Exon	SP	72.4%	71%	70%
		SN	61%	62%	57%
	Gene	SP	48%	47%	40%
		SN	34.7%	33%	29%
h178	Base	SP	96%	97%	89%
		SN	87%	86%	91%
	Exon	SP	82.7%	83%	66%
		SN	74.5%	75%	75%
	Gene	SP	38.5%	40%	14%
		SN	37%	36%	15%
sag178	Base	SP	93%	94%	89%
		SN	83.2%	64%	78%
	Exon	SP	67.4%	68%	67%
		SN	61%	45%	60%
	Gene	SP	20%	18%	17%
		SN	22%	14%	17%

We measured the gene prediction accuracy with the sensitivity and specificity. A predicted exon is considered correct if both splice sites are at the annotated position of an exon. A predicted gene is considered correct if all exons predicted are correctly and no additional exons are predicted. Predicted partial genes were counted as predicted genes. For each data set these measures were computed globally. For comparing we choose GENESCAN and GENEID. We took GENSCAN as it is the most commonly used gene prediction program and as it is considered one of the best programs for humans. Our method considers memory efficient which is considering GENESCAN. We used GENEID (version 1.1) as there is a special Drosophila parameter set available for it and as it uses a different approach not modeling the lengths. GENEID first finds splice site candidates, then exon candidates are using the splice site candidates and then genes using the exon candidates.

By combining both measures we use the f-measure, a good indicator of overall precision and recall of the algorithm. F-measure (Figure 11) indicates the positive predictive value of a data set.

$$F - measure = \frac{2 * SP * SN}{SP + SN} \tag{7}$$

Internal exon prediction is important for gene prediction. Internal exons also have flanking splicing boundaries: the acceptor splicing sites at the 5′ end and the donor sites at the 3′end. Potentially all of the selected donor site and acceptor site candidates can be paired to form exon boundaries. The number

Figure 11. F-.Measurement of gene prediction for different method; for different types of genome fragmentation Euler path based on de Brujin graphs gives the better result. Genemarker generates the more accurate result rather the GeneId algorithm.

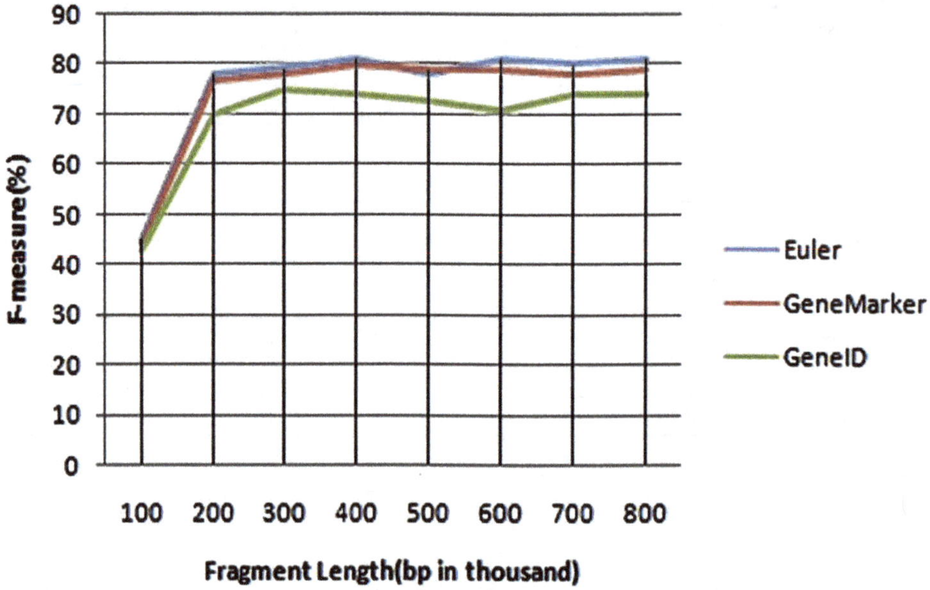

of internal exons in a gene is one less than the number of introns. In our learning data set, there are only 125 internal exons. When we paired 348 selected donor site candidates and 607 selected acceptor site candidates, we had got another set of 314 pseudo exons, The final internal exon prediction combined all the features of donor sites and acceptor sites, with the in-frame hexamer preferences and the log of exon length. The optimal discriminate function had the performance in Table 2.

The Sensitivity and Specificity measure the estimate of the program capability of detecting reads that contains gene. Coefficient indicates the accuracy of gene detection. The Genome Analyzer can generate paired reads with a length of 150 bp and more. There are, however, alternate technologies such as sequencing that produce longer unpaired reads. In this experiment, we investigate the influence of read length on an assembly.We simulated paired reads of 150 bp length (with a 450 bp fragment size) and 400 bp unpaired reads from the E. coli genome and human chromosome 20, respectively. All reads were simulated as error-free and at 50× base coverage. We used Velvet with a k-mer size of 31 to assemble all four data sets.

Table 2. Internal Exon measurement based on sensitivity, specificity, coefficient co-relation

Measurement	Total Number	Accuracy		
		SP	SN	CC
Base Pair	145	94.1%	87.2%	92.1%
Exon	325	91.0%	87.1%	87.1%

The contig sizes for each assembly. The assemblies using the 150 bp paired reads yield far larger contigs as compared to the 450 bp single read assemblies (Table 3). This is in part due to the way a de Bruijn graph assembler such as Velvet works: the reads are split into smaller pieces, the k-mers. In this experiment, we used a k-mer size of 35 which is the maximum for Velvet . Therefore we compared in principle k-mers of length 35 with and without pairing information. The strong impact of read pairs as opposed to single ended reads is evident (Figure 12).

To examine how long inserts can improve the assembly we sequenced E. coli with different base pair size(6kb to 10 kb). All of the de novo assemblers that we tested have the ability to use long-insert size (Table 4). Table 4 shows results obtained using De Brujin graph with a variety of long insert libraries. The 6 kb inserts already help bridge most of the repeats in E. coli if combined with the short insert sequence, and result in an assembly with an N50 of 1,403,330 bp. The two largest contigs cover a region of 2,348,095 bp, which corresponds to 68% of the E. coli genome. The rest of the genome is contained in smaller contigs (Figure 12).

The use of graph reduction rules to store a de Bruijn graph is straightforward and memory efficient. The expected false positive rate can be tuned based on desired memory usage, yielding a wide range of possible storage efficiencies . Optimized de bruijn graph is more efficient in time and space than the other assembler tools. We find out optimal euler path by using optimized de bruijn graph for gene annotation

Table 3. Effect of read length for different E.Coli sample with different base pair

Sample	N50 Contig Size	Largest Contig	Genome Coverage
E. coli, 150 bp pe	122,776 bp	326,886 bp	97.07%
E. coli, 450 bp sr	21,405 bp	127,976 bp	96.27%
Chr. 20, 150 bp pe	56,744 bp	401,312 bp	89.59%
Chr. 20, 450 bp sr	2,214 bp	23,423 bp	91.05%

Figure 12. Genome accuracy analysis by using de brujin graph for four data set (E.coli, 150 bp pe, E. coli, 450 bp sr, Chr. 20, 150 bp pe, Chr. 20, 450 bp sr); we find better accuracy for E.coli, 150 bp.

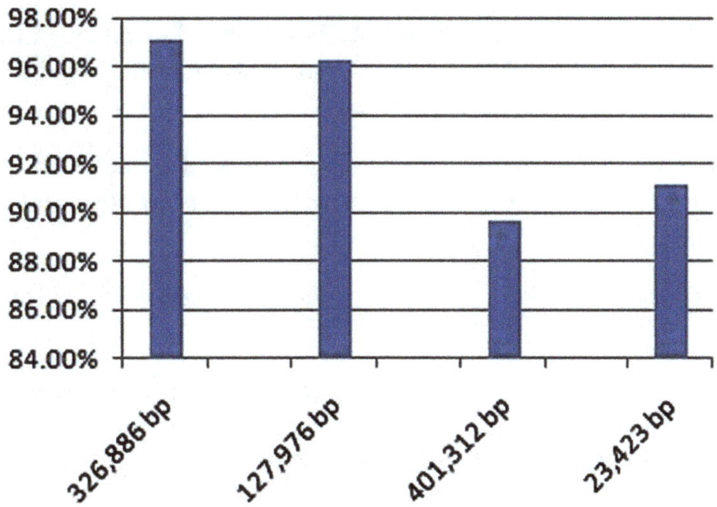

Table 4. Effect of insert size for different super contig

Inserts	Reads (bp)	Coverage	N50 Super Contig	Largest Super Contig	Genome Coverage
200 bp	2×75	50×	94 kb	224 kb	98.88%
200 bp	2×75	50×	1.1 Mb	1.9 Mb	97.17%
200 bp	2×75	50×	4.2 Mb	4.2 Mb	98.59%

CONCLUSION

In this research, we have observed that graph theory gives better accuracy than other two models. Our method is a robust that continuously vacant the memory storage, especially the proposed algorithm truly stands out when the data set of DNA segments are increased. In fact, our simulation result indicates that is more accurate in large data set. It performs relatively well on the task of assembling exons to genes because programs with a similar exon level accuracy often have a lower gene level accuracy. This means those programs more often combine the exons to a wrong gene structure for example by splitting or joining genes. With the growing number of sequenced species, the possibilities of finding approximate possible exons and genome assembly by cross-species alignments of homologue genomic sequences also increase. This leaves the task of assembling possible exons or pattern to genes. In future, we shall consider this concept for finding possible introns analysis.

REFERENCES

Arthur, D., Kirsten, B., Edwin, P., & Steven, S. (2007). Identifying bacterial genes and endosymbiont dna with glimmer. *Bioinformatics (Oxford, England)*, *23*, 7. PMID:17237039

Besemer, J., & Borodovsky, M. (1999). Heuristic approach to deriving models for gene finding. *Nucleic Acids Research*, *27*(19), 3911–3920. doi:10.1093/nar/27.19.3911 PMID:10481031

Brown, T. A. (2002). *Genomes 2*. John Wiley & Sons Inc.

Butler, J., MacCallum, I., Kleber, M., Shlyakhter, I. A., Belmonte, M. K., Lander, E. S., & Jaffe, D. B. et al. (2008). AllPaths: De novo assembly of whole-genome shotgun microreads. *Genome Research*, *18*(5), 810–820. doi:10.1101/gr.7337908 PMID:18340039

Chang, Z., Li, G., Li, J., Zhang, Y., Ashby, C., Liu, D., & Huang, X. et al. (2015). Bridger: A new framework for de novo transcriptome assembly using RNA-seq data. *Genome Biology*, *16*(1), 30. doi:10.1186/s13059-015-0596-2 PMID:25723335

Christopher, B. B. (1997). *Identification of genes in human genomicdna*. (Ph.D. Thesis). Stanford University, Stanford, CA.

Dalevi, D., Ivanova, N. N., Mavromatis, K., Hooper, S. D., Szeto, E., Hugenholtz, P., & Markowitz, V. M. et al. (2008). Annotation of metagenome short reads using proxygenes. *Bioinformatics (Oxford, England)*, *24*(16), i713. doi:10.1093/bioinformatics/btn276 PMID:18689842

Ehrenfeucht, A., Harju, T., Petre, I., Prescott, D. M., & Rozenberg, G. (2004). *Computation in Living Cells: Gene Assembly in Ciliates*. Springer. doi:10.1007/978-3-662-06371-2

Ewan, B., Michele, C., & Richard, D. (2004). *Gene wise and genome wise*. Genome Res.

Fryer, R. M., Randall, J., Yoshida, T., Hsiao, L., Blumenstock, J., Jensen, K. E., & Gullansa, S. R. et al. (2002). Global Analysis of Gene Expression:Methods, Interpretation, and Pitfalls. *Experimental Nephrology*, *10*(2), 64–74. doi:10.1159/000049901 PMID:11937753

Gens, P., Enrique, B., & Roderic, G. (2000). Geneid in drosophila. *Genome Research*, *10*(4), 511–515. doi:10.1101/gr.10.4.511 PMID:10779490

Green, P., Lipman, D., Hillier, L., Waterston, R., States, D., & Claverie, J. M. (1993). Ancient conserved regions in new gene sequences and the protein databases. *Science*, *259*(5102), 1711–1716. doi:10.1126/science.8456298 PMID:8456298

Greenblum, S., Turnbaugh, P. J., & Borenstein, E. (2011). Metagenomic systems biology of the human gut microbiome reveals topological shifts associated with obesity and inflammatory bowel disease. *Proceedings of the National Academy of Sciences of the United States of America*, *109*(2), 594–599. doi:10.1073/pnas.1116053109 PMID:22184244

Handelsman, J. (2007). *Committee on Metagenomics*. Challenges and Functional Applications The National Academies Press.

Hoff, K. J., Lingner, T., Meinicke, P., & Tech, M. (2009). Orphelia:predicting genes in metagenomic sequencing reads. *Nucleic Acids Research*, *37*(Web Server), 101–105. doi:10.1093/nar/gkp327 PMID:19429689

Huttenhower, C., Gevers, D., Knight, R., Abubucker, S., Badger, J. H., Chinwalla, A. T., & White, O. et al. (2012). Structure, function and diversity of the healthy human microbiome. *Nature*, *486*(7402), 207–214. doi:10.1038/nature11234 PMID:22699609

Kanehisa, M., Goto, S., Sato, Y., Furumichi, M., & Tanabe, M. (2012). KEGG for integration and interpretation of large-scale molecular data sets. *Nucleic Acids Research*, *40*(D1), 109–114. doi:10.1093/nar/gkr988 PMID:22080510

Karim, R., Khaliluzzaman, M., & Mahmud, S. (2014). A Review of Image Analysis Techniques for Gene Spot Identification in cDNA Microarray Images. *International Journal of Artificial Intelligence & Application*, *5*, 1–7.

Karlsson, F. H., Tremaroli, V., Nookaew, I., Bergstrom, G., & Behre, C. J. (2013). Gut metagenome in European women with normal, impaired and diabetic glucose control. *Nature*, 4–10. PMID:23719380

Leila, T., Oliver, R., Saurabh, G., Alexander, S., Michael, B., Serafim, B., & Burkhard, M. (2003). Agenda: Homology-based gene prediction. *Bioinformatics (Oxford, England)*, *19*(12), 1575–1577. doi:10.1093/bioinformatics/btg181 PMID:12912840

Ley, R. E., Hamady, M., Lozupone, C., Turnbaugh, P. J., Ramey, R. R., Bircher, J. S., & Gordon, J. I. et al. (2008). Evolution of mammals and their gut microbes. *Science*, *320*(5883), 1647–1651. doi:10.1126/science.1155725 PMID:18497261

Mardis, E. R. (2008). The impact of next-generation sequencing technology on genetics. *Trends in Genetics*, *24*(3), 133–141. doi:10.1016/j.tig.2007.12.007 PMID:18262675

Margulies, M., Eghol, M., Altman, W. E., Attiya, S., Bader, J. S., Bemben, L. A., & Rothberg, J. M. et al. (2005). Genome sequencing in microfabricated high-density picolitre reactors. *Nature*, *437*, 376–378. PMID:16056220

Mario, S., & Stephan, W. (2003). Gene prediction with a hidden markov model and a new intron submodel. Oxford University Press.

Martin, G., David, K., Hari, T., & David, H. (2000). Genie–gene finding in drosophila melanogaster. *Genome Research*, 529–538.

Miller, J. R., Koren, S., & Sutton, G. (2010). Assembly algorithms for nextgeneration sequencing data. *Genomics*, *95*(6), 315–327. doi:10.1016/j.ygeno.2010.03.001 PMID:20211242

Mohammad, I. K., Sarwar, K., & Linkon, C. (2015). MSuPDA: A Memory Efficient Algorithm for Sequence Alignment. *Interdisciplinary Sciences Computational Life Sciences*, *6*, 1.

Morgan, X. C., Segata, N., & Huttenhower, C. (2012). Biodiversity and functional genomics in the human microbiome. *Trends in Genetics*, 1–8. PMID:23140990

Nimmy, S. F., & Kamal, M. S. (2015). Next generation sequencing under de novo genome assembly. *International Journal of Biomathematics*, *8*(05), 5. doi:10.1142/S1793524515300018

Nimmy, S. F., & Rahman, M. S. (2014). Algorithms for global protein–protein interaction network alignment. *Netw Model Anal Health Inform Bioinformatics*, *3*(1), 65. doi:10.1007/s13721-014-0065-y

Noguchi, H., Park, J., & Takagi, T. (2006). MetaGene: Prokaryotic gene finding from environmental genome shotgun sequences. *Nucleic Acids Research*, *34*(19), 5623–5630. doi:10.1093/nar/gkl723 PMID:17028096

Noguchi, H., Taniguchi, T., & Itoh, T. (2008). Meta Gene Annotator: Detecting Species- Specific Patterns of Ribosomal Binding Site for Precise Gene Prediction in Anonymous Prokaryotic and Phage Genomes. *DNA Research*, *15*(6), 387–396. doi:10.1093/dnares/dsn027 PMID:18940874

Peng, Y., Henry, C. M., Yiu, S. M., & Francis, Y. L. (2011). T-IDBA: A de novo iterative de Bruijn graph assembler for transcriptome. In Research in Computational Molecular Biology, Vancouver, Canada.

Powell, S., Szklarczyk, D., Trachana, K., Roth, A., Kuhn, M., Muller, J., & Bork, P. et al. (2012). eggnog v3.0: Orthologous groups covering 1133 organisms at 41 different taxonomic ranges. *Nucleic Acids Research*, *40*(D1), 284–289. doi:10.1093/nar/gkr1060 PMID:22096231

Qin, J., Li, R., Raes, J., Arumugam, M., Burgdorf, K. S., Manichanh, C., & Wang, J. et al. (2010). A human gut microbial gene catalogue established by metagenomic sequencing. *Nature*, *464*(7285), 59–65. doi:10.1038/nature08821 PMID:20203603

Qin, J., Li, Y., Cai, Z., Li, S., Zhu, J., Zhang, F., & Wang, J. et al. (2012). A metagenome-wide association study of gut microbiota in type 2 diabetes. *Nature*, *490*(7418), 55–60. doi:10.1038/nature11450 PMID:23023125

Rusch, D. B., Halpern, A. L., Sutton, G., Heidelberg, K. B., Williamson, S., Yooseph, S., & Venter, J. C. et al. (2007). The Sorcerer II Global Ocean Sampling expedition: Northwest Atlantic through eastern tropical Pacific. *PLoS Biology*, *5*(3), e77. doi:10.1371/journal.pbio.0050077 PMID:17355176

Schmidt, B., Sinha, R., Beresford, B., & Puglisi, S. J. (2009). A fast hybrid short read fragment assembly algorithm. *Bioinformatics (Oxford, England)*, *25*(17), 2279–2280. doi:10.1093/bioinformatics/btp374 PMID:19535537

Simpson, J.T., Wong, K., Jackman, K., Schein, J.E., Jones, S.J., & Birol, I. (2009), A parallel assembler for short read sequence data, Res. ABySS.

Tatusov, R. L., Fedorova, N. D., Jackson, J. D., Jacobs, A. R., Kiryutin, B., Koonin, E. V., & Natale, D. A. et al. (2003). The COG database: An updated version includes eukaryotes. *BMC Bioinformatics*, *4*(1), 41. doi:10.1186/1471-2105-4-41 PMID:12969510

Tyson, G. W., Chapman, J., Hugenholtz, P., Allen, E. E., Ram, R. J., Richardson, P. M., & Banfield, J. F. et al. (2004). Community structure and metabolism through reconstruction of microbial genomes from the environment. *Nature*, *428*(6978), 37–43. doi:10.1038/nature02340 PMID:14961025

Wang, S., Cho, H., Zhai, C. X., Berger, B., & Peng, J. (2015). Exploiting ontology graph for predicting sparsely annotated gene function. *Bioinformatics (Oxford, England)*, *31*(12), i357–i364. doi:10.1093/bioinformatics/btv260 PMID:26072504

Wilke, A., Harrison, T., Wilkening, J., Field, D., Glass, E. M., Kyrpides, N., & Meyer, F. et al. (2012). The M5nr: A novel non-redundant database containing protein sequences and annotations from multiple sources and associated tools. *BMC Bioinformatics*, *13*(1), 141. doi:10.1186/1471-2105-13-141 PMID:22720753

Wu, D., Wu, M., Halpern, A., Rusch, D. B., Yooseph, S., Frazier, M., & Eisen, J. A. et al. (2011). Stalking the fourth domain in metagenomic data: Searching for, discovering, and interpreting novel, deep branches in marker gene phylogenetic trees. *PLoS ONE*, *6*(3), e18011. doi:10.1371/journal.pone.0018011 PMID:21437252

Xu, L., Chen, H., Hu, X., Zhang, R., Zhang, Z., & Luo, Z. W. (2006). Average Gene Length Is Highly Conserved in Prokaryotes and Eukaryotes and Diverges Only Between the Two Kingdoms. *Molecular Biology and Evolution*, *23*(6), 1107–1108. doi:10.1093/molbev/msk019 PMID:16611645

Yatsunenko, T., Rey, F. E., Manary, M. J., Trehan, I., & Dominguez, M. G. (2012). Human gut microbiome viewed across age and geography. *Nature*, 10. PMID:22699611

W.Yinan, D. W. Renner, I. Albert, & M. L.SzparaL.(2015).VirAmp: a galaxy-based viral genome assembly pipeline GigaScience 4,19.

Yuzhen, Y., & Haixu, T. (2015). Utilizing de Bruijn graph of metagenome assembly for metatranscriptome analysis. *Bioinformatics (Oxford, England)*, 1–8.

Zerbino, D. R., & Birney, E. (2008). Velvet: Algorithms for de novo short read assembly using de Bruijn graphs. *Genome Research*, *18*(5), 821–829. doi:10.1101/gr.074492.107 PMID:18349386

Zhang, Z., Schwartz, S., Wagner, L., & Miller, W. (2000). A greedy algorithm for aligning DNA sequences. *Journal of Computational Biology*, *7*(1-2), 203–214. doi:10.1089/10665270050081478 PMID:10890397

KEY TERMS AND DEFINITIONS

De Brujin Graph: A generalized de Bruijn graph is a directed graph, where an edge exists from all nodes of form $V=(v_{1,}\ v_2 \ldots\ldots\ v_n)$ to $U=(u_1 u_{2\ldots\ldots} u_n)$ with U being a left-shifted version of V, or $u_1=v_2$, $u_2=v_3, \ldots u_{n-1}=v_n$.

DNA Fragmentation: DNA fragmentation is the breaking of DNA molecules into smaller pieces. Fragmentation of DNA is an early step in next generation sequencing workflows, as well in the creation of DNA inserts for expression libraries.

Euler Path and Circuit: An Euler path is a path that uses every edge of a graph exactly once. An Euler circuit is a circuit that uses every edge of a graph exactly once path.

Exons: A segment of a DNA or RNA molecule containing information coding for a protein or peptide sequence.

Gene: A linear sequence of nucleotides along a segment of DNA that provides the coded instructions for synthesis of RNA which, when translated into protein, leads to the expression of hereditary character.

Gene Annotation: Annotation is the process by which relevant information about these raw DNA sequences is added to the genome databases. This involves describing different regions of the code and identifying which regions can be called genes.

Gene Assembly: Genome assembly algorithms are sets of well defined procedures for reconstructing DNA sequences from large numbers of shorter DNA sequence fragments.

Genome: The total amount of genetic information in the chromosomes of an organism, including its genes and DNA sequences.

Introns: A segment of a DNA or RNA molecule that does not code for proteins and interrupts the sequence of genes.

Metagenomic Gene: Metagenomics is the study of a collection of genetic material (genomes) from a mixed community of organisms. Metagenomics usually refers to the study of microbial communities.

Signed Graph: A signed graph is a graph in which each edge has a positive or negative sign. Formally, a signed graph Σ is a pair (G, s) that consists of a graph G = (V, E) and a sign mapping or signature s from E to the sign group {+,−}.

Chapter 13
Classification of Surface Electromyogram Signals Acquired from the Forearm of a Healthy Volunteer

Uvanesh K.
National Institute of Technology, Rourkela, India

Suraj Kumar Nayak
National Institute of Technology, Rourkela, India

Biswajeet Champaty
National Institute of Technology, Rourkela, India

Goutam Thakur
Manipal Institute of Technology, India

Biswajit Mohapatra
Vesaj Patel Hospital, India

D. N. Tibarewala
Jadavpur University, India

Kunal Pal
National Institute of Technology, Rourkela, India

ABSTRACT

Surface EMG (sEMG) signals from the palmaris longus, flexor carpi radialis and flexor carpi ulnaris muscles were recorded using an in-house developed EMG signal acquisition system. The bandwidth of the acquisition system was 1500 Hz. The extracted sEMG signal was processed using Discrete Wavelet Transform (DWT). The features of the extracted and the wavelet processed signals were determined and were used for probable classification using Artificial Neural Network (ANN). A classification efficiency of more than 90% was achieved using ANN classifiers. The results suggested that the sEMG may be successfully used for designing efficient control system.

DOI: 10.4018/978-1-5225-0140-4.ch013

INTRODUCTION

In recent years, the use of biosignals associated with the residual functional capability of the incapacitated persons has gained much importance for controlling assistive or rehabilitative devices/ aids (Allison, et al., 2012; Barea, Boquete, Mazo, & López, 2002; Chen & Newman, 2004; Moon, Lee, Chu, & Mun, 2005; Tanaka, Matsunaga, & Wang, 2005). This is of utmost importance for such patients because the biosignal controlled devices may provide better independence. Amongst the various biosignals, electromyogram (EMG), electrooculogram (EOG) and electroencephalogram (EEG) signals have been extensively studied (Mukherjee, Dey, Dey, & Dey, 2015; Neto, Celeste, & Martins, 2006; Oskoei & Hu, 2007; Ubeda, Ianez, & Azorín, 2011). Even though EOG and EEG-based control systems are quite efficient, the patient compliance during signal acquisition might be very low. This is due to the fact that the EOG signal acquisition system needs electrodes to be placed around the eyes and hence, might be inconvenient for the patients. But the main advantage of the EOG signals is its stability, even in the severely motor-incapacitated patients. Hence, EOG based control systems have been found useful for the patients suffering from progressive neuro-motor degenerative diseases (Ubeda, et al., 2011; Usakli, Gurkan, Aloise, Vecchiato, & Babiloni, 2010). Similar to the EOG signals, the EEG electrodes are placed on the scalp across the head. Additionally, analysis of the EEG signals is comparatively complex as compared to the EOG and the EMG signals. This is because of the fact that the EEG electrodes acquire the signals from the underlying group of neurons (located within the cortex of the brain) from a specific area of the scalp. The signals, which are represented over the surface of the scalp, are due to addition of the electrical potentials of the groups of neurons present in the underlying area. Proper analysis of the EEG signals can divulge information about the physical and mental state of the persons. The analysis of the EEG signals has found extensive applications in cognitive learning, disorders related to the nervous system of the brain and development of the control systems for neuroprosthetics (Lauer, Peckham, & Kilgore, 1999; Laufs, et al., 2003; Neto, et al., 2006).

EMG signals are the biopotential signals, which are generated due to the activity of the neuro-muscular junctions (Criswell, 2010). The muscles may be excited either voluntarily by the volunteer or by applying an electrical stimulus. The excitation of the muscles induces contraction of the muscles, which is due to the collective contraction of the muscle fibres. These signals are manifested at the surface of the skin. The acquisition of these surface signals, due to the activity of the muscles, is regarded as "surface electromyogram" (sEMG) (Gerdle, Karlsson, Day, & Djupsjöbacka, 1999). The main advantage of acquisition of the sEMG is that the signal may be acquired in a non-invasive manner (Merletti & Parker, 2004). These EMG signals appear as random signals, but the sEMG signals of similar profiles can be generated by activating a specific group of muscles. Similar sEMG profiles are repetitively generated until and unless the muscle becomes fatigued or any physiological changes occur in the muscle. This helps in the analysis of the neural drive, which excites the muscles. Usually, the sEMG signals have amplitude in the range of 0 and 10 $mV_{p\text{-}p}$ (Reaz, Hussain, & Mohd-Yasin, 2006). The frequency of the sEMG signal lies mainly in the range of 5 and 500 Hz (Merletti & Di Torino, 1999; Van Boxtel, 2001). EMG signals have gained the attention of the researchers as the most preferable physiological signals due to their ability to provide information on both clinical and engineering aspects. These signals have been explored for diagnosing diseased conditions of not only muscles but also of the bones with which the muscles are attached (Drost, Stegeman, van Engelen, & Zwarts, 2006; Hogrel, 2005; Zwarts & Stegeman, 2003). Apart from the clinical investigation, the sEMG signals may be acquired from the limb amputees for extracting information about the voluntary muscular contraction with typical sEMG features. The classification of the sEMG signals may help in generating control signals for controlling rehabilitation devices/ aids (e.g. prosthetics and myoelectric control systems) (Reaz, et al., 2006). The emergence of artificial intelligence as a tool for classification has improved the efficiency of the biosignal classification to a great extent (Park & Lee, 1998). But, like the two sides of a coin, artificial intelligence based biosignal classification is quite complex and may slow down the processing speed of the control system processor. To avoid this, there is a need for high-speed processors, which may increase the cost of the rehabilitation devices/ aids.

As mentioned in the previous paragraph, the sEMG signals look like random signals. Hence, the analysis of the sEMG signals using the normal signal processing techniques is very difficult. In general, the statistical features of the sEMG signals are calculated for analysis. In the recent years, Wavelet based signal processing has gained extensive attention for analysing biosignals including sEMG signals and has become a common signal processing tool (Dickhaus & Heinrich, 1996; Gyaw & Ray, 1993). Discrete Wavelet Transform (DWT) is a collection of a series of Low pass and High pass filters. These filters allow decomposing the signals into various sub-bands depending on the frequency components of the signal. DWT is a joint time-frequency domain analysis technique, which can be successfully used for the analysis of the non-stationary signals. All the biosignals (including ECG, EEG and EMG) are non-stationary signals. The frequency components of the non-stationary signals change with time unlike stationary signals (e.g. sinusoidal, triangular and square waves) whose frequency components remain same throughout the time period. The analysis of the biosignals in the joint time- frequency domain has been found to be quite useful in in-depth analysis of the complex biological processes. The main disadvantage of the wavelet- based analysis of the biosignals is the lack of appropriate mother wavelets. But many authors have reported the successful use of the lower order Daubechies (db1 to db20) wavelet basis functions for the analysis of the biosignals (Adeli, Zhou, & Dadmehr, 2003).

In the present study, the statistical features of the sEMG signals and the wavelet processed signals were calculated. The features were used for probable classification using artificial neural network (ANN). ANN has found applications in developing assistive devices using cognitive processes for the motor- incapacitated patients. The use of the ANN tools has been found to allow quick adaptation of the motor- incapacitated patients in controlling rehabilitation devices/ aids. This is important as the process of adaptation of the patients to the rehabilitation devices/ aids might be quite long and frustrating for the patients and trainers. Due to this reason, many patients have been found to lose hope during the training period. ANN based tool may help in quick learning with good classification accuracy. Good classification efficiency is essentially required for designing control systems for rehabilitative devices.

BACKGROUND

The tissues are generally categorized either as excitable or non-excitable, based on their excitability(Bourne, 2012).The excitable tissues have neuronal innervations which make the tissues respond to a stimulus. On the contrary, the non-excitable tissues have glial cells, which do not respond to any stimuli. Structurally, the neurons can be divided into three parts, namely, soma (cell body), dendrites and axon. The neurons consist of only one axon, but it may have multiple dendrites. The potential flows in a unidirectional manner from axon to dendrite. In other words, the axon terminal of the neuron picks up the stimuli and transmits the stimuli towards the dendrites for stimulating the next neuron or the tissues. The excitation of the axon (second neuron) for transferring the potential from the previous neuron (first neuron) occurs by the interaction of the chemicals (neurotransmitters; e.g. acetylcholine) released by the dendrites of the first neuron and the chemical receptors present in the axon of the second neuron. As the stimuli reach the neuron-tissue interface, the released neurotransmitters induce the excitation of the tissues by interacting with the cellular receptors (Marieb & Hoehn, 2007). The excitation of the excitable tissues results in the generation of signals, which are associated with the physiological processes. Such signals are regarded as biosignals.

In the last decade, there has been an exponential increase in the use of biosignals for manipulating the functioning of the machines. With the advent of advancements in the field of robotics technology, it has been possible to use the technology for improving the lifestyle of not only the incapacitated persons but also the elderly persons. Such robotic machines are controlled using signals associated with the physiological processes (biosignals) (Rechy-Ramirez & Hu, 2014). Since such machines have an interface between human and the machine, they are broadly categorized as the human- machine interface (HMI) based devices. The use of biosignals for controlling the rehabilitative devices has opened up a new arena for research. The commonly used biosignals, which have been used for devising HMI devices include EOG, EMG, EEG and eye gazing. This has allowed the researchers to develop rehabilitative devices/ aids, which are user- friendly in nature. This, in turn, has allowed not only improving the quality of life of the incapacitated persons to a great extent but also has ensured the safety of the users. The increased safety of the users of the HMI devices is ensured as the system uses information encoded within the biosignals, which are voluntarily generated by the users. The decoding of the information is done by extracting the statistical features of the signals and subsequently classifying the signals.

The EOG signals are generated by the movement of the eyes (Bronzino, 1999). There is a natural difference in the potential of the cornea and the retina of the eye. The cornea is relatively positive as compared to the retina. This potential difference results in the generation of a natural dipole moment. As the EOG measuring electrodes are across the eyes, the movement of the eye (and hence the cornea) results in the movement of the positive end of the dipole towards a specific electrode. This results in the electrode to assume a positive charge as compared to the other active electrode. The differential potential is amplified to obtain EOG signals. Movement of the eye towards the second electrode results in the generation of the signals with opposite polarity. The main disadvantage of the EOG signals is that they are easily corrupted by the EMG signals associated with the movement of the head and the neck.

The EEG signals are recordings of the post-synaptic potentials, which are generated within the cortex (which forms the inner core of the brain). The generated potential travels through the skull and represents itself on the scalp. Hence, the signal which is represented on the scalp is due to the neuronal activity of a group of neurons and not from a single neuron. Due to the above- mentioned reasons, the signal- to- noise ratio of the EEG signals is very poor. Apart from this, the topographical resolution of the EEG signals is also poor. The above- mentioned reasons make the processing of the EEG signals a bit difficult. The analysis of the EEG signals has been explored for determining the mood of the persons (Horlings, Datcu, & Rothkrantz, 2008). Also, it is possible to predict what the person is thinking. Suitable signal processing techniques have been employed to decode the thinking information of the person. Once the EEG signals are decoded to extract the information, they can be used to control the functioning of the rehabilitation devices/ aids. The HMI devised using EEG is also regarded as BCI (brain- computer interface) (Leuthardt, Schalk, Moran, Wolpaw, & Ojemann, 2006; Vallabhaneni, Wang, & He, 2005). Slow cortical potential, P300 potentials and mu and beta rhythms are some of the typical EEG signal types, which have been explored for developing control systems of the rehabilitation devices/ aids for the severely disabled. Like EOG signals, EEG signals can also be acquired in a non- invasive manner.

The EMG signals are generated due to the neuromuscular activities, which result in the contraction of the muscles (Criswell, 2010). Muscles consist of a large number of muscle fibres, self-organized in groups. Each muscle is innervated with a single motor neuron that has the ability to stimulate muscle fibres to undergo contraction. All the muscle fibres within a muscle contract simultaneously to bring a contraction of the whole muscle. The action potential generated due to the contraction of the muscle can be acquired directly from the muscles using needle electrodes or from the surface of the skin just above the muscle. The EMG signal which represents itself on the surface of the skin is regarded as surface EMG, also known as sEMG (Gerdle, et al., 1999).The sEMG signals appear as noise. This is because all the muscle fibres are oriented in a 3- dimensional space. This results in the time delay as the signal travels to the surface of the skin. Since the action potentials are additive in nature, the action potentials from different muscle fibres add up. This results in the appearance of the signal similar to a noise. This is the disadvantage of using the sEMG signals for analysis. But fortunately, the sEMG signals are repetitive in nature. This means, if the muscles are stimulated with a stimulus of particular characteristics, the nature of the sEMG signals remains same until and unless the muscle becomes fatigued. Care must be taken to ensure that the stimuli are not given within the refractory period (absolute or relative). In that case, the muscle may either fail to respond to the stimuli or will respond with the generation of action potentials of lower intensities. It is also important to keep in mind that the muscles contract in a single axis and hence it is possible to detect the isometric contraction of the muscles if the electrodes are placed at suitable locations. The use of the sEMG signals for probable applications in rehabilitation and HMI devices has gained much importance in the last three decades (Barreto, Scargle, & Adjouadi, 2000; Gomez-Gil, San-Jose-Gonzalez, Nicolas-Alonso, & Alonso-Garcia, 2011; Oskoei & Hu, 2007). The control of the peripheral equipments has been achieved using the sEMG signals associated with the hand gestures (e.g. movement of the fingers, wrists and upper arm) (Shenoy, Miller, Crawford, & Rao, 2008). A classification efficiency of >90% has already been achieved using the processed sEMG signals from the hand gestures (Crawford, Miller, Shenoy, & Rao, 2005). Hand gesture controlled speech system for the non- vocal persons and prosthesis control for motor- disabled persons have already been proposed. The classification of the sEMG signals is a great challenge. Artificial intelligence based signal classification is being explored with success. Artificial neural network based signal classification has been extensively studied in this regard (Soares, Andrade, Lamounier, & Carrijo, 2003). The other artificial intelligence (e.g. genetic algorithm, fuzzy logic and neuro- fuzzy logic) based algorithms are being tested for improving the classification efficiency of the sEMG signals (Ajiboye, 2005; Soares, et al., 2003).

MAIN FOCUS OF THE CHAPTER

The main focus of the chapter is to study the ability of the artificial neural network based algorithms (multi-layer perceptron (MLP) and radial basis function (RBF)) for the classification of the sEMG signals generated by different hand gestures. The statistical features of the sEMG signals were used as the input features for probable classification using the artificial neural networks. The classification analysis using artificial neural network is important because it can provide us with information whether the generated EMG signals may be efficiently classified and hence, may be used for developing control systems for rehabilitative devices/ aids.

METHODS

The sEMG signals were recorded by placing the active electrodes (Ag/AgCl disposable electrodes, BPL India) on the surface of the skin, just above palmaris longus, flexor carpi radialis and flexor carpi ulnaris muscles. The use of Ag/ AgCl electrodes was preferred because their half-cell potential values are low and remain steady. A low and steady half-cell potential is desirable as it helps in reducing the offset. The volunteer was trained to generate similar sEMG signals by index finger flexion, ring finger flexion, all fingers flexion (<1sec) and all fingers flexion (>2sec). After the successful training of the volunteer, the volunteer was advised to initiate the movement of the specific fingers for 10 times to generate sEMG signals. Each sEMG signal was saved in a text file. The acquisition of the signals was done using an in- house developed sEMG amplifier. The gain of the amplifier was 2501. The amplifier was made using an INA128P instrumentation amplifier. The INA128P instrumentation amplifier was preferred for developing the sEMG amplifier circuit because of its very low offset (null), presence of an in- built filter to eliminate the 50Hz power line interference and a very high CMRR value. The output of the amplifier circuit was filtered using a low- pass filter having cut- off frequency of 1.59 Hz.

The recorded sEMG signals were processed using a LabVIEW program developed in- lab so as to extract the sEMG signals. The statistical features of these extracted sEMG signals were calculated using another LabVIEW based program (developed in- lab). The extracted sEMG signals were further processed using Discrete Wavelet Transform (DWT). Each extracted sEMG signal was decomposed using db07 wavelet at the level of 9 and reconstruction was achieved using D3+D4+D5 sub-bands. The statistical parameters of the reconstructed signal were also calculated.

The features of the sEMG signals were initially processed using linear (analysis of variance (ANOVA)) and non-linear (classification and regression tree (CART), boosted tree (BT) and random forest (RF)) classifiers. Using the above- mentioned classifiers, the important predictors were identified. The important predictors were used as the inputs for probable classification using artificial neural networks (ANNs) in order to determine the best classification efficiency. An ANN is a data processing model inspired by the structure and functioning of biological neural networks. It possesses processing nodes (similar to neurons) having multiple connections like the dendrites and axons. Each connection has adaptable parameters that alter the signal passing through it. Various types of neural networks have been developed for solving different types of problems like pattern recognition, classification and prediction of the evolution of dynamic systems (Bailer-Jones, Gupta, & Singh, 2001).

RESULTS AND DISCUSSION

Acquisition of the sEMG Signals

The representative signals were obtained by the flexion of index finger, flexion of ring finger, flexion of all the fingers (<1sec) and flexion of all the fingers (>2sec). The sEMG signals were categorized as signal A (SA), signal B (SB), signal C (SC) and signal D (SD), respectively (Figure 1). A preliminary analysis of the sEMG signals suggested that the duration of the movement may allow us to generate sEMG signals having significantly different features. All the sEMG signals showed that there was an amplitude variation across the baseline, even though, there was no muscular activity. This may be at-

Figure 1. Waveforms of the representative signals used for further processing: (a) signal A (b) signal B (c) signal C and (d) signal D

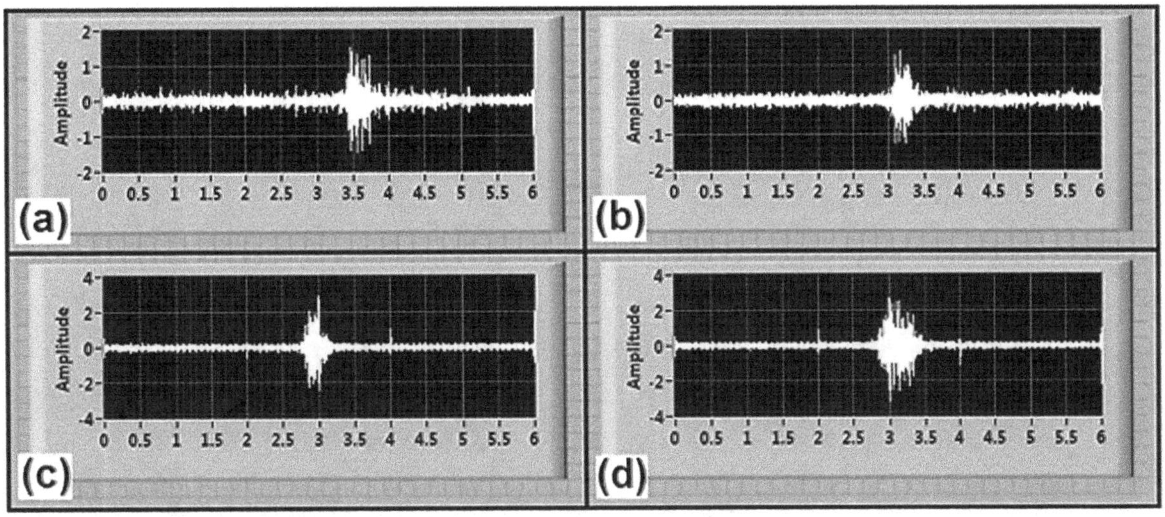

tributed to the EMG associated with the basal muscular activity. The basal EMG signals are produced due to the muscular activity required to maintain the tone of the muscles.

The sEMG signals obtained during the motor activity were extracted using a LabVIEW program. Figure 2 shows the waveforms of the sEMG signals and their corresponding extracted signals. The algorithm used for extracting the sEMG signals and their classification using artificial neural network has been shown as a flowchart in Figure 3.

The extracted signal was further processed using Discrete Wavelet Transform (DWT). DWT has emerged as one of the essential tools for the analysis of the non- stationary signals like sEMG signals. It is a time- frequency analysis method that enables the generation and subsequent use of the useful frequency components (or scales) of the desired signal instead of using all the frequency components (or scales) (Phinyomark, Limsakul, & Phukpattaranont, 2011). The extracted sEMG signals were decomposed using db07 wavelet at level 9. The sub- bands D3, D4 and D5 were used for reconstructing the sEMG signal. Figure 4 shows the sEMG sub-bands D3, D4, D5 and the reconstructed signal of the representative sEMG signal. The features of the extracted sEMG signal and the reconstructed signal were calculated using a LabVIEW program. The calculated features of the sEMG signal include Arithmetic Mean (AM), Root Mean Square (RMS), Standard Deviation (SD), Variance, Kurtosis, Mode, Summation, Skewness, Median, Energy Density (ED), Entropy and Signal Length (SL). These features can be quickly and easily calculated as they do not need any transformation. There has been wide spread use of these features in both medical and engineering researches (Reaz, et al., 2006). The description and mathematical expressions of the sEMG signal features have been given in Table 1.

Classification of Extracted sEMG Signal

The statistical features obtained from the program were tabulated in the trial version of Statistica worksheet (Ver. 12.6, Statsoft, Inc, Oklahoma, USA). Initially, the features were statistically analysed using ANOVA. ANOVA is a linear classifier that helps in comparing the mean of three or more groups. The

Figure 2. Waveforms of the sEMG signals and their corresponding extracted signals

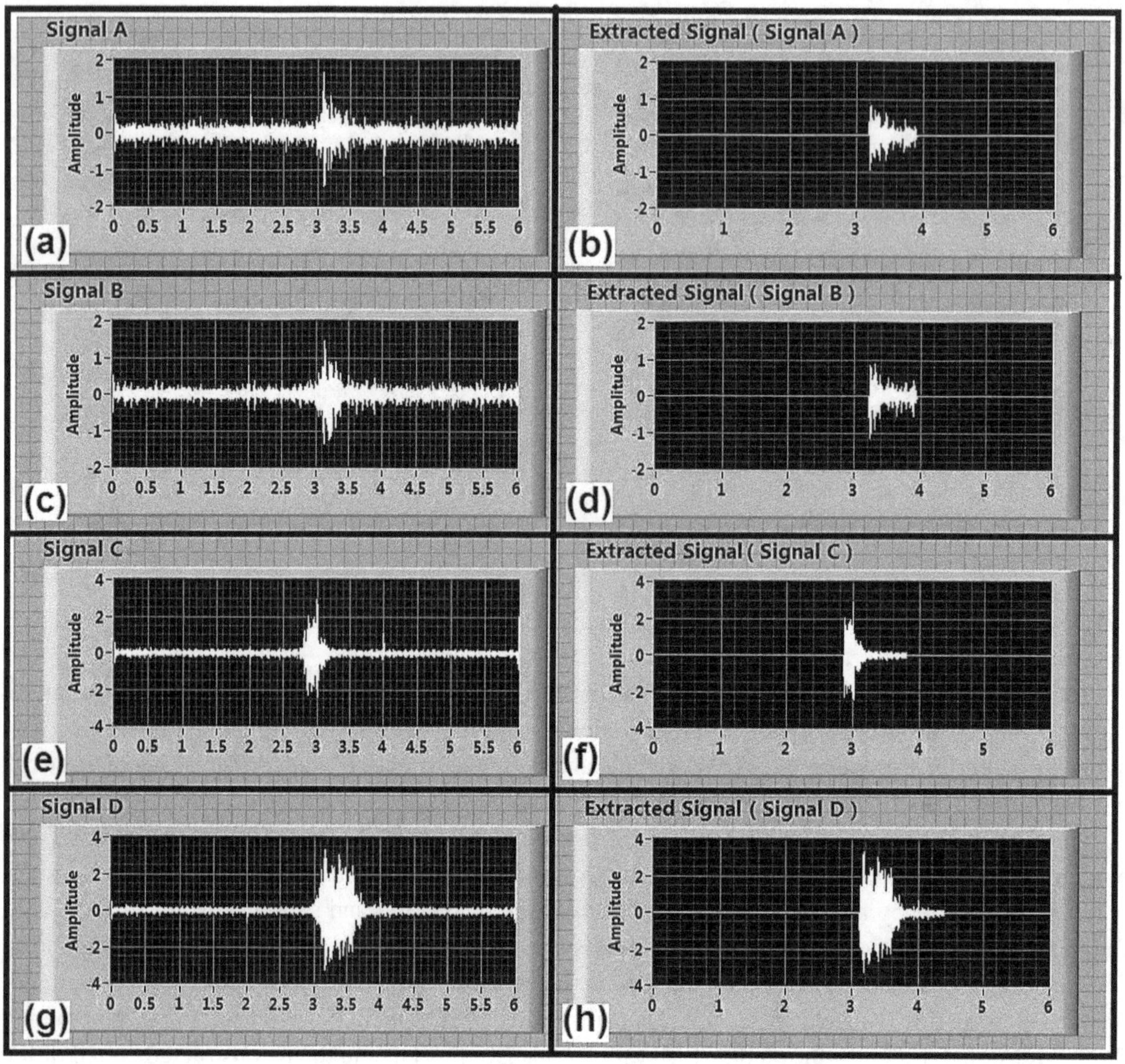

features were regarded as important if the mean of the groups were statistically significant. The means were regarded as significant if the p-value was <0.05 (5% error was considered as acceptable). The analysis of the features suggested that RMS, standard deviation (SD), Variance, Signal Length (SL) and Kurtosis were the important predictors.

The features were further classified using decision tree classifiers (CART, boosted tree and random forest classifiers). CART is the one of the basic decision tree classifiers. Each node of the decision tree has only two outgoing edges. Boosted tree is similar to the CART with some modifications. Each tree in boosted tree classifier is generated using the residuals of the previous trees. On the other hand, Random Forest classifier employs a number of tree predictors. The accuracy of the Random Forest classifier has been reported to be highest followed by Boosted tree and CART classifiers, respectively (Breiman, 2001; Liaw & Wiener, 2002; Prasad, Iverson, & Liaw, 2006; Strobl, Malley, & Tutz, 2009).

Figure 3. Flowchart for extraction of the sEMG signal components and classification of the signals using artificial neural network

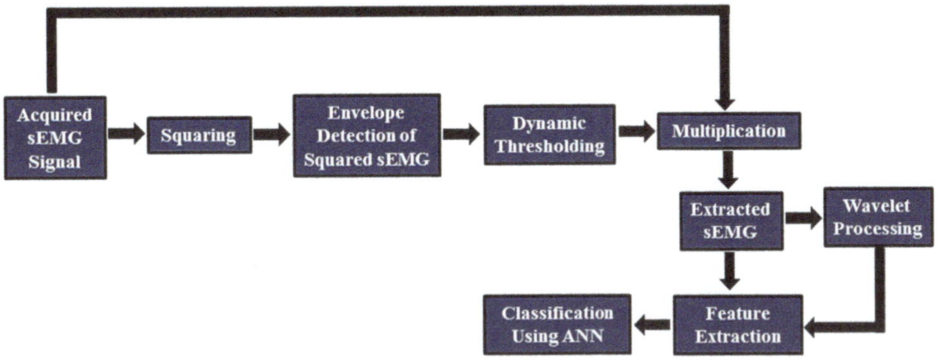

Figure 4. (a) Representative sEMG signal (b) D3 decomposed signal (c) D4 decomposed signal (d) D5 decomposed signal (e) reconstructed signal (D3+D4+D5) (f) wavelet transform and subband selection window

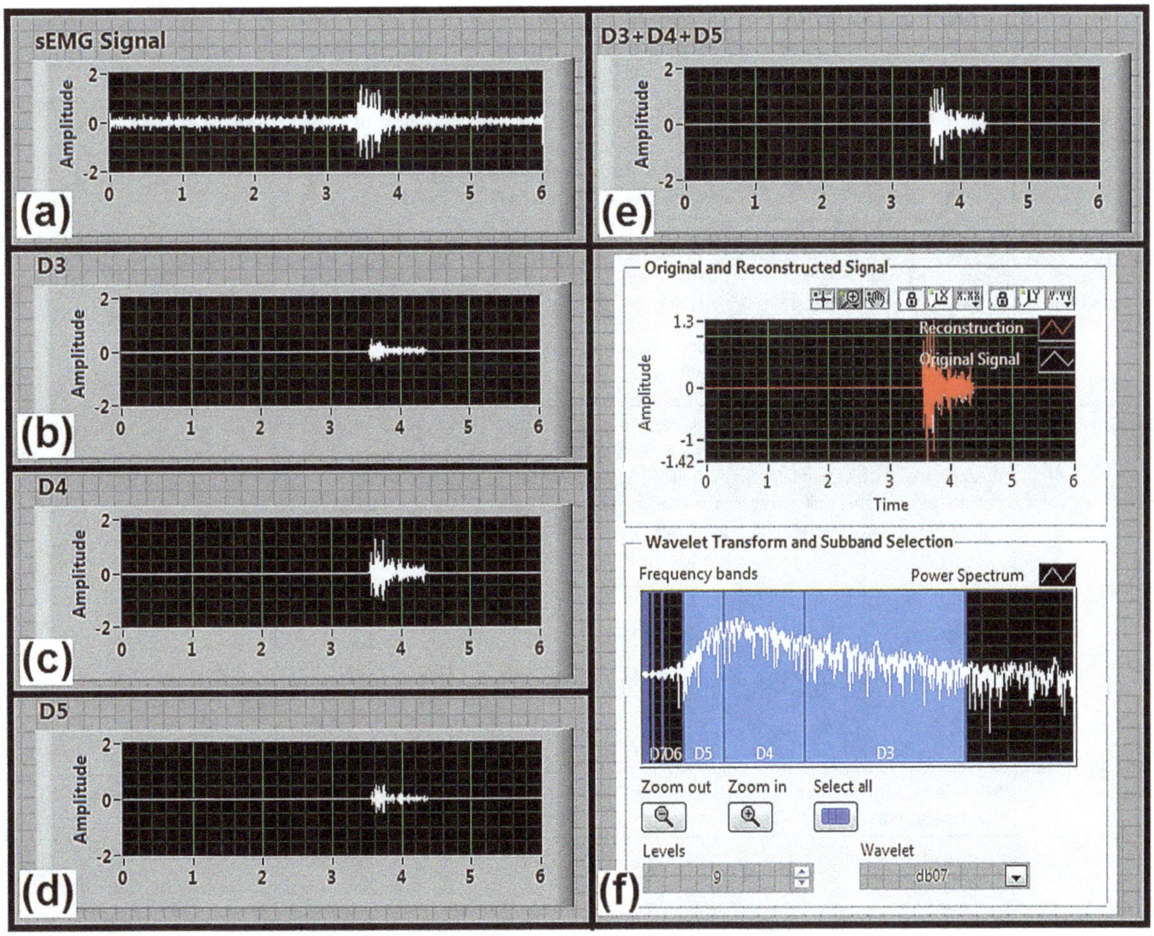

Table 1. Description and mathematical expressions of the sEMG signal features

Parameter	Description	Reference
Arithmetic Mean (AM)	The arithmetic mean of a sequence or signal segment can be defined as the average of values of the sequence or segment. It is a measure of central tendency, i.e., it provides an idea where the center of a set of values lies. $Arithmatic\ Mean = \frac{1}{L}\sum_{m=1}^{L} x_m$ where L represents the length of the sequence or signal segment and x_m corresponds to the values of the sequence or signal segment.	(Dunlop & Tamhane, 2000)
Root Mean Square (RMS)	The root mean square value of a sequence or signal segment can be defined as the square root of the average of squared values of the sequence or segment. $RMS = \sqrt{\frac{1}{L}\sum_{m=1}^{L} x_m^2}$ where L represents the length of the sequence or segment and x_m corresponds to the values of the sequence or segment.	(Phinyomark, Phukpattaranont, & Limsakul, 2012)
Variance	Variance is a measure of dispersion of the values of a sequence (sample) or signal segment from its mean value. It can be defined as the average of squared deviations of the values of the sequence or segment from its mean value. $Variance = \frac{1}{L-1}\sum_{m=1}^{L}\left(x_m - \overline{x}\right)^2$ where L represents the length of the sequence or segment, x_m corresponds to the values of the sequence or segment and $\overline{x}$ is its mean value. Variance of a signal provides a measure of its power.	(Dixon & Massey, 1969; Oskoei & Hu, 2008; Zardoshti-Kermani, Wheeler, Badie, & Hashemi, 1995)
Standard Deviation (SD)	Standard deviation of a sequence or signal segment is an important measure of dispersion of the values of the sequence or signal segment from its mean value. It can be defined as the square root of the average of squared deviations of the values of the sequence or segment from its mean value. In other words, standard deviation is the square root on the variance. $SD = \sqrt{\frac{1}{L-1}\sum_{m-1}^{L}\left(x_m - \overline{x}\right)^2}$ where L represents the length of the sequence or segment, x_m corresponds to the values of the sequence or segment and $\overline{x}$ is its mean value.	(Dixon & Massey, 1969; Zardoshti-Kermani, et al., 1995)
Median	Median is a measure of central tendency like the mean value. It is less prone to skewed distributions and provides better representation of the central tendency than mean in sequences with skewed distribution of the values. Median of a sequence can be defined as the value that separates the sequence into two equal halves when all the values of the sequence have been arranged in an ascending order. $Median = \begin{cases} x_{\frac{n+1}{2}}; & n\ is\ odd \\ 0.5\left(x_{\frac{n}{2}} + x_{\frac{n}{2}+1}\right); & n\ is\ even \end{cases}$ where n is the number of values in the sequence	(Dunlop & Tamhane, 2000)
Mode	Mode is a useful measure of central tendency. The mode of a sequence is the value of the sequence that has the highest frequency.	(Dunlop & Tamhane, 2000)

continued on following page

Table 1. Continued

Parameter	Description	Reference
Kurtosis	Kurtosis is a measure of the peakedness of the probability distribution function of a random variable. It is calculated as the ratio of fourth cumulant of the random variable to square of its second cumulant. $$Kurtosis_x = \frac{E[x^4]}{E[x^2]^2} - 3$$ where *x* is the random variable and *E*[ ] represents the statistical expectation operator.	(Nazarpour, Al-Timemy, Bugmann, & Jackson, 2013)
Skewness	Skewness measures the asymmetry or irregularity of the distribution of a random variable or sequence from the normal distribution. Skewness can be positive or negative depending on whether the values of the random variable or sequence are skewed to the left or right of the mean. Skewness of a random variable *x* (Skew(*x*)) is defined as the third moment of the standard score of *x* $$Skew(X) = E\left[\left(\frac{x-\mu}{\sigma}\right)^3\right]$$ where *E*[ ] represents the statistical expectation operator and $\frac{x-\mu}{\sigma}$ denotes the standard score of *x*.	(Phinyomark, et al., 2013)
Summation	Summation is the addition of all the values present in a sequence. $$Summation = \sum_{i=1}^{n} x_i$$ where x_i represents the *i*th value of a *n* valued sequence.	
Signal Length	Signal length can be defined as the total or cumulative length of the waveform of a signal over the time segment. It represents the waveform complexity. $$SL = \sum_{m=1}^{N} \left\|x_{m-1} - x_m\right\|$$ where x_m denotes the *m*th value of the *N*- valued signal.	(Hudgins, Parker, & Scott, 1993)
Energy Density (ED)	Energy density of a signal represents the distribution of the signal energy among all frequency bands with time.	(Junsheng, Dejie, & Yu, 2005)
Entropy	Entropy (Shannon Entropy) represents the randomness or unpredictable information present in a signal. Entropy of a discrete random variable *x* with probability mass function P(*x*) can be defined as the expected value of the negative logarithm of the probability distribution of the random variable. $$H(x) = E\left[-\ln(P(x))\right]$$ where *E*[ ] represents the statistical expectation operator.	(Won-Young, 2014; Zhao, et al., 2006)

The CART analysis of the extracted sEMG signals suggested that RMS, SD, Variance, Kurtosis and SL are the important predictors. Boosted tree classifier suggested that RMS, SD and Variance were the important predictors. Random forest suggested that only RMS was the important predictor. The mean values of the features along with their predictor importance have been tabulated Table 2.

The significant features obtained from the linear and the non-linear classifiers were used in various combinations as inputs for probable classification using artificial neural network. Multilayer perceptron (MLP) and Radial basis function (RBF) algorithms were used for the analysis. Previous studies have

Table 2. Important features of extracted sEMG signal

Classifiers	Features	Mean ± SD				p-Value	Predictor Importance
		Signal A	Signal B	Signal C	Signal D		
ANOVA	RMS	0.067± 0.015	0.065± 0.008	0.138± 0.021	0.242±0.049	0.000	--
	SD	0.067± 0.015	0.065± 0.008	0.138 ± 0.021	0.242±0.049	0.000	--
	Variance	0.004± 0.002	0.004± 0.001	0.019 ± 0.006	0.061±0.024	0.000	--
	SL	3625.4± 328.58	3631.2±256.342	4448.6±160.148	5437.7±278.631	0.000	--
	Kurtosis	74.343± 29.329	95.583±28.841	100.541±31.401	59.961±16.197	0.006	--
CART	RMS	0.067 ± 0.015	0.065± 0.008	0.138 ± 0.021	0.242±0.049	--	1.000
	SD	0.067 ± 0.015	0.065± 0.008	0.138 ± 0.021	0.242±0.049	--	1.000
	Variance	0.004 ± 0.002	0.004± 0.001	0.019± 0.006	0.061±0.024	--	1.000
	SL	3625.4±328.585	3631.2±256.342	4448.6±160.148	5437.7±278.631	--	1.000
Boosted Tree	RMS	0.067 ± 0.015	0.065± 0.008	0.138 ± 0.021	0.242±0.049	--	1.000
	SD	0.067 ± 0.015	0.065± 0.008	0.138 ± 0.021	0.242±0.049	--	1.000
	Variance	0.004 ± 0.002	0.004± 0.001	0.019 ± 0.006	0.061±0.024	--	1.000
Random Forest	RMS	0.067 ± 0.015	0.065± 0.008	0.138 ± 0.021	0.242±0.049	--	1.000

suggested that the classification using RBF algorithm gives better classification efficiency as compared to the MLP algorithm (S. K. Nayak, et al., 2015). In contradiction to the previous report, here we found that the MLP algorithm provided better classification efficiency as compared to the RBF algorithm. The best classification was obtained when RMS, SD, Variance and SL were used as the inputs to the classifier. The best classification efficiency of 97.5% was achieved using MLP (4-10-4) ANN classifier. The details of the classifier have been shown in Table 3. The confusion matrix for the classification has been tabulated in Table 4. As per the literature, a classification efficiency of ≥80% is considered as efficient

Table 3. Summary of the MLP (4-10-4) network

Networks	Classification Efficiency	Algorithm	Error Function	Hidden Act.	Output Act.
MLP 4-10-4	97.500	BFGS 51	CE	Tanh	Softmax

Table 4. Confusion matrix of the MLP (4-10-4) network

	Category-SA	Category-SB	Category- SC	Category- SD	Result
Total	10.000	10.000	10.000	10.000	40.000
Correct	9.000	10.000	10.000	10.000	39.000
Incorrect	1.000	0.000	0.000	0.000	1.000
Correct (%)	90.000	100.000	100.000	100.000	97.500
Incorrect (%)	10.000	0.000	0.000	0.000	2.500

for ANN based classification (S. Nayak, Sahoo, Champaty, & Pal, 2014). The results suggested that the extracted sEMG signal features can be used to efficiently classify different sEMG signals for generating control signals that can be used in various assistive devices.

Classification of Wavelet Processed sEMG Signal

Similar to the analysis of the extracted sEMG signal using the linear and non-linear classifiers, wavelet processed signals also showed the same features as the important predictors, which are tabulated in Table 5. The analysis of the wavelet processed sEMG signals using artificial neural network classification technique showed a classification efficiency of 90% using MLP algorithm. The detail of the MLP ANN classifier has been tabulated in Table 6. The confusion matrix for the classification has been tabulated in Table 7.

Table 5. Important features of wavelet processed sEMG signal

Classifiers	Features	Mean ± SD				p-Value	Predictor Importance
		Signal A	Signal B	Signal C	Signal D		
ANOVA	RMS	0.061±0.015	0.062±0.008	0.128±0.021	0.228±0.047	0	--
	SD	0.061±0.015	0.062±0.008	0.128±0.021	0.228±0.047	0	--
	Variance	0.004±0.002	0.004±0.001	0.017±0.006	0.054±0.022	0	--
	Kurtosis	67.559±24.953	91.505±25.302	104.427±38.171	60.079±15.831	0	--
	SL	3625.400± 328.585	3631.200± 256.343	4448.600 ± 160.149	5437.700± 278.632	0.003	--
CART	RMS	0.06±0.015	0.062±0.008	0.128±0.021	0.228±0.047	--	1
	SD	0.061±0.015	0.062±0.008	0.128±0.021	0.228±0.047	--	1
	Variance	0.004±0.002	0.004±0.001	0.017±0.006	0.054±0.022	--	1
	SL	3625.400± 328.585	3631.200±256.342	4448.600 ± 160.148	5437.700±278.631	--	0.978
Boosted Tree	RMS	0.061±0.015	0.062±0.008	0.128±0.021	0.228±0.047	--	1
	SD	0.061±0.015	0.062±0.008	0.128±0.021	0.228±0.047	--	1
	Variance	0.004±0.002	0.004±0.001	0.017±0.006	0.054±0.022	--	1
Random Forest	RMS	0.061±0.015	0.062±0.008	0.128±0.021	0.228±0.047	--	1

Table 6.Summary of Summary of the MLP (4-6-4) network

Networks	Classification Efficiency	Algorithm	Error Function	Hidden Act.	Output Act.
MLP 4-6-4	90.0000	BFGS 33	CE	Logistic	Softmax

Table 7.Confusion matrix of the MLP (4-6-4) ANN algorithm

	Category-SA	Category-SB	Category- SC	Category- SD	Result
Total	10.00000	10.00000	10.00000	10.0000	40
Correct	7.00000	9.00000	10.00000	10.0000	36
Incorrect	3.00000	1.00000	0.00000	0.0000	4
Correct (%)	70.00000	90.00000	100.00000	100.0000	90
Incorrect (%)	30.00000	10.00000	0.00000	0.0000	10

FUTURE RESEARCH DIRECTIONS

The current study focused on achieving the efficient classification of sEMG signals (acquired from the palmaris longus, flexor carpi radialis and flexor carpi ulnaris muscles through the flexion of fingers in different combinations and durations) using artificial neural network so that the sEMG signals can be utilized for designing control systems. Future research can be performed using other artificial intelligence algorithm (e.g. genetic algorithm, fuzzy logic and neuro- fuzzy logic) based classification of sEMG signals so that the best classification method can be determined. Future studies can be done by acquiring sEMG signals from other muscles of the body so as to obtain the best site for sEMG signal recording with minimal artifacts. Future studies can further explore new domains of application of sEMG signals.

CONCLUSION

The current study discusses about the classification of the sEMG signal recorded from the skin surface just above the palmaris longus, flexor carpi radialis and flexor carpi ulnaris muscles by flexing fingers in different combinations and durations. The sEMG signals were subsequently extracted and their features were calculated. The extracted sEMG signals were further processed using discrete wavelet transform. Each extracted sEMG signal was decomposed using db07 wavelet at the level of 9 and reconstruction was achieved using D3+D4+D5 sub-bands. Similar to the extracted sEMG signals, the features of the wavelet processed sEMG signals were also calculated. The features of extracted sEMG signals and wavelet processed sEMG signals were analysed by various linear (ANOVA) and non-linear (CART, BT, RF) classifiers so as to determine the important predictors, which were subsequently used for probable classification using RBF and MLP artificial neural networks. The classification efficiency was found to be higher when MLP algorithms were used against RBF algorithm. Classification efficiency of ≥90% was achieved using MLP networks for both extracted sEMG signals and wavelet processed sEMG signals. From the above results, it may be concluded that the features of the extracted sEMG signal were efficient enough for the classification of the sEMG signals.

REFERENCES

Adeli, H., Zhou, Z., & Dadmehr, N. (2003). Analysis of EEG records in an epileptic patient using wavelet transform. *Journal of Neuroscience Methods*, *123*(1), 69–87. doi:10.1016/S0165-0270(02)00340-0 PMID:12581851

Ajiboye, A. B. (2005). A heuristic fuzzy logic approach to EMG pattern recognition for multifunctional prosthesis control. *Neural Systems and Rehabilitation Engineering. IEEE Transactions on, 13*(3), 280–291.

Allison, B., Leeb, R., Brunner, C., Müller-Putz, G., Bauernfeind, G., Kelly, J., & Neuper, C. (2012). Toward smarter BCIs: Extending BCIs through hybridization and intelligent control. *Journal of Neural Engineering, 9*(1), 013001. doi:10.1088/1741-2560/9/1/013001 PMID:22156029

Bailer-Jones, C. A., Gupta, R., & Singh, H. P. (2001). *An introduction to artificial neural networks.* arXiv preprint astro-ph/0102224

Barea, R., Boquete, L., Mazo, M., & López, E. (2002). System for assisted mobility using eye movements based on electrooculography. *Neural Systems and Rehabilitation Engineering. IEEE Transactions on, 10*(4), 209–218.

Barreto, A. B., Scargle, S. D., & Adjouadi, M. (2000). A practical EMG-based human-computer interface for users with motor disabilities. *Journal of Rehabilitation Research and Development, 37*(1), 53–64. PMID:10847572

Bourne, G. (2012). *Anatomy and physiology* (Vol. 1). Elsevier.

Breiman, L. (2001). Random forests. *Machine Learning, 45*(1), 5–32. doi:10.1023/A:1010933404324

Bronzino, J. D. (1999). *Biomedical engineering handbook* (Vol. 2). CRC press.

Chen, Y., & Newman, W. S. (2004). *A human-robot interface based on electrooculography.* Paper presented at the Robotics and Automation, 2004. Proceedings. ICRA'04. 2004 IEEE International Conference on.

Crawford, B., Miller, K., Shenoy, P., & Rao, R. (2005). *Real-time classification of electromyographic signals for robotic control.* Paper presented at the AAAI.

Criswell, E. (2010). *Cram's introduction to surface electromyography.* Jones & Bartlett Publishers.

Dickhaus, H., & Heinrich, H. (1996). Classifying biosignals with wavelet networks [a method for noninvasive diagnosis]. *Engineering in Medicine and Biology Magazine, IEEE, 15*(5), 103–111. doi:10.1109/51.537066

Dixon, W. J., & Massey, F. J. (1969). *Introduction to statistical analysis* (Vol. 344). McGraw-Hill New York.

Drost, G., Stegeman, D. F., van Engelen, B. G., & Zwarts, M. J. (2006). Clinical applications of high-density surface EMG: A systematic review. *Journal of Electromyography and Kinesiology, 16*(6), 586–602. doi:10.1016/j.jelekin.2006.09.005 PMID:17085302

Dunlop, D. D., & Tamhane, A. C. (2000). *Statistics and data analysis: from elementary to intermediate.* Prentice Hall.

Gerdle, B., Karlsson, S., Day, S., & Djupsjöbacka, M. (1999). *Acquisition, processing and analysis of the surface electromyogram. In Modern techniques in neuroscience research* (pp. 705–755). Springer. doi:10.1007/978-3-642-58552-4_26

Gomez-Gil, J., San-Jose-Gonzalez, I., Nicolas-Alonso, L. F., & Alonso-Garcia, S. (2011). Steering a tractor by means of an EMG-based human-machine interface. *Sensors (Basel, Switzerland), 11*(7), 7110–7126. doi:10.3390/s110707110 PMID:22164006

Gyaw, T., & Ray, S. (1993). The wavelet transform as a tool for recognition of biosignals. *Biomedical Sciences Instrumentation, 30*, 63–68. PMID:7948651

Hogrel, J.-Y. (2005). Clinical applications of surface electromyography in neuromuscular disorders. *Neurophysiologie Clinique. Clinical Neurophysiology, 35*(2), 59–71. doi:10.1016/j.neucli.2005.03.001 PMID:16087069

Horlings, R., Datcu, D., & Rothkrantz, L. J. (2008). *Emotion recognition using brain activity.* Paper presented at the 9th international conference on computer systems and technologies and workshop for PhD students in computing.

Hudgins, B., Parker, P., & Scott, R. N. (1993). A new strategy for multifunction myoelectric control. *Biomedical Engineering. IEEE Transactions on, 40*(1), 82–94.

Junsheng, C., Dejie, Y., & Yu, Y. (2005). Time–energy density analysis based on wavelet transform. *NDT & E International, 38*(7), 569–572. doi:10.1016/j.ndteint.2005.02.002

Lauer, R. T., Peckham, P. H., & Kilgore, K. L. (1999). EEG-based control of a hand grasp neuroprosthesis. *Neuroreport, 10*(8), 1767–1771. doi:10.1097/00001756-199906030-00026 PMID:10501572

Laufs, H., Krakow, K., Sterzer, P., Eger, E., Beyerle, A., Salek-Haddadi, A., & Kleinschmidt, A. (2003). Electroencephalographic signatures of attentional and cognitive default modes in spontaneous brain activity fluctuations at rest. *Proceedings of the National Academy of Sciences of the United States of America, 100*(19), 11053–11058. doi:10.1073/pnas.1831638100 PMID:12958209

Leuthardt, E. C., Schalk, G., Moran, D. W., Wolpaw, J. R., & Ojemann, J. G. (2006). Brain computer interface: Google Patents.

Liaw, A., & Wiener, M. (2002). Classification and regression by randomForest. *R News, 2*(3), 18-22.

Marieb, E. N., & Hoehn, K. (2007). *Human anatomy & physiology.* Pearson Education.

Merletti, R., & Di Torino, P. (1999). Standards for reporting EMG data. *Journal of Electromyography and Kinesiology, 9*(1), 3–4.

Merletti, R., & Parker, P. A. (2004). *Electromyography: physiology, engineering, and non-invasive applications* (Vol. 11). John Wiley & Sons. doi:10.1002/0471678384

Moon, I., Lee, M., Chu, J., & Mun, M. (2005). *Wearable EMG-based HCI for electric-powered wheelchair users with motor disabilities.* Paper presented at the Robotics and Automation, 2005. ICRA 2005.

Mukherjee, A., Dey, G., Dey, M., & Dey, N. (2015). *Web-Based Intelligent EEG Signal Authentication and Tamper Detection System for Secure Telemonitoring. In Brain-Computer Interfaces* (pp. 295–312). Springer.

Nayak, S., Sahoo, S., Champaty, B., & Pal, K. (2014). *Effect of horror clips on the physiology of ANS & heart using ECG signal classification.* Paper presented at the Control, Instrumentation, Communication and Computational Technologies (ICCICCT), 2014 International Conference on. doi:10.1109/ICCICCT.2014.6993010

Nayak, S. K., Panda, I., Champaty, B., Bagh, N., Pal, K., & Tibarewala, D. (2015). *Automated Neural Network Based Classification of HRV and ECG Signals of Smokers: A Preliminary Study. In Advancements of Medical Electronics* (pp. 271–279). Springer.

Nazarpour, K., Al-Timemy, A. H., Bugmann, G., & Jackson, A. (2013). A note on the probability distribution function of the surface electromyogram signal. *Brain Research Bulletin*, *90*, 88–91. doi:10.1016/j.brainresbull.2012.09.012 PMID:23047056

Neto, A. F., Celeste, W. C., & Martins, V. R. (2006). *Human-machine interface based on electro-biological signals for mobile vehicles.* Paper presented at the Industrial Electronics, 2006 IEEE International Symposium on. doi:10.1109/ISIE.2006.296086

Oskoei, M. A., & Hu, H. (2007). Myoelectric control systems—A survey. *Biomedical Signal Processing and Control*, *2*(4), 275–294. doi:10.1016/j.bspc.2007.07.009

Oskoei, M. A., & Hu, H. (2008). Support vector machine-based classification scheme for myoelectric control applied to upper limb. *Biomedical Engineering. IEEE Transactions on*, *55*(8), 1956–1965.

Park, S.-H., & Lee, S.-P. (1998). EMG pattern recognition based on artificial intelligence techniques. *Rehabilitation Engineering. IEEE Transactions on*, *6*(4), 400–405.

Phinyomark, A., Limsakul, C., & Phukpattaranont, P. (2011). Application of wavelet analysis in EMG feature extraction for pattern classification. *Measurement Science Review*, *11*(2), 45–52. doi:10.2478/v10048-011-0009-y

Phinyomark, A., Phukpattaranont, P., & Limsakul, C. (2012). Feature reduction and selection for EMG signal classification. *Expert Systems with Applications*, *39*(8), 7420–7431. doi:10.1016/j.eswa.2012.01.102

Phinyomark, A., Quaine, F., Charbonnier, S., Serviere, C., Tarpin-Bernard, F., & Laurillau, Y. (2013). EMG feature evaluation for improving myoelectric pattern recognition robustness. *Expert Systems with Applications*, *40*(12), 4832–4840. doi:10.1016/j.eswa.2013.02.023

Prasad, A. M., Iverson, L. R., & Liaw, A. (2006). Newer classification and regression tree techniques: Bagging and random forests for ecological prediction. *Ecosystems (New York, N.Y.)*, *9*(2), 181–199. doi:10.1007/s10021-005-0054-1

Reaz, M., Hussain, M., & Mohd-Yasin, F. (2006). Techniques of EMG signal analysis: Detection, processing, classification and applications. *Biological Procedures Online*, *8*(1), 11–35. doi:10.1251/bpo115 PMID:16799694

Rechy-Ramirez, E. J., & Hu, H. (2014). A Flexible Bio-Signal Based HMI for Hands-Free Control of an Electric Powered Wheelchair. *International Journal of Artificial Life Research*, *4*(1), 59–76. doi:10.4018/ijalr.2014010105

Shenoy, P., Miller, K. J., Crawford, B., & Rao, R. P. (2008). Online electromyographic control of a robotic prosthesis. *Biomedical Engineering. IEEE Transactions on, 55*(3), 1128–1135.

Soares, A., Andrade, A., Lamounier, E., & Carrijo, R. (2003). The development of a virtual myoelectric prosthesis controlled by an EMG pattern recognition system based on neural networks. *Journal of Intelligent Information Systems, 21*(2), 127–141. doi:10.1023/A:1024758415877

Strobl, C., Malley, J., & Tutz, G. (2009). An introduction to recursive partitioning: Rationale, application, and characteristics of classification and regression trees, bagging, and random forests. *Psychological Methods, 14*(4), 323–348. doi:10.1037/a0016973 PMID:19968396

Tanaka, K., Matsunaga, K., & Wang, H. O. (2005). Electroencephalogram-based control of an electric wheelchair. *Robotics. IEEE Transactions on, 21*(4), 762–766.

Ubeda, A., Ianez, E., & Azorín, J. M. (2011). Wireless and portable EOG-based interface for assisting disabled people. *Mechatronics, IEEE/ASME Transactions on, 16*(5), 870-873.

Usakli, A. B., Gurkan, S., Aloise, F., Vecchiato, G., & Babiloni, F. (2010). On the use of electrooculogram for efficient human computer interfaces. *Computational Intelligence and Neuroscience, 2010*, 1. doi:10.1155/2010/630649 PMID:19841687

Vallabhaneni, A., Wang, T., & He, B. (2005). *Brain—computer interface. In Neural engineering* (pp. 85–121). Springer. doi:10.1007/0-306-48610-5_3

Van Boxtel, A. (2001). Optimal signal bandwidth for the recording of surface EMG activity of facial, jaw, oral, and neck muscles. *Psychophysiology, 38*(1), 22–34. doi:10.1111/1469-8986.3810022 PMID:11321618

Won-Young, H. (2014). A Coherent View on Entropy. *Natural Science, 6*(7), 540–544. doi:10.4236/ns.2014.67053

Zardoshti-Kermani, M., Wheeler, B. C., Badie, K., & Hashemi, R. M. (1995). EMG feature evaluation for movement control of upper extremity prostheses. *Rehabilitation Engineering. IEEE Transactions on, 3*(4), 324–333.

Zhao, J., Xie, Z., Jiang, L., Cai, H., Liu, H., & Hirzinger, G. (2006). *EMG control for a five-fingered underactuated prosthetic hand based on wavelet transform and sample entropy.* Paper presented at the Intelligent Robots and Systems, 2006 IEEE/RSJ International Conference on. doi:10.1109/IROS.2006.282425

Zwarts, M. J., & Stegeman, D. F. (2003). Multichannel surface EMG: Basic aspects and clinical utility. *Muscle & Nerve, 28*(1), 1–17. doi:10.1002/mus.10358 PMID:12811768

KEY TERMS AND DEFINITIONS

Arithmetic Mean: The "arithmetic mean" or simply "mean" value of a given input sequence or segment is nothing but finding the average value for the segment. The mean value is the measure of a central or typical value of a random segment. The mean is calculated by summing all the variables present in a segment and dividing it by the number of variables or samples present in that segment. It is an important feature of sEMG signals.

Entropy: Entropy is a measure of the randomness or unpredictable information present in the signal. It can be determined from a finite set of values of a signal using various algorithms. Entropy has widespread application in field of signal processing for separating the desired signal from the interfering noise.

Median: The median separates the higher half of the data sequence from the lower half of the data sequence, which is done by arranging all the data of a sequence in an orderly manner from lowest value to highest value and sorting out the midpoint or middle value is from the sequence. The median is useful for making qualitative analysis of whether the central value has the highest priority or importance.

Root Mean Square (RMS): The root man square (RMS) value of a given input sequence or segment can be calculated by taking the square root of the squared input variable or segment or sequence. RMS can be regarded as a measure of the constant force applied or non-fatiguing contraction of muscle.

Skewness: Skewness is a measure of the asymmetry or irregularity present in a set of real-valued random variables or a sequence about the mean of a given signal.

Standard Deviation (SD): The standard deviation (SD) of an input sequence or segment is used to define the amount of variation or dispersion occurred. In general standard deviation is nothing but the square root on the variance. Standard deviation is used to find the threshold level of the muscle contraction activity.

Variance: Variance is used to measure the dispersion or spreadability of a variable present in a segment with respect to the mean. The variance will always have a non-negative value because squares are always positive and non-zero, unless and until all the variables present in the sequence or segment have the same value as the mean. The variance for an input sequence or segment is equal to the mean of the sum of the squared deviations from the mean of that sequence or segment. Variance uses the power of the signal as a feature. It can be used to find measure of the consistency.

Section 6
Wireless Systems for Healthcare

Chapter 14
Development of a Surface EMG-Based Control System for Controlling Assistive Devices:
A Study on Robotic Vehicle

Uvanesh K.
National Institute of Technology, Rourkela, India

Suraj Kumar Nayak
National Institute of Technology, Rourkela, India

Biswajeet Champaty
National Institute of Technology, Rourkela, India

Goutam Thakur
Manipal Institute of Technology, India

Biswajit Mohapatra
Vesaj Patel Hospital, India

D. N. Tibarewala
Jadavpur University, India

Kunal Pal
National Institute of Technology, Rourkela, India

ABSTRACT

The current study discusses about the development of an EMG based wireless control system for the patients suffering from high-level motor disability. Surface EMG (sEMG) signals were processed in the time domain and using discrete wavelet transforms (DWT). The statistical features of the signals (sEMG, envelope of the squared sEMG and wavelet processed sEMG) were determined and analyzed. The analysis of the features suggested that the features of the envelope of the squared sEMG signals were sufficient to be used for high-efficiency classification and control signal generation. A hall-effect sensor based switching mechanism was introduced for controlling the duration of the activation of the device. The control signals were wirelessly transmitted to the assistive device (robotic vehicle). The training and the subsequent use of the developed control system were easy.

DOI: 10.4018/978-1-5225-0140-4.ch014

INTRODUCTION

Biosignals may be defined as the electric potentials associated with the physiological functioning of the tissues and the organs (Sanei & Chambers, 2013). The biosignals are time-variant signals and can be described using signal amplitude, frequency and phase, like any other electronic signals (Semmlow & Griffel, 2014). Unlike the electronic signals, whose existence is due to the flow of electrons, the biosignals are associated with the flow of ions (sodium, potassium and chloride). Hence, the potential associated with the biosignals are ionic in nature. The generation of the biosignals is due to flow of ions across the cell membrane and hence, results in the electrochemical activity. Some of the common biosignals include electrocardiogram (ECG), electroencephalogram (EEG), electrooculogram (EOG) and electromyogram (EMG).

Recent years have seen a rise in the development of biosignal controlled assistive devices/aids. This has been made possible due to the advancements in the technology related to the biosignal acquisition and transmission. The use of biosignals for controlling the functions of the assistive devices has opened up a new research area, which is regarded as "Body-Computer Interface" (BCI) or "Human-Machine Interface" (HMI). This field of study uses the residual signals of the incapacitated persons for controlling the machines (assistive devices). Such devices have been reported to improve the quality of the life of the incapacitated persons and drastically reduce their dependence on the caretakers. Amongst the various biosignals, the use of EEG, EOG and EMG has received much attention for devising HMI control systems (Allison et al., 2012; Rafael Barea, Luciano Boquete, Manuel Mazo, & Elena López, 2002a; Chen & Newman, 2004; Moon, Lee, Chu, & Mun, 2005; Tanaka, Matsunaga, & Wang, 2005). As per the reported literature, the use of EMG and EOG biosignals are comparatively easier for devising HMI control systems as compared to the EEG biosignal. This is due to the fact that the processed EMG and EOG biosignals represent themselves with definite patterns.

The EEG biosignals are acquired by placing the measuring electrodes over the scalp. The frequency of the EEG biosignal range is normally in between 0.1 Hz and 100 Hz (Lim & Hong, 2009). The generation of the EEG biosignals is due to the neuronal activity within the cerebral cortex region of the brain. Unfortunately, the signals perceived by the electrodes are due to the neuronal activity of a number of neurons beneath the electrode and not due to the activity of a single neuron. Hence, the analysis of the EEG signals is quite complicated. Another problem associated with the measurement of the EEG biosignals is the placement of the electrodes due to the presence hair. This increases the chances of incorporation of the artifacts. Even though the EEG signal can be acquired in a non-invasive manner, due to the above reasons the use of EEG signal based human-computer interface (HCI) system is not preferably used for the development of control system for the assistive devices (Ferreira et al., 2008; Ferreira, Silva, Celeste, Bastos Filho, & Sarcinelli Filho, 2007). But with the advent of advancements in the rehabilitative technology front, many researchers are trying to develop human-machine interface (HMI) systems for the neuromuscular incapacitated patients using EEG signals (Raya et al., 2015; Sellers, Ryan, & Hauser, 2014).

The generation of the EOG biosignals is due to the natural existence of corneo-retinal potential difference. The potential difference is usually in the range of 0.05 mV and 3.5 mV (Dey, Biswas, Das, Das, & Chaudhuri, 2012). The corneal tissue is relatively positive in nature as compared to the retinal tissue. This results in the formation of a dipole. The movement of the eyes in different directions consequently results in the movement of the dipole in different directions. The EOG signals are acquired by placing 2 electrodes vertically (orbital positions: below and above the orbit) and 2 electrodes horizontally (canthus position: on the lateral sides of the eyes). Movement of the eye towards a particular electrode makes the electrode relatively positive as compared to the oppositely placed electrode. The potential sensed by the other two electrodes are negligible. Control systems for the rehabilitative aids (e.g. wheelchair and robotic arm) can be designed easily in a non-invasive manner using EOG signals. The frequency of the EOG biosignal lies in the range of 0.1 Hz and 100 Hz (Rafael Barea, Luciano Boquete, Manuel Mazo, & E López, 2002b). Hence, special care has to be taken during the designing of the EOG signal amplifier such that a very high gain of amplification is achieved, but with very low levels of offset voltage. This may lead to the increase in the complexity of the hardware and the signal processing techniques (Barea, Boquete, Bergasa, López, & Mazo, 2003; Barea et al., 2002a).

EMG signal is generated due to the contraction and the relaxation of the muscle fibers (Mendez-Villanueva, Edge, Suriano, Hamer, & Bishop, 2012). The main advantage of the EMG signal is its ability to manifest itself on the surface of the skin (Seo et al., 2013). This allows the acquisition of the signals in a non-invasive manner. The strength of the EMG signal is dependent on the anatomical positioning of the surface electrodes (placement of electrode) and the physiological properties of the muscle (Watanabe, Kouzaki, Merletti, Fujibayashi, & Moritani, 2012). Also, it is easier to train the patient to generate specific biosignals with similar profiles. The frequency components of the EMG signal mainly lie in the range of 5 Hz and 500 Hz (Merletti & Di Torino, 1999; Van Boxtel, 2001). The major disadvantage of the acquisition of the EMG signal using surface electrodes is the recording of the EMG signals from a collective motor units of the muscle (Cescon et al., 2014). Even though the surface EMG signal is a marker of a collective motor unit of a muscle, it can divulge information about the clinical pathology of the muscles and different kind of motor activities (Hourigan et al., 2015). Due to this reason, EMG signal analysis has found applications not only in clinical diagnosis, but also for biomedical applications (Gooch et al., 2014).

EMG signals of different patterns may be produced by performing different motor activities. This leads to the alteration in the EMG signal features. This property of the EMG signals has been widely explored to design control systems for assistive devices (Nurhanim et al., 2014). As mentioned previously, the field of study dealing with the development of the control systems for the assistive devices is regarded as HMI (Yin, Fan, & Xu, 2012). A thorough literature survey suggested that EMG signal has been used to control devices like wheelchair, robotic manipulator, user-selected intentional movements and hand gesture control (Chapin, Moxon, Markowitz, & Nicolelis, 1999; Erik Scheme MSc & Kevin Englehart PhD, 2011; Fukuda, Tsuji, Ohtsuka, & Kaneko, 1998; Momen, Krishnan, & Chau, 2007). Also, residual EMG signals have been used for controlling the motion of the artificial limb (Wu, Song, Ling, Wang, & Tian, 2014). The HMI device amplifies the acquired EMG signals and processes the signals for extracting the features. The extracted features of the EMG signals are used for designing a control system for controlling the movement of the rehabilitation aids.

In this study, the development of a control system using EMG signal features for decision making has been reported. The envelope of the squared EMG signal was extracted and the statistical features (arithmetic mean, root mean square (RMS), standard deviation, variance, kurtosis, mode, summation, skewness, median, energy density, entropy and log entropy) were calculated. Similarly, the EMG signals were extracted and the above-mentioned statistical features were calculated. The extracted EMG signal was further processed using discrete wavelet transform (DWT) and their statistical features were also calculated. The above features were analyzed using analysis of variance (ANOVA) and the statistically significant features were identified. Out of the significant features, three features (arithmetic mean, mode and summation) were selected for classifying the EMG signals into the four classes/categories (left, right, forward and backward). Once the features were selected, in-range logic was developed for development of a control system. The developed control system was tested using an in-house developed robotic vehicle as the representative assistive device.

BACKGROUND

The word "electromyogram" has been derived from 3 words: "electro" (electrical activity), "myo" (muscle) and "gram" (recording). Combining all the 3 words, we get the term "electromyogram" (EMG). Hence, EMG stands for the electrical activity associated with the muscular movements. Like all other excitable cells, muscle cells (fibre) also show electrical activity. The electrical activity is due to the depolarization of the muscle cells. The motor endplate within a muscle fibre is innervated with the nerve cells, which are responsible for the initiation of the depolarization of the muscle cells. A motor unit is a collection of muscle fibres, which are innervated with a single motor neuron. Each muscle is the collection of a number of motor units. A collective activity of each of the motor units results in the particular action of the muscle. Since each motor unit of the muscles is innervated by single nerve cell, during the activation of the motor units all the muscle fibres, present in the particular muscle, will either contract or remain relaxed. The electrical potential generated during the contraction can be recorded by placing a needle electrode into the motor units, but the disadvantage of this method is that the method is invasive in nature.

In general, when a muscle is contracted, the combination of electrical activity of each of the motor unit is combined and is manifested on the skin surface. The electrical potential that is manifested over the skin is regarded as the "surface electromyogram" (sEMG). The surface electromyogram can be acquired by placing surface electrodes over a particular muscle (Criswell, 2010). This provides information about the physiological state of that particular muscle and can be recorded for study. The recording of the surface EMG has gained a lot of importance among the researchers and the clinicians due to its non-invasive nature. To study the physiological state of any particular muscle, surface EMG can be used to find "the state of physiology of that particular muscle". In case of any pathological conditions, there is a reduction in the amplitude of the EMG signals (Farina, Cescon, & Merletti, 2002). Also, different activities may result in the activation of the muscles in the different manner. This results in the generation of the EMG signals with different properties.

There are many diseased conditions that lead to the motor impairment. The degree of impairment dictates whether the EMG signal from the particular muscle may be used for classifying the feature and subsequent analysis. Based on the results of the analysis, the EMG signal from that particular muscle may be used for developing the control system for rehabilitative aids. The use of EMG signal for developing HCI system is not advisable for patients suffering from progressive motor-neuron degenerative diseases. This kind of system has been used in persons suffering from injuries (like spinal cord injury), which may leave the patient even with little (only head and/or shoulders) muscle activity. In other physiological conditions, (e.g. paraplegic, hemiplegic, etc.) the residual muscular activity of the remaining limb has been explored to a greater extent.

In recent years, advancements in the field of robotics have allowed to use the robotic technologies for improving the lifestyle of the motor disabled persons. Such devices have improved the independence of these (motor-disabled) patients. The use of robotic technologies for the betterment of the lifestyle of the disabled person is possible by means of integrating machine/computer with the human body. This integrity is termed as human-machine interface (HMI)/human-computer interface (HCI) (Neto, Celeste,

& Martins, 2006). The main aim for using HMI based system is to provide a device, which helps the physically disabled persons to do their day-to-day activities with minimal help from others. The HMI system collects input from the physiological actions and converts it into the machine commands using appropriate signal processing techniques. The signal processing techniques mainly contain pre-processing, feature extraction and control signal generation algorithm. Normally pre-processing is done to eliminate the noise due to artifacts, power line interference and impedance mismatch of the circuits. Additionally, pre-processing also help in nullifying offset voltage and current, if any, within the circuit. This step ensures that the biosignals can be amplified without or minimal noise. This preprocessing can be done using an EMG amplifier circuit (EMG-DAQ) (Biswal, Uvanesh, Champaty, Ray, & Pal, 2014). Feature extraction is an important process to determine the statistical parameters of the signals. The features are helpful in categorizing the biosignals into their known categories. The classified signals are used for the generation of the control signals.

Patient suffering from the paralysis of the lower extremities are advised to use wheelchair (Bajd, Kralj, Štefančič, & Lavrač, 1999). The operation of the conventional wheelchairs needs assistants. Unfortunately, the hiring of the assistant is a costly affair. To solve this problem, the electrically powered wheelchairs were introduced, which are controlled using joysticks or some kind of mechanical switches (Ding & Cooper, 2005). But in many cases, the use of these control systems is not possible (e.g. paraplegic patients). For providing assistance to such patients, biosignal based control systems have been proposed by many researchers. Most of the developed control systems use a complex algorithm (classification using the neural network, processing of signal using wavelets etc.) (Felzer & Freisleben, 2002; Karlsson & Gerdle, 2001; Kuribayashi, Shimizu, Okimura, & Taniguchi, 1993; Pope et al., 2000; Subasi, Yilmaz, & Ozcalik, 2006; Zennaro, Wellig, Koch, Moschytz, & Läubli, 2003). Cheng *et al.* (2008) reported the use of discrete wavelet transform (DWT) for processing of surface EMG (sEMG) signals and back propagation neural network for classification of the wavelet processed sEMG signals to identify different emotion patterns for potential application in emotion mouse, emotion toy, stress detection systems etc. (Cheng & Liu, 2008). Though these methods have been reported to improve the movement accuracy by improving the efficiency of the control system, there is an increased burden on the processors. To reduce the burden on the processor, the use of high performance processor has been proposed. But the increased performance is associated with the increase in the cost of the wheelchairs (Ohnishi, Weir, & Kuiken, 2007).

MAIN FOCUS OF THE CHAPTER

In this current study, a simple method to generate control signals for assistive devices has been proposed. For this purpose, the envelope of the squared EMG signal has been used. It is expected that this process will allow the development of a real-time control system with improved efficiency and accuracy. Additionally, "Boolean Change State Logic" has been introduced into the system to avoid unintentional activation of the assistive device. The logic has two Boolean inputs. As per this logic, there will be a high output signal when both the inputs are in the high states. The output of the logic will continue to be in the high state until and unless both the inputs become low. This is particularly of importance because the motor unit action potential trains (MUAPT) for EMG signals are generally of the duration 1 to 10 sec (De Luca, 1979). Hence, under normal conditions the EMG signal will activate the assistive device for a particular period of time. This might lead to either undershooting or overshooting the target position.

The use of the "Boolean Change State Logic" will allow the user to control the duration of generation of the control signals for controlling the wheelchair towards the target position. This was achieved using a Hall-effect sensor as a switching device, whose output was used as the one of the inputs for the "Boolean Change State Logic". The schematic diagrams of the program logic and the corresponding outputs have been shown in Figure 1.

METHODS

Volunteer

A 24 years old healthy volunteer was selected for the study. Institute ethical clearance was taken for the acquisition of the biosignals (including EMG) vide permit no. NITRKL/IEC/FORM-1 dated 13/12/2013. The volunteer was advised to move specific fingers as per the instructions. The corresponding EMG signal generated in the forearm muscles (flexor carpi radialis and palmaris longus) was recorded. The features of the acquired EMG signal were calculated. The volunteer was trained to generate similar kind of EMG signals using the developed device and was subsequently asked to control the movement of the in-house developed robotic vehicle.

Figure 1. (a) LabVIEW program of proposed Boolean change state logic, and (b-e) outputs of Boolean change state logic

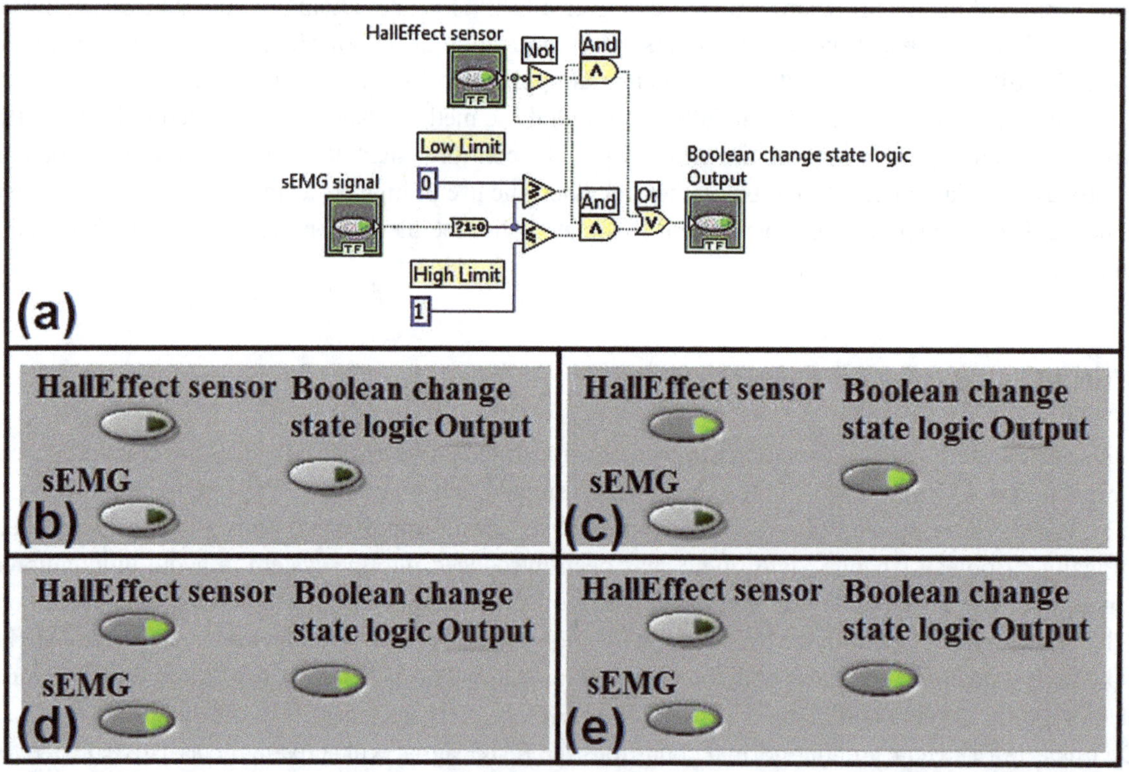

Acquisition of the EMG Signal

An EMG signal amplifier was developed as per the previously reported literature by our group with some modifications (Biswal et al., 2014). The developed EMG amplifier had a gain of ~2500. An integrator with a cut-off frequency of about 15.9 Hz was introduced in the circuit for removing the DC offset. To eliminate the high frequency components present within the EMG signal, a low-pass filter (LPF) was used (cut-off frequency = 1591 Hz). The output of the signal amplifier was acquired The EMG amplifier was developed as per the circuit diagram given in Figure 2 (a). A PCB layout was designed in Ultiboard(Ver. 13.0, National Instruments, USA). The layout was used to develop a PCB board using one sided copper-cladded board by carbon transfer method followed by ferric chloride ($FeCl_3$) etching process, as reported in the literature (li et al., 2015). A 3D PCB layout of the amplifier has been shown in Figure 2 (b). Since the surface EMG signals can manifest itself on the surface of the skin, two active electrodes were placed on the forearm muscle (flexor carpi radialis and palmaris longus) of the left hand,

Figure 2. (a) Circuit diagram of the EMG amplifier circuit, and (b) 3D layout of the EMG amplifier

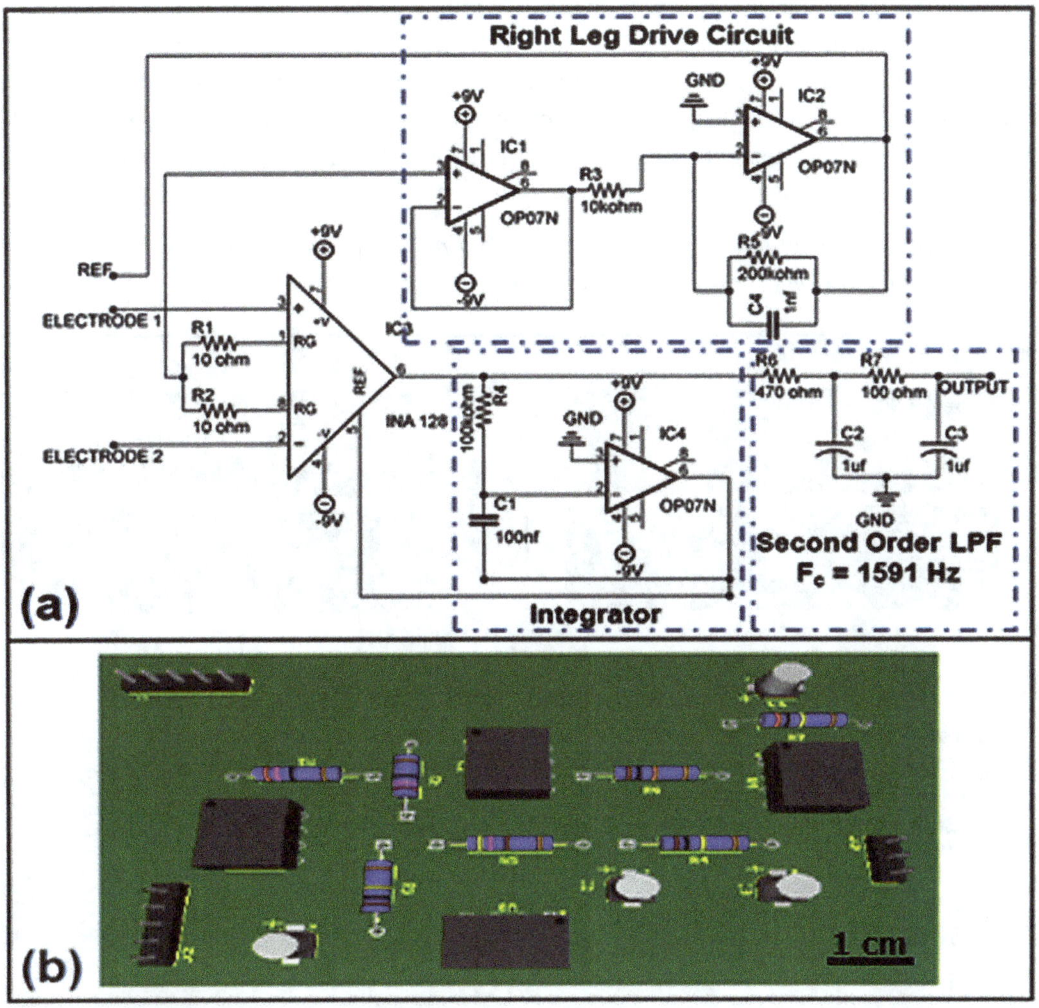

whereas, the ground electrode was placed on the wrist (Ulna) of the right hand. The active electrodes (surface electrode) were placed approximately 1 cm apart. Commercially available dry electrodes (Ag/AgCl, BPL Pvt. Ltd., India) were used for the acquisition of the EMG signals. The volunteer was asked to flex index finger, ring finger and all fingers (for two different time durations). The EMG signals generated corresponding to the finger movement activity of the volunteer was recorded into a laptop (working in the battery mode) using a data acquisition system (NI USB 6008, National Instruments, USA). The combination of the amplifier and USB 6008 was regarded as EMG-DAQ. A LabVIEW (Ver. 2010, National Instruments, USA) program was developed to record the data in the laptop. The volunteer was trained until he was able to generate EMG signals of similar profiles. Figure 3 shows the EMG profiles due to the movement of the different fingers.

Signal Processing

The recorded EMG signal was processed using a custom-made LabVIEW program in whichthe acquired EMG signals were squared so as to rectify the EMG signals. This allowed shifting the negative potentials to the positive side. Thereafter, the envelope of the squared signal was determined using smoothening filter (Rectangular moving average filter with a half-width of 2000). The envelope of the EMG signal was thresholded to obtain a pulse. The pulse, so obtained, had a time duration equal to the length of the duration of the EMG signal generated. The multiplication of the pulse with the original signal resulted in the extraction of the original EMG signal and rejection of the unwanted signal. Later the extracted EMG signal was further processed using Discrete Wavelet transform (DWT). The flowchart of the processing

Figure 3. EMG profiles generated by the movement of the fingers: (a) index finger flexion, (b) ring finger flexion, (c) all finger flexion (<1 sec) and (d) all finger flexion (>2 sec)

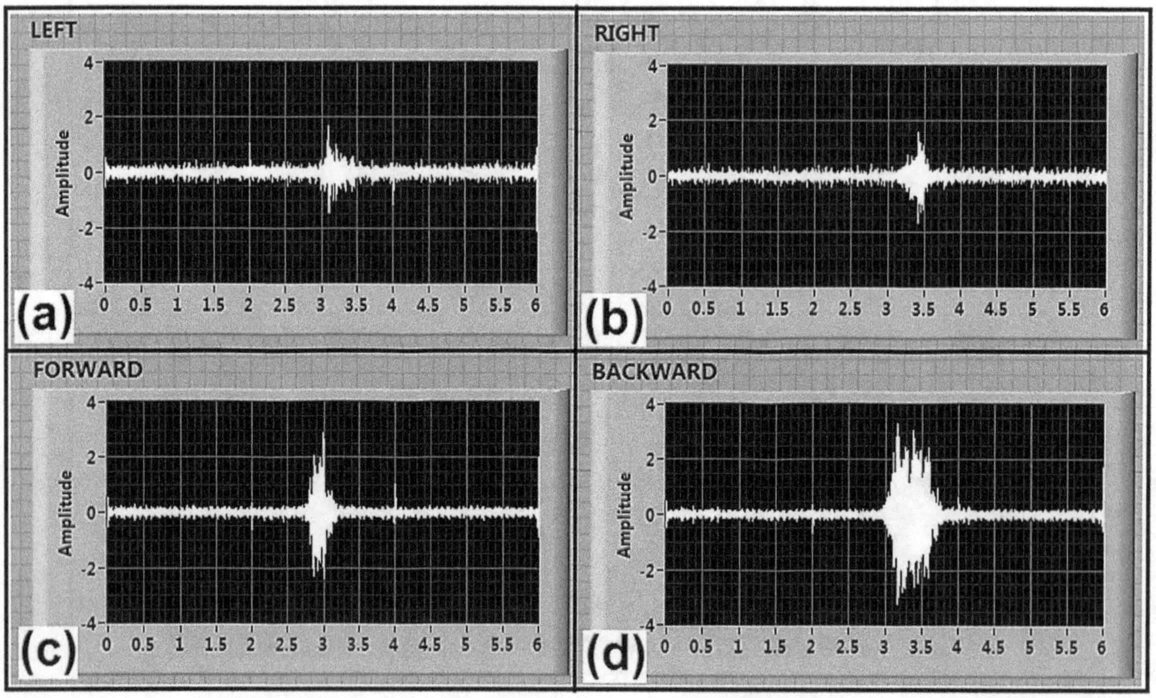

of the EMG signal has been shown in Figure 4. The program was capable of calculating the statistical features like arithmetic mean, median, mode, summation, standard deviation, variance, kurtosis, skewness, root mean square, entropy, log entropy, energy density and was able to save the corresponding results in a text file. The features of the signals were further analyzed using ANOVA for determining significantly different features.

Control System Development

Feature extraction and selection is the important part in designing a control system. Features of a signal can be extracted using a combination of statistical analysis and signal processing techniques. Here, thebasic statistical features have been used, which are mentioned in the previous section as features for probable classification. The important criterion in selecting the best feature depends on the repeatability or reproducing same type of signals. Three different features were selected depending upon their importance and a series of in-range logic was applied to generate control signals. Designing a control system using in-range logic reduces the complexity of the processing for classifying biosignals. In addition to the in-range logic, a hall-effect sensor was used as a switching device to avoid false activation of the robotic vehicle and also to keep it in motion as per the wish of the user.

Figure 4. Flowchart depicting the processing of the EMG signal

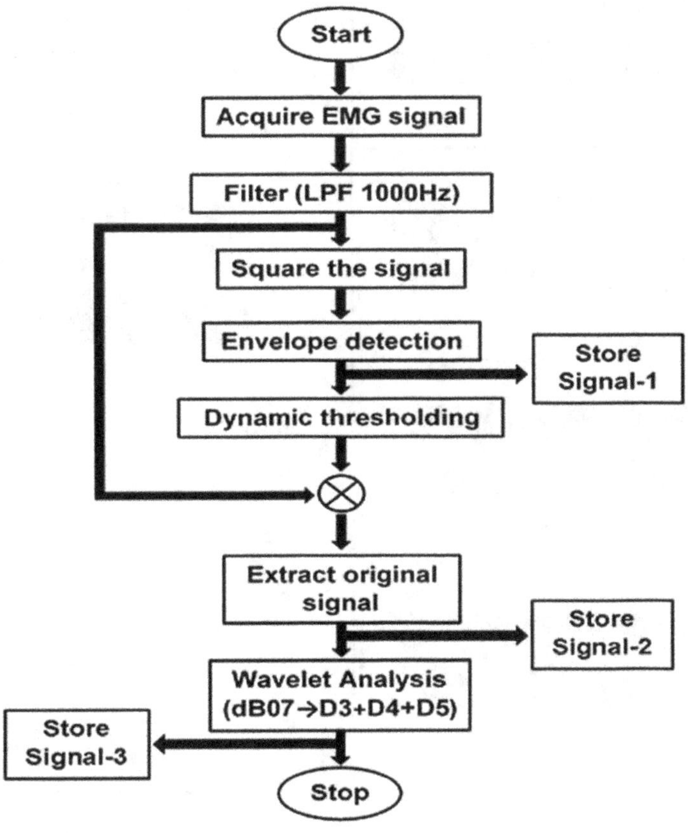

RESULTS AND DISCUSSION

The statistical features (arithmetic mean, median, mode, summation, standard deviation, variance, kurtosis, skewness, root mean square, entropy, log entropy and energy density) of the envelope of the EMG signals were calculated using the statistical palette of LabVIEW and the customized Matlab Script palette. Similarly, the statistical features of the extracted EMG signal were also calculated. The extracted EMG signal was further decomposed using db07 wavelet at level 9. The db07 wavelet function was used for decomposition of the sEMG signal, as it provides the highest value of RES index (the ratio of a Euclidean distance to a standard deviation index) of the mean absolute value (MAV) of the sEMG signal in comparison to other wavelets (Phinyomark, Limsakul, & Phukpattaranont, 2011). The reconstruction of the EMG signals was done using D3, D4 and D5 sub-bands (Figure 5). This was done to eliminate any unwanted noise present in the EMG signal. The statistical features of the reconstituted EMG signals were determined in the similar manner as described above. Figure 6 shows the representative original EMG signal, its envelope, extracted EMG signal and wavelet transformed EMG signal.

Figure 5. (a) Representative EMG signal, (b-d) wavelet decomposed EMG signal, (e) reconstructed signal, and (f) wavelet transform and sub-band selection window

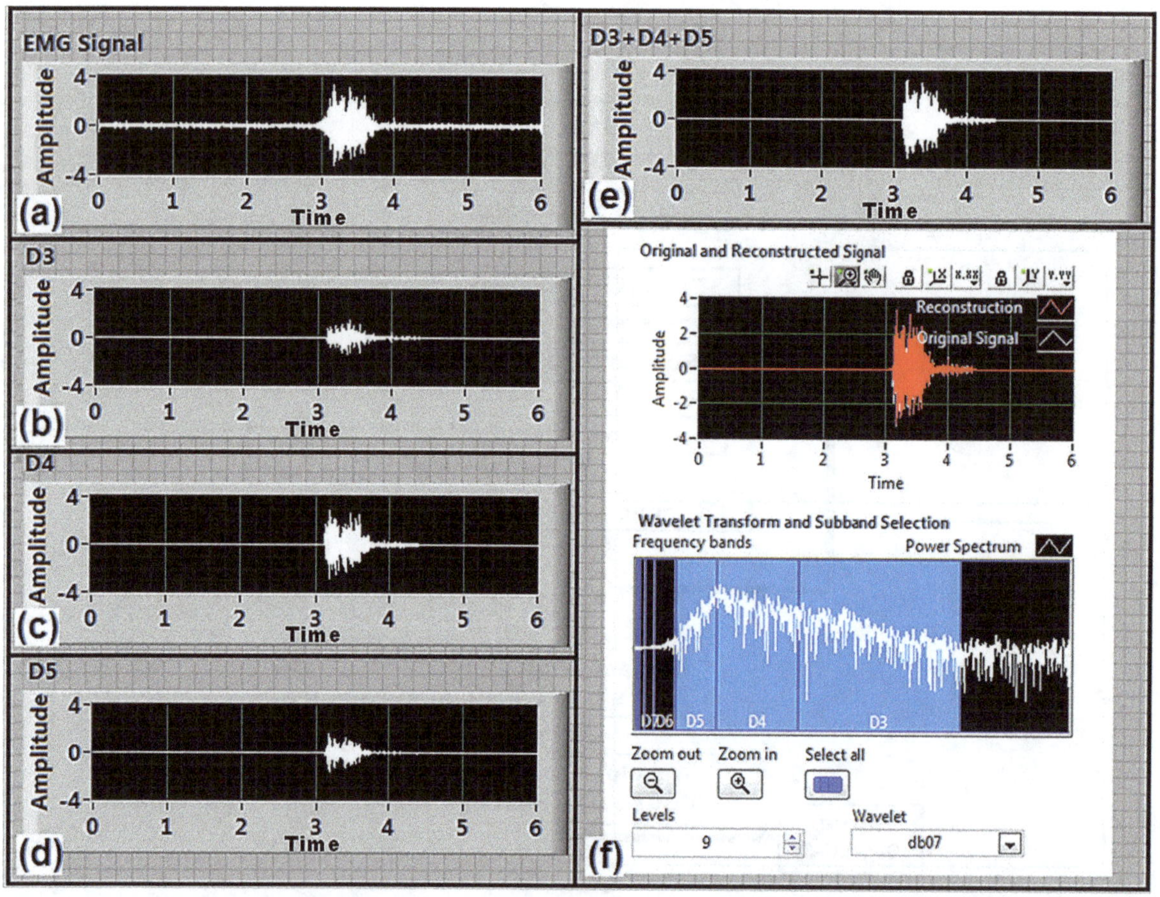

Figure 6. (a) Original EMG signal, (b) envelope of the EMG signal, (c) extracted EMG signal and (d) wavelet transformed EMG signal

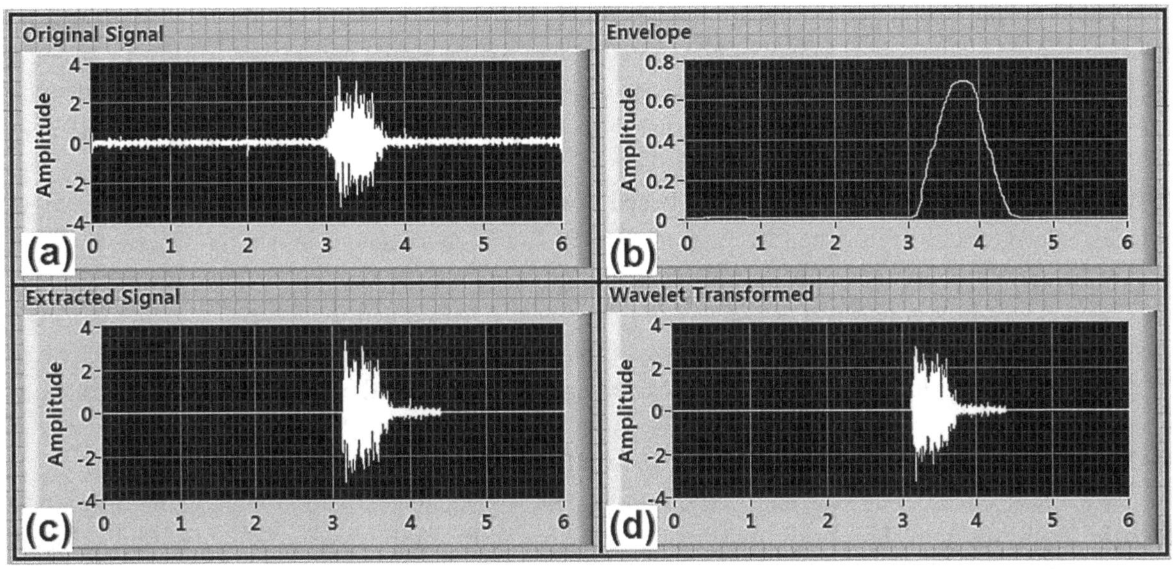

The statistical features of the EMG signal envelope, so obtained, were analyzed using analysis of variance (ANOVA). ANOVA is a statistical tool used to compare the means of more than two groups. The summary of the analysis of the features has been tabulated in Table 1. It was observed that all the twelve features, which were calculated, of the EMG signal envelope were significantly different. The accepted limit of the error was <5% ($p < 0.05$). Thereafter, the statistical features of the extracted EMG signals and the wavelet processed EMG signals were also analyzed using ANOVA. The results of the

Table 1. Important features of the EMG signals envelope calculated from ANOVA

Features	Mean ± SD				p-Value
	Left	Right	Forward	Backward	
AM	0.018±0.002	0.015±0.001	0.027±0.004	0.071±0.024361	0.000000
RMS	0.027±0.005	0.026±0.002	0.059±0.009759	0.165±0.059621	0.000000
SD	0.020±0.005	0.021±0.001	0.05±0.008952	0.149±0.054451	0.000000
Variance	0.000±0.000	0.0004±0.000	0.002±0.000953	0.025±0.017472	0.000000
Kurtosis	5.377±0.164	5.514±0.107	5.750±0.030	5.754±0.034369	0.000000
Mode	0.009±0.001	0.006±0.001	0.005±0.0009	0.004±0.001432	0.000001
Summation	566.55±68.59	477.91±43.25	831.42±120.00	2144.44±730.83	0.000000
Skewness	1.957±0.076	2.033±0.048	2.131±0.009	2.106±0.021	0.000000
Median	0.010±0.001	0.007±0.001	0.005±0.000	0.005±0.000	0.000000
ED	0.0002±0.000	0.00009±0.000	0.0001±0.000	0.00006±0.00003	0.000000
Entropy	0.002±0.0005	0.0008±0.0002	0.001±0.0002	0.0005±0.0003	0.000000
Log Entropy	-8.355±0.342	-9.331±0.290	-8.944±0.267	-9.857±0.659	0.000000

ANOVA analysis have been tabulated in Table 2 and Table 3. The results indicated that root mean square (RMS), standard deviation (SD), variance and kurtosis were statistically different in both extracted signal and wavelet processed extracted signal. Arithmetic mean (AM), mode and summation of the squared EMG signal envelope were selected for classification and control signal generation. This is because the signal processing steps for obtaining the envelope of the EMG signal is much simpler as compared to the extraction of the EMG signal and/or processing the extracted signal in the joint time-frequency domain using discrete wavelet transformation (DWT).

Once the features (arithmetic mean, mode and summation) were selected, necessary in-range logic was developed for classifying the EMG signals into the four classes/categories (left, right, forward and backward). The in-range logic was chosen because designing a control system using in-range logic reduces the complexity of the processing for classifying biosignals. A Boolean logic classification algorithm using X-OR and AND gates was developed. Boolean X-OR gate generates a high output when only one of its inputs is high. Hence, the X-OR gate may be used to verify whether there is any dual activation. In the event of dual activation, the output of the X-OR gate generates a low output. The output of the X-OR gate was used as one of the inputs for the AND gate. The second input of the AND gate was a binary output from the initial in-range logic system. The AND gate generates a high output only when both the inputs are high. This helps in preventing false activation of the system. Classification using all the three features was achieved in the first stage. The flowchart of the classification process in the first stage has been shown in Figure 7 (a). The classified (binary) outputs from all the three features were used as input for a three terminal AND gate logic. The AND gate produced a high output only when all the three features were in agreement during classification in the first stage. The output of the AND gate was again compared with the output of the other three classes using X-OR gate, which produced a high output when it received a high input from only one classification channel. The classified signals were

Table 2. Important features of the extracted EMG signals calculated from ANOVA

Features	Mean ± SD				p-Value
	Left	Right	Forward	Backward	
RMS	0.067±0.015	0.065±0.008	0.138±0.021	0.242±0.049	0.0000
SD	0.067±0.015	0.065±0.008	0.138±0.021	0.242±0.049	0.0000
Variance	0.004±0.002	0.004±0.001	0.019±0.006	0.061±0.024	0.0000
Kurtosis	74.34±29.32	95.58±28.84	100.54±31.40	59.961±16.197	0.0061

Table 3. Important features of the wavelet transformed EMG signals calculated from ANOVA

Features	Mean±SD				p-Value
	Left	Right	Forward	Backward	
RMS	0.061±0.014	0.061±0.008	0.128±0.020	0.227±0.047	0.0000
SD	0.061±0.014	0.061±0.008	0.128±0.020	0.227±0.047	0.0000
Variance	0.003±0.001	0.003±0.001	0.016±0.005	0.053±0.021	0.0000
Kurtosis	67.55±24.95	91.50±25.30	104.42±38.17	60.078±15.831	0.0025

Figure 7. Flowchart for the classification of the EMG signals: (A1/B1/C1/D1: control signals generated using arithmetic mean feature in stage-1; A2/B2/C2/D2: control signals generated using mode feature in stage-1; and A3/B3/C3/D3: control signals generated using summation feature in stage-1)

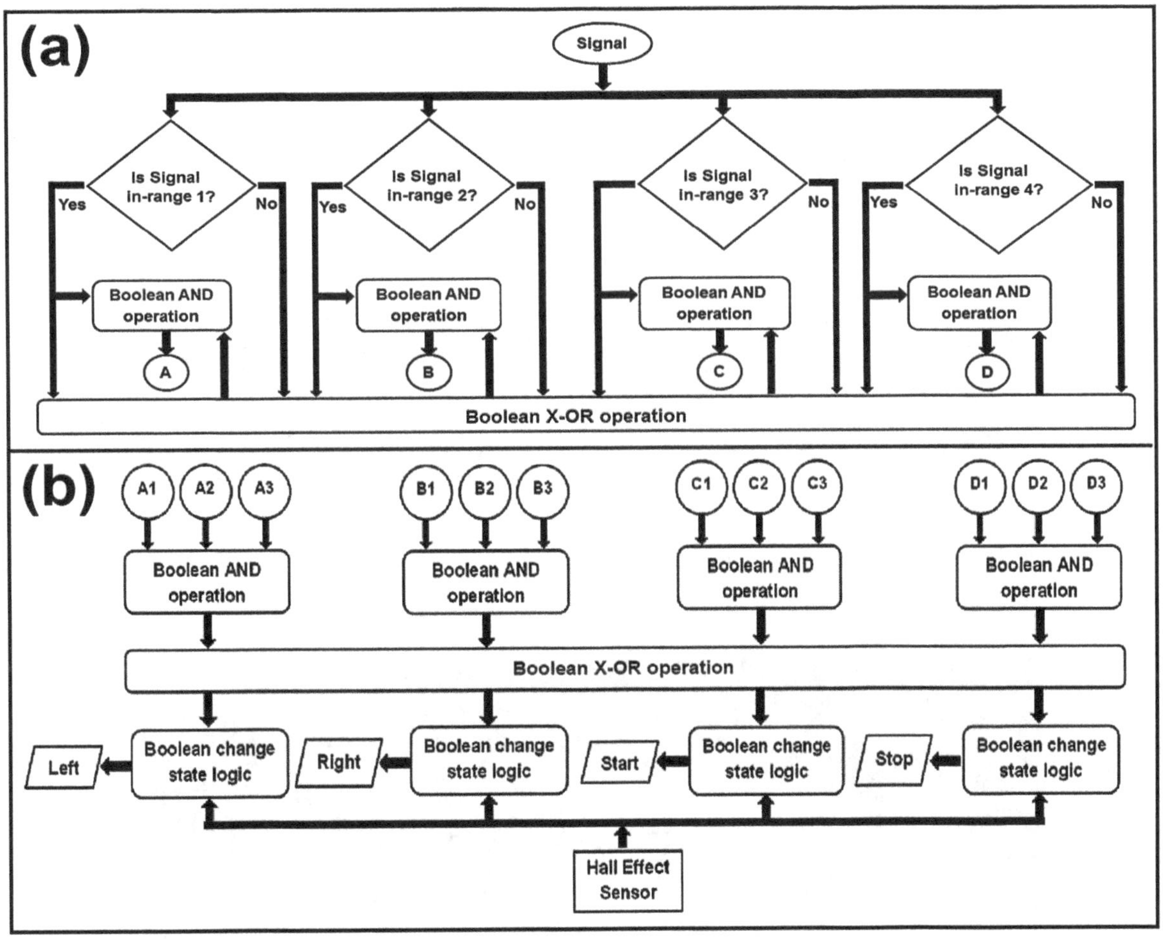

used for driving the robotic vehicle. A Hall- effect sensor based switching was incorporated in the control system for two reasons. The primary reason was to prevent any unintended activation of the robotic vehicle as the device will only be activated when the Hall-effect sensor was on a high state. Hence, the classified signals were able to generate control signals only when the Hall-effect was on a high state. The second reason being, the output of the Hall-effect sensor was a determinant of the distance and angle of rotation of the robotic vehicle. A "Boolean change state logic" was employed to achieve this. The "Boolean change state logic" helped keeping the robotic vehicle in motion even after the cessation of the EMG signals until the Hall- Effect sensor generated a low output signal. The logic of this classification has been in Figure 7 (b).

The control signals were used to power a LED panel (Figure 8). The training of the volunteer was done using this LED panel. This is because the LED panel provided a visual feedback, which in turn, helped the volunteer to generate similar EMG profiles. The generated signals were wirelessly communicated to the robotic vehicle. A pair of XBee (S1) was used for the transmission of the control signals to the

Figure 8. Generation of the control signals during training

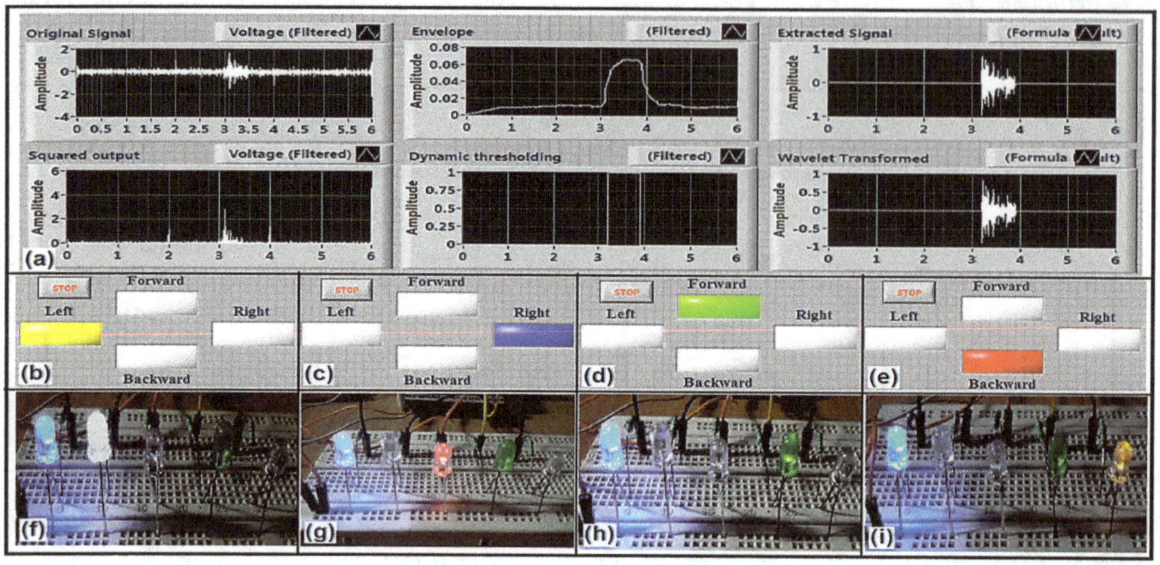

Figure 9. (a) The control signal generation set-up along with the robotic vehicle and (b-e) movement of the robotic vehicle in different directions

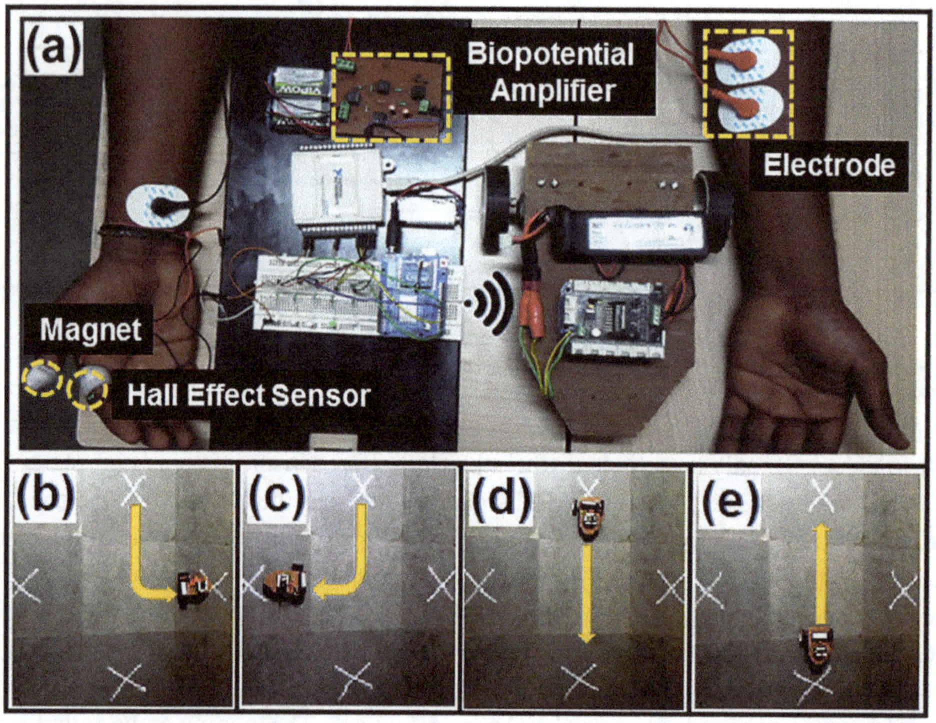

robotic vehicle. The device was tested and was found to satisfactorily perform as per the expectation without any false activation (Figure 9).

The direction of the robotic vehicle was controlled by controlling the direction of the movement of the right and the left motors, which were attached to the rear wheels of the robotic vehicle. The direction of the movement of the motors during the different classes of movement has been tabulated in Table 4.

FUTURE RESEARCH DIRECTIONS

The current study proposes the development of a EMG based control system having potential application in assistive devices for incapacitated persons. The EMG signals were acquired from the forearm muscles (flexor carpi radialis and palmaris longus). Future research can be carried out by acquiring EMG signals from other muscles (triceps, pectoralis major, latissimus dorsi and external oblique etc.) of the body so that the best site for EMG signal can be reported. The present study utilized the Boolean logic for the generation of control signals. Future studies can be performed using other methods of control signal generation. Also, the proposed EMG based control system can be utilized during future studies in other domains of application.

CONCLUSION

The motor disabled persons often find it difficult to control the movement of the rehabilitation aids. To help these people, many researchers are working on the development of control systems, which can improve the independent mobility. The paraplegic patients lose the functionality of the lower extremities (paralysis). Conventional electric powered wheelchairs use joystick for controlling the movement of the wheelchair. But in many cases (e.g. spinal cord injury and quadriplegia), it has been reported that the patients are not able to control the joystick. In this study, we report a simple surface EMG based control system, which can be used for controlling the movement of not only the wheelchair but also other rehabilitative devices. For improving the safety and the convenience of the patients, a Hall-effect sensor based switching mechanism was introduced for avoiding unintentional activation of the assistive device and controlling the direction of the device.

Table 4. Finger flexion and direction of the movement of the robotic vehicle

Finger Movement	Movement Intended	Direction Of Gearing The DC Motor	
		Left Side Motor (Rotor Direction)	Right Side Motor (Rotor Direction)
Index finger flexion	Left	0	+
Ring finger flexion	Right	+	0
All finger flexion (<1 sec)	Forward	+	+
All finger flexion (>2 sec)	Backward	-	-

(+) Clockwise rotation, (-) Anticlockwise rotation and (0) Neutral

REFERENCES

Allison, B., Leeb, R., Brunner, C., Müller-Putz, G., Bauernfeind, G., Kelly, J., & Neuper, C. (2012). Toward smarter BCIs: Extending BCIs through hybridization and intelligent control. *Journal of Neural Engineering*, *9*(1), 013001. doi:10.1088/1741-2560/9/1/013001 PMID:22156029

Bajd, T., Kralj, A., Štefančič, M., & Lavrač, N. (1999). Use of functional electrical stimulation in the lower extremities of incomplete spinal cord injured patients. *Artificial Organs*, *23*(5), 403–409. doi:10.1046/j.1525-1594.1999.06360.x PMID:10378929

Barea, R., Boquete, L., Bergasa, L. M., López, E., & Mazo, M. (2003). Electro-oculographic guidance of a wheelchair using eye movements codification. *The International Journal of Robotics Research*, *22*(7-8), 641–652. doi:10.1177/027836490302207012

Barea, R., Boquete, L., Mazo, M., & López, E. (2002a). System for assisted mobility using eye movements based on electrooculography. *Neural Systems and Rehabilitation Engineering. IEEE Transactions on*, *10*(4), 209–218.

Barea, R., Boquete, L., Mazo, M., & López, E. (2002b). Wheelchair guidance strategies using EOG. *Journal of Intelligent & Robotic Systems*, *34*(3), 279–299. doi:10.1023/A:1016359503796

Biswal, D., Uvanesh, K., Champaty, B., Ray, S. S., & Pal, K. (2014). *Development of an ambulatory universal bio potential recording device.* Paper presented at the Control, Instrumentation, Communication and Computational Technologies (ICCICCT), 2014 International Conference on. doi:10.1109/ICCICCT.2014.6993130

Cescon, C., Raimondi, E. E., Začesta, V., Drusany-Starič, K., Martsidis, K., & Merletti, R. (2014). Characterization of the motor units of the external anal sphincter in pregnant women with multichannel surface EMG. *International Urogynecology Journal and Pelvic Floor Dysfunction*, *25*(8), 1097–1103. doi:10.1007/s00192-014-2356-3 PMID:24623258

Chapin, J. K., Moxon, K. A., Markowitz, R. S., & Nicolelis, M. A. (1999). Real-time control of a robot arm using simultaneously recorded neurons in the motor cortex. *Nature Neuroscience*, *2*(7), 664–670. doi:10.1038/10223 PMID:10404201

Chen, Y., & Newman, W. S. (2004). *A human-robot interface based on electrooculography.* Paper presented at the Robotics and Automation, 2004.

Cheng, B., & Liu, G.-Y. (2008). *Emotion recognition from surface EMG signal using wavelet transform and neural network.* Paper presented at the 2nd International Conference on Bioinformatics and Biomedical Engineering (ICBBE). doi:10.1109/ICBBE.2008.670

Criswell, E. (2010). *Cram's introduction to surface electromyography.* Jones & Bartlett Publishers.

De Luca, C. J. (1979). Physiology and mathematics of myoelectric signals. *Biomedical Engineering, IEEE Transactions on,* (6), 313-325.

Dey, N., Biswas, S., Das, P., Das, A., & Chaudhuri, S. S. (2012). *Feature analysis for the reversible watermarked electrooculography signal using low distortion prediction-error expansion.* Paper presented at the Communications, Devices and Intelligent Systems (CODIS), 2012 International Conference on. doi:10.1109/CODIS.2012.6422280

Ding, D., & Cooper, R. (2005). Electric powered wheelchairs. *Control Systems, IEEE, 25*(2), 22–34. doi:10.1109/MCS.2005.1411382

Farina, D., Cescon, C., & Merletti, R. (2002). Influence of anatomical, physical, and detection-system parameters on surface EMG. *Biological Cybernetics, 86*(6), 445–456. doi:10.1007/s00422-002-0309-2 PMID:12111273

Felzer, T., & Freisleben, B. (2002). *HaWCoS: the hands-free wheelchair control system.* Paper presented at the fifth international ACM conference on Assistive technologies. doi:10.1145/638249.638273

Ferreira, A., Celeste, W. C., Cheein, F. A., Bastos-Filho, T. F., Sarcinelli-Filho, M., & Carelli, R. (2008). Journal of NeuroEngineering and Rehabilitation. *Journal of Neuroengineering and Rehabilitation, 5*, 10. doi:10.1186/1743-0003-5-10 PMID:18366775

Ferreira, A., Silva, R., Celeste, W., Bastos Filho, T. F., & Sarcinelli Filho, M. (2007). *Human–machine interface based on muscular and brain signals applied to a robotic wheelchair.* Paper presented at the Journal of Physics: Conference Series.

Fukuda, O., Tsuji, T., Ohtsuka, A., & Kaneko, M. (1998). *EMG-based human-robot interface for rehabilitation aid.* Paper presented at the Robotics and Automation, 1998. doi:10.1109/ROBOT.1998.680978

Gooch, C. L., Doherty, T. J., Chan, K. M., Bromberg, M. B., Lewis, R. A., & Stashuk, D. W. (2014). Motor unit number estimation: A technology and literature review. *Muscle & Nerve, 50*(6), 884–893. PMID:25186553

Hourigan, M. L., McKinnon, N. B., Johnson, M., Rice, C. L., Stashuk, D. W., & Doherty, T. J. (2015). Increased motor unit potential shape variability across consecutive motor unit discharges in the tibialis anterior and vastus medialis muscles of healthy older subjects. *Clinical Neurophysiology, 126*(12), 2381–2389. doi:10.1016/j.clinph.2015.02.002 PMID:25727901

Karlsson, S., & Gerdle, B. (2001). Mean frequency and signal amplitude of the surface EMG of the quadriceps muscles increase with increasing torque—a study using the continuous wavelet transform. *Journal of Electromyography and Kinesiology, 11*(2), 131–140. doi:10.1016/S1050-6411(00)00046-8 PMID:11228426

Kuribayashi, K., Shimizu, S., Okimura, K., & Taniguchi, T. (1993). A discrimination system using neural network for EMG-controlled prostheses-Integral type of EMG signal processing. Paper presented at the Intelligent Robots and Systems' 93, IROS'93.

Li, w., Liu, J., Zhang, S., He, W., Chen, S., & Li, Z. (2015). Study on process technique of PCBs with ladder conductive lines. *Circuit World, 41*(1). doi: doi:10.1109/IROS.1993.583873

Lim, C. T., & Hong, J. G. C. (2009). *13th International Conference on Biomedical Engineering: ICBME 2008* (Vol. 23). Springer Science & Business Media.

Mendez-Villanueva, A., Edge, J., Suriano, R., Hamer, P., & Bishop, D. (2012). The recovery of repeated-sprint exercise is associated with PCr resynthesis, while muscle pH and EMG amplitude remain depressed. *PLoS ONE*, *7*(12), e51977. doi:10.1371/journal.pone.0051977 PMID:23284836

Merletti, R., & Di Torino, P. (1999). Standards for reporting EMG data. *Journal of Electromyography and Kinesiology*, *9*(1), 3–4.

Momen, K., Krishnan, S., & Chau, T. (2007). Real-time classification of forearm electromyographic signals corresponding to user-selected intentional movements for multifunction prosthesis control. *Neural Systems and Rehabilitation Engineering. IEEE Transactions on*, *15*(4), 535–542.

Moon, I., Lee, M., Chu, J., & Mun, M. (2005). *Wearable EMG-based HCI for electric-powered wheelchair users with motor disabilities.* Paper presented at the Robotics and Automation, 2005.

Neto, A. F., Celeste, W. C., & Martins, V. R. (2006). *Human-machine interface based on electro-biological signals for mobile vehicles.* Paper presented at the Industrial Electronics, 2006 IEEE International Symposium on. doi:10.1109/ISIE.2006.296086

Nurhanim, K., Elamvazuthi, I., Vasant, P., Ganesan, T., Parasuraman, S., & Khan, M. A. (2014). Joint Torque Estimation Model of Surface Electromyography (sEMG) Based on Swarm Intelligence Algorithm for Robotic Assistive Device. *Procedia Computer Science*, *42*, 175–182. doi:10.1016/j.procs.2014.11.049

Ohnishi, K., Weir, R. F., & Kuiken, T. A. (2007). Neural machine interfaces for controlling multifunctional powered upper-limb prostheses. *Expert Review of Medical Devices*, *4*(1), 43–53. doi:10.1586/17434440.4.1.43 PMID:17187470

Phinyomark, A., Limsakul, C., & Phukpattaranont, P. (2011). Application of wavelet analysis in EMG feature extraction for pattern classification. *Measurement Science Review*, *11*(2), 45–52. doi:10.2478/v10048-011-0009-y

Pope, M., Aleksiev, A., Panagiotacopulos, N., Lee, J., Wilder, D., Friesen, K., & Goel, V. K. et al. (2000). Evaluation of low back muscle surface EMG signals using wavelets. *Clinical Biomechanics (Bristol, Avon)*, *15*(8), 567–573. doi:10.1016/S0268-0033(00)00024-3 PMID:10936428

Raya, R., Rocon, E., Urendes, E., Velasco, M. A., Clemotte, A., & Ceres, R. (2015). *Assistive Robots for Physical and Cognitive Rehabilitation in Cerebral Palsy. In Intelligent Assistive Robots* (pp. 133–156). Springer.

Sanei, S., & Chambers, J. A. (2013). *EEG signal processing*. John Wiley & Sons.

Scheme, E., & Englehart, K. (2011). Electromyogram pattern recognition for control of powered upper-limb prostheses: State of the art and challenges for clinical use. *Journal of Rehabilitation Research and Development*, *48*(6), 643. doi:10.1682/JRRD.2010.09.0177 PMID:21938652

Sellers, E. W., Ryan, D. B., & Hauser, C. K. (2014). Noninvasive brain-computer interface enables communication after brainstem stroke. *Science Translational Medicine*, *6*(257).

Semmlow, J. L., & Griffel, B. (2014). *Biosignal and medical image processing*. CRC Press.

Seo, S.-H., Jeon, I.-H., Cho, Y.-H., Lee, H.-G., Hwang, Y.-T., & Jang, J.-H. (2013). Surface EMG during the push-up plus exercise on a stable support or swiss ball: Scapular stabilizer muscle exercise. *Journal of Physical Therapy Science*, *25*(7), 833–837. doi:10.1589/jpts.25.833 PMID:24259864

Subasi, A., Yilmaz, M., & Ozcalik, H. R. (2006). Classification of EMG signals using wavelet neural network. *Journal of Neuroscience Methods*, *156*(1), 360–367. doi:10.1016/j.jneumeth.2006.03.004 PMID:16621003

Tanaka, K., Matsunaga, K., & Wang, H. O. (2005). Electroencephalogram-based control of an electric wheelchair. *Robotics. IEEE Transactions on*, *21*(4), 762–766.

Van Boxtel, A. (2001). Optimal signal bandwidth for the recording of surface EMG activity of facial, jaw, oral, and neck muscles. *Psychophysiology*, *38*(01), 22–34. doi:10.1111/1469-8986.3810022 PMID:11321618

Watanabe, K., Kouzaki, M., Merletti, R., Fujibayashi, M., & Moritani, T. (2012). Spatial EMG potential distribution pattern of vastus lateralis muscle during isometric knee extension in young and elderly men. *Journal of Electromyography and Kinesiology*, *22*(1), 74–79. doi:10.1016/j.jelekin.2011.09.010 PMID:21996320

Wu, C., Song, A., Ling, Y., Wang, N., & Tian, L. (2014). *A Control Strategy with Tactile perception Feedback for EMG Prosthetic Hand*. Academic Press.

Yin, Y. H., Fan, Y. J., & Xu, L. D. (2012). EMG and EPP-integrated human–machine interface between the paralyzed and rehabilitation exoskeleton. *Information Technology in Biomedicine. IEEE Transactions on*, *16*(4), 542–549.

Zennaro, D., Wellig, P., Koch, V. M., Moschytz, G. S., & Läubli, T. (2003). A software package for the decomposition of long-term multichannel EMG signals using wavelet coefficients. *Biomedical Engineering. IEEE Transactions on*, *50*(1), 58–69.

ADDITIONAL READING

Ahsan, M. R., Ibrahimy, M. I., & Khalifa, O. O. (2009). EMG signal classification for human computer interaction: A review. *European Journal of Scientific Research*, *33*(3), 480–501.

Andreasen, D., Alien, S., & Backus, D. (2005). *Exoskeleton with EMG based active assistance for rehabilitation*. Paper presented at the Rehabilitation Robotics, 2005. ICORR 2005. 9th International Conference on. doi:10.1109/ICORR.2005.1501113

Ariga, Y., Maeda, D., Pham, H. T., Uemura, M., Hirai, H., & Miyazaki, F. (2012). *Novel equilibrium-point control of agonist-antagonist system with pneumatic artificial muscles: II. Application to EMG-based human-machine interface for an elbow-joint system*. Paper presented at the Intelligent Robots and Systems (IROS), 2012 IEEE/RSJ International Conference on.

Barreto, A. B., Scargle, S. D., & Adjouadi, M. (2000). A practical EMG-based human-computer interface for users with motor disabilities. *Journal of Rehabilitation Research and Development*, *37*(1), 53–64. PMID:10847572

Bos, D. P.-O., Reuderink, B., van de Laar, B., Gürkök, H., Mühl, C., & Poel, M. (2010). *Brain-computer interfacing and games Brain-Computer Interfaces* (pp. 149–178). Springer.

Cannan, J., & Hu, H. (2011). Human-Machine Interaction (HMI): A Survey. *University of.*

Choi, C., & Kim, J. (2007). *A real-time EMG-based assistive computer interface for the upper limb disabled.* Paper presented at the Rehabilitation Robotics, 2007. ICORR 2007. IEEE 10th International Conference on. doi:10.1109/ICORR.2007.4428465

Felzer, T., & Freisleben, B. (2002). *HaWCoS: the hands-free wheelchair control system.* Paper presented at the Proceedings of the fifth international ACM conference on Assistive technologies. doi:10.1145/638249.638273

Ferreira, A., Celeste, W. C., Cheein, F. A., Bastos-Filho, T. F., Sarcinelli-Filho, M., & Carelli, R. (2008). Journal of NeuroEngineering and Rehabilitation. *Journal of Neuroengineering and Rehabilitation*, *5*, 10. doi:10.1186/1743-0003-5-10 PMID:18366775

Ferreira, A., Silva, R., Celeste, W., Bastos Filho, T. F., & Sarcinelli Filho, M. (2007). *Human–machine interface based on muscular and brain signals applied to a robotic wheelchair.* Paper presented at the Journal of Physics: Conference Series.

Fukuda, O., Tsuji, T., Kaneko, M., & Otsuka, A. (2003). A human-assisting manipulator teleoperated by EMG signals and arm motions. *Robotics and Automation. IEEE Transactions on*, *19*(2), 210–222.

Gomez-Gil, J., San-Jose-Gonzalez, I., Nicolas-Alonso, L. F., & Alonso-Garcia, S. (2011). Steering a tractor by means of an EMG-based human-machine interface. *Sensors (Basel, Switzerland)*, *11*(7), 7110–7126. doi:10.3390/s110707110 PMID:22164006

Jatupaiboon, N., Pan-ngum, S., & Israsena, P. (2013). Real-time EEG-based happiness detection system. *The Scientific World Journal*, 2013. PMID:24023532

Leeb, R., Sagha, H., Chavarriaga, R., & Millán, J. R. (2011). A hybrid brain–computer interface based on the fusion of electroencephalographic and electromyographic activities. *Journal of Neural Engineering*, *8*(2), 025011. doi:10.1088/1741-2560/8/2/025011 PMID:21436524

Marchal-Crespo, L., & Reinkensmeyer, D. J. (2009). Review of control strategies for robotic movement training after neurologic injury. *Journal of Neuroengineering and Rehabilitation*, *6*(1), 20. doi:10.1186/1743-0003-6-20 PMID:19531254

Moon, I., Lee, M., Chu, J., & Mun, M. (2005). *Wearable EMG-based HCI for electric-powered wheelchair users with motor disabilities.* Paper presented at the Robotics and Automation, 2005. ICRA 2005. Proceedings of the 2005 IEEE International Conference on.

Müller, K.-R., Tangermann, M., Dornhege, G., Krauledat, M., Curio, G., & Blankertz, B. (2008). Machine learning for real-time single-trial EEG-analysis: From brain–computer interfacing to mental state monitoring. *Journal of Neuroscience Methods*, *167*(1), 82–90. doi:10.1016/j.jneumeth.2007.09.022 PMID:18031824

Neto, A. F., Celeste, W. C., & Martins, V. R. (2006). *Human-machine interface based on electro-biological signals for mobile vehicles*. Paper presented at the Industrial Electronics, 2006 IEEE International Symposium on. doi:10.1109/ISIE.2006.296086

Son, J., Hwang, S., & Kim, Y. (2010). An EMG-based muscle force monitoring system. *Journal of mechanical science and technology, 24*(10), 2099-2105.

Tsui, C. S. L., Jia, P., Gan, J. Q., Hu, H., & Yuan, K. (2007). *EMG-based hands-free wheelchair control with EOG attention shift detection*. Paper presented at the Robotics and Biomimetics, 2007. ROBIO 2007. IEEE International Conference on.

Tuga, M. R., Rupp, R., Liebetanz, D., Mikut, R., & Reischl, M. (2013). *Concept of a Co-Adaptive Training Environment for Human-Machine Interfaces Based on EMG-Control*. Biomedical Engineering/ Biomedizinische Technik.

Xu, X., Zhang, Y., Luo, Y., & Chen, D. (2013). Robust bio-signal based control of an intelligent wheelchair. *Robotics*, *2*(4), 187–197. doi:10.3390/robotics2040187

Yi, Z., Lingling, D., Yuan, L., & Huosheng, H. (2011). *Design of a surface EMG based human-machine interface for an intelligent wheelchair.* Paper presented at the Electronic Measurement & Instruments (ICEMI), 2011 10th International Conference on.

KEY TERMS AND DEFINITIONS

Electromyogram (EMG): A measure of the electrical activity associated with the muscles at rest and during contraction. It is helpful in determining the cause of muscle weakness, paralysis and pain in the various parts (e.g. leg, hand, feet and face etc.) of the body.

Energy Density: Energy Density is a measure of the amount of energy stored per unit volume of the signal.

Kurtosis: Kurtosis is a measure of the peakedness of a real-valued random variable present in a given signal.

Mode: A measure of the repeated occurrence of a value in an input sequence.

Signal Length or Waveform Length: It measures the total or cumulative length of a waveform or signal over a given time interval.

Summation: The sum of the values present in an input sequence.

Surface Electromyogram (sEMG): The electrical potential manifested on the skin surface due to the muscle contraction is regarded as surface electromyogram.

Chapter 15
Development of Bluetooth, Xbee, and Wi-Fi-Based Wireless Control Systems for Controlling Electric-Powered Robotic Vehicle Wheelchair Prototype

Biswajeet Champaty
National Institute of Technology, Rourkela, India

Suraj Kumar Nayak
National Institute of Technology, Rourkela, India

Goutam Thakur
Manipal Institute of Technology, India

Biswajit Mohapatra
Vesaj Patel Hospital, India

D. N. Tibarewala
Jadavpur University, India

Kunal Pal
National Institute of Technology, Rourkela, India

ABSTRACT

In this study, multiple control systems were developed using commonly used wireless communication protocols like Bluetooth, Xbee, and Wi-Fi. Mechanical switch based control systems were initially designed using Xbee and Bluetooth protocols. Further, Android application based control systems were developed using Bluetooth and Wi-Fi protocols. A robotic vehicle was used as an electric-powered wheelchair prototype. Ultrasonic sensors and infrared sensors were integrated with the robotic vehicle for obstacle and pothole detection, respectively. The control systems were tested in an L-shaped corridor for identifying the suitable wireless communication protocol to efficiently guide the robotic vehicle through a scheduled navigational pathway. Both Xbee and Wi-Fi technology based control systems were able to guide the robotic vehicle through the corridor. But the implementation of Xbee communication protocol is economic. However, for shorter distances, Bluetooth technology may be used for cost-effective implementation.

DOI: 10.4018/978-1-5225-0140-4.ch015

INTRODUCTION

In the current day world, there is a dramatic increase in the job, family and social commitments of the people. Due to these reasons, most of the people find it difficult to arrange time for their health and well-being activities. Patients suffering from neurodegenerative diseases (e.g. Amyotrophic lateral sclerosis (ALS), spinal cord injuries, multiple sclerosis, paraplegia and quadriplegia) become heavily dependent on the family members. These patients lose their muscular activity very rapidly, which results in the total body paralysis, inability in speech formation, swallowing and respiratory failure (Simmons, 2005). Hence, these patients are considered as burden to their family members (Coco et al., 2005; Zarit, Reever, & Bach-Peterson, 1980). Due to this reason, many of the families, who are economically stable, hire the services of specialized caregivers. But in developing countries like India, Bangladesh, Pakistan, Sri Lanka, Myanmar, and many African countries etc., most of the people are economically challenged to hire the services of the specialized caregivers for long period. It has been reported in literature that the care rendered to the patients on their deathbed decide whether the patients will receive a better death or a worse death (Soros & Madrick, 1999). Keeping this in mind, many researchers across the globe are trying to improve the quality of life of such severely disabled persons. The quality of life has also been related with the non-medical activities of the patients which include level of independence, social association, personal beliefs and psychological states of the patients (Simmons, 2005). These factors are highly hampered in the severely motor-disabled persons. Though mental strength and intelligence remain intact, they find it difficult to manipulate the conventional wheelchairs. This has led to the conceptualization of motorized wheelchairs, which have helped in drastically improving the self-assisted mobility of these patients. Various scientists have reported the use of intelligent sensors for acquiring information around the immediate environment of the patients (Cowan et al., 2012; Sevillano et al., 2009; R. Simpson, LoPresti, Hayashi, Nourbakhsh, & Miller, 2004; Tomari, Kobayashi, & Kuno, 2012). These sensors can divulge information about any adversities around the patients. The main disadvantage of these wheelchairs is the complex hardware architecture. The complexities can be minimized to some extent using certain wireless control systems. The simplistic nature of the wireless controlled electric-powered wheelchairs can considerably reduce the physical labor of the caregivers and enhance the autonomy of these patients. These advantages have been reported to improve the social integration of such disabled patients (R. C. Simpson, 2005).

Keeping a note of the above, in this present study, we propose a mechatronic approach for designing an economically assembled archetype (robotic vehicle). The proposed approach is helpful in realizing the directional control of a motorized wheelchair using various wireless protocols (Bluetooth, Xbee, and Wi-Fi). In addition to responding to the auxiliary controls (activation, deactivation and stop), the robotic vehicle was programmed to navigate in four different directions (forward, backward, left and right). The commands were wirelessly relayed to the robotic vehicle from the peripheral remote controllers. The remote controllers were designed using pushbutton switches, joystick and Android application. To identify the optimum wireless protocol for probable multitasking use in wheelchair control, home automation and robotic arm movement control; a comparative study was performed using the above mentioned wireless technologies.

BACKGROUND

Since the late eighties, researchers have been trying to develop affordable assistive technologies for the severely disabled persons. Amongst the various assistive technologies, the control of electric-powered wheelchairs has gained much attention of these scientists (Levine et al., 1999; R. Simpson et al., 2004; R. C. Simpson, 2005). This is because, the use of wheelchairs improves the mobility and hence the autonomous travelling potency of such persons (Matsumoto, Komoriya, Hatase, & Nishimura, 2006). Apart from this, these wheelchairs reduce the physical toil of the caregivers, responsible for moving the patients from one place to other in both domestic and hospital environments (Wu, Jen, & Huang, 2011). Usually, such electric-powered wheelchairs use mechanical switching systems (pedals, joysticks and levers) for controlling the movement (Zhang, Zhang, & Luo, 2011). But the patients suffering from severe motor disabilities find it difficult to operate the mechanical switching arrangements using the residual physiological activities (Fehr, Langbein, & Skaar, 2000). For such patients, biosignal controlled rehabilitation aids have been proposed. The main advantage of using such devices is the drastic improvement in the ability of the disabled persons. This correspondingly decreases the workload on the caregivers. These wheelchairs have been found to improve the mobility of the physically handicapped persons. Various biosignals like speech (Fezari & Bousbia-Salah, 2007; Kurtzberg & Lew, 2000; Pačnik, Benkič, & Brečko, 2005; Rockland & Reisman, 1998), electrooculogram (EOG) (Barea, Boquete, Mazo, & López, 1999; Barea, Boquete, Mazo, & López, 2002; Champaty, Jose, Pal, & Thirugnanam, 2014; Wijesoma et al., 2005; Yathunanthan, Chandrasena, Umakanthan, Vasuki, & Munasinghe, 2008), electromyogram (EMG) (Han, Bien, Kim, Lee, & Kim, 2003; Moon, Lee, Chu, & Mun, 2005; Mulroy, Gronley, Newsam, & Perry, 1996; Tsui, Jia, Gan, Hu, & Yuan, 2007) and electroencephalogram (EEG) (Choi & Cichocki, 2008; Lin, Chen, & Yang, 2010; Rebsamen et al., 2006; Rebsamen et al., 2007; Tanaka, Matsunaga, & Wang, 2005) have been proposed for maneuvering the wheelchairs. While using these biosignals, the rehabilitation engineer has to assess the stability of the physiological process during longer time durations. This is due to the fact that if the rehabilitation devices are controlled using biosignals, whose physiological process will tend to degrade in near future, then the rehabilitation device will become useless for the disabled persons. Hence, attempts should always be made so as to use biosignals associated with the physiological processes, which will tend to remain stable during the remaining life-time of the disabled persons. To improve the interactions of the persons with the immediate environment of the disabled persons, wheelchairs integrated with ultrasonic sensors and video cameras have been proposed (Sevillano et al., 2009). At the initial stages, the hardware was made with wired communication protocol. Due to the use of wires for transferring the information, encoded within biosignals, to the control unit of the rehabilitation devices, the hardware architecture was quite complex. To simplify the hardware architecture complexity, wireless communication protocols are being proposed. The use of wireless communication protocols drastically reduced the hardware architecture complexity. The additional benefit of such devices is that the physically disabled persons remain completely isolated from the rehabilitation device hardware. This helps in improving the independence of the patients. Though various wireless technologies like Bluetooth, Wi-Fi, and Xbee protocols are available, not much work has been progressed to establish their efficiency in controlling rehabilitation devices.

MAIN FOCUS OF THE CHAPTER

In general, automated wheelchair systems are broadly categorized into three major categories. The categories include autonomous controlled wheelchair, semi-autonomous controlled wheelchair and shared controlled wheelchair (Perrin, 2009). Research has revealed that the semi-autonomous controlled wheelchairs are the optimal alternative for the patients suffering from motor neuron disorders (Lopes, Nunes, & Vaz, 2010; Parikh, Grassi Jr, Kumar, & Okamoto Jr, 2005). In semi-autonomous control systems, the patient has to generate the commands and the corresponding tasks are carried out by the computers or the controllers. The on-board sensors generate a real-time local map of the environment through continuous scanning, which enables the safe mobility of the wheelchair (Tomari et al., 2012). Based on the above findings, a simple mechatronic approach is presented in this study to realize the wireless control of the movement of a semi-autonomic motorized wheelchair. A robotic vehicle was designed as the representative rehabilitative device. Pushbutton assembly board, joystick shield and Android mobile applications were used for devising the control systems. The control signals generated using the aforesaid interfaces were wirelessly transferred to the robotic vehicle via Bluetooth, Xbee and Wi-Fi wireless technologies. All these three wireless protocols are of IEEE (Institute of Electrical and Electronics Engineers) standards. A comparative study of the aforementioned control systems were carried out to identify the optimum wireless technology for controlling the robotic vehicle movement.

COMMONLY USED IEEE WIRELESS PROTOCOLS

Wireless technology enables the devices to transfer/receive data from matched devices and the web without using any physical connection. The IEEE (Institute of Electrical and Electronics Engineers) wireless standards followed in our study are described under IEEE 802.11 and 802.15 families. Basically, the IEEE 802 family of standards deals with the local area networks (LAN) and metropolitan area networks (MAN); maintained by IEEE 802 LAN/MAN Standards Committee (LMSC). The IEEE 802.11 standard describes the protocol for Wireless Local Area Network (WLAN) and Mesh Network (Wi-Fi certification). The IEEE 802.15 describes the protocol for wireless personal area networks (WPANs), which include Bluetooth (IEEE 802.15.1), IEEE 802.15 & IEEE 802.11 coexistence (IEEE 802.15.2), High-Rate WPAN (IEEE 802.15.3), Low-Rate WPAN (IEEE 802.15.4), Mesh networking for WPAN (IEEE 802.15.5), Body Area Network (IEEE 802.15.6) and visible light communication (IEEE 802.15.7). Each of these wireless IEEE protocol has its own characteristic advantages and limitations depending upon the mode of communication, speed of communication, point of communication and power consumption. Generally, these WPANs speak to portable microcontrollers and mobile computing devices like PCs, computer peripherals, mobile phones, home appliances and different microcontrollers wirelessly and let these devices to communicate with one another.

IEEE 802.11: Wi-Fi

Wi-Fi, otherwise known as Wireless Fidelity, is a wireless digital communication protocol that supports unicasting and broadcasting of data between devices. Following the decision of United States Federal Communications Council (USFCC) to use some bands of wireless spectrum without any license fee, the IEEE 802 standard was extended to 802.11. The license free bands are categorized as industrial, scientific and medical (ISM) radio bands. In the beginning, the Wi-Fi was lunched with 2.5 GHz frequency and a data transmission rate of 1-2 Mbps. In the present day, Wi-Fi uses distinct frequency ranges like 3.6 GHz, 4.9 GHz, 5 GHz and 5.9 GHz bands with enhanced data transmission rates, which may reach up to 54 Mbps. The unlicensed spectrums can also be shared by other users. Hence, the system has to be resilient to interference. The 802.11 standard uses different variants of different bands. The band ranges for different 802.11 standards are tabulated in Table 1.

The data transmission in Wi-Fi can be described in 3 phases. The data is prepared and made ready for transmission in phase 1. The procedures include data encoding and changing into frames. The frequency for transmitting the data is selectively decided based on the wireless data transmission techniques. The data is propagated in air in phase 2, whereas, the data is received, retrieved (decoded) and acknowledged in phase 3.

A basic service set (BSS) is formed when two or more wireless client devices (also called, stations or STAs) wirelessly speak to each other through an Access Point (AP) forming a WLAN. The Access Point creates a wireless distribution system (WDS) to connect two or more BSSs. The interconnection of set of one or more BSSs is called as Extended Service Set (ESS) having a common service set identifier (SSID). Each STA may receive a signal from several APs and can manually or automatically select the network. As a part of ESS, multiple APs may share the same SSID. The discrepancies can be avoided by network and security settings of each AP. The virtual area where the members of a BSS are connected to each other is termed as Basic Service Area (BSA). The conceptual boundary of a BSA may be up to tens of meters. Two or more BSSs can be collocated with each other through their BSA without impeding their functional capacity. This is possible through a temporary user controlled ad-hoc networking. The Wi-Fi architecture has been shown in Figure 1. Two major Wi-Fi security standards are ubiquitously used to achieve the privacy of data over Wi-Fi. The protocols are Wireless Equivalent Privacy (WEP) and Wi-Fi Protected Access (WPA). Currently, the WPA has been upgraded to WPA-2 to provide better security over Wi-Fi communication.

Beyond accessing the web, the Wi-Fi is used extensively in industries, household, office, enterprise, institutes, and public areas etc. It is possible to easily convert the devices (like smart phones and laptops) into a virtual Wi-Fi router. Hence, the smart phones are tethered to PCs or laptops to access internet.

Table 1. Different 802.11 standards and their frequency bands

IEEE 802.11 Variant	Frequency Bands Used
802.11a	5GHz
802.11b	2.4GHz
802.11g	2.4GHz
802.11n	2.4, 4.9 & 5 GHz
802.11j	4.9 GHz
802.11y	3.65 GHz
802.11p	5.9 GHz
802.11ac	5, 4.9 & 3.65 GHz
802.11ad	Up to 60 GHz
802.11af	White-Fi and Super Wi-Fi (54 and 790 MHz)
802.11ah	0.9 GHz

Figure 1. Wi-Fi architecture

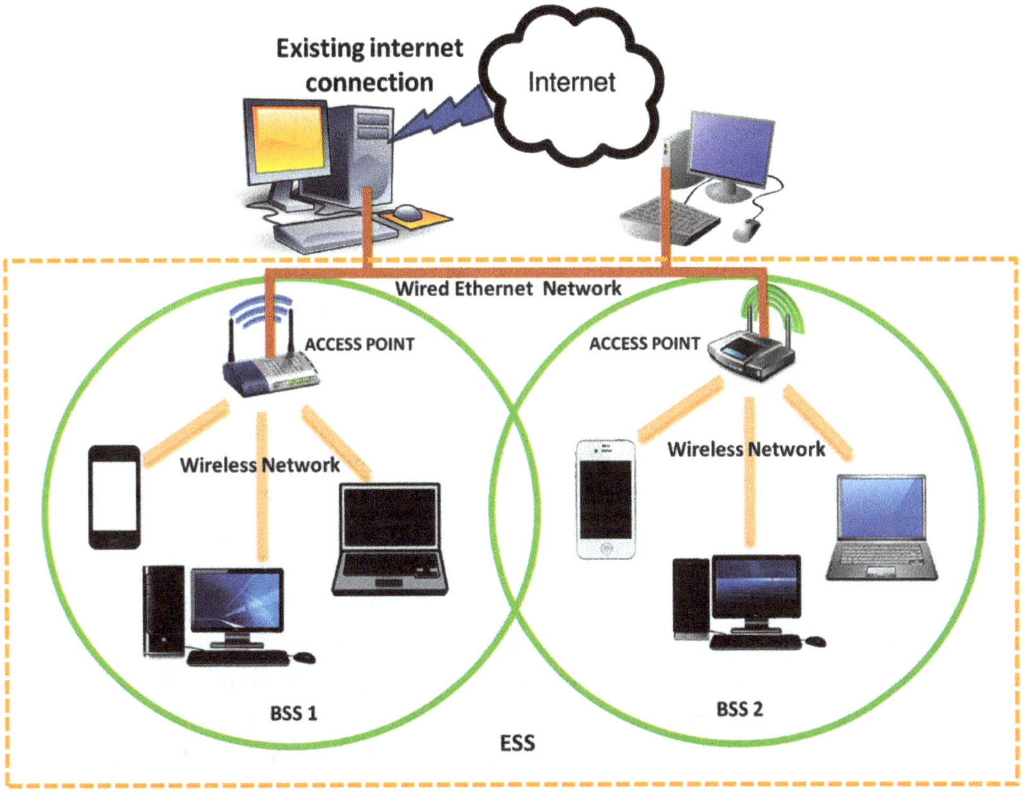

The computer peripherals (like printers and scanners) are remotely accessed from any PC or smartphone through Wi-Fi. The Wi-Fi supported TVs or media devices can stream HD videos within the Wi-Fi network coverage area of the device. Any files can be shared between computers or other devices at a high speed. Likewise, the Wi-Fi is found to be advantageous in medical sectors. The physiological signals, acquired from the patients, are transferred to the health caregivers for online health monitoring and diagnosis (Silva, Lourenço, & Paz, 2011).

IEEE 802.15.1: Bluetooth Protocol

Bluetooth has pioneered the wireless technology these days with a tag line of "wireless communication made easy". This technology provides a way to connect a variety of fixed or mobile devices for transmission and sharing of data using radio waves. The working range of Bluetooth is 15-50 feet. This wireless standard endeavors short-range wireless communication along with diminutive size, ease of use, data security, minimal power consumption and cost-effective. The rapid progress using Bluetooth technology is found in gadgets ranging from mobile phones and computers to medical devices and home appliances for short range connectivity. In medical sectors, the Bluetooth technology is being used to transfer physiological signals like electrocardiogram (ECG) (LV, ZHAO, XV, & JIN, 2007), photoplethysmogram (PPG) (Tafa & Stojanovic, 2006), EEG (Gargiulo et al., 2010) etc. to nearby nursing stations for round the clock health monitoring. Starting from the Version 1.0 (draft version of Bluetooth) till Version 1.2

was standardized under IEEE 802.15.1 protocol. These days, the marketed Bluetooth products are certified by Bluetooth Special Interest group (SIG).

In brief, Bluetooth transmits and receives data to/from another Bluetooth device through special radio frequency. All Bluetooth supported devices come with an inbuilt Bluetooth adapter (transceiver) which can both send and receive data. One Bluetooth adapter can pair with another adapter, if the later is present within the range of the former one. The pairing of two Bluetooth device is carried out in several steps. Initially, one Bluetooth device search for another Bluetooth device to confirm the availability within the range. Subsequently, the type of device (like mobile phone, headset etc.) is recognized along with its device name. The device name can be allocated by the user or the manufacturer. The device recognition is followed by exchange of passkey (default '1234') between the devices. Upon successful verification of passkeys, a Bluetooth pairing is established to exchange the information. The pairing is remembered by the device once it is setup. Hence, there is no need of user intervention to re-pair the same device on subsequent use. The pairing can be undone by the user. Theoretically, during the process of pairing of the two devices, they search for a common frequency through which they can speak. When such a frequency is discovered, the devices are found to each other. Connecting of two devices does not obstruct the connecting of two other devices due to the use of dissimilar frequency channels.

The Bluetooth transceiver operates in the ISM 2.45 GHz (varies across the countries) frequency band. Like Wi-Fi, Bluetooth uses the Frequency-Hopping Spread Spectrum (FHSS) technique. This technique splits the frequency band of 2.402-2.480 GHz into 79 channels (called hops), each 1MHz wide. The operation of any Bluetooth device is based on a master/slave mode. These master/slave connection is maintained till they are disconnected either by the user or due to poor radio link (devices going out of range of each other). Bluetooth technology allows two or more devices to share their information at the same time. When two or more Bluetooth devices come along into the process of pairing for data sharing, they form a virtual micro-network termed as "piconet". A single piconet can accommodate maximum of seven devices. Up to ten piconets can coexist within a single coverage area. Under a single piconet, one device acts like a master to initiate communication. The other connected devices are known as slaves. One master can speak to seven active slaves at a time within a piconet. Any Bluetooth device can either act as the Master or as the Slave, depending upon the application and condition. A device can enter a piconet (through pairing) and leave a piconet (manually or poor connectivity). Two or more piconets join together to form a wider network, termed a "scatternet". The data transfer rate of Bluetooth devices vary as per their versions. The data transfer rate for Version 1.2, Version 2.0 and Version 3.0 are 1 Mbit/s, 3 Mbit/s, and 24 Mbits/s, respectively. Bluetooth protocol comprises of four types of protocols like telephony control protocol, Bluetooth core protocol, cable replacement protocol and adopted protocols.

IEEE 802.15.4: Zigbee Technology

ZigBee is another wireless networking standard which comes under IEEE 802.15.4 standard. The IEEE 802.15.4 standard is intended to work on controlling and monitoring applications mainly in the areas where relatively low levels of data throughput are needed along with the requirement of low power consumption, remote operation and battery powered sensor applications. The Zigbee Alliance created the low-cost and low-power driven Zigbee for the ubiquitous use in devices with low data rate and long battery sustainability to realize control and monitoring applications through WPANs. Typically, the Zigbee devices are integrated with radios and microcontrollers with minimum 60-256 KB flash memory.

Zigbee operates in the standard ISM 2.4 GHz frequency band. The data rates vary from 20 kbps to 250 kbps depending on the frequency bands.

Zigbee devices can form networks with Mesh, Star and Generic Mesh topologies among themselves (Figure 2). The network can be expanded as a cluster of smaller networks. A ZigBee network can have three types of nodes: Zigbee Coordinator (ZBC), Zigbee router (ZBR) and Zigbee End Device (ZBE), each having some unique property. Zigbee protocol is mostly used in home automation systems, industrial machinery coordination systems, sensor networking, hospital alerting systems etc. Physiological signals like ECG (Kitayoshi, Sawaya, & Kuwano, 2013), EEG (Simms, 2014), EMG (Kobayashi, 2011), EOG (Sung, Chen, & Chang, 2013) can be acquired wirelessly to design patient care monitoring systems (Mamatha, 2015). These biosignals can also be processed and classified to generate control commands for designing real-time assistive rehabilitative devices (Mageswari & Selvavinayagam, 2013; Pereira et al., 2015; Shaheen & Umamakeswari, 2013; Simms, 2014).

MATERIALS

Hardware Requirements

Arduino UNO (Arduino, Italy), Arduino Mega ADK (Arduino, Italy), Arduino Xbee shield (Arduino, Italy), Arduino compatible Motor Shield V1.0 (Seeed Studio, China), Arduino Wi-Fi shield (Arduino, Italy), joystick shield V1.A (Funduino, China), Bluetooth Transceiver HC-05 TTL (Robomart, India), Xbee S1 transceiver module (Digi International, Bangalore, India), 300 RPM 12 V DC gear motor (Robomart, India), 2200 mAh 3 Cell Li-Po battery (Turnigy, India) and in-lab developed robotic vehicle were used in this study.

Figure 2. Zigbee network

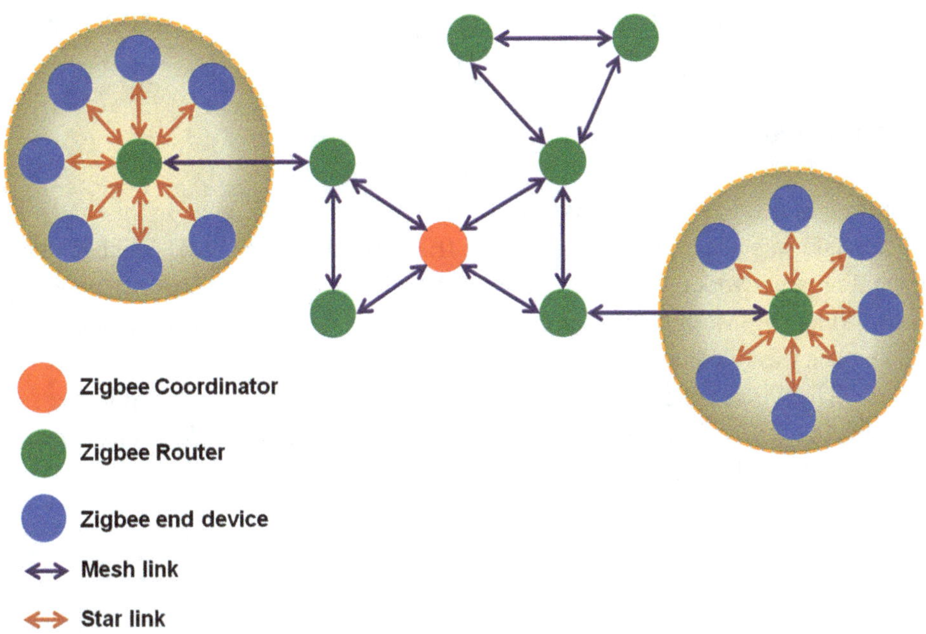

Hardware Requirements

Two open-source software, namely, Arduino IDE 1.0.5 and Tera Term Pro terminal emulator were used in this study.

BRIEF DESCRIPTION OF THE MAJOR COMPONENTS AND SOFTWARES

HC-05 Bluetooth Breakout Board

The HC-05 Bluetooth breakout board is ubiquitously used for setting up the wireless serial communication. The breakout board is a transceiver which supports both master and slave modes. The board is Class 2, v2.0+EDR (enhanced data rate) version of the Bluetooth. It can operate in both 2 Mbps and 3 Mbps modulation within the baseband of 2.4 GHz. The board has its own default settings like baud rate (9600, which can go up to 1382400), device name (HC-05), password ('1234'). All the default settings can be changed as per the user by AT commander. The HC-05 modules serve as slaves by default.

Arduino Wi-Fi Shield

Arduino Wi-Fi shield can be used for designing the Wi-Fi wireless control system. The Wi-Fi shield enables the Arduino Mega ADK to connect to the wireless network operating at 802.11b and 802.11g specifications. The HDG204 quad flat package (QFP) IC in the Wi-Fi shield provides a low cost, ultra low power and feature-rich high performance client solution to address the proliferation of Wi-Fi technology into embedded devices. The data transmission rate of the HDG204 is up to 54 Mbps (in Orthogonal frequency-division multiplexing (OFDM) mode) and up to 11 Mbps (in direct-sequence spread spectrum /complementary code keying (DSSS/CCK) mode). The 32-bit AT32UC3 embedded microcontroller in the Wi-Fi shield provides a way to perform very high speed communication. The communication library includes the complete package of TCP/IP stack which supports IP, TCP, UDP, ICMP, DHCP, PPP, ARP, FTP server, HTTP web server, SMTP client, and POP3 client.

Xbee-S1 Transceiver

Zigbee technology can be employed to design an effective RF wireless system. In this study, Xbee (series 1) transceiver module was used. It works as per the IEEE 802.15.4 standard, which supports low-rate wireless personal area networks. Xbee can be loaded with various firmwares to support Zigbee and DigiMesh networking. DigiMesh is the improved alternative of ZigBee, which provides a very reliable, simple and convenient way of communication between microcontrollers, computers, sensor networks and complex systems. The wireless device supports point-to-point, star and mesh topologies. The module operates in the ISM 2.4 GHz frequency band with a data transfer rate of 250 Kbps. The transmission range varies from 30 m (indoor) to 100 m (outdoor).

Arduino Wireless Proto Shield

Arduino wireless proto shield is used for accommodating Xbee and other wireless modules with similar footprints. The wireless proto shield can be stacked on the Arduino board through its wire-wrap female pin headers. An onboard single pole double throw (SPDT) serial select slide switch allows toggling between "USB" mode and "MICRO" mode. When the MICRO mode is selected, the wireless proto shield board allows communication of the wireless module with the microcontroller. The DIN and DOUT pins of the wireless module are connected with the Tx and Rx pins of the microcontroller, respectively. Hence, any data, which is originated by the microcontroller can be transmitted to the computer via USB port and transmitted to the wireless module, simultaneously. It may be kept in mind that the microcontroller can't be programmed when the SPDT switch is toggled to MICRO mode. When the SPDT switch is toggled to USB mode, the DIN and the DOUT pins of the wireless module are connected with the Rx and Tx pins of the microcontroller, respectively. In this mode, the microcontroller is completely bypassed. If we intend to use the shield in USB mode, either the microcontroller should be removed from the board or may be programmed with an empty sketch. The microcontroller can be programmed via USB in this mode. In gist, the serial select switch in USB mode is used to upload the code into the microcontroller and transfer of serial data from the computer to the microcontroller. In MICRO mode, the serial data from the microcontroller is available for wireless transmission. The working of the serial select switch is shown in Figure 3.

HC-SR04 Ultrasonic Sensor

The HC-SR04 ultrasonic sensor is used to determine the distance of an object. This is an excellent non-contact range finder with a range of 2 cm to 400 cm. The unit comes with an ultrasonic transmitter, receiver and a control circuit in an easy-to-use package. The sensor gives high accuracy and a stable reliable reading. The range of the ultrasonic sensor is reasonably fair to be used in robotics and automation applications. The performance of the sensor is found to be the best with a measuring angle of 30°. The minimum surface area of the object (closest detectable object in front of the sensor) to be detected should

Figure 3. Working of the serial select switch

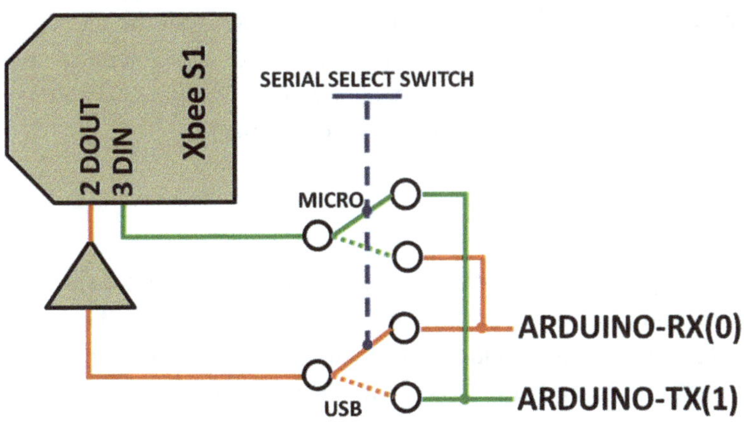

be 0.5 m^2 (Kepa & Abaid, 2015). The sensor operates at +5 V DC supply and is capable of producing an ultrasound wave of 40 KHz. Three HC-SR04 ultrasonic sensors were used at the front end and sideways of the prototype. The sensor has four pins, namely, Vcc, Gnd, Trig (pulse input) and Echo (pulse output). The sensor provides distance information by "time of flight" method. The Arduino sends a short pulse of 10 μs to the Trig pin and waits for the Arduino to start a pulseIn () function. At the same time, the transmitter of the ultrasonic sensor sends an 8 cycle burst of ultrasound at 40 KHz (square wave) to the air and sends a feedback high signal to the microcontroller. The feedback signal remains high till the receiver detects the echo that bounces off from an object. After the reception of the echo, the Echo pin is set to high, which in turn, converts the high feedback signal to low. The pulseIn() function stores the time duration of the feedback signal, i.e. the time duration for which the sensor transmitted high signal. The duration (in μs) between sending trigger signal and receiving echo signal can be used to calculate the distance by the following formulae.

$$Distance\left(cm\right) = \frac{\left(time\ duration\ /\ 2\right)}{29} = \frac{time\ duration}{58} \tag{1}$$

$$Distance\left(inch\right) = \frac{\left(time\ duration\ /\ 2\right)}{74} = \frac{time\ duration}{148} \tag{2}$$

In the advent of absence of obstacle, the time duration is nearly 38 ms (Kepa & Abaid, 2015). Otherwise, the time duration depends on the distance and is in the range 150 μs to 25 ms (Kepa & Abaid, 2015). To detect obstacles having surface area < 0.5 m^2, photoelectric sensors or laser sensors may be used.

Infrared Sensor

A simple infrared distance sensor has poor resolution (up to 5 inch or 13 cm), but is capable of successfully detecting potholes. The sensor breakout board consists of infrared transmitting LED, infrared receiving photodiode, a comparator IC (LM 358), resistors and a potentiometer (10 KΩ). The IR transmitter LED constantly emits the IR light. The light, when reflected back from any obstacle, falls on the IR receiver LED (black in color). Based on the intensity of the IR light received, the output of the sensor varies. An on-board comparator processes the input from the IR receiver and generates a logical HIGH output, if any obstacle is encountered. The range of the sensor can be fine-tuned with the potentiometer. The module fails to work properly when it comes across a black object.

Joystick Shield

An Arduino UNO R3 compatible joystick shield was used to design a remote controller. The shield has seven momentary push buttons (four big buttons, two small pushbuttons and one joystick select button) and a two-axis joystick. The joy stick provides movement in eight directions like Up, Down, Left, Right, Right-Up, Right-Down, Left-Up, and Left-Down. The rocker of the shield is connected with two potentiometers. When the rocker moves in X or Y coordinate directions, the respective potentiometers read the twisted angles in analog form. The analog reading is acquired by the Arduino UNO microcontroller. The threshold limits were set for all possible rocker movements so that the movement can be detected.

MIT App Inventor Version 2 (MIT AI2)

MIT App Inventor Version 2 (MIT AI2) is an Android application development platform that uses drag-and-drop visual graphical objects to design software applications that run in Android operating system. The physical layout of the application can be designed in the Designer window. This window includes various palettes like User Interface, Layout, Media, Drawing and Animation, Sensors, Social, Storage and Connectivity. These palettes carry visible components and non-visible components under them. Along with all the components of User Interface palette and Layout palette, other components like EmailPicker, PhoneNumberPicker, ContactPicker, Canvas, ImagePicker are treated as visible components, which can be placed directly on the simulated screen. Except the components listed under visible components, all other components are non-visible or hidden components. Non-visible components are listed below the simulated screen. The program logic can be created in the BLOCKS EDITOR window by logically connecting blocks. The MIT AI2 enables real-time debugging on connected devices through USB and Wi-Fi.

METHODOLOGY

In this study, wireless control systems were developed using Bluetooth, Xbee, and Wi-Fi wireless communication protocols. An in-lab developed robotic vehicle was used as a representative rehabilitation device for the testing of the developed wireless control system. To improve the safety of the robotic vehicle, ultrasonic range finder and infrared based pothole detection systems were integrated with the robotic vehicle. The details of the methodology are given in the following subsections.

Designing of the Robotic Vehicle

A robotic vehicle was developed in lab. The Robotic vehicle was used as a prototype for automated wheelchair. The chassis of the robotic vehicle was made using a wooden platform. At the rear end of the wooden chassis, two L-shaped metallic clamps were attached. To the metallic clamps, two motors (12 V DC center shaft gear motors with 300 revolutions per minute) were fixed. The shafts of the motors were attached with two robotic wheels (Diameter: 70 mm, Thickness: 19 mm, Bore: 6 mm). At the front end of the wooden platform, a round castor wheel was attached. An Arduino Mega ADK microcontroller was used for implementing the directional and the movement control of the robotic vehicle via a motor shield, which was instilled into it. The motor shield enabled the Arduino board to drive the DC motors for directional control. An audio-visual (AV) panel was developed, which provided indication about the direction and the movement of the robotic vehicle. The AV panel consisted of seven groups of LEDs and one buzzer. Table 2 summarizes the various movement information and the corresponding AV panel outputs.

An external 11.1 V DC Li-Po battery was used for powering the Arduino Mega ADK, which in turn, powered the DC motors, motor shield, and AV panel. The different components which were used for

Table 2. Movement information and the output of the AV panel

Movement Information	Output	
	LED Status	Buzzer Sound
Activate	$[1_3][2_3][3_3][4_3][5_3][6_3][7_3]$	$[Beep_3]$
Stop	$[1_c][2_c][5_c]$	$[Long_1]$
Pause	$[3_c][4_c][6_c][7_c]$	$[Short_1]$
Forward	$[3_c]$	No
Backward	$[7_c]$	No
Left	$[4_c]$	No
Right	$[6_c]$	No

$[X_Y]$: X= LED number/ type of buzzer sound, Y= No. of times the LED flashes/ No. of times the buzzer sounds, c=continuous

designing the robotic vehicle are shown in Figure 4. Figure 5 shows the pictograph of the developed robotic vehicle without the attachment of the external sensors.

Environment screening features, like pothole detection and obstacle detection, were integrated with robotic vehicle. Infrared distance sensor and ultrasonic sensors were used for the purpose. The arrangement of the sensors on the robotic vehicle is schematically given in Figure 6.

Two infrared sensors were placed at the front and the rear ends to detect any potholes during forward and backward movements (Figure 6). The robotic vehicle has to undergo the primary pothole detection test prior to other associated functions (like obstacle detection and movement in different directions). The infrared sensors were calibrated and the threshold for pothole detection was set to 7 cm (with 0.5 cm tolerance). The actual distance between the infrared sensor and a plane surface was 6.5 cm. The wheels of the robotic vehicle were capable to move through a pothole of < 0.5 cm. During the initiation of the control commands for the movement of the robotic vehicle, the infrared sensors instigated scanning the

Figure 4. Parts of the proposed prototype: (a) wooden chassis, (b) motor shield, (c) round caster wheel, (d) wheel, (e) L-clamp, (f) center shaft DC gear motor, (g) 11.1 V DC battery, and (h) Arduino Mega ADK

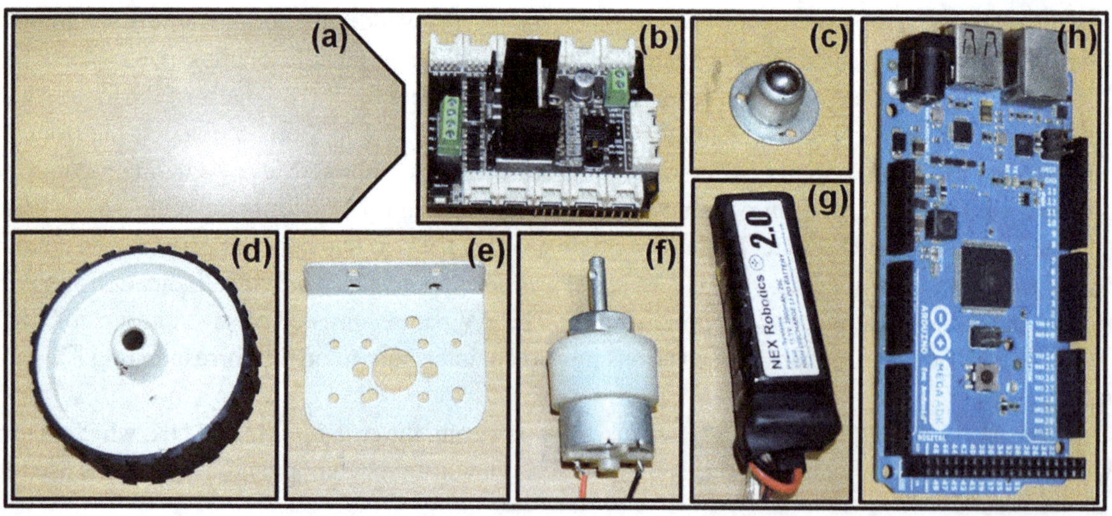

Figure 5. Assembled robotic vehicle without the attachment of external sensors: (a) top view, (b) side view, (c) front view, and (d) rear view

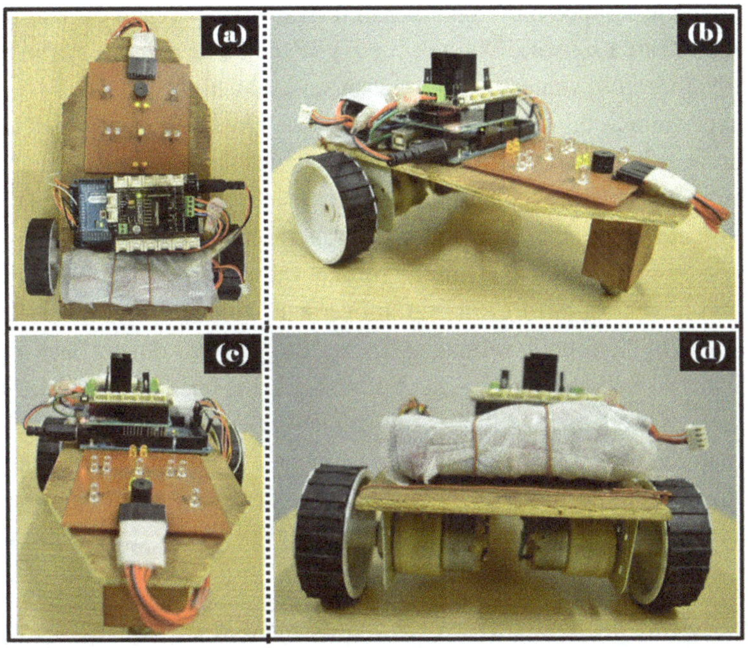

Figure 6. Arrangement of four ultrasonic sensors and two infrared sensors on the robotic vehicle

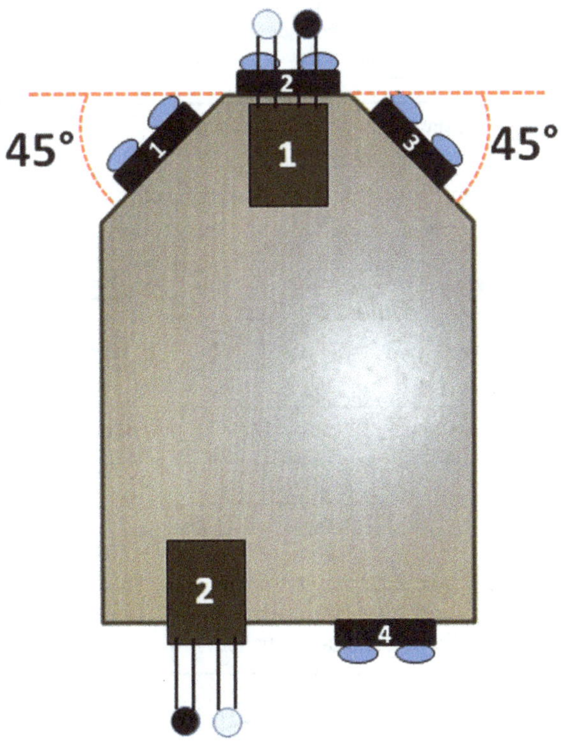

terrain properties. If the distance estimated by the infrared sensor was > 7 cm, the sensor sent a low signal to the microcontroller which was interpreted as detection of pothole. As long as the sensor output was low, the robotic vehicle stopped moving either in forward or backward direction (depending on the output of the localized infrared sensor). On the contrary, if the distance read by the infrared sensor was less than or equal to the threshold value, the infrared sensor sent a high signal to the microcontroller stating that there was no pothole in the path. The flowchart for detecting the potholes is given in Figure 7. The pothole detection was followed by obstacle detection which was realized by four ultrasonic sensors. Three ultrasonic sensors were placed at the front and sideways of the vehicle. While one of the ultrasonic sensors was placed to detect obstacles in front of the robotic vehicle, the other two ultrasonic sensors were placed at an angle of 45°, on either side of the robotic vehicle, to detect obstacles either on the right or left side of the robotic vehicle during sideway movements (Figure 6). The fourth ultrasonic sensor was placed at the rear end of the robotic vehicle to determine obstacles during backward movement. The threshold for obstacle detection was set to 20 cm. According to the need of the hardware designer and the types of ultrasonic sensors used, the threshold limit can be varied. If the distance read by the ultrasonic sensor was greater than the threshold value, the ultrasonic sensors kept on scanning obstacles around. On the contrary, in the event of confronting an obstacle, the distance estimated by the ultrasonic sensor was less than the threshold value. As soon as an obstacle was detected, the robotic vehicle temporarily

Figure 7. Flowchart showing the mechanism for pothole detection

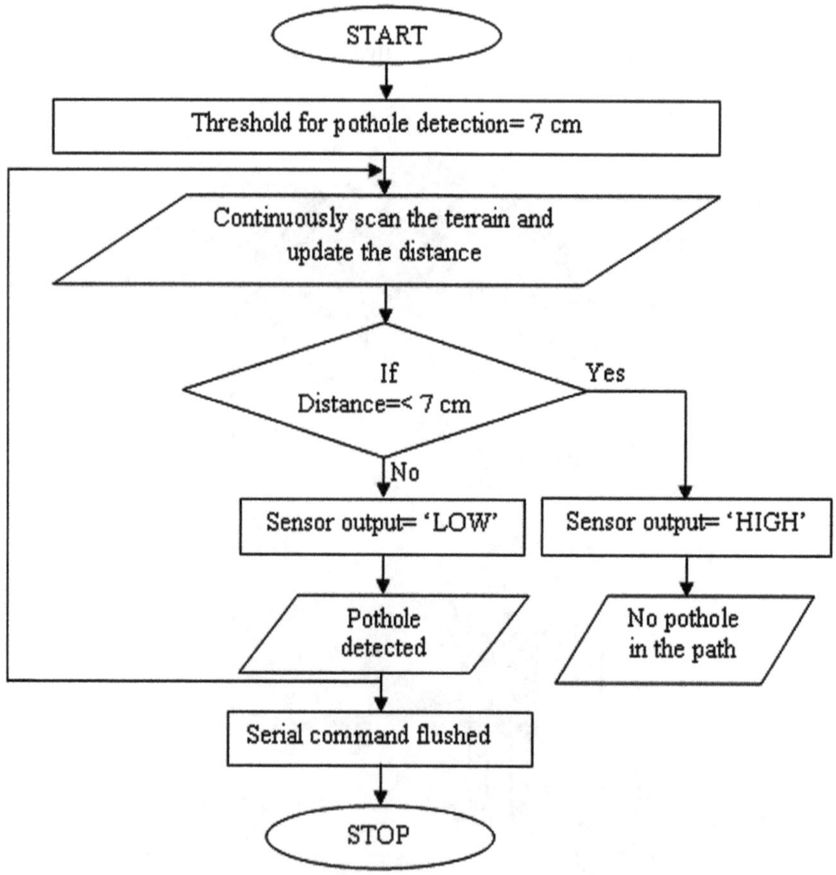

halted for 2 seconds, considering the object to be non-stationary. If the object was moved within the 2 seconds, the robotic vehicle resumed its movement. Otherwise, it stopped permanently and the serial command was flushed from the memory. The flowchart for detecting the obstacles is given in Figure 8. The AV panel indicated the detection of any obstacle or pothole by selective flashing of LEDs and beeping of buzzer as described in Table 3.

Designing of Wireless Control Systems

The wireless control system comprised of both the transmitter and the receiver sections operating in wireless modes, namely, Bluetooth, Xbee and Wi-Fi. Three different types of remote controllers were developed using pushbutton assembly, joystick shield and Android applications. The signals from the transmitters were wirelessly transmitted to the robotic vehicle, which was considered as the receiver unit. Figure 9 shows the block diagrams of the developed wireless control systems, remote controllers and the customized robotic vehicle.

A pair of HC-05 Bluetooth modules was configured by Tera Term software and Arduino integrated development environment (IDE) to behave as master and slave, respectively. Both the units were configured to work at a baud rate of 38400. The master Bluetooth module was connected to the transmitter units designed by pushbutton assembly and joystick shield to send serial commands, whereas, the slave module was connected to the robotic vehicle to receive the serial commands. The host Arduino Mega ADK (at the receiver end) retrieved the information and used that command signals to control the movement of the robotic vehicle. In order to enhance the usability of the Bluetooth based wireless control system for smartphone users, another Bluetooth based control system was developed in which the master Bluetooth module was replaced by a Bluetooth supported Android device. An Android application was designed to send serial commands to the slave Bluetooth module. By default, the marketed HC-05 Bluetooth modules are slaves. The configuration of the Bluetooth module was not required when Android application was used. The slave module was paired with the Bluetooth of the Android device through the default pass code ('1234'). The pairing was a onetime process. The Android device remembered the address of the slave and connected automatically when the Bluetooth was switched on. It allowed the most suitable way of pairing and communicating with the microcontroller. The flowchart for the operation of the Bluetooth based Android application is given in Figure 10.

A pair of XBee S1 transceiver antenna was used to design the Xbee wireless network. The Xbee modules were instilled into the Arduino wireless proto shields, which were stacked on the microcontroller

Table 3. Status of AV panel in accordance environment monitoring

Types of Environment Detected	LED Status	Buzzer Sound
Obstacle at the front	$[1_c][2_c]$	$[Beep_2]$
Obstacle at the rear	$[5_c]$	$[Beep_2]$
Obstacle at the left	$[1_c]$	$[Beep_2]$
Obstacle at the right	$[2_c]$	$[Beep_2]$
Pothole at the front	$[1_c][2_c]$	$[Beep_2]$
Pothole at the rear	$[5_c]$	$[Beep_2]$

$[X_Y]$: X= LED number/ type of buzzer sound, Y= No. of times the LED flashes/ No. of times the buzzer sounds, c=continuous

Figure 8. Flowchart showing the mechanism for obstacle detection

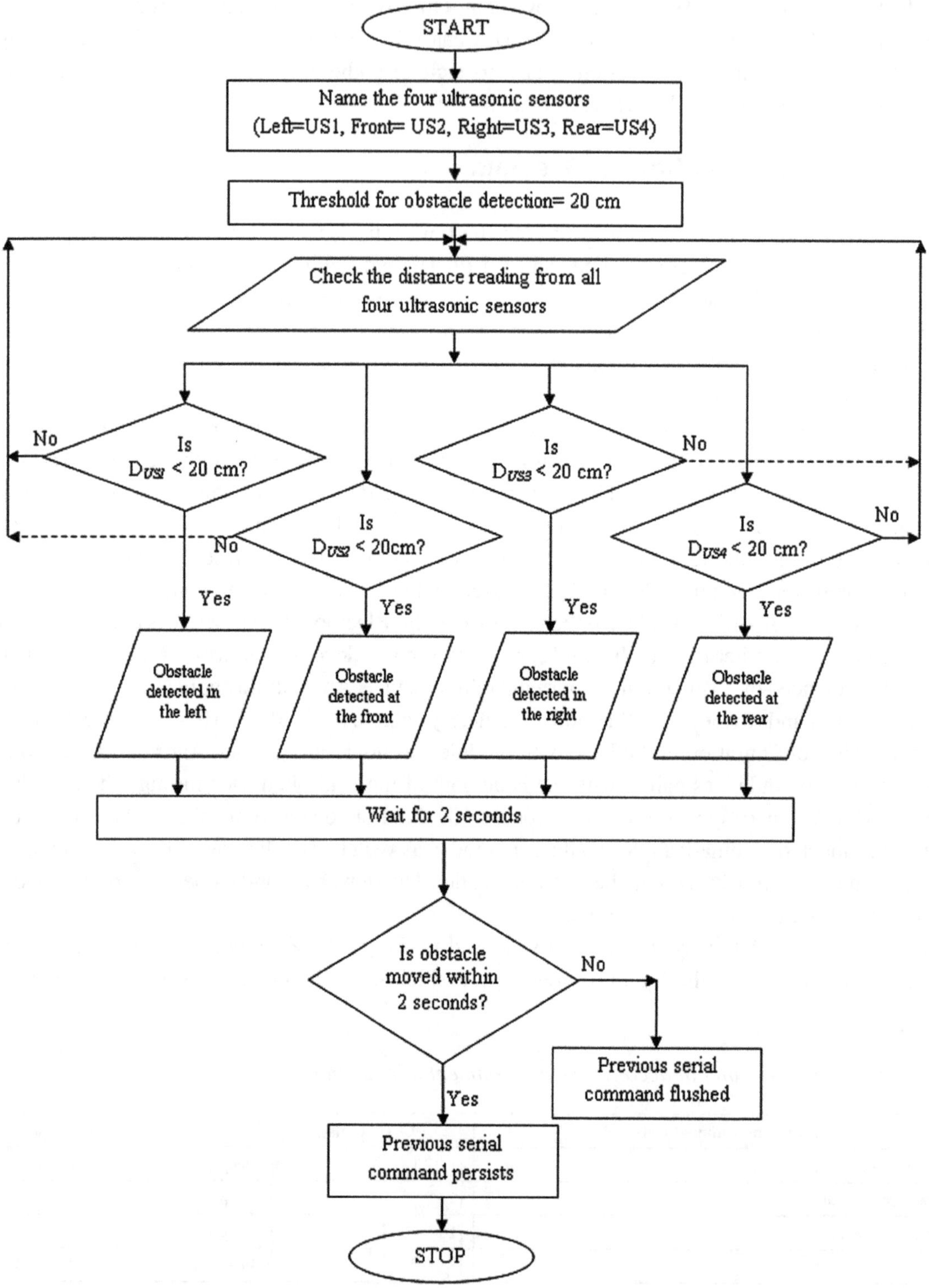

Figure 9. Block diagrams showing the interconnectivity of the components of the control systems and the robotic vehicle: (a) Xbee mode, (b) Bluetooth mode, (c) Bluetooth Android App mode, and (d) Wi-Fi Android App mode

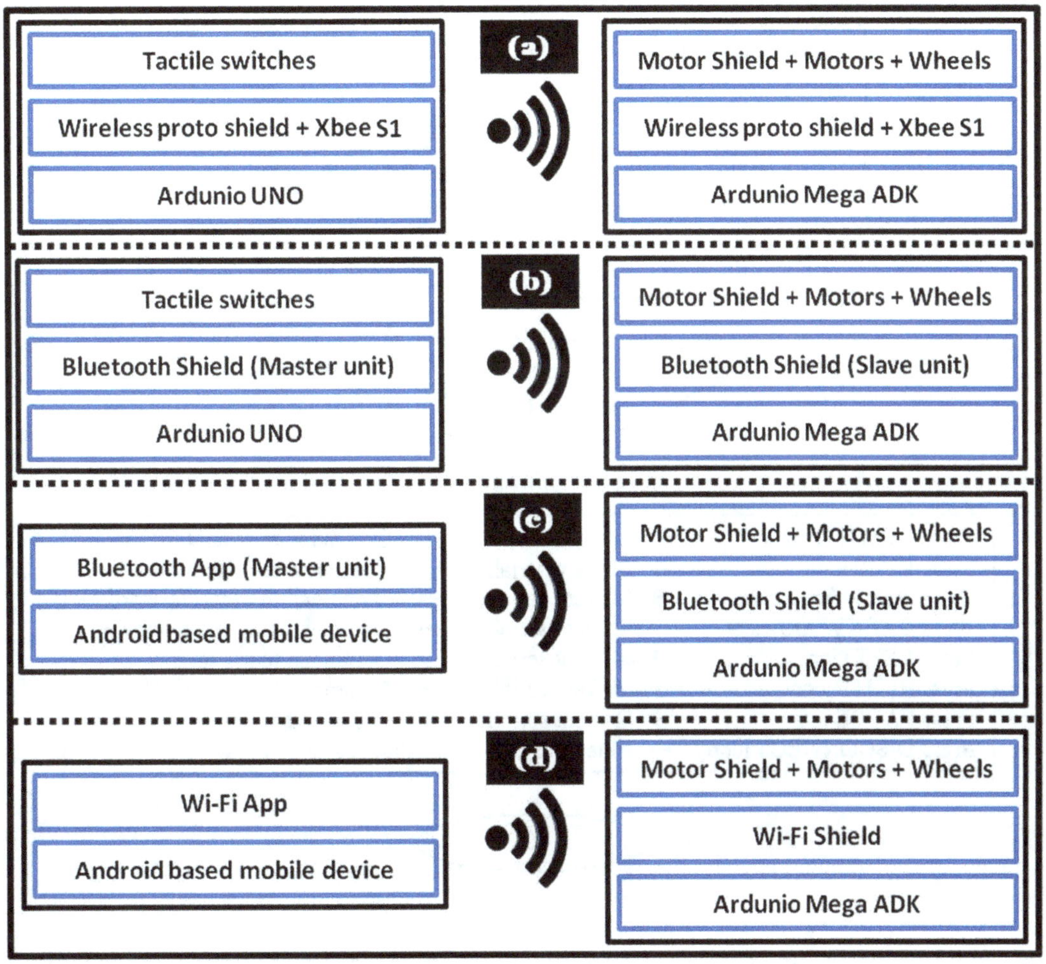

boards. The baud rate was set to 9600 for wireless serial data transmission. The Xbee module used at the transmitter end was considered as the coordinator, whereas the Xbee module used at the receiver end (with the robotic vehicle) was considered as the router. Besides the router on the robotic vehicle, four additional routers were used in a mesh network to enhance the performance of the wireless control system which has been discussed later. While implementing this technology, the pushbutton and the joystick interfaces were made Xbee compatible to serve as transmitter units.

For designing of the Wi-Fi wireless system, a Wi-Fi shield was stacked on the top of the Arduino Mega ADK board (at the receiver end) through the extended wire-wrap headers of the shield. The Wi-Fi shield communicated with the microcontroller through Digital pin 7. Using the Wi-Fi library, a sketch was drafted in Arduino IDE to connect the shield to the internet wirelessly. The Wi-Fi shield supports IEEE 802.11 b/g standards and was connected to the cyberom wireless local area network (WLAN) via a wireless router (D-link). A Wi-Fi based Android application was designed to send serial control

Figure 10. Flowchart showing the operations of the Bluetooth based Android application

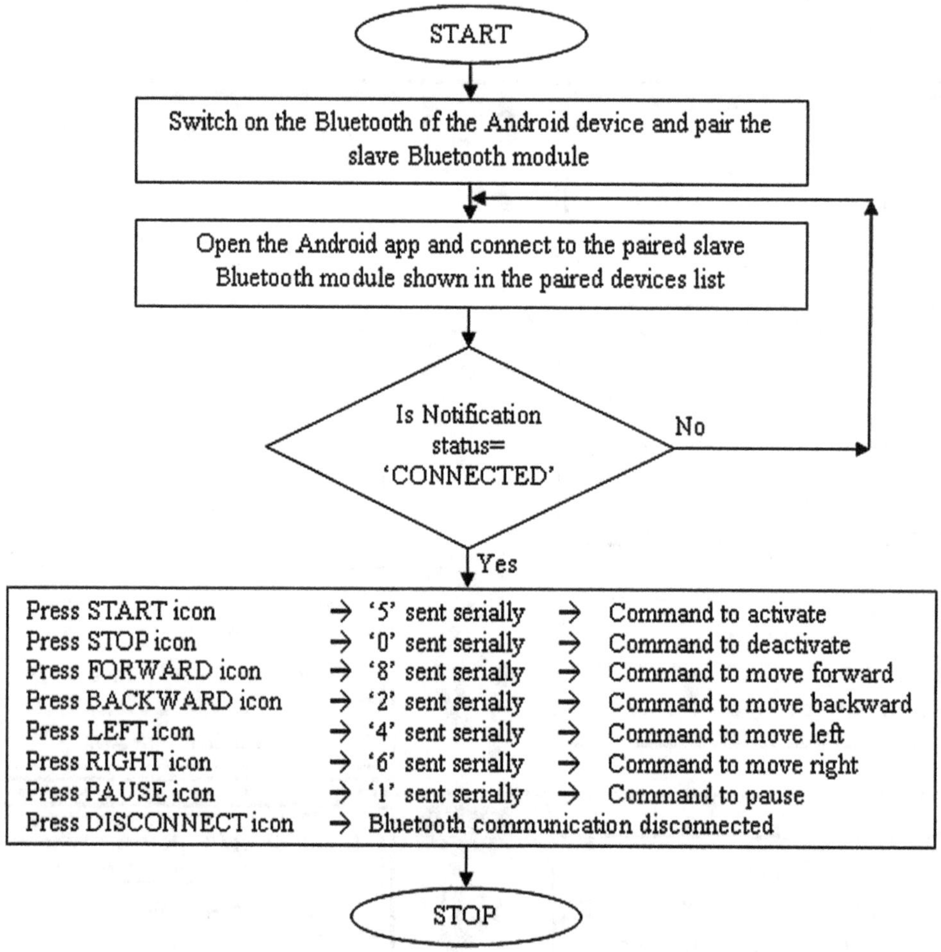

commands to the robotic vehicle and served as the transmitter unit. The Wi-Fi wireless network was established with the data transfer rate of 12 Mbps. The flowchart for the operation of the Wi-Fi based android application is given in Figure 11.

Testing of the Controllers

The testing of the developed controllers was achieved in an L-shaped corridor as shown in Figure 12. The two sides of a rectangular corridor were selectively chosen based on the availability of the Wi-Fi network. The dimensions of the L-shaped corridor were pre-defined. The outer dimension of the corridor was 45 m (L) X 35 m (B). One end of the corridor was considered as the starting point (A) and the other end was regarded as the ending point (C) which passed through an intermediate point (B). The distance between A to B was 30 m and from B to C was 40 m. Hence, the total navigational distance of the corridor was 70 m. The pathway between A to B and B to C were intended for line-of-sight communication, whereas, the path between A to C was intended for non-line-of-sight communication. All the three transmitting remote controllers remained stationary at the starting point. The range of the

Figure 11. Flowchart showing the operations of the Wi-Fi based Android application

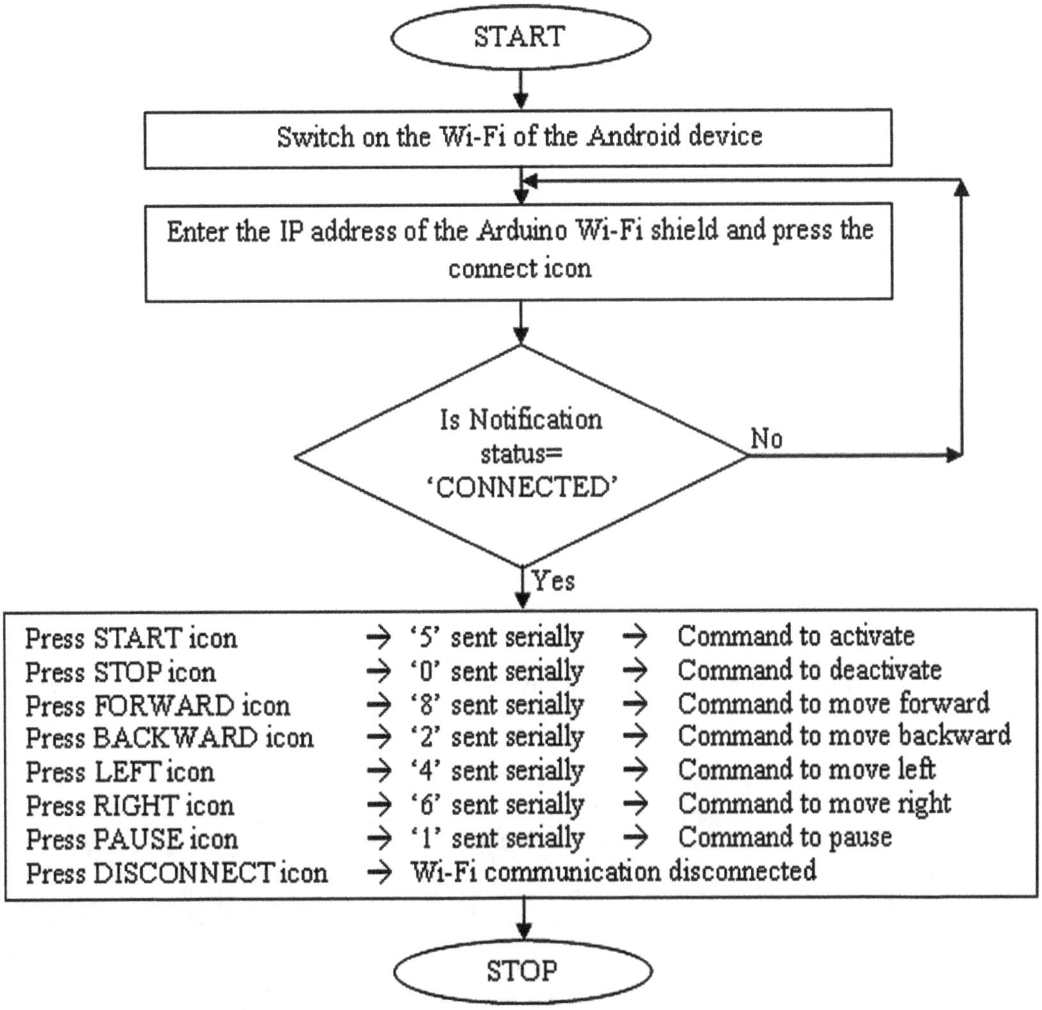

Wi-Fi router, installed at the starting point, was found to cover the described corridor. The efficiency of the controllers to manipulate the movement of the robotic vehicle along the entire corridor was judged.

RESULTS AND DISCUSSION

Designing of the Robotic Vehicle

A three-legged robotic vehicle, equipped with external sensors, was developed. The pictograph of the fully-fledged developed vehicle is shown in Figure 13. The robotic vehicle consisted of two wheels connected to the rear end. The wheels were powered using two independent DC motors, which were controlled using a motor shield. The front wheel was a round caster wheel, which enabled the directional movements of the robotic vehicle based on the changing direction of the movement of the wheels. The

Figure 12. Pictograph of the proposed L-shaped corridor for testing the controllers

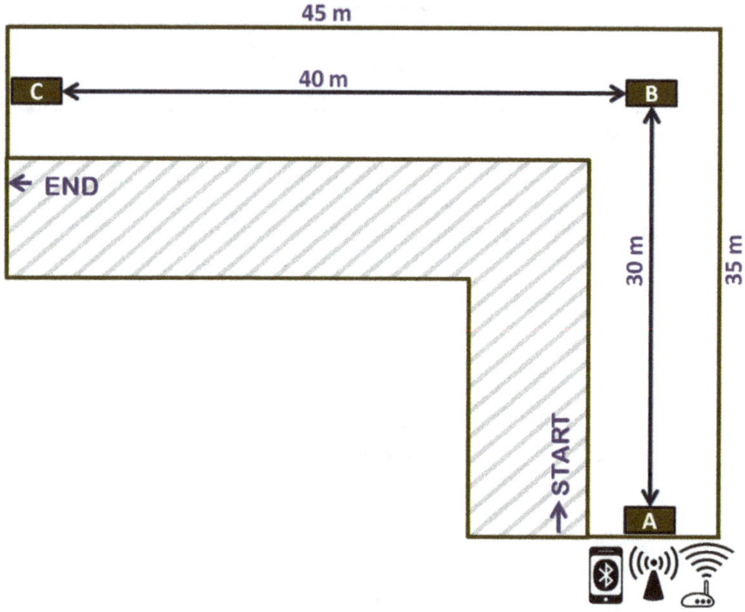

Figure 13. Final assembled prototype: (a) top view, (b) front view, (c) rear view, (d) left view, and (e) right view

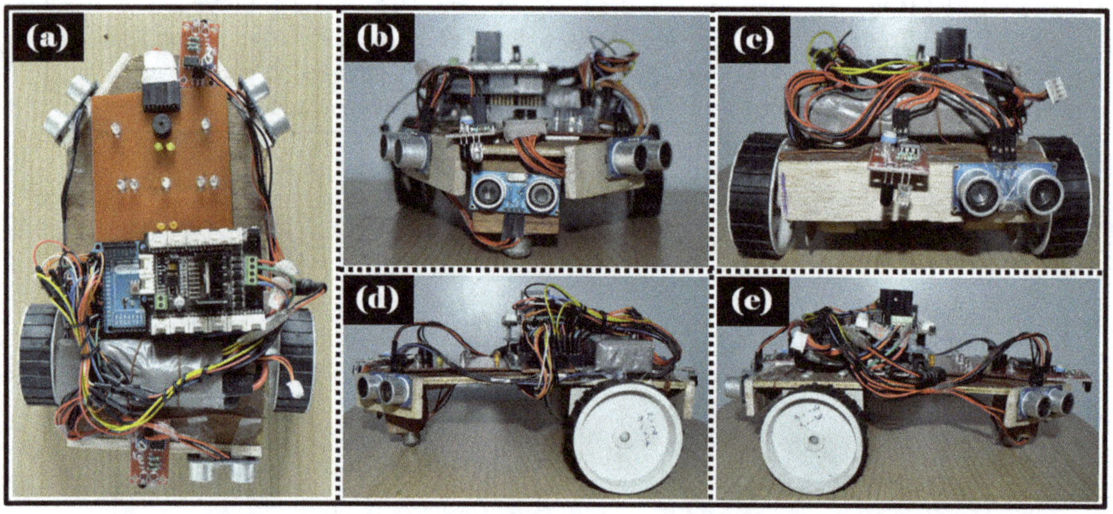

robotic vehicle was further attached with four ultrasonic sensors for obstacle detection. Three ultrasonic sensors were put at the front end of the robotic vehicle to detect in-front and sideways obstacles. One ultrasonic sensor was put at the rear end to detect obstacles at the rear position of the robotic vehicle. Two pothole detection sensors, one at the front and the other at the rear, were also integrated with the robotic vehicle. The motor shield, the obstacle detection sensors and the pothole detection sensors were controlled using the Arduino Mega ADK board. The microcontroller of the Arduino Mega ADK board was programmed with the logic given in Figure 14. The program, which was installed, was a universal program to be accessed by all the developed remote controllers. The pictographs of the developed remote controllers are given in Figure 15.

Set of Serial Commands for Directional Control and Navigation

A set of serial commands were defined for controlling the movement of the robotic vehicle. The remote controllers were programmed to send these serial commands wirelessly to the robotic vehicle, where as the Arduino Mega ADK of the robotic vehicle was solely programmed to direct the motor shield to move the DC motors in various directions as per the serial commands received. The set of serial commands, their corresponding operations, and the direction of the DC motors are given in Table 4. Figure 16 and 17 show the execution of the primary commands (Forward, backward, left and right) and the auxiliary commands (activate, deactivate and pause), respectively.

Testing the Robotic Vehicle for Detecting Environmental Conditions

Figure 18 shows the pictographs of the robotic vehicle when it was confronted with obstacles at different locations. Similarly, pothole detection sensors were also tested by taking the robotic vehicle to the edges of a table. Both the front and the rear infrared sensors were verified to detect the potholes at their respective paths (Figure 19). The testing of the device revealed that the movement of the robotic vehicle was paused for 2 seconds, if the obstacle was within 20 cm of the obstacle detectors. After 2 seconds, the obstacle detector again screened the environment. If the obstacle was moved away or removed within the 2 seconds time frame, the robotic vehicle continued to proceed along the same path before the system was paused. In an unlikely event of the obstacle remaining at the same position even after 2 seconds, the previous command was flushed out of the buffer and the user had to provide a new command to move the robotic vehicle. In the event of the robotic vehicle moved to the edges of the table, which emulated

Table 4. List of serial commands and their proposed tasks

Serial Commands	Operations Performed by the Prototype	Movement of the DC Motors							
		Left			Right			Enable Pins	
		M1+	M1-	Direction	M2+	M2-	Direction	EA	EB
'5'	Activate	-	-	-	-	-	-	HIGH	HIGH
'0'	Deactivate	-	-	-	-	-	-	LOW	LOW
'1'	Pause	LOW	LOW	X	LOW	LOW	X	HIGH	HIGH
'4'	Left movement	LOW	LOW	X	HIGH	LOW	CW	HIGH	HIGH
'6'	Right movement	HIGH	LOW	CW	LOW	LOW	X	HIGH	HIGH
'2'	Backward movement	LOW	HIGH	ACW	LOW	HIGH	ACW	HIGH	HIGH
'8'	Forward movement	HIGH	LOW	CW	HIGH	LOW	CW	HIGH	HIGH

(CW: Clockwise, ACW: Anticlockwise, X: No Movement)

Figure 14. Flowchart showing the logic for driving the robotic vehicle in forward, left, right, and backward directions

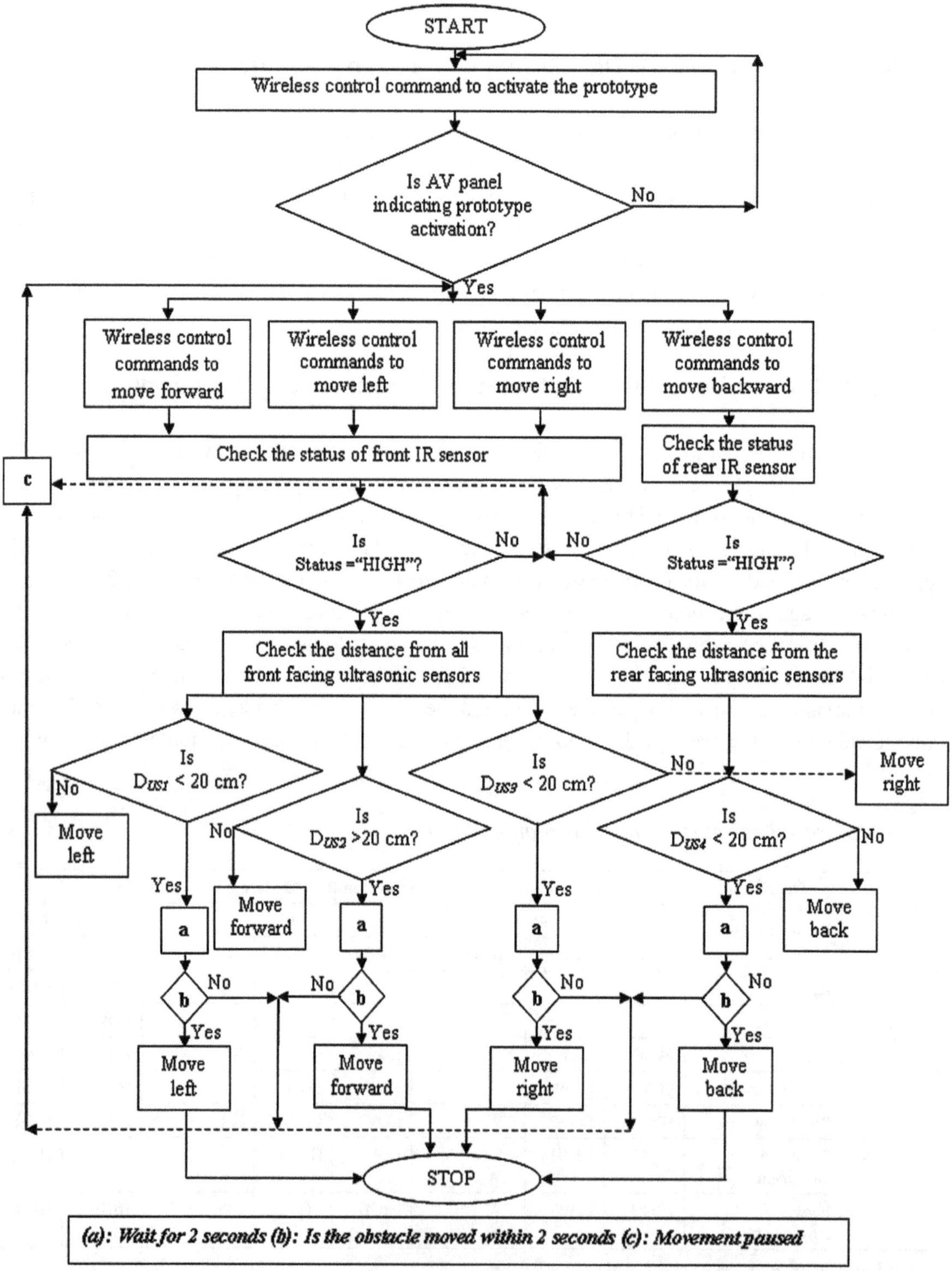

Figure 15. Pictograph of pushbutton based remote controller: (a) front side with switches labeled (b) Bluetooth shield stacked on Arduino UNO and fixed to the back, and (c) Xbee shield stacked on Arduino UNO and fixed to the back side; pictograph of joystick based remote controller: (d) joystick shield stacked on wireless proto shield and Arduino UNO, and (b) joystick shield stacked on Arduino UNO and grooved with Bluetooth module; pictograph of Android applications based remote controller: (a) bluetooth based Android application, and (b) Wi-Fi based Android application

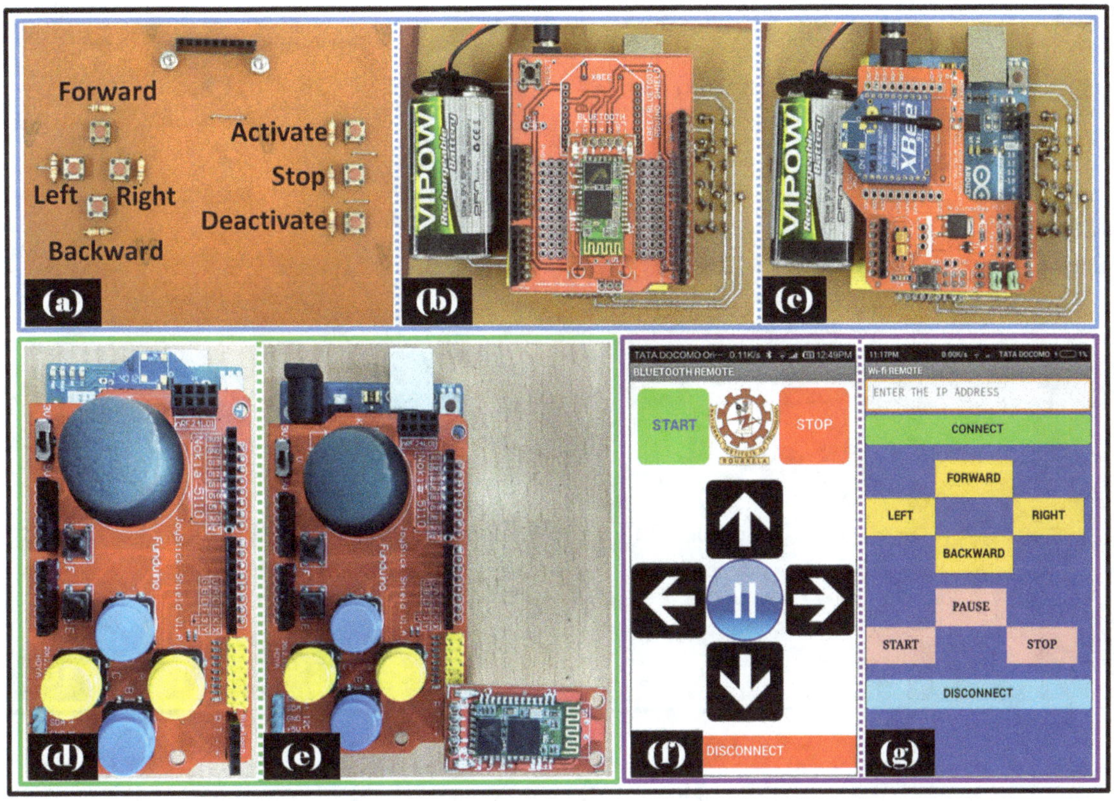

the pothole condition, the infrared sensor sent a logical low signal to the microcontroller. This resulted in the halting of the robotic vehicle and reinitiated the control panel to receive fresh serial commands so as to move the robotic vehicle in other directions.

Testing of The Wireless Control Systems

The assembled pushbutton remote controller was used for guiding the robotic vehicle in the L-shaped corridor. Initially, the robotic vehicle was guided in the Bluetooth mode. It was found that the Bluetooth controller was not able to guide the robotic vehicle after it reached a distance of 13.3 m (along the line-of-sight). Subsequently, the remote controller and the robotic vehicle were configured with the Xbee wireless transceivers. In this mode, the controller was able to guide the robotic vehicle up to a distance of 23 m. To enhance the range of functioning of the controller unit, four Xbee nodes (excluding the co-

Figure 16. Execution of primary commands: (a) left movement, (b) backward movement, (c) right movement, (d) forward movement, and (e) no movement

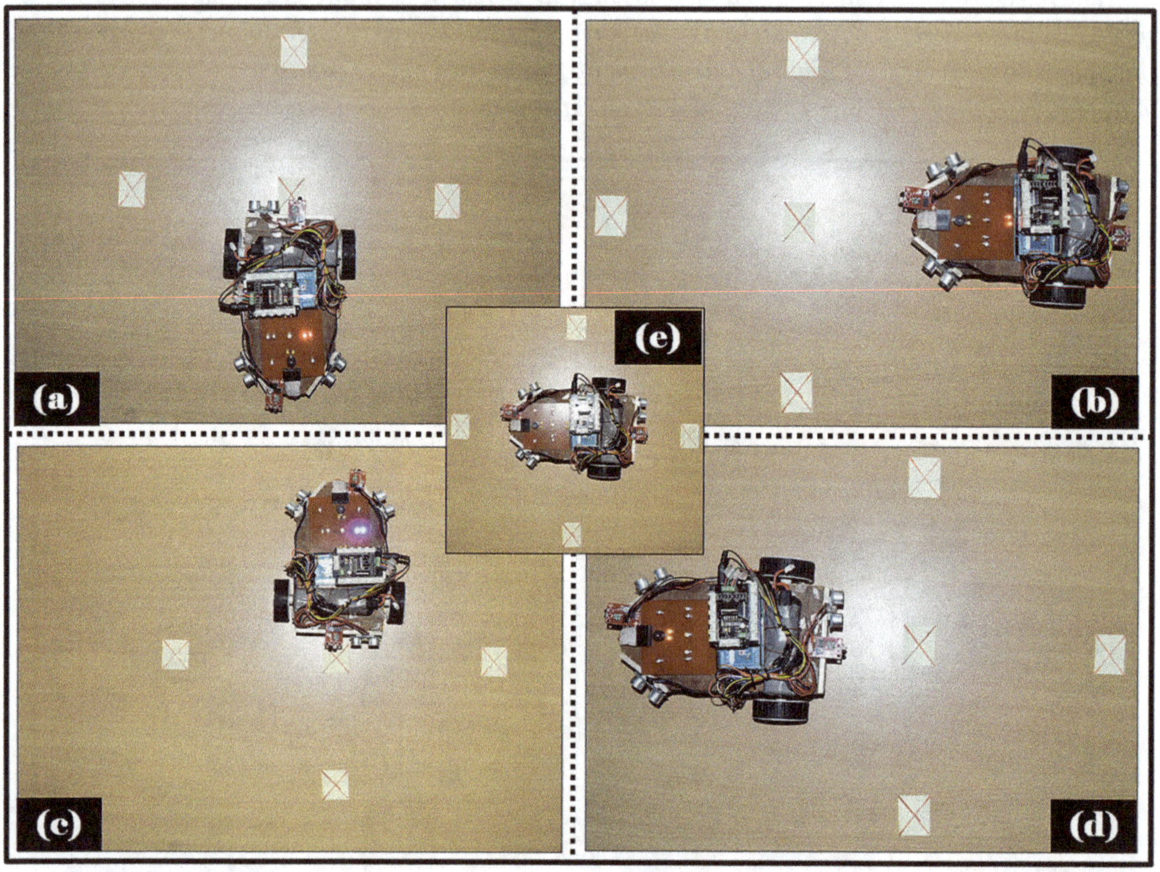

Figure 17. Execution of secondary commands: (a) prototype activated (b) prototype paused, and (c) prototype deactivated

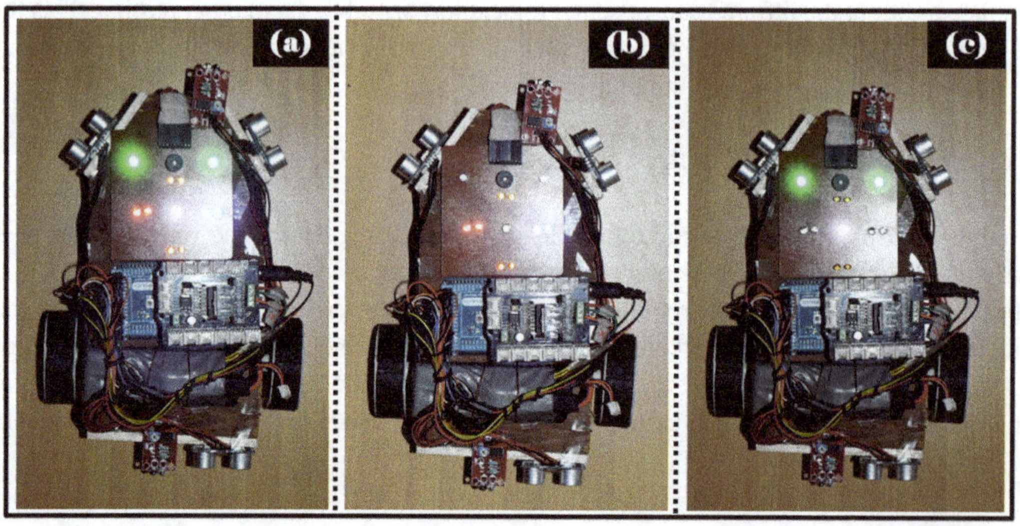

Figure 18. Obstacle detection: (a) at front side (b) at right side, (c) at rear side, and (d) at left side

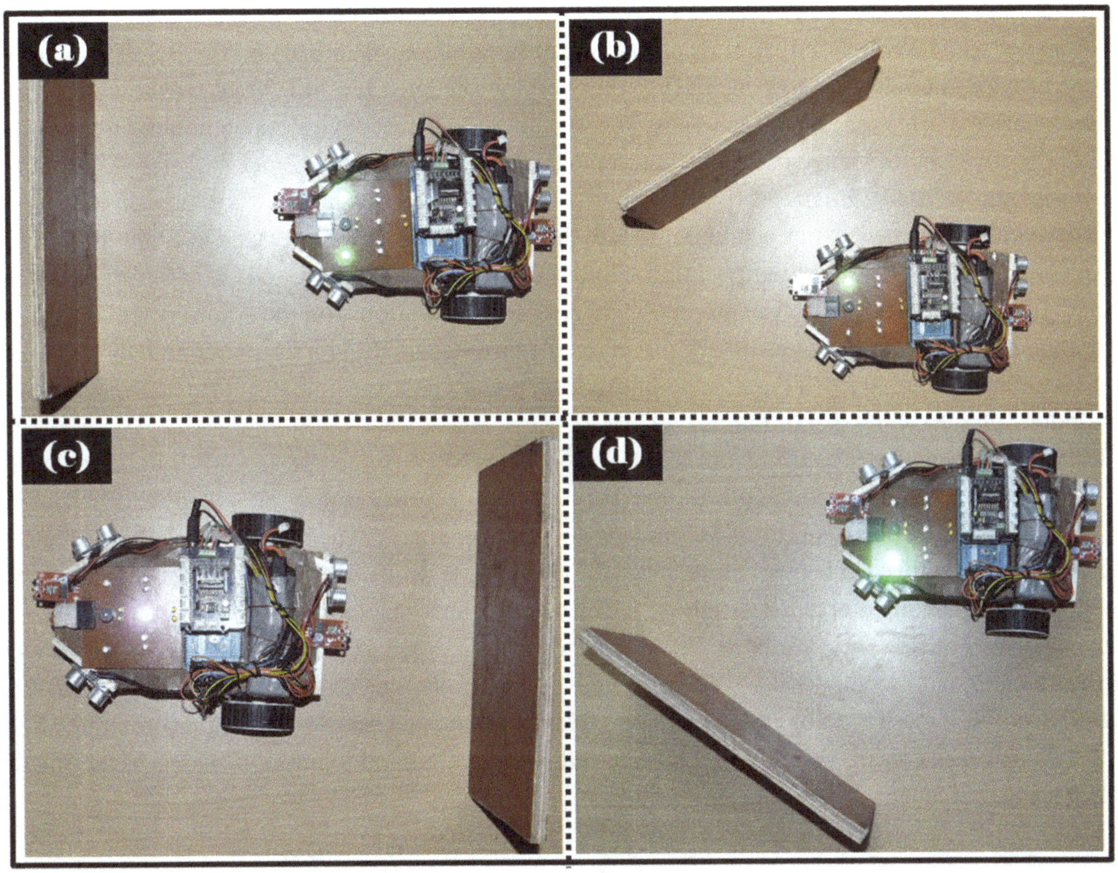

Figure 19. Pothole detection: (a) at front side, and (b) at rear side

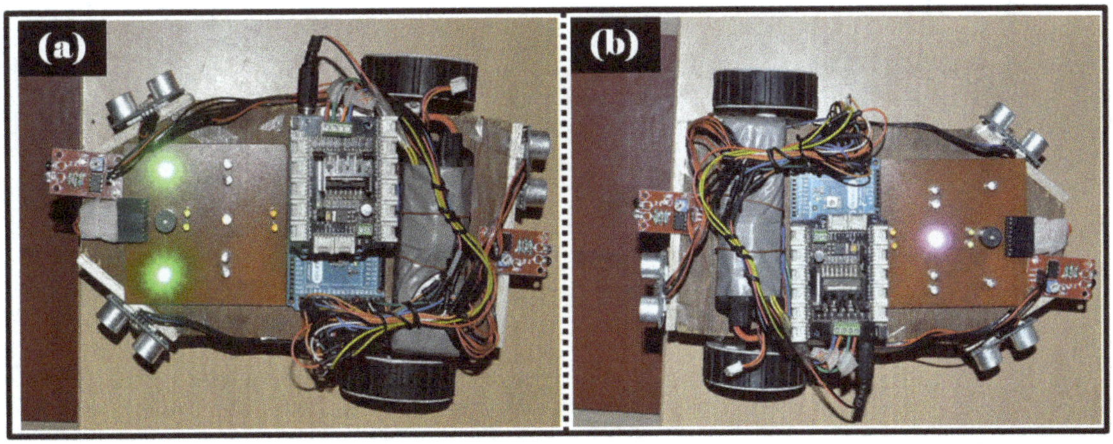

ordinator) were installed at an interval of 20 m throughout the corridor (Figure 20). The installed nodes created a mesh network to guide the robotic vehicle along the entire length of the corridor. This is the advantage of using Xbee based wireless communication protocols. The Bluetooth wireless technology doesn't provide the advantage of increasing the working distance like the Xbee technology. Similar results were also achieved by implementing the Bluetooth and Xbee wireless technology via joystick shield. The main disadvantage of the pushbutton based controller was the quick fatigue of the fingers. The mitigating effect of fatigue of the fingers was not evidenced during the operation of guiding the robotic vehicle using the joystick shield. Similar to the testing of the pushbutton and joystick shield based remote controllers; the Android application based controllers were also tested. It was also found that when the Bluetooth communication protocol was used in combination with the Android application, the movement of the robotic vehicle was controlled up to a distance of 13.3 m. On the other hand, when the Wi-Fi wireless technology was employed, the Android application was able to control the movement of the robotic vehicle till the end of the passage.

It can be inferred that the Bluetooth technology presented an economic way of designing wireless communication for short range applications. This economic criterion may be suited well because of the exponential usage of Android based mobile devices these days. The installation of the Bluetooth Android application would be enough to serve the purpose. Even if, the Wi-Fi and Xbee technologies were found efficient in completing the tasks, the installation and maintenance of Wi-Fi router is a costly affair. The Wi-Fi network is not power efficient too. On the other hand, the implementation of Xbee wireless technology is cheap and power efficient. Multiple nodes can be incorporated in a single Xbee network forming a mesh topology for long distance line-of-sight and near-line-of-sight communications. Hence, Xbee based control system may be preferred, if there is a need for controlling home automation system located at longer distances.

Figure 20. Proposed area for testing the navigation of the robotic vehicle using wireless control systems

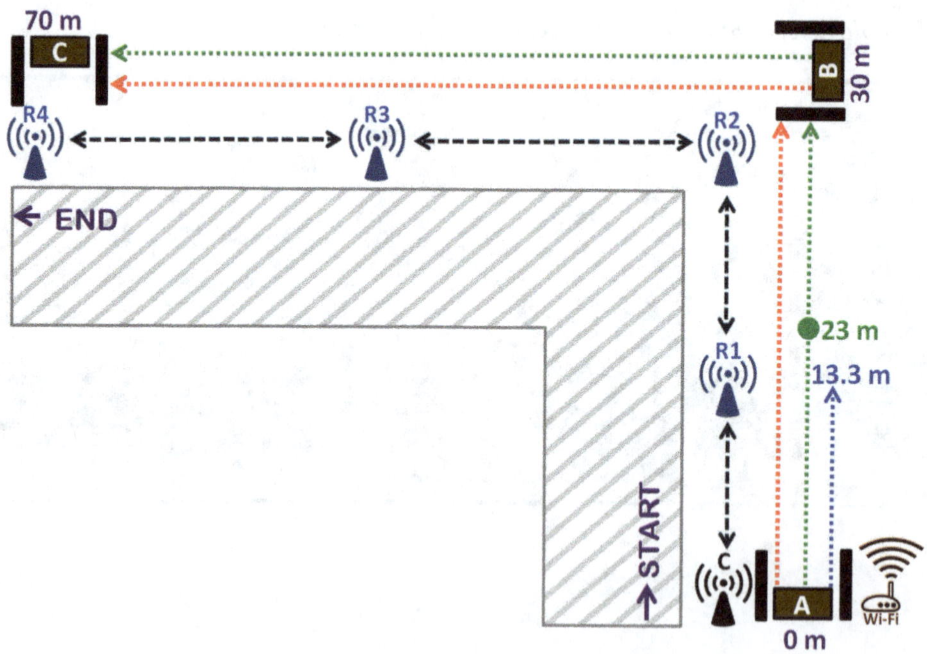

FUTURE RESEARCH DIRECTION

The current study was mainly focused on the development of wireless control systems using various wireless communication protocols, namely, Bluetooth, Xbee, and Wi-Fi. The proper functioning of the control systems were tested successfully by wirelessly controlling the operation of an in-lab developed prototype wheelchair (robotic vehicle). Future research can be performed using the developed control systems to design multitasking interfaces that can accommodate wheelchair navigation, home automation, robotic arm control, and mobile communication simultaneously. Further, the control systems can be modified by the implementation of biosignals (e.g. EOG, EMG and EEG) in place of the conventional mechanical switches (e.g. joystick, push button), so as to make the device accessible to motor-disabled persons. The prototype can be upgraded to a wheelchair that can handle a reasonable weight along with a robotic arm.

CONCLUSION

In the recent years, wireless communication protocols have gained popularity due to their robustness, low-cost, easy installation, and mobility. The short-range wireless communication protocols mainly include Bluetooth, Xbee, and Wi-Fi. Each of these technologies has its own advantages and disadvantages depending on the type of applications and environmental conditions. In the current study, different wireless control systems have been proposed for wireless control of the operation of a prototype wheelchair (robotic vehicle). The testing of the Bluetooth and the Xbee based control systems for guiding the movement of the robotic vehicle suggested that the Xbee based control system provided a longer communication range as compared to the Bluetooth based control system. The Xbee based control system also provided the facility of further enhancement in the communication range through the installation of additional Xbee nodes, which formed mesh networks. This suggested that the Xbee based control system can be preferred, if wireless control of devices, located at long distances, is necessary. In order to transmit the wireless serial commands to the robotic vehicle, remote controllers like the pushbutton assembly, joystick shield and Android Applications were used. The use of a pushbutton board as the remote controller for controlling the movement of the robotic vehicle resulted in the quick fatigue of the fingers. The use of a joystick shield as the remote controller resolved the mitigating effect of the quick fatigue of the fingers. An Android application based remote controller, in conjunction with Bluetooth communication protocol was also tested for controlling the movement of the robotic vehicle. This control system failed to guide the robotic vehicle to reach the destination. On the other contrary, when Wi-Fi communication protocol was used in combination with an Android application, the robotic vehicle successfully covered the entire navigational pathway. Though the Wi-Fi technology was found to be efficient, the maintenance of the Wi-Fi router is costly which may limit the use of Wi-Fi for developing wireless control systems. Therefore, it may be concluded that for short distance communication, the implementation of Bluetooth wireless technology is efficient and cost-effective; whereas, for long distance communication, the implementation of Xbee wireless technology is economic.

REFERENCES

Barea, R., Boquete, L., Mazo, M., & López, E. (1999). *Guidance of a wheelchair using electrooculography.* Paper presented at the 3rd IMACS International Multiconference on Circuits, Systems, Communications and Computers (CSCC'99).

Barea, R., Boquete, L., Mazo, M., & López, E. (2002). Wheelchair guidance strategies using EOG. *Journal of Intelligent & Robotic Systems, 34*(3), 279–299. doi:10.1023/A:1016359503796

Champaty, B., Jose, J., Pal, K., & Thirugnanam, A. (2014). *Development of EOG based human machine interface control system for motorized wheelchair.* Paper presented at the Emerging Research Areas: Magnetics, Machines and Drives (AICERA/iCMMD), 2014 Annual International Conference on. doi:10.1109/AICERA.2014.6908256

Choi, K., & Cichocki, A. (2008). *Control of a wheelchair by motor imagery in real time. In Intelligent Data Engineering and Automated Learning–IDEAL 2008* (pp. 330–337). Springer. doi:10.1007/978-3-540-88906-9_42

Coco, G. L., Coco, D. L., Cicero, V., Oliveri, A., Verso, G. L., & Piccoli, F. (2005). Individual and health-related quality of life assessment in amyotrophic lateral sclerosis patients and their caregivers. *Journal of the Neurological Sciences, 238*(1), 11–17. doi:10.1016/j.jns.2005.05.018 PMID:16109426

Cowan, R. E., Fregly, B. J., Boninger, M. L., Chan, L., Rodgers, M. M., & Reinkensmeyer, D. J. (2012). Recent trends in assistive technology for mobility. *Journal of Neuroengineering and Rehabilitation, 9*(1), 20. doi:10.1186/1743-0003-9-20 PMID:22520500

Fehr, L., Langbein, W. E., & Skaar, S. B. (2000). Adequacy of power wheelchair control i terfaces for persons with severe disabilities: A clinical survey. *Journal of Rehabilitation Research and Development, 37*(3), 353–360. PMID:10917267

Fezari, M., & Bousbia-Salah, M. (2007). Speech and sensor in guiding an electric wheelchair. *Automatic Control and Computer Sciences, 41*(1), 39–43. doi:10.3103/S0146411607010063

Gargiulo, G., Bifulco, P., Cesarelli, M., Jin, C., McEwan, A., & van Schaik, A. (2010). Wearable dry sensors with Bluetooth connection for use in remote patient monitoring systems. *Studies in Health Technology and Informatics, 161*, 57–65. PMID:21191158

Han, J.-S., Bien, Z. Z., Kim, D.-J., Lee, H.-E., & Kim, J.-S. (2003). *Human-machine interface for wheelchair control with EMG and its evaluation.* Paper presented at the Engineering in Medicine and Biology Society.

Kepa, K., & Abaid, N. (2015). *Development of a frequency-modulated ultrasonic sensor inspired by bat echolocation.* Paper presented at the SPIE Smart Structures and Materials+ Nondestructive Evaluation and Health Monitoring.

Kitayoshi, H., Sawaya, K., & Kuwano, H. (2013). *Ultra low power wireless ECG sensor tag with wearable antenna.* Paper presented at the SENSORS, 2013 IEEE. doi:10.1109/ICSENS.2013.6688381

Kobayashi, H. (2011). *A ZigBee based wireless EMG/ECG streaming system for the universal interface.* Paper presented at the IECON 2011-37th Annual Conference on IEEE Industrial Electronics Society.

Kurtzberg, J. M., & Lew, J. S. (2000). *Voice-controlled motorized wheelchair with sensors and displays.* Google Patents.

Levine, S. P., Bell, D., Jaros, L., Simpson, R. C., Koren, Y., & Borenstein, J. (1999). The NavChair assistive wheelchair navigation system. *Rehabilitation Engineering. IEEE Transactions on, 7*(4), 443–451.

Lin, J.-S., Chen, K.-C., & Yang, W.-C. (2010). *EEG and eye-blinking signals through a Brain-Computer Interface based control for electric wheelchairs with wireless scheme.* Paper presented at the New Trends in Information Science and Service Science (NISS), 2010 4th International Conference on.

Lopes, A. C., Nunes, U., & Vaz, L. (2010). *Assisted navigation based on shared-control, using discrete and sparse human-machine interfaces.* Paper presented at the Engineering in Medicine and Biology Society (EMBC), 2010 Annual International Conference of the IEEE. doi:10.1109/IEMBS.2010.5626221

Lu, H.-Y., Zhao, Q.-S., Xu, M.-Z., & Jin, T.-H. (2007). ECG monitoring module based on Bluetooth technology. *Chinese Medical Equipment Journal, 9*, 9.

Mageswari, D. U., & Selvavinayagam, G. (2013). Wheelchair Motion Control Guide Using Eye Movement Based on EEG Signals. *International Journal of Engineering Sciences & Research Technology.*

Mamatha, M. (2015). *Development of Novel Architectures for Patient Care Monitoring System and Diagnosis. In Advancements of Medical Electronics* (pp. 333–342). Springer.

Matsumoto, O., Komoriya, K., Hatase, T., & Nishimura, H. (2006). *Autonomous Traveling Control of the "TAO Aicle" Intelligent Wheelchair.* Paper presented at the Intelligent Robots and Systems, 2006 IEEE/RSJ International Conference on.

Moon, I., Lee, M., Chu, J., & Mun, M. (2005). *Wearable EMG-based HCI for electric-powered wheelchair users with motor disabilities.* Paper presented at the Robotics and Automation.

Mulroy, S. J., Gronley, J. K., Newsam, C. J., & Perry, J. (1996). Electromyographic activity of shoulder muscles during wheelchair propulsion by paraplegic persons. *Archives of Physical Medicine and Rehabilitation, 77*(2), 187–193. doi:10.1016/S0003-9993(96)90166-5 PMID:8607745

Pačnik, G., Benkič, K., & Brečko, B. (2005). *Voice operated intelligent wheelchair-VOIC.* Paper presented at the Industrial Electronics.

Parikh, S. P., Grassi, V., Jr., Kumar, V., & Okamoto, J., Jr. (2005). *Usability study of a control framework for an intelligent wheelchair.* Paper presented at the Robotics and Automation. doi:10.1109/ROBOT.2005.1570853

Pereira, F., Barros, C., Carvalho, V., Machado, J., Leão, C., & Soares, F. (2015). *Ambient Assisted Living Platform for Remote Monitoring of Bedridden People. In New Trends in Mechanism and Machine Science* (pp. 573–581). Springer.

Perrin, X. (2009). *Semi-autonomous navigation of an assistive robot using low throughput interfaces.* (Diss.). Eidgenössische Technische Hochschule ETH Zürich.

Rebsamen, B., Burdet, E., Guan, C., Zhang, H., Teo, C. L., & Zeng, Q. (2006). *A brain-controlled wheelchair based on P300 and path guidance.* Paper presented at the Biomedical Robotics and Biomechatronics, 2006. BioRob 2006. The First IEEE/RAS-EMBS International Conference on. doi:10.1109/BIOROB.2006.1639239

Rebsamen, B., Teo, C. L., Zeng, Q., Ang, M. H. Jr, Burdet, E., & Guan, C. (2007). Controlling a wheelchair indoors using thought. *IEEE Intelligent Systems*, *22*(2), 18–24. doi:10.1109/MIS.2007.26

Rockland, R. H., & Reisman, S. (1998). *Voice activated wheelchair controller.* Paper presented at the Bioengineering Conference.

Sevillano, J. L., Cascado, D., Cagigas, D., Vicente, S., Lujan, C., & Rio, F. (2009). *A real-time wireless sensor network for wheelchair navigation.* Paper presented at the Computer Systems and Applications, 2009. AICCSA 2009. IEEE/ACS International Conference on. doi:10.1109/AICCSA.2009.5069311

Shaheen, S., & Umamakeswari, A. (2013). Intelligent Wheelchair For People With Disabilities. *IACSIT International Journal of Engineering and Technology*, *5*(1), 391–397.

Silva, H., Lourenço, A., & Paz, N. (2011). *Real-time Biosignal Acquisition and Telemedicine Platform for AAL based on Android OS.* Paper presented at the AAL.

Simmons, Z. (2005). Management strategies for patients with amyotrophic lateral sclerosis from diagnosis through death. *The Neurologist*, *11*(5), 257–270. doi:10.1097/01.nrl.0000178758.30374.34 PMID:16148733

Simms, A. P. (2014). *Reading and Wirelessly Sending EEG Signals Using Arduinos and XBee Radios to Control a Robot.* Academic Press.

Simpson, R., LoPresti, E., Hayashi, S., Nourbakhsh, I., & Miller, D. (2004). The smart wheelchair component system. *Journal of Rehabilitation Research and Development*, *41*(3b3B), 429–442. doi:10.1682/JRRD.2003.03.0032 PMID:15543461

Simpson, R. C. (2005). Smart wheelchairs: A literature review. *Journal of Rehabilitation Research and Development*, *42*(4), 423. doi:10.1682/JRRD.2004.08.0101 PMID:16320139

Soros, G., & Madrick, J. (1999). The international crisis: An interview. *The New York Review of Books*, *46*, 36–37.

Sung, W.-T., Chen, J.-H., & Chang, K.-Y. (2013). ZigBee based multi-purpose electronic score design and implementation using EOG. *Sensors and Actuators. A, Physical*, *190*, 141–152. doi:10.1016/j.sna.2012.11.028

Tafa, Z., & Stojanovic, R. (2006). Bluetooth-based approach to monitoring biomedical signals. *WSEAS Transactions on Business and Economics*, *2*(3), 75–80.

Tanaka, K., Matsunaga, K., & Wang, H. O. (2005). Electroencephalogram-based control of an electric wheelchair. *Robotics. IEEE Transactions on*, *21*(4), 762–766.

Tomari, M. R. M., Kobayashi, Y., & Kuno, Y. (2012). Development of smart wheelchair system for a user with severe motor impairment. *Procedia Engineering*, *41*, 538–546. doi:10.1016/j.proeng.2012.07.209

Tsui, C. S. L., Jia, P., Gan, J. Q., Hu, H., & Yuan, K. (2007). *EMG-based hands-free wheelchair control with EOG attention shift detection.* Paper presented at the Robotics and Biomimetics, 2007. ROBIO 2007. IEEE International Conference on.

Wijesoma, W. S., Wee, K. S., Wee, O. C., Balasuriya, A. P., San, K. T., & Soon, L. K. (2005). *EOG based control of mobile assistive platforms for the severely disabled.* Paper presented at the Robotics and Biomimetics (ROBIO). 2005 IEEE International Conference on. doi:10.1109/ROBIO.2005.246316

Wu, B.-F., Jen, C.-L., & Huang, T.-W. (2011). *Intelligent radio based positioning and fuzzy based navigation for robotic wheelchair with wireless local area networks.* Paper presented at the Robot, Vision and Signal Processing (RVSP), 2011 First International Conference on. doi:10.1109/RVSP.2011.61

Yathunanthan, S., Chandrasena, L., Umakanthan, A., Vasuki, V., & Munasinghe, S. (2008). *Controlling a wheelchair by use of EOG signal.* Paper presented at the Information and Automation for Sustainability, 2008. ICIAFS 2008. 4th International Conference on. doi:10.1109/ICIAFS.2008.4783987

Zarit, S. H., Reever, K. E., & Bach-Peterson, J. (1980). Relatives of the impaired elderly: Correlates of feelings of burden. *The Gerontologist, 20*(6), 649–655. doi:10.1093/geront/20.6.649 PMID:7203086

Zhang, Y., Zhang, J., & Luo, Y. (2011). *A novel intelligent wheelchair control system based on hand gesture recognition.* Paper presented at the Complex Medical Engineering (CME), 2011 IEEE/ICME International Conference on. doi:10.1109/ICCME.2011.5876761 doi:10.1109/ICCME.2011.5876761

KEY TERMS AND DEFINITIONS

AT Commander: AT Commander is a software application that allows configuring any external Bluetooth module as master or slave. It also enables to send AT Commands to a phone over Bluetooth.

Conventional Wheelchair: A conventional wheelchair is an ergonomically designed chair fitted with wheels at the front and rear side. The front wheels are castor wheels meant for swift direction control. The rear wheels are assembled with breaks and hand rims. The wheelchair may be driven actively (by the occupant) or passively.

Motorized Wheelchair: The motorized wheelchair is a battery powered joystick driven electro-mechanical up gradation of conventional wheelchair.

Wireless Communication: Wireless communication is an umbrella term that facilitates all techniques and means of connecting and communicating between two or more devices to transfer information over a distance without the help of any electrical conductors.

Chapter 16

Wireless Body Area Networks Combined with Mobile Cloud Computing in Healthcare: A Survey

Srijan Goswami
WEBEL Informatics Ltd., Bashirhat College, India

Nilanjan Dey
Techno India College of Technology, India

Payel Roy
St. Mary's Technical Campus, India

Sayan Chakraborty
Bengal College of Engineering, India

ABSTRACT

This chapter introduces the combination of wireless body area network and mobile cloud computing in healthcare. The increased growth of low-power integrated circuits, physiological sensors and wireless communication has introduced a new generation of wireless sensor networks. Cloud computing is on high demand, whereas in case of mobile cloud computing the device is much more user friendly to manage the information. The combination of wireless body area network (WBAN) and mobile cloud computing (MCC) promises a better performance to the users immediately. It is more feasible to wire a sensor which performs the required medical tests and provides the information through devices like mobile phones and tablets. In this chapter, a theoretical study on the combination of WBAN and mobile cloud computing has been done.

INTRODUCTION

Wireless Body Area Network (WBAN) and Healthcare

A Body Area Network (BAN) also known as Wireless Body Area Network (WBAN) are wearable computing devices based on wireless sensor network technology.

The network comprises of several mini Body Sensor Units (BSUs). Advancement of physiological sensors, wireless communication technology and low power integrated circuits have given rise to a new

DOI: 10.4018/978-1-5225-0140-4.ch016

generation of wireless sensor networks. WBAN is interdisciplinary fields which allow low cost and uninterrupted health monitoring along with real time updates of medical data through Internet. Several perceptive physiological sensors have been implemented into wireless body area network which is wearable and applicable for computer – aided recovery or advance diagnosis of medical state. This technology is based on the achievability of introducing miniaturized biosensors inside human system that doesn't interfere with their normal activity. Implanted sensors in human's system gather different physiological changes for monitoring the health status regardless of their location. The data gathered are transmitted to an external processing unit via wireless network. The device immediately transfers all data in real time to the healthcare personnel throughout the world. When an emergency is detected, alarm or caution signals along with relevant information are sent to the subject by the healthcare personnel. This is a promising technology which is expected to revolutionize the healthcare system.

Mobile Cloud Computing (MCC) and Healthcare

Mobile Cloud Computing (MCC) is the integration of Cloud computing technology and mobile networks. It is slowly becoming promising technology with the ability of providing versatile stack of huge computing, storage and software based services in a virtualized process at affordable cost.

In this paper some underlying aspects of these technologies for providing the patients with advanced and reliable healthcare facilities has been described. Following topics like basic idea behind this field of research, literature reviews, statistical reports, target users, possible solutions and recommendations and future scope of this technology has been covered.

Main Objective

The main objective is integrating the wireless body area network with mobile cloud computing technology to revolutionize the field of medical sciences and healthcare.

In MCC enabled WBAN systems, wearable miniaturized biosensors coupled with wireless body area network are implanted into human body. This technology can be used for computer aided recovery or advance diagnosis of medical state. These miniaturized biosensors gathers physiological signals like changes in blood pressure, body temperature, changes in insulin level, nerve impulses etc. occurring in human body in real time regardless of the person's location. The physiological information gathered will be transmitted to external processing unit via wireless network. The physiological data received through wireless network are processed in the cloud and transmitted to the users selectively on their mobile devices. Here we will consider this concept based on three major possibilities.

- **Patients in Hospital Environment:** Wireless biosensor gathers the changes in physiological signals occurring in the patient's body which are transmitted to the cloud sever through wireless network. As soon as it receives the signals from the sensors it analyses the data and decides whether the patient needs immediate treatment or not. In case there is need for immediate treatment doctors, healthcare staffs and family are notified automatically with an emergency alarm along with all relevant information and rescue operation can be carried out. If the situation is not critical then, doctors get the patient's information, location and physiological data. Camera video, GIS and GPS systems are coupled with this technology.

- **Patients at Home:** If the patients at home require immediate treatment then doctors, healthcare staffs and family are notified with emergency alarm along with all relevant information so that rescue operation can be carried out. On the contrary, if the patient does not require immediate treatment then the doctors, healthcare staffs gets the information about the location and current physiological state of the patient via wireless communication.
- **Patients in Outdoor Environment:** In this case, smart phones are used for receiving and transmitting patient's physiological signals to the cloud network to the outdoor patients. If any accidents take place doctors, healthcare staffs and family members are informed with the alarm signal and patient can be rescued according to the GPS location.

Motivations and limitations for various related work is introduced in Table 1.

SYSTEM ARCHITECTURE

WBAN Architecture

- **Network Architecture:** The network architecture of WBAN can be classified into two main categories- Flat architecture and multi tier architecture. Flat architectures contains of a single data-gathering unit which sends its records to a personal computer or a personal server application which is running on a PDA. Jovanov *et al.* (2001) described the use of wireless intelligent breathing telemetry sensor (WIBRATE) to observe the breathing patterns. This is a point-to-point network of a single client server.
- In Figure 1 in three tiers can be observed. In first tier, data are gathered as multiple physiological signals through multiple nodes (implantable or wearable). Afterwards, a gateway at the second tier acts as an interface between first tier and a server mean the third tier (personal server). It holds patient authenticated information and it is configured with the medical server IP address to create an interface among the medical services. If the medical server's communication channel is available, the PS makes a secure communication to the server and sends reports that can be merged with the patient's medical record. Khan *et al.* (2008) described the architecture which is a prototypical WBAN which is multitier architecture.

The interface to the WBAN contains the network configuration and management also. The network configuration performs the following tasks: sensor node registration, initialization, customization and a secure communication setup. Once it is configured, the personal server handles the network, taking care of channel sharing, data retrieval and processing, fusion of the data and time synchronization. Based on the data from multiple medical sensors the PS application can determine the user's state and his or her current health status and also provide feedback through a user friendly and graphical or audio user interface.

The WBAN nodes must satisfy the requirements for minimal weight, low-power consumption to permit prolonged monitoring, miniature form-factor, standards based interface protocols, seamless integration into WBAN and the patient-specific calibration and customization. The wireless sensor

Table 1. Motivations and limitations for various related work

SN.	Paper Title	Authors Name	Motivation	Limitation
1	MobiSense: Mobile Body Sensor Network for Ambulatory Monitoring	Waluyo *et al.* (2010)	In this article MobiSense, a mobile body sensor network for ambulatory monitoring is presented. It can Track wearers' activities and display in the form of human animation on the user screen. It is also equipped with reconfiguration schemes and resource management.	Here the proposed system is incorporate with additional sensors such as SPO2 and BP sensor, and merge the data from respective sensors to determine the fitness level of a user in real time at the given time.
2	An Overview of Body Sensor Networks in Enabling Perva-sive Healthcare and Assistive Environments	Liolios *et al.* (2010)	It is a comprehensive review of the promising field through a survey of WBAN research projects and technologies, including applications, sensors, and interconnection of WBANs.	WBAN technologies provide a reliable and promising platform to perform ubiquitous communications. Here several open issues are still need to be mentioned.
3	KNOWME: An Energy-Efficient Multimodal Body Area Network for Physical Activity Monioring	Thatte *et al.* (2012)	Here a prototype is implemented of the KNOWME Network which is energy-efficient health care monitoring system that can detect physical activity.	For an upcoming field trial the integrated optimal sampling protocols and high-dimensional classifiers are implemented on the mobile device.
4	CRHIS: Cloud based Rural Healthcare Information System	Patra *et al.* (2012)	In this work the need for an information system to facilitate rural healthcare has been highlighted. The proposed cloud based solution is aimed at providing a cost effective way of dealing with the patient information for remotely located areas in India.	In this work the issue of data security and quality of service is not addressed which is a challenging area of research in cloud computing and WBAN.
5	e-Health Cloud: Opportunities and Challenges	AbuKhousa *et al.* (2012)	A literature review of e-Health Cloud issues are presented here with emphasis on the importance of the concepts which are involved in this issue, challenges and implementations. Also described the major technical and non-technical challenges which the researchers and users are facing in the e-Health Cloud. The discussion of several proposed solutions to address the challenges and emphasized on the security and privacy issues in e-Health Cloud as those are the biggest challenges.	The models are discussed in this paper which offers the beginnings of more comprehensive approaches that will satisfy the need of the healthcare providers. But there are still many more approaches have been left.
6	Cloud-Enabled Wireless Body Area Networks for Pervasive Healthcare	Wan *et al.* (2013)	The functionality, reliability and availability of MCC services. It also suggests some future scope to improve performance and cloud-enabled WBANs.	
7	Modeling of WBAN and Cloud Integration for Secure and Reliable Healthcare	Divi, K., & Liu (2013)	This paper proposes a secure and reliable WBAN-cloud for healthcare, called FTTT Secure Architecture. It provides a platform to fulfill security goals for various medical services.	The Further work includes demonstration of simulation of the effectiveness of FTTT Secure Architecture. It has not also the prototype of the Architecture to securely access the information of the patient.
8	Cloud Based Mental State Monitoring System for Suicide Risk Reconnaissance Using Wearable Bio-sensors	Alam *et al.* (2014)	Predicted the mental states using some small sensors and cloud computing technology to monitor patients' suicide risk and mental disorders. Some minimal setup in home, clinic or hospital can performs the task.	The sensors are not integrated with Mobile Cloud Computing so that we can get the data in an easier way.

Figure 1. MCC coupled WBAN architecture

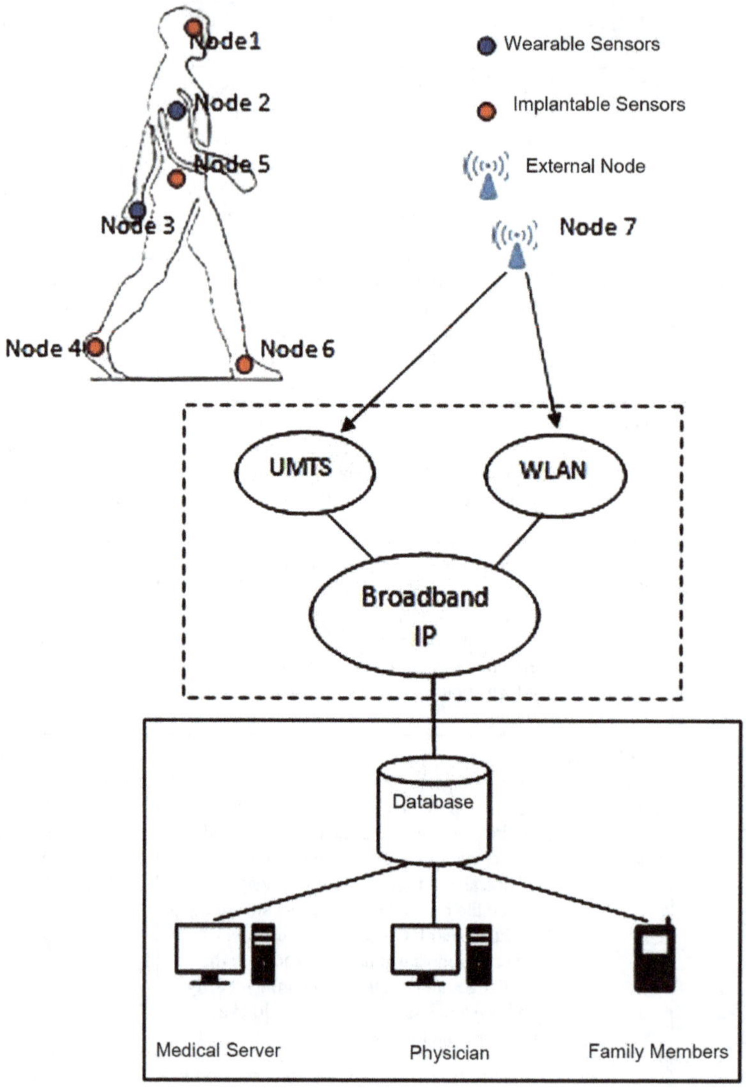

nodes can also be implemented as tiny patches or implanted into clothes or shoes. The network nodes continuously gather and process the raw data, then store them locally, and finally send processed event alarms to the personal server.

Jovanov *et al.* (2001) presented general system architecture for WBANs. According to this architecture:

1. A system for activity sensing (multi tier system architecture of artificial intelligent physiological sensor) at base tier.
2. A personal server on the second tier.
3. A medical server or the internet the last or third tier.

- **Routing:** A Wireless Body Area Network (WBAN) that needs the design of a routing protocol which are frequent network partitioning. It causes postural mobility of the body sensors, low transmission power of sensors, high propagation loss throughout the human body and low reliability of end-to-end path. Natarajan *et al.* (2009) observed the Link layer behavior of WBANs at 2.4 GHz. Here they noticed the following:
    - Increasing transmission power at specific regions with low multipath increases the PDR more.
    - Average packet delivery ratio (PDR) is directly proportional to the transmission power.
    - Environments have an effect on PDR.

Whereas it has been observed that channel symmetry is more effective in environments having better surfaces.

- **MCC Architecture:** Mobile Cloud Computing uses computational task. Through this approach resource-constraint mobile devices can use computational resources of many cloud-based resources. Saeid *et al.* (2013) described that in MCC, there are four types of cloud-based resources are available- proximate immobile computing entities, proximate mobile computing entities, distant immobile clouds and hybrid (combination of the other models). Fernando *et al.* (2013) proposed a giant cloud like Amazon EC2 which is the distant immobile groups whereas the cloudlet is a member of proximate immobile computing. Smartphone's, tablets and wearable devices which can compute are part of the third group.

WBAN collects various important signal information like body temperature, heat rate etc from wearable and implantable sensors. The collected data are processed in the clod and then selectively sent to the specific users. They can receive the collected monitored data through even any mobile devices. Figure 1 illustrates the MCC Coupled WBAN architecture.

BRIEF OVERVIEW OF MCC COUPLED WBAN SYSTEM ARCHITECTURE

The system is composed of four major elements:

1. Wireless Body Area Networks (WBANs).
2. Wireless transmission.
3. Cloud services.
4. End users.

WBAN senses and collects crucial physiological signals such as changes in body temperature, fluctuation in insulin levels or heart rate with the help of implantable or wearable sensors. The data generated based on the physiological signals are processed in the cloud and selectively conveyed to the users. Cloud servers consists of sophisticated resources like central processing unit (CPU), memory, band width, for providing all kinds of cloud services which includes automatic diagnosis and alarm signals, geographical information system services (GIS), medical decision making (MDM) and location based services. Different users such as researchers, doctors, hospitals, clinics and patients receives multiple cloud services through a variety of interfaces like personal computer and mobile phones.

For implementing the architecture the following three aspects should be considered:

1. **Standard of Communication:** The crucial issue in WBANs is their low power consumption which creates some problems in the standards of communication. Several protocols and standards are available for different tiny sensors in WBAN such as Bluetooth over IEEE 802.15.1, Zigbee over IEEE 802.15.4, UWB over IEEE 802.15.6, RuBee, ANT, Z-wave, and Insteon.
2. **Hybrid Clouds:** Hybrid cloud architecture can speed up the relocation from present/existing Information Technology resources at hospital to cloud computing, fully utilizes WBAN resources and cuts down the cost. Crucial medical data or application like GIS can be sent on a private cloud to assure its security.
3. **Implementation of Social Networks:** MCC-WBAN system is progressively integrating the social networks. This helps in advancement in the field of medical research such as epidemiological studies, disease prevention, diagnosis of mental health, drug therapy and monitoring of healthcare systems and organization.

HEALTH CARE APPLICATIONS

The wireless sensors are spatially distributed to monitor physical or environmental conditions to cooperatively inform their data through the network to a main location. The medical applications of the sensors can be of two types: wearable and implanted. Wearable sensors are used on the body surface of human or just kept very close to the user. The implantable medical devices are inserted inside human body. Hooda *et al.* (2013) discussed the wireless communications for both medical and consumer electronics applications using WBAN. Here are some examples:

- **ECG:** The electrocardiogram (ECG) is a waveform which represents the propagation of electric waves through our heart muscle with respect to time. The ECG waveform provides a non-invasive heart function. Standard ECG measurements perform twelve observations of the electrical activity of the heart. However, ECG using wireless sensors is generally for ambulatory applications. Fulford-Jones *et al.* (2004) designed an ECG measurement sensor which is supported by a Mica2 mote hardware platform. The sensor used two electrodes to produce only one ECG signal. This sensor is another node in the CodeBlue medical sensor network platform. Kario *et al.* (2003) described about the development of a wireless single-lead ECG sensor, where ECG signal is measured across both of two Ag/AgCl electrodes by the Human++ research program. Cao *et al.* (2010) also have developed a wireless three-pad ECG system (W3ECG).
- **EEG:** Electroencephalography (EEG) is a wireless sensor which records the electrical activity along scalp. It also measures voltage fluctuations. This fluctuation is the result of ionic current flows within the neurons of the brain.

Jovanov *et al.* (2001) have introduced Wireless Intelligent SEnsor (WISE) which is designed by them for EEG signal acquisition applications. This sensor is a microcontroller-based system which is capable of low-level real-time signal processing, analog signal conditioning, data acquisition and wireless communication. Farshchi *et al.* (2006) have also proposed a wireless neural interface, which contain Mica2 and Mica2dot systems as the wireless sensor networks that can perform using two channels of EEG data.

- **EMG:** Basmajian *et al.* (1985) described Electromyography (EMG) as a sensor which can observes the muscle function through the monitoring of the electrical signals which is emitted from the muscle. When a surface electrode is kept on the skin above a muscle while it is contracting, it will receive the electrical signal which is emitted from several muscle fibers associated with the different motor units.

Bonato *et al.* (2003) stated that data-mining technique which was used to cluster EMG data achieved over a 24-hour period of day. These clustered data was used to check the accuracy of function of neuromuscular mechanisms associated with specific biomechanical activities.

- **Motion Detector:** A motion detector is a device which detects moving objects, especially people. A motion detector is often considered as a component of a system that automatically performs or alerts a user of motion in a particular area.

Kusserow *et al.* (2009) introduced BodyANT which is equipped an accelerometer. Their observation revealed the effectiveness of this device in long-term activity in monitoring applications. Keijsers *et al.* (2003) described one of the main applications of these motion detectors which can monitor the uncontrolled body movements, experienced by sufferers of Parkinson's disease while under a levodopa treatment regime.

- **Blood Pressure:** Blood Pressure is the pressure which is exerted at the time of circulating blood on the walls of blood vessels. During every heartbeat, blood pressure varies between a maximum (systolic) and a minimum (diastolic) pressure. Kario *et al.* (2003) observed that ambulatory BP is more closely effective to target organ damage and cardiovascular events than BP readings taken in a clinical and home environment. In 2011 after this incidence Carr *et al.* (2001) create wireless BP sensor. The AMON system has a BP sensor which uses expansive cuff around the wrist and obtains the data of systolic and diastolic reading through oscillometric method.
- **Cancer Detection:** It represents one of the major concerns in healthcare. Nowadays, one of biggest disease for human life is cancer. In 2008, National Center for Health Statistics described the second leading cause of death in US with increasing numbers every year. The observations are saying that cancer cells exude nitric oxide, which affects the blood in the particular area which is surrounding a tumor. Researchers are trying to place a sensor on a needle, which enabling physicians to diagnose tumors without a biopsy. Schwiebert *et al.* (2001) introduced the sensors those are used in this device can differentiate between several types of cells, identifying cancerous.
- **Glucose Monitoring:** Basmajian *et al.* (1985) introduced an implantable sensor. It provides the real-time continuous blood glucose data which will assist in reducing hyperglycemic excursions for diabetes of type 1. By placing an implantable sensor which is covered with a multilayered membrane in the subcutaneous tissue of abdomen Continuous monitoring was enabled.

- **Target Users:** The main purpose here is easy accessibility of patient's physiological condition to the doctor, healthcare personnel, and hospitals irrespective of the location so that they would be able to take the required actions at appropriate time, which will help saving the valuable time in case of emergency.

Based on the proposed scenario there are four major classes of users:

1. **Care Seekers:** The care seekers are the patient themselves suffering from certain diseases.
2. **Care Takers:** This group of users includes Doctors or nurses, healthcare personnel, medical emergency vehicles, nearest hospitals and family members. This way care takers can stay aware about the physiological conditions of care seekers.
3. **Administrators:** This group of users is those who have the authority to add remove or modify information about care seekers and care takers.
4. **Other Users:** This group of users includes researchers, network service providers, and software and biomedical engineering companies.

SECURITY IN WBAN AND MOBILE CLOUD COMPUTING IN HEALTHCARE

The WBAN and mobile cloud computing must implement the security operations which guaranteed the data integrity, security, privacy and confidentiality of the patients' medical data. In case of privacy issues, it must be ensured that the Health Insurance Portability and Accountability Act of 1996 are noticed.

- **Data Integrity:** This is also needed to prevent the altering of data traversing into the communication paths between nodes.
- **Authentication:** This is necessary to ensure that the WBAN and the mobile device to validate network nodes and prevent network compromise.
- **Confidentiality:** The network and the mobile device should be able to guarantee the privacy of message exchange among nodes.
- **Privacy:** The patients' medical and personal records should not be disclosed to unauthorized persons.
- **Availability:** Because the network carries highly sensitive and important life-saving information, it is the most importance that the network resources should be available at all times.

CHALLENGES

Integrating the wireless body area network and mobile cloud computing itself is a challenge. So there are many problems arising whenever we try merging both the devices. In case of MCC, the mobile computing, cloud computing, and communication network creates several challenges like Mobile Computation Seamless Connectivity, Context-Processing, Energy Constraint, Offloading, Mobility Management, Long WAN Latency, Data Lock-in, Privacy, Elasticity that suppressing MCC. There are some challenges also regarding WBAN. Here are some examples:

- **Validation of Sensors:** Ubiquitous sensing devices are subject to limitation of internet communication and hardware along with unreliable wired/wireless network links, intervention and finite power reserves. This may result in inaccurate datasets being transmitted to the end user. It is the greatest consequence particularly within the healthcare domain that all sensor records and readings are validated. According to Donoghue *et al.* (2012) this will help reducing false alarm generation and also identify possible weaknesses within the software and hardware design.
- **Data Consistency:** Information from multiple mobile devices and wireless patient networks need to be gathered/collected and analyzed in a seamless manner. Within body area networks, important patient datasets may be distributed over a number of nodes and across a large number of networked PCs, Laptops or the other monitoring devices. The quality of patient care may degenerate if medical practitioner's mobile device does not hold all required information.
- **Interference:** The wireless link which is used for body sensor networks should minimize the intervention and expand the coexistence of sensor nodes with other network systems available in the environment. This is mainly important for wide range implementation of WBAN devices.
- **Data Management:** As WBANs generate huge amount of data, there is a need to manage and maintain these data sets of utmost importance. So, the database which dedicated for this purpose is required.

Besides hardware challenges, there are some human-centric challenges also. These issues should be considered for practical WBAN development. The issues include cost, consistent performance, constant monitoring and constrained deployment.

- **Node Accuracy:** There is another challenge regarding limited node number with every node required to be accurate and robust.
- **Organizational Change:** In Mobile Cloud enabled WBAN technology requires significant changes to business and clinical processes and also to the organizational barriers in the healthcare industry.
- **Data Ownership:** The ownership of data in healthcare industry basically an area with no specific guidelines.

The major challenge in integrating MCC and WBAN is security. So in this portion we recommend some Security Solutions. The light weight, small size and integrated function are mainly desirable for sensor devices. The sensor design complies with the requirements and then provides comfort to the user. It is challenging to develop smaller, lighter and integrated sensing functions. A memory unit that integrated into a wearable device can be used to store data of the sensor device locally. Actually it works when a specific communication channel can't be established with the gateway. Kusserow *et al.* (2009) proposed sleep mechanism and an adaptive listens to reduce the energy consumption. The mechanism creates a tree structure among body sensors to ensure a collision free access to the wireless medium It also route the data towards the WBAN gateway. Keijsers *et al.* (2003) checked the energy management mechanism and a dynamic power control scheme which performed adaptive body posture inference for optimal power assignments.

TinySecas is a security solution and recommendation in biomedical sensor network to achieve link-layer encryption and authentication of data. Karlof *et al.* (2004) introduced it as software based security architecture. It is an official component of the TinyOS. Leonardo *et al.* (2007) stated that it is very popular in the wireless sensors and has been implemented on a various custom hardware. There are also several securities can be implemented under IEEE 802.15.4. In 2001, the National institute of Standards and Technology classified it in two basic modes- Secured mode and unsecured mode. The unsecure mode means no security suite has been specified. Tiny Tate is a lightweight Identity-Based Encryption (IBE) security solution for traditional wireless sensor networks. Tan *et al.* (2008) proposed an Identity-Based cryptographic security solution for WBAN. They used the sensor nodes to compute public keys through a hash function.

In case of MCC until, the assets were difficult to access due to fragmentation and technical limitations. The application developers would have to connect to multiple networks in a given area, with differing technical interfaces (APIs), meaning they have to create several versions of the same application.

CONCLUSION

To overcome the challenges is the utmost future research direction in Mobile cloud computing enabled Wireless body area network field. Some approaches are undergoing also. There are already Some protocols exist that take care of the networking layer and the data link layer, this specific area still has a lots of open research issues. On data link layer, more WBAN specified MAC-protocols need to be implemented that observes the mobility of the nodes, more low-power features, the use of the human movements like heart beat to ensure time synchronization and many more. Whereas in case of the network layer, a promising research field is combination of thermal routing with much more energy efficient mechanisms. More efficient QoS-mechanisms are also needed. The other interesting open research areas are mobility support which is embedded in the protocol, security and so on. To introduce a globally optimal system, it is necessary to unite all of these mechanisms and many more in a cross layer protocol.

However Mobile Cloud Computing (MCC) and Wireless Body Area Network (WBAN) in the domain of medical sciences and healthcare management is still growing, these two technologies when integrated together holds the potential to become an essential infrastructure component in remotely supervised rehabilitation of patients. This new technology will be able to deliver better healthcare services in a reliable and cost effective manner. In this chapter we have mentioned the MCC and WBAN technologies individually and together in healthcare in brief. MCC coupled WBAN will monitor the patient's health continuously and accurately. Continuous monitoring with early detection has the ability to provide patients with an increasing level of confidence which may improve the quality of life. Combining MCC with tiny sensors and computers will give rise to new applications that will influence the change in daily lifestyle of the citizens. Also offers insights into disease evolution process and drug therapy.

REFERENCES

AbuKhousa, E., Mohamed, N., & Al-Jaroodi, J. (2012). e-Health cloud: Opportunities and challenges. *Future Internet*, *4*(3), 621–645. doi:10.3390/fi4030621

Alam, M. G. R., Cho, E. J., Huh, E. N., & Hong, C. S. (2014, January). Cloud based mental state monitoring system for suicide risk reconnaissance using wearable bio-sensors. In *Proceedings of the 8th International Conference on Ubiquitous Information Management and Communication* (p. 56). ACM. doi:10.1145/2557977.2558020

Bonato, P., Mork, P. J., Sherrill, D. M., & Westgaard, R. H. (2003). Data Mining of Motor Patterns Recorded with Wearable Technology. *IEEE Engineering in Medicine and Biology Magazine*, *22*(3), 110–119. doi:10.1109/MEMB.2003.1213634 PMID:12845827

Braem, B., Moerman, I., & Blondia, C. (2007). A Low Delay Protocol for Multihop Wireless Body Area Networks. *Fourth Annual International Conference on Mobile and Ubiquitous Systems: Networking & Services (MobiQuitous)*.

Cao, H., Li, H., Stocco, L., & Victor, C. M., Leung (2010). Demonstration of A Novel Wireless Three-pad ECG System for Generating Conventional 12-lead Signals. *5th Annual International ICST Conference on Body Area Networks*. doi:10.1145/2221924.2221931

Devaul, R. W., Sung, M., Gips, J., & Pentland, S. (2003). MIThril 2003: Applications and architecture. In *Proceedings of the International Semantic Web Conference (SWC)*.

Divi, K., & Liu, H. (2013, September). Modeling of wban and cloud integration for secure and reliable healthcare. In *Proceedings of the 8th International Conference on Body Area Networks* (pp. 128-131). ICST (Institute for Computer Sciences, Social-Informatics and Telecommunications Engineering). doi:10.4108/icst.bodynets.2013.253706

Doukas, C., Pliakas, T., & Maglogiannis, I. (2010). Mobile Healthcare Information Management utilizing Cloud Computing and Android OS. In *Proc. IEEE Eng. Med. Bio. Soc.*

Farshchi, S., Nuyujukian, P. H., Pesterev, A., Mody, I., & Judy, J. W. (2006). A TinyOS-Based Wireless Neural Interface. *Proceedings of the 26th Annual International Conference of the IEEE EMBS*, *53*(7), 1416-1424.

Fernando, N., Seng, W. L., & Wenny, R. (2013). Mobile cloud computing: A survey. *Future Generation Computer Systems*, *29*(1), 84–106. doi:10.1016/j.future.2012.05.023

Fulford-Jones, T. R. F., Wei, & Welsh, M. (2004). A Portable, Low-Power & Wireless Two-Lead EKG System. *26th Annual International Conference of the IEEE EMBS*. doi:10.1109/IEMBS.2004.1403627

Hooda, A., Sharma, S., & Sharma, A. (2013). Wireless body area network. *International Journal of Electronics, Communication & Instrumentation Engineering Research and Development*, *3*(1), 203–210.

Jovanov, E., Milenkovic, A., Otto, C., & Piet, C. G. (2005). A wireless body area network of intelligent motion sensors for computer assisted physical rehabilitation. *Journal of Neuroengineering and Rehabilitation*, 2–6. PMID:15740621

Jovanov, E., Raskovic, D., Price, J., Chapman, J., Moore, A., & Krishnamurthy, A. (2001). Patient Monitoring Using Personal Area Networks of Wireless Intelligent Sensors. *Biomedical Sciences Instrumentation*, 373–378. PMID:11347420

Kario, K., Yasui, N., & Yokoi, H. (2003). Ambulatory Blood Pressure Monitoring for Cardiovascular Medicine. *IEEE Engineering in Medicine and Biology Magazine*, *22*(3), 81–88. doi:10.1109/MEMB.2003.1213630 PMID:12845823

Karlof, C., Sastry, N., & Wagner, D. (2004). TinySec:A Link Layer Security Architecture for Wireless Sensor Networks. *Second ACM Conference on Embedded Networked Sensor Systems (SenSys '04)*. doi:10.1145/1031495.1031515

Keijsers, N. L. W., Horstink, M. W. I. M., & Gielen, S. C. A. M. (2003). Online Monitoring of Dyskinesia in Patients with Parkinson's Disease. *IEEE Engineering in Medicine and Biology Magazine*, *22*(3), 96–103. doi:10.1109/MEMB.2003.1213632 PMID:12845825

Khan, J. Y., Yuce, M. R., & Karami, F. (2008). Performance evaluation of a wireless body area sensor network for remote patient monitoring. *30th Annual International Conference of the IEEE Engineering in Medicine and Biology Society (EMBS)*. doi:10.1109/IEMBS.2008.4649394

Kusserow, M., Amft, O., & Tröster, G. (2009). BodyANT: Miniature wireless sensors for naturalistic monitoring of daily activity. *4th Annual International ICST Conference on Body Area Networks*. doi:10.4108/ICST.BODYNETS2009.5899

Leonardo, B. O., Diego, F. A., Eduardo, M., Felipe, D., Julio, L., & Ricardo, D. (2007). TinyTate:Identity-Based Encryption for Sensor Networks. *NCA*, *2007*(020), 318–323.

Li, H. B., Takizawa, K. I., Zhen, B., & Kohno, R. (2007). Body area network and its standardization at IEEE 802.15.MBAN. 16th IST on mobile and wireless communications summit.

Liolios, C., Doukas, C., Fourlas, G., & Maglogiannis, I. (2010, June). An overview of body sensor networks in enabling pervasive healthcare and assistive environments. In *Proceedings of the 3rd International Conference on PErvasive Technologies Related to Assistive Environments* (p. 43). ACM. doi:10.1145/1839294.1839346

Meingast, M., Roosta, T., & Sastry, S. (2006). Security and Privacy Issues with Health Care Information Technology. *28th Annual International Conference of the IEEE Engineering in Medicine and Biology Society (EMBS 06)*. doi:10.1109/IEMBS.2006.260060

Natarajan, A., De Silva, B., Yap, K. K., & Motani, M. (2009). Link Layer Behavior of Body Area Networks at 2.4 GHz. In *15th Annual International Conference on Mobile Computing and Networking(MobiCom '09)*.

O'Donoghue, J., & Herbert, J. (2012). Data management within mHealth environments: Patient sensors, mobile devices, and databases. *Journal of Data and Information Quality*, *4*(1), 1–20. doi:10.1145/2378016.2378021

O'Donoghue, J., Herbert, J., & Fensli, R. (2006). Sensor Validation within a Pervasive Medical Environment. In *Proceedings of IEEE Sensors*.

Patra, M. R., Das, R. K., & Padhy, R. P. (2012, October). CRHIS: cloud based rural healthcare information system. In *Proceedings of the 6th International Conference on Theory and Practice of Electronic Governance* (pp. 402-405). doi:10.1145/2463728.2463805

Schwiebert, L., Gupta, S. S., & Weinmann, J. (2001). Research Challenges in Wireless Networks of Biomedical Sensors. *7th Annual International Conference on Mobile Computing and Networking*.

Sergio, G. V., Xuedong, L., Cao, H., Min, C., & Leung, V. C. M. (2011). Body Area Networks: A Survey. *Springer Mobile Networks and Applications*, *16*(2), 171–193. doi:10.1007/s11036-010-0260-8

Tan, C. C., & Wang, H. (2008). Body Sensor Network Security: An Identity-Based Cryptography Approach. In *FristACM Conference on Wireless Network Security (WiSec '08)*. doi:10.1145/1352533.1352557

Thatte, G., Li, M., Lee, S., Emken, A., Narayanan, S., Mitra, U., & Annavaram, M. et al. (2012). Knowme: An energy-efficient multimodal body area network for physical activity monitoring. *ACM Transactions on Embedded Computing Systems*, *11*(S2), 48. doi:10.1145/2331147.2331158

Waluyo, A. B., Yeoh, W. S., Pek, I., Yong, Y., & Chen, X. (2010). Mobisense: Mobile body sensor network for ambulatory monitoring. *ACM Transactions on Embedded Computing Systems*, *10*(1), 13. doi:10.1145/1814539.1814552

Wan, J., Zou, C., Ullah, S., Lai, C. F., Zhou, M., & Wang, X. (2013). Cloud-enabled wireless body area networks for pervasive healthcare. *IEEE Network*, *27*(5), 56–61. doi:10.1109/MNET.2013.6616116

Zohreh, S., Saeid, A., Abdullah, G., & Rajkumar, B. (2013). Heterogeneity in Mobile Cloud Computing: Taxonomy and Open Challenges. *IEEE Communications Surveys and Tutorials*, (99): 1–24.

ADDITIONAL READING

Baronti, P., Pillai, P., Chook, V., Chessa, S., Gotta, A., & Hu, Y. F. (2007). Wireless sensor networks: A survey on the state of the art and the 802.15.4 and zigbee standards. *Computer Communications*, *30*(7), 1665–1695. doi:10.1016/j.comcom.2006.12.020

Basmajian, J. V., & Deluca, C. (1985). *Muscles Alive* (5th ed.). Baltimore: Williams & Wilkins.

Benny, L., Fani, D., & Yang, G. Z. (2006). Source Recovery for Body Sensor Network. *IEEE proceedings of the International Workshop on Wearable and Implantable Body Sensor Networks*, 199-202.

Bhargava, A., & Zoltowski, M. (2003). Sensors and wireless communication for medical care. *14th international workshop on database and expert systems applications*, 956–960.

Carr, J. J., & Brown, J. M. (2001). *Introduction to Biomedical Equipment Technology*. Prentice- Hall.

Cavalcanti, D., Schmitt, R., & Soomro, A. (2007). Performance analysis of 802.15.4 and 802.11e for body sensor network applications. *In 4th International workshop on wearable and implantable Body Sensor Networks (BSN 2007),Berlin: Springer*, 9–14.

Chow, R., Golle, P., Jakobsson, M., Shi, E., Staddon, J., Masuoka, R., & Molina, J. (2003). Controlling Data in the Cloud: Outsourcing Computation without Outsourcing Control. *2009 ACM Workshop on Cloud Computing Security*, Chicago, IL, USA, 85–90.

Drude, S. (2007). Requirements and application scenarios for body area networks. 16th IST on Mobile and wireless communications summit, Budapest, Hungary, 1–5.

Farella, E., Pieracci, A., Benini, L., & Acquaviva, A. (2006). A wireless body area sensor network for posture detection. *ISCC '06: Proceedings of the 11th IEEE symposium on computers and communications*. 454–459. doi:10.1109/ISCC.2006.21

Heile, B., Gifford I. &Siep, T. (1999). Wireless Personal Area Networks: An Overview of the IEEE P802.15 Working Group. *IEEE Netw.,* vol.(4), 4–5.

Huynh, T., Blanke, U., & Schiele, B. (2007). Scalable recognition of daily activities with wearable sensors. *Proceedings of the 3rd International Conference on Location and Context Awareness.* Lecture Notes in Computer Science, vol. 4718, Springer, Berlin, 50-67. doi:10.1007/978-3-540-75160-1_4

Milenkovic, A., Otto, C., & Jovanov, E. (2006). Wireless sensor networks for personal health monitoring: Issues and an implementation. *Computer Communications, Wireless Sensor Networks and Wired/ Wireless Internet Communications*, 29(13), 2521–2533.

Nguyen. D.K., Lelli, F., Papazoglou, M.P. & van den Heuvel, W.J. (2012) Blueprinting Approach in Support of Cloud Computing. *Future Internet*, 322–346.

Niedermeyer, E., & da Silva, F. L. (2004). *Electroencephalography: Basic Principles, Clinical Applications, and Related Fields.* Lippincot Williams & Wilkins.

Olugbara, O. O., Adigun, M. O., Ojo, S. O., & Mudali, P. (2007). Utility grid computing and body area network as enabler for ubiquitous rural e-healthcare service provisioning. *9th International conference on e-Health networking, application and services, Taipei, Taiwan*, 202–207. doi:10.1109/ HEALTH.2007.381630

Rayport, J.F. & Heyward, A. (2009) Envisioning the Cloud: The Next Computing Paradigm. A MarketspaceNext Point of View.*Introduction to Cloud Computing Architecture.*1-57.

Sriram, I., & Khajeh-Hosseini, A. (2010). Research Agenda in Cloud Technologies. *1st ACM Symposium on Cloud Computing, SOCC 2010*, Indianapolis, USA, 1-11.

KEY TERMS AND DEFINITIONS

Cloud Computing: Cloud computing is the computing of service along with shared data, resources, software and information which is provided to computers and other devices over a network.

MCC: Mobile cloud computing is the combination of cloud computing and mobile networks to give benefits for mobile users, network operators, and for the cloud computing providers.

Medical Test: A medical test is a medical procedure to detect, diagnose, monitor diseases and determine the course of treatment.

Sensor: A sensor is a converter that measures physical quantity of respective organ and converts the data into a signal that can be read by an instrument or by an observer.

WBAN: A wireless body area network (WBAN) is a wireless network of wearable computing devices. WBAN devices may be embedded inside the body or may be mounted on the surface of the body or implanted in respective position.

Compilation of References

Abd-ElGawad, E. A., Ibraheem, M. A., & Fouly, E. H. (2013). Evaluation of supraspinatus muscle tears by ultrasonography and magnetic resonance imaging in comparison with surgical findings. *The Egyptian Journal of Radiology and Nuclear Medicine*, *44*(4), 829–834. doi:10.1016/j.ejrnm.2013.08.001

Abramovich, T. S., & Silverman, B. W. (1998). Wavelet thresholding via a Bayesian approach. *Journal of the Royal Statistical Society. Series B. Methodological*, *60*(4), 725–749. doi:10.1111/1467-9868.00151

AbuKhousa, E., Mohamed, N., & Al-Jaroodi, J. (2012). e-Health cloud: Opportunities and challenges. *Future Internet*, *4*(3), 621–645. doi:10.3390/fi4030621

Adeli, H., Zhou, Z., & Dadmehr, N. (2003). Analysis of EEG records in an epileptic patient using wavelet transform. *Journal of Neuroscience Methods*, *123*(1), 69–87. doi:10.1016/S0165-0270(02)00340-0 PMID:12581851

Agarwal, A., & Triggs, B. (2006). *Hyperfeatures - Multilevel local coding for visual recognition.* Paper presented at the Conference on Computer Vision. doi:10.1007/11744023_3

Agarwal, M., & Maheshwari, R. P. (2012). *Content Based Image Retrieval Based on Log Gabor Wavelet Transform. Advanced Materials Research.* Switzerland: Trans Tech Publications.

Ahmed, M. M., & Mohamad, D. B. (2008). Segmentation of brain MR images for tumor extraction by combining C-means clustering and Perona-Malik anisotropic diffusion model. *International Journal of Image Processing*, *2*(1), 27–34.

Ahuja, A. T., Ying, M., Ho, S. Y., Antonio, G., Lee, Y. P., & King, A. D. (2008). Ultrasound of malignant cervical lymph nodes. *Cancer Imaging; the Official Publication of the International Cancer Imaging Society*, *8*, 48–56. PMID:18390388

Ahumada, A. J., & Null, C. H. (1993). *Digital images and human vision. chapter Image quality: a multidimensional problem.* Cambridge, MA: MIT Press.

Ajiboye, A. B. (2005). A heuristic fuzzy logic approach to EMG pattern recognition for multifunctional prosthesis control. *Neural Systems and Rehabilitation Engineering. IEEE Transactions on*, *13*(3), 280–291.

Akgul, C., Rubin, D., Napel, S., Beaulieu, C., Greenspan, H., & Acar, B. (2011). Content-based image retrieval in radiology: Current status and future directions. *Journal of Digital Imaging*, *24*(2), 208–222. doi:10.1007/s10278-010-9290-9 PMID:20376525

Al-Ameen, Sulong & Johar. (2012). Fast Deblurring Method for Computed Tomography Medical Images Using a Novel Kernels Set. *International Journal of Bio-Science and Bio-Technology*, *4*(3), 9–20.

Alam, M. G. R., Cho, E. J., Huh, E. N., & Hong, C. S. (2014, January). Cloud based mental state monitoring system for suicide risk reconnaissance using wearable bio-sensors. In *Proceedings of the 8th International Conference on Ubiquitous Information Management and Communication* (p. 56). ACM. doi:10.1145/2557977.2558020

Aljabar, P., Wolz, R., & Rueckert, D. (2012). Manifold Learning for Medical Image Registration, Segmentation, and Classification. In K. Suzuki (Ed.), *Machine Learning in Computer-Aided Diagnosis: Medical Imaging Intelligence and Analysis*. IGI Global. doi:10.4018/978-1-4666-0059-1.ch017

Allison, B., Leeb, R., Brunner, C., Müller-Putz, G., Bauernfeind, G., Kelly, J., & Neuper, C. (2012). Toward smarter BCIs: Extending BCIs through hybridization and intelligent control. *Journal of Neural Engineering*, *9*(1), 013001. doi:10.1088/1741-2560/9/1/013001 PMID:22156029

Al-Marzouqi, H., & Al Regib, G. (2014). Texture similarity using periodically extended and adaptive curvelets. In *Signal and Information Processing (GlobalSIP),2014 IEEE Global Conference*. doi:10.1109/GlobalSIP.2014.7032261

Altschuler, I. (2001). A psychiatrist's experience with music as a therapeutic agent. *Nordic Journal of Music Therapy*, *10*(1), 69–76. doi:10.1080/08098130109478019

Alzu'bi, A., Jaber, T., & Amira, A. (2014). The effectiveness of LSI-based CBIR with image noise using wavelet-based texture. In *Image Processing Theory, Tools and Applications (IPTA), 2014 4th International Conference*. DOI: doi:10.1109/IPTA.2014.7001969

Amira, S. A., & Sourav, S. (2015). Computed Tomography Image Enhancement Using Cuckoo Search: A Log Transform Based Approach. *Journal of Signal and Information Processing*, *6*(03), 244–257. doi:10.4236/jsip.2015.63023

Amiri, S., Movahedi, M. M., Kazemi, K., & Parsaei, H. (2013). An automated MR image segmentation system using multi-layer perceptron neural network. *Journal of Biomedical Physics & Engineering*, *3*(4), 115–122. PMID:25505757

Anju, T. A., & Chandy, D. A. (2014). Brain image retrieval using Local Ternary Co-Occurrence Pattern and CDF 9/7 wavelet. In *Electronics and Communication Systems (ICECS),2014 International Conference*. DOI: doi:10.1109/ECS.2014.6892540

Antani, S., Xue, Z., Long, L. R., Bennett, D., & Ward, S. Thoma and G.R. (2011): *Is there a need for biomedical CBIR systems in clinical practice: Outcomes from a usability study*. Paper presented at the SPIE. doi:10.1117/12.878268

Anter, E., Tschabrunn, C. M., & Josephson, M. E. (2015). High-resolution mapping of scar-related atrial arrhythmias using smaller electrodes with closer interelectrode spacing. *Circulation: Arrhythmia and Electrophysiology*, *8*(3), 537–545. doi:10.1161/CIRCEP.114.002737 PMID:25792508

Antonie Maintz, J. B., & Max Viergerer, A. (1998). A survey of medical image registration. *Medical Image Analysis*, *2*(1), 1–36. doi:10.1016/S1361-8415(01)80026-8 PMID:10638851

Araki, T., Ikeda, N., Dey, N., Chakraborty, S., Saba, L., Kumar, D., & Suri, J. S. et al. (2015). A comparative approach of four different image registration techniques for quantitative assessment of coronary artery calcium lesions using intravascular ultrasound. *Computer Methods and Programs in Biomedicine*, *118*(2), 158–172. doi:10.1016/j.cmpb.2014.11.006 PMID:25523233

Arifin, A. Z., & Asano, A. (2006). Image segmentation by histogram thresholding using hierarchical cluster analysis. *Pattern Recognition Letters*, *27*(13), 1515–1521. doi:10.1016/j.patrec.2006.02.022

Arora, S., Acharya, K., Verma, A., & Panigrahi, P. K. (2006). Multilevel thresholding for image segmentation through a fast statistical recursive algorithm. *Pattern Recognition Letters*, *29*(2), 119–125. doi:10.1016/j.patrec.2007.09.005

Arthur, L., Zhou, J., & Do Minh, N. (2006). Nonsubsampled Contourlet Transform: Filter design and applications in denoising. In *Proceedings of the 12th IEEE International Conference on Image Processing*, (pp. 749–752). IEEE.

Arthur, D., Kirsten, B., Edwin, P., & Steven, S. (2007). Identifying bacterial genes and endosymbiont dna with glimmer. *Bioinformatics (Oxford, England)*, *23*, 7. PMID:17237039

Arthur, L, Zhou, & Do. (2005). Nonsubsampled Contourlet Transform: Theory, Design, and Applications. *IEEE Transactions on Image Processing*, *159*(10), 3089–3101. PMID:17022272

Awe, J.-H., Philips, W., Pizunca, A., & Lemahieu, I. (2001). A Novel Method for Adaptive Enhancement and unsupervised Segmentation of MRI Brain Image. *International Conference on Accoustics, speech and signal processing(ICASSP)*. IEEE.

Azar, J. C., Simonsson, M., Bengtsson, E., & Hast, A. (2015). Automated Classification of Glandular Tissue by Statistical Proximity Sampling. *International Journal of Biomedical Imaging*, *2015*, 1–11. doi:10.1155/2015/943104

Babu, G.R. & Sivakumar. (2013). Automatic 3D Brain Image Registration - Survey. *International Journal of Innovation. Management and Technology*, *4*(5), 502–505.

Bailer-Jones, C. A., Gupta, R., & Singh, H. P. (2001). *An introduction to artificial neural networks.* arXiv preprint astro-ph/0102224

Bajd, T., Kralj, A., Štefančič, M., & Lavrač, N. (1999). Use of functional electrical stimulation in the lower extremities of incomplete spinal cord injured patients. *Artificial Organs*, *23*(5), 403–409. doi:10.1046/j.1525-1594.1999.06360.x PMID:10378929

Balla-Arabé, S., & Gao, X. (2013). A multiphase entropy-based level set algorithm for MR breast image segmentation using lattice boltzmann model. In *Proc. Sino, Foreign, Interchange Workshop Intell. Sci. Intell. Data Eng*. doi:10.1007/978-3-642-36669-7_2

Balla-Arabe, S., & Gao, X. (2012). Image multi-thresholding by combining the lattice Boltzmann model and a localized level set algorithm. *Neurocomputing*, *93*, 106–114. doi:10.1016/j.neucom.2012.04.019

Balla-Arabé, S., Gao, X., & Wang, B. (2012). A fast and robust level set method for image segmentation using fuzzy clustering and lattice Boltzmann method. *IEEE Transactions on Systems, Man, and Cybernetics. Part B, Cybernetics*, *99*, 1–11. PMID:23076068

Balla-Arabe, S., Gao, X., & Wang, B. (2013). GPU Accelerated Edge-Region Based Level Set Evolution Constrained By 2D Gray-scale Histogram. *IEEE Transactions on Image Processing*, *10*(1), 1–11. PMID:23549895

Balla-Arabé, S., Wang, B., & Gao, X.-B. (2011). Level set region based image segmentation using lattice Boltzmann method. In *Proc. 7th Int. Conf. Comput. Intell. Security*. doi:10.1109/CIS.2011.257

Banhan, M., & Katsaggelos, A. K. (1997). Digital image restoration. *IEEE Signal Processing Magazine*, *14*(2), 24–41. doi:10.1109/79.581363

Barbhaiyam, C. R., Kumar, S., Ng, J., Tedrow, U., Koplan, B., John, R., & Michaud, G. F. et al. (2014). Overdrive pacing from downstream sites on multielectrode catheters to rapidly detect fusion and to diagnose macroreentrant atrial arrhythmias. *Circulation*, *129*(24), 2503–2510. doi:10.1161/CIRCULATIONAHA.113.008494 PMID:24812357

Barea, R., Boquete, L., Mazo, M., & López, E. (1999). *Guidance of a wheelchair using electrooculography.* Paper presented at the 3rd IMACS International Multiconference on Circuits, Systems, Communications and Computers (CSCC'99).

Barea, R., Boquete, L., Bergasa, L. M., López, E., & Mazo, M. (2003). Electro-oculographic guidance of a wheelchair using eye movements codification. *The International Journal of Robotics Research*, *22*(7-8), 641–652. doi:10.1177/02783649030227012

Barea, R., Boquete, L., Mazo, M., & López, E. (2002). System for assisted mobility using eye movements based on electrooculography. *Neural Systems and Rehabilitation Engineering. IEEE Transactions on*, *10*(4), 209–218.

Barea, R., Boquete, L., Mazo, M., & López, E. (2002b). Wheelchair guidance strategies using EOG. *Journal of Intelligent & Robotic Systems, 34*(3), 279–299. doi:10.1023/A:1016359503796

Barisci, N., & Hardalaç, F. (2007). Application of an adaptive neuro-fuzzy inference system for classification of behcet disease using the fast Fourier transforms method. *Expert Systems: International Journal of Knowledge Engineering and Neural Networks, 24*(2), 123–130. doi:10.1111/j.1468-0394.2007.00424.x

Barreto, A. B., Scargle, S. D., & Adjouadi, M. (2000). A practical EMG-based human-computer interface for users with motor disabilities. *Journal of Rehabilitation Research and Development, 37*(1), 53–64. PMID:10847572

Bauer, S., Fejes, T., Slotboom, J., Weist, R., Nolte, L. P., & Reyes, M. (2012). Segmentation of brain tumor images based on integrated hierarchical classification and regularization.*Proceedings MICCAI-BRATS.*

BBC News. (2012, May 31). Retrieved from http://www.bbc.com/news/health-18238356

Beckerman, B., Patton, R., Symons, C., McMillan, A., Gleason, S., Kerekes, R., . . . Nishikawa, R. (2009). *An Overview of the Data Analytics for Medicine Using Semi-Supervised learning (DAMSEL) Program.* Paper presented at the First Annual ORNL Biomedical Science & Engineering Conference, Chicago, IL.

Begelrnan, G., Gur, E., Rivli, E., Rudzsky, M., & Zalevsky, Z. (2004, October). Cell nuclei segmentation using fuzzy logic engine.*2004 International Conference on Image Processing, ICIP'04, 5*, 2937-2940. doi:10.1109/ICIP.2004.1421728

Berger, M. O. (1990). Snake Growing. In *Computer Vision Proc. First EuropeanConference on Computer Vision (ECCV'90).*

Bernardi, L., Porta, C., & Sleight, P. (2006). Cardiovascular, cerebrovascular, and respiratory changes induced by different types of music in musicians and non-musicians: The importance of silence. *Heart (British Cardiac Society), 92*(4), 445–452. doi:10.1136/hrt.2005.064600 PMID:16199412

Bernsen, J. (1986). Dynamic thresholding of gray level images. In *Proceedings of the 8th International Conference on Pattern Recognition*, (pp. 1251– 1255). Paris, France.

Besemer, J., & Borodovsky, M. (1999). Heuristic approach to deriving models for gene finding. *Nucleic Acids Research, 27*(19), 3911–3920. doi:10.1093/nar/27.19.3911 PMID:10481031

Beukema, R. J., Elvan, A., Smit, J. J., Delnoy, P. P., Misier, A. R., & Reddy, V. (2012). Pulmonary vein isolation to treat paroxysmal atrial fibrillation: Conventional versus multi-electrode radiofrequency ablation. *Journal of Interventional Cardiac Electrophysiology, 34*(2), 143–152. doi:10.1007/s10840-011-9653-2 PMID:22354772

Bezdek, J. C. (1981). *Pattern recognition with fuzzy objective function algorithms*. New York, NY: Plenum Press. doi:10.1007/978-1-4757-0450-1

Bharath, A. (1998). Steerable filters from Erlang functions.*Proc. 9th British Machine Vision Conference*, (pp. 144–153).

Bhatt, P., Rusiya, P., & Birchha, V. (2014). WAGBIR: Wavelet and Gabor Based Image Retrieval Technique for the Spatial-Color and Texture Feature Extraction Using BPN in Multimedia Database. In *Computational Intelligence and Communication Networks (CICN),2014 International Conference*. DOI: doi:10.1109/CICN.2014.71

Bibicu, D., Moraru, L., & Biswas, A. (2013). Thyroid nodule recognition based on feature selection and pixel classification methods. *Journal of Digital Imaging, 26*(1), 119–128. doi:10.1007/s10278-012-9475-5 PMID:22546981

Bibicu, D., Moraru, L., & Biswas, A. (2015). Efficient segmentation using active contours embedded in an image feature. *Journal of Medical Imaging and Health Informatics, 5*(2), 241–247. doi:10.1166/jmihi.2015.1379

Bilchick, K. C., & Berger, R. D. (2006). Heart rate variability. *Journal of Cardiovascular Electrophysiology, 17*(6), 691–694. doi:10.1111/j.1540-8167.2006.00501.x PMID:16836727

Billman, G. E. (2013). The LF/HF ratio does not accurately measure cardiac sympatho-vagal balance. *Frontiers in Physiology, 4*.

Binh, N. T., & Dien, T. A. (2013). Object Detection and Tracking in Contourlet Domain. *Context-Aware Systems and Applications*, *109*, 192–200. doi:10.1007/978-3-642-36642-0_20

Binh, N. T., & Khare, A. (2010). Multilevel threshold based image denoising in curvelet domain. *Journal of Computer Science and Technology*, *25*(3), 632–640. doi:10.1007/s11390-010-9352-y

Binh, N. T., & Khare, A. (2013). *Image Denoising, Deblurring and Object Tracking, A new Generation wavelet based approach*. Lap Lambert Academic Publishing.

Binh, N. T., Tuyet, V. T. H., & Vinh, P. C. (2015). Increasing the quality of medical images based on the combination of filters in ridgelet domain. *Nature of Computation and Communication, Springer*, *144*, 320–331. doi:10.1007/978-3-319-15392-6_30

Binitha, S., & Sathya, S. S. (2012). A survey of bio inspired optimization algorithms. *International Journal of Soft Computing and Engineering*, *2*(2), 137–151.

Bishop, C. M. (2006). *Pattern Recognition and Machine Learning*. Springer.

Biswal, D., Uvanesh, K., Champaty, B., Ray, S. S., & Pal, K. (2014). *Development of an ambulatory universal bio potential recording device*. Paper presented at the Control, Instrumentation, Communication and Computational Technologies (ICCICCT), 2014 International Conference on. doi:10.1109/ICCICCT.2014.6993130

Bloch, I., Gousseau, Y., Maître, H., Matignon, D., Schmitt, F., Sigelle, M., & Tupin, F. (2005). *Le traitement des images*. Département TSI – Télécom-Paris.

Bonato, P., Mork, P. J., Sherrill, D. M., & Westgaard, R. H. (2003). Data Mining of Motor Patterns Recorded with Wearable Technology. *IEEE Engineering in Medicine and Biology Magazine*, *22*(3), 110–119. doi:10.1109/MEMB.2003.1213634 PMID:12845827

Bourne, G. (2012). *Anatomy and physiology* (Vol. 1). Elsevier.

Bouslimi, R., Messaoudi, A., & Akaichi, J. (2013). Using a bag of words for automatic medical image annotation with a latent semantic. *International Journal of Artificial Intelligence & Applications*, *4*(3), 51–60. doi:10.5121/ijaia.2013.4305

Bradley, D., & Roth, G. (2007). Adaptive thresholding using the integral image. *Journal of Graphics, GPU, and Game Tools*, *12*(2), 13–21. doi:10.1080/2151237X.2007.10129236

Braem, B., Moerman, I., & Blondia, C. (2007). A Low Delay Protocol for Multihop Wireless Body Area Networks. *Fourth Annual International Conference on Mobile and Ubiquitous Systems: Networking & Services (MobiQuitous)*.

Breiman, L. (2001). Random forests. *Machine Learning*, *45*(1), 5–32. doi:10.1023/A:1010933404324

Breiman, L., Friedman, J. H., Olshen, R. A., & Stone, C. J. (1984). *Classification and Regression Trees*. Chapman & Hall.

Brimelow, A. (2012). *Trial of "touchless" gaming technology in surgery*. Academic Press.

Bronzino, J. D. (1999). *Biomedical engineering handbook* (Vol. 2). CRC Press.

Brownlee, J. (2013). *A Tour of Machine Learning Algorithms*. Retrieved from http://machinelearningmastery.com/a-tour-of-machine-learning-algorithms/

Brown, T. A. (2002). *Genomes 2*. John Wiley & Sons Inc.

Buch, E., & Shivkumar, K. (2015). Catheter Ablation of Atrial Fibrillation: Advent of Second-Generation Technologies. *Journal of the American College of Cardiology*, *66*(12), 1361–1363. doi:10.1016/j.jacc.2015.07.056 PMID:26383723

Bui, A. A. T., & Taira, R. K. (Eds.). (2010). *Medical imaging informatics*. New York: Springer. doi:10.1007/978-1-4419-0385-3

Bullmore, E., & Sporns, O. (2009). Complex brain networks: Graph theoretical analysis of structural and functional systems. *Nature Reviews. Neuroscience*, *10*(3), 186–198. doi:10.1038/nrn2575 PMID:19190637

Burns, T., Rogers, S., Ruck, D., & Oxley, M. (1994). Discrete, spatiotemporal, wavelet multiresolution analysis method for computing optical flow. *Optical Engineering (Redondo Beach, Calif.)*, *33*(7), 2236–2247. doi:10.1117/12.172250

Butler, J., MacCallum, I., Kleber, M., Shlyakhter, I. A., Belmonte, M. K., Lander, E. S., & Jaffe, D. B. et al. (2008). AllPaths: De novo assembly of whole-genome shotgun microreads. *Genome Research*, *18*(5), 810–820. doi:10.1101/gr.7337908 PMID:18340039

Cai, T. W., Kim, J., & Feng, D. D. (2008). *Content-based medical image retrieval in Biomedical Information Technology*. Burlington: Academic Press.

Camargo, J. E., Caicedo, J. C., & Gonzalez, F. A. (2013). A kernel-based framework for image collection exploration. *Journal of Visual Languages and Computing*, *24*(1), 53–57. doi:10.1016/j.jvlc.2012.10.008

Campbell, M. (2012). Kinect imaging lets surgeons keep their focus. *New Scientist*. Retrieved from https://www.newscientist.com/article/mg21428655.200-kinect-imaging-lets-surgeons-keep-their-focus

Candemir, S., Jaeger, S., Palaniappan, K., Musco, J. P., Singh, R. K. Xue, Z., … McDonald, C.J. (2014). Lung Segmentation in Chest Radiographs Using Anatomical Atlases With Nonrigid Registration. IEEE Transactions on Medical Imaging, 33(2), 577-590. DOI: doi:10.1109/TMI.2013.2290491

Candes & Donoho. (1999). *Curvelets: A surprisingly effective nonadaptive representation of objects with edges* (pp. 123–143). Nashville, TN: Vanderbilt University Press.

Candes, E. J. (1998). *Ridgelets: Theory and Applications*. (PhD thesis). Department of Statistics, Stanford University.

Candes, E.J. & Donoho, D.L (1999). Ridgelets: a Key to Higher- Diemensional Intermittency?. *Philosophical Transactions of the Royal Society A: Mathematical, Physical & Engineering Sciences, 357*(1760), 2495-2509

Candes, E. J. (1998). *Ridgelets: Theory and Applications*. Stanford University.

Candes, E. J. (1999). *Monoscale ridgelets for the representation of images with edges. Dept. Statist., Stanford Univ.* Stanford, CA: Technical Representation.

Candes, E. J., Demanet, L., Donoho, D. L., & Ying, L. (2006). Fast Discrete Curvelet Transforms. *Multiscale Modeling & Simulation*, *5*(3), 861–899. doi:10.1137/05064182X

Candes, E. J., & Donoho, D. L. (2000). Curvelets - A Surprisingly Effective Nonadaptive Representation for Objects with Edges. In *Curves and Surface Fitting* (pp. 105–120). Saint-Malo: Vanderbilt University Press.

Candes, J., & Demanet, L. (2005). The curvelet representation of wave propagators is optimally sparse. *Communications on Pure and Applied Mathematics*, *58*(11), 1472–1528. doi:10.1002/cpa.20078

Cao, H., Li, H., Stocco, L., & Victor, C. M., Leung (2010). Demonstration of A Novel Wireless Three-pad ECG System for Generating Conventional 12-lead Signals.*5th Annual International ICST Conference on Body Area Networks*. doi:10.1145/2221924.2221931

Caputo, B., Muller, H., Syeda-Mahmood, T., Duncan, J., Wang, F., & Kalpathy-Cramer, J. (Eds.). Medical Content-Based Retrieval for Clinical Decision Support, Vol. 5853 of Lecture Notes in Computer Science. Berlin: Springer. doi:10.1007/978-3-642-11769-5

Caputo, B., Syeda-Mahmood, T., & Wang, F. (2010). *Overview of the first workshop on medical content- based retrieval for clinical decision support*. MICCAI 2009.

Cardiology, T. F. E. S. (1996). Heart rate variability standards of measurement, physiological interpretation, and clinical use. *European Heart Journal*, *17*(3), 354–381. doi:10.1093/oxfordjournals.eurheartj.a014868 PMID:8737210

Cardiology, T. F. E. S., & Cardiology, T. F. E. S. (1996). the North American Society of Pacing and Electrophysiology. Heart rate variability: Standards of measurement, physiological interpretation and clinical use. *Circulation*, *93*(5), 1043–1065. doi:10.1161/01.CIR.93.5.1043 PMID:8598068

Carneiro, G., Georgescu, B., & Good, S. (2008). *Knowledge-based Automated Fetal Biometrics*. SIEMENS White Paper.

Carneiro, G., Georgescu, B., Good, S., & Comaniciu, D. (2007). Automatic fetal measurements in ultrasound using constrained probabilistic boosting tree. *Med Image Comput Comput Assist Interv*, *10*(Pt 2), 571–579. PMID:18044614

Carneiro, G., Georgescu, B., Good, S., & Comaniciu, D. (2008). Detection and Measurement of Fetal Anatomies from Ultrasound Images using a Constrained Probabilistic Boosting Tree. Medical Imaging. *IEEE Transactions on*, *27*(9), 1342–1355.

Carvalho, T. D., Pastre, C. M., de Godoy, M. F., Fereira, C., Pitta, F. O., & de Abreu, L. C. (2011). Fractal correlation property of heart rate variability in chronic obstructive pulmonary disease. *International Journal of Chronic Obstructive Pulmonary Disease*, *6*, 23. doi:10.2147/COPD.S15099 PMID:21311690

Caselles, V., Catte, F., Coll, T., & Dibos, F. (1993). *A geometric model for active contours in image processing*. Numerical Math.

Caselles, V., Catte, F., Coll, T., & Dibos, F. (1993). *A geometric model for active contours*. Numerische Mathematik.

Caselles, V., Kimmel, R., & Sapiro, G. (1995). Geodesic active contours. In *Proceedings of IEEE international conference on computer vision*. doi:10.1109/ICCV.1995.466871

Caselles, V., Kimmel, R., & Sapiro, G. (1997). Geodesic active contours. *International Journal of Computer Vision, No.*, *1*(1), 61–79. doi:10.1023/A:1007979827043

Cauvin, J. M. (2003). Computer-assisted diagnosis system in digestive endoscopy.*IEEE Transaction on Information Technology in Biomedicine*, *7*(4), 256-262.

Ceresnak, S. R., Nappo, L., Janson, C. M., & Pass, R. H. (2015). Tricking CARTO: Cryoablation of Supraventricular Tachycardia in Children with Minimal Radiation Exposure Using the CARTO3 System. *Pacing and Clinical Electrophysiology*, *28*(Sep). doi: doi:10.1111/pace.12754 PMID:26412504

Cescon, C., Raimondi, E. E., Začesta, V., Drusany-Starič, K., Martsidis, K., & Merletti, R. (2014). Characterization of the motor units of the external anal sphincter in pregnant women with multichannel surface EMG. *International Urogynecology Journal and Pelvic Floor Dysfunction*, *25*(8), 1097–1103. doi:10.1007/s00192-014-2356-3 PMID:24623258

Chae, S., Oral, H., Good, E., Dey, S., Wimmer, A., Crawford, T., & Chugh, A. et al. (2007). Atrial tachycardia after circumferential pulmonary vein ablation of atrial fibrillation: Mechanistic insights, results of catheter ablation, and risk factors for recurrence. *Journal of the American College of Cardiology*, *50*(18), 1781–1787. doi:10.1016/j.jacc.2007.07.044 PMID:17964043

Champaty, B., Jose, J., Pal, K., & Thirugnanam, A. (2014). *Development of EOG based human machine interface control system for motorized wheelchair.* Paper presented at the Emerging Research Areas: Magnetics, Machines and Drives (AICERA/iCMMD), 2014 Annual International Conference on. doi:10.1109/AICERA.2014.6908256

Chandhok, C., Chaturvedi, S., & Khurshid, A. A. (2012). An approach to image segmentation using k-means clustering algorithm. *International Journal of Information Technology*, *1*(1), 11–17.

Chang, H., & Valentino, D. (2006). Image segmentation using a charged fluid method. *Journal of Electronic Imaging*, *15*(2).

Chang, H., & Valentino, D. (2008). An electrostatic deformable model for medical image segmentation. *Computerized Medical Imaging and Graphics*, *32*(1), 22–35. doi:10.1016/j.compmedimag.2007.08.012 PMID:17933492

Chang, Z., Li, G., Li, J., Zhang, Y., Ashby, C., Liu, D., & Huang, X. et al. (2015). Bridger: A new framework for de novo transcriptome assembly using RNA-seq data. *Genome Biology*, *16*(1), 30. doi:10.1186/s13059-015-0596-2 PMID:25723335

Chan, T., & Vese, L. (2001). Active contours without edges. *IEEE Transactions on Image Processing*, *10*(2), 266–277. doi:10.1109/83.902291 PMID:18249617

Chapelle, O. A. (Ed.). (2006). *Semi-Supervised Learning*. MIT Press.

Chapin, J. K., Moxon, K. A., Markowitz, R. S., & Nicolelis, M. A. (1999). Real-time control of a robot arm using simultaneously recorded neurons in the motor cortex. *Nature Neuroscience*, *2*(7), 664–670. doi:10.1038/10223 PMID:10404201

Chawla, N. V. (2002). Synthetic Minority Over-sampling Technique. *Journal of Artificial Intelligence Research*, *16*, 321–357.

Chen, C.-M., Lu, H. Y. H.-S., & Han, K.-C. (2000). A textuel approch based on gabor fonctions for texture edge detection in ultrasound images. Institute of Biomedical Engineering, National Taiwan University and Institute of Statistics, National Chiao-Tung University.

Chen, X., Hu, X., & Shen, X. (2009). *Spatial weighting for bag-or-visual-words and its application in content-based image retrieval.* Paper presented at the Pacific-Asia Conference on Knowledge Discovery and Data Mining. doi:10.1007/978-3-642-01307-2_90

Chen, Y., & Newman, W. S. (2004). *A human-robot interface based on electrooculography.* Paper presented at the Robotics and Automation, 2004.

Chen, Y., & Newman, W. S. (2004). *A human-robot interface based on electrooculography.* Paper presented at the Robotics and Automation, 2004. Proceedings. ICRA'04. 2004 IEEE International Conference on.

Cheng, B., & Liu, G.-Y. (2008). *Emotion recognition from surface EMG signal using wavelet transform and neural network.* Paper presented at the 2nd International Conference on Bioinformatics and Biomedical Engineering (ICBBE). doi:10.1109/ICBBE.2008.670

Cheng, G., Han, J., Guo, L., Liu, Z., Bu, S., & Ren, J. (2015). Effective and Efficient Midlevel Visual Elements-Oriented Land-Use Classification Using VHR Remote Sensing Images. IEEE Transactions on Geoscience and Remote Sensing, 53(8). DOI: doi:10.1109/TGRS.2015.2393857

Chen, S. A., Tai, C. T., Chiang, C. E., Ding, Y. A., & Chang, M. S. (1998). Focal atrial tachycardia: Reanalysis of the clinical and electrophysiologic characteristics and prediction of successful radiofrequency ablation. *Journal of Cardiovascular Electrophysiology*, *9*(4), 355–365. doi:10.1111/j.1540-8167.1998.tb00924.x PMID:9581952

Chen, S., Chiang, C., Yang, C., Cheng, C., Wu, T., Wang, S., & Chang, M. S. et al. (1994). Sustained atrial tachycardia in adult patients. Electrophysi- ological characteristics, pharmacological response, possible mechanisms, and effects of radiofrequency ablation. *Circulation, 90*(3), 1262–1278. doi:10.1161/01.CIR.90.3.1262 PMID:8087935

Chen, Y. (2012). Microscopic Image Segmenting and Classification with RBF Neural Network.*2012 International Symposium on Information Science and Engineering (ISISE)*. doi:10.1109/ISISE.2012.78

Choi, C., Choi, Y. K., & Park, C. C. (2004). The color retrieval system with color component analysis. *Imaging Systems and Techniques, 2004. (IST).2004 IEEE International Workshop*. doi:10.1109/IST.2004.1397277

Choi, K., & Cichocki, A. (2008). *Control of a wheelchair by motor imagery in real time. In Intelligent Data Engineering and Automated Learning–IDEAL 2008* (pp. 330–337). Springer. doi:10.1007/978-3-540-88906-9_42

Christopher, B. B. (1997). *Identification of genes in human genomicdna*. (Ph.D. Thesis). Stanford University, Stanford, CA.

Chui, M. Feng, Wang, Li & Xu. (2012). Image Denoising Method with Adaptive Bayes threshold in Nonsubsampled Contourlet Domain. American Applied Science Research Institute, 1, 512 – 518.

Chunming, L., Rui, H., Zhaohua, D., Gatenby, J. C., Metaxas, D. N., & Gore, J. C. (2011). A Level Set Method for Image Segmentation in the Presence of Intensity Inhomogeneities With Application to MRI. Image Processing. *IEEE Transactions on, 20*(7), 2007–2016.

Clausi, D.A., & Jernigan, M.E. (1999). *Designing Gabor Filters for optimal texture separability*. Department of Systems Design Engineering, University of Waterloo.

Clonda, J.-M. L., & Goulard, B. (2004). Complex Daubechies wavelets: Properties and statistical image modeling. *Signal Processing, 84*(1), 1–23. doi:10.1016/j.sigpro.2003.06.001

Cobzas, D., Birkbeck, N., Schmidt, M., Jagersand, M., & Murtha, A. (2007). 3D variational brain tumor segmentation using a high dimensional feature set. *IEEE 11th International Conference on Computer Vision.*

Cobzas, D., Birkbeck, N., Schmidt, M., Jagersand, M., & Murtha, A. (2007). *3D variational brain tumor segmentation using a high dimensional feature set*. Computer Vision. doi:10.1109/ICCV.2007.4409130

Coco, G. L., Coco, D. L., Cicero, V., Oliveri, A., Verso, G. L., & Piccoli, F. (2005). Individual and health-related quality of life assessment in amyotrophic lateral sclerosis patients and their caregivers. *Journal of the Neurological Sciences, 238*(1), 11–17. doi:10.1016/j.jns.2005.05.018 PMID:16109426

Cohen, L. D. (1991). On Active Contour Models and Balloons. *CVGIP. Image Understanding, 53*(2), 211–218. doi:10.1016/1049-9660(91)90028-N

Cohen, L. D., & Cohen, I. (1993). Finite Element Methods for Active Contour models and Balloons for 2D and 3D Images. *IEEE Transactions on Pattern Analysis and Machine Intelligence, 15*(11), 1131–1147. doi:10.1109/34.244675

Collins, M., Schapire, R. E., & Singer, Y. (2002). Logistic regression, AdaBoost and Bregman distances. *Machine Learning, 48*(1/3), 253–285. doi:10.1023/A:1013912006537

Comaniciu, D., Meer, P., & Foran, D. J. (1999). Image-guided decision support system for pathology. *International Journal of Machine Vision and Applications., 11*(4), 213–224. doi:10.1007/s001380050104

Conti, G., Ucelli, G., & De Amicis, R. (2005). Automatic extraction of semantic information for a context sensitive multimodal framework for VR. In *Cyberworlds, 2005.International Conference*. doi:10.1109/CW.2005.25

Corrado, D., Basso, C., Leoni, L., Tokajuk, B., Bauce, B., Frigo, G., & Thiene, G. et al. (2005). Three-dimensional electroanatomic voltage mapping increases accuracy of diagnosing arrhythmogenic right ventricular cardiomyopathy/dysplasia. *Circulation, 111*(23), 3042–3050. doi:10.1161/CIRCULATIONAHA.104.486977 PMID:15939822

Corso, J. J., Yuille, A. L., Sicotte, N. L., & Toga, A. W. (2007). Detection and segmentation of pathological structures by the extended graph shifts algorithm. *Medical Image Computing and Computer Aided Intervention, 1*, 985–994. PMID:18051154

Costa Oliveira, M., & Raniery Ferreira, J. (2013). A Bag-of-Tasks approach to speed up the lung nodules retrieval in the BigData age. In *e-Health Networkg, Applications & Services (Healthcom), 2013 IEEE 15th International Conference*. DOI: doi:10.1109/HealthCom.2013.6720753

Costianes, P. J., & Plock, J. B. (2010). Gray-level co-occurrence matrices as features in edge enhanced images. In *Applied Imagery Pattern Recognition Workshop (AIPR), 2010 IEEE 39th*. doi:10.1109/AIPR.2010.5759705

Cowan, R. E., Fregly, B. J., Boninger, M. L., Chan, L., Rodgers, M. M., & Reinkensmeyer, D. J. (2012). Recent trends in assistive technology for mobility. *Journal of Neuroengineering and Rehabilitation, 9*(1), 20. doi:10.1186/1743-0003-9-20 PMID:22520500

Cozman, F., & Cohen, I. (2006). Risks of Semi-Supervised Learning. In O. Chapelle, B. Schölkopf, & A. Zien (Eds.), *Semi-Supervised Learning, September 2006*. MIT Press.

Crawford, B., Miller, K., Shenoy, P., & Rao, R. (2005). *Real-time classification of electromyographic signals for robotic control.* Paper presented at the AAAI.

Criminisi, A., Robertson, D., Konukoglu, E., Shotton, J., Pathak, S., White, S., & Siddiqui, K. (2013). Regression Forests for Efficient Anatomy Detection and Localization in Computed Tomography Scans. In *Medical Image Analysis (MedIA)*. Elsevier.

Criswell, E. (2010). *Cram's introduction to surface electromyography*. Jones & Bartlett Publishers.

Crosby, J. (2014). Mayo seeks to dominate with data. *Star Tribune*. Retrieved from http://www.startribune.com/mayo-seeks-to-dominate-with-data/285132621/

Csurka, G., Dance, C., Fan, L., Willamowski, J., & Bray, C. (2004). *Visual categorization with bags of keypoints.* Paper presented at the ECCV'04 workshop on Statistical Learning in ComputerVision.

Cunha, L. D., Zhou, J., & Do, M. N. (2006). The Nonsubsampled Contourlet Transform: Theory, Design, and Applications. *IEEE Transactions on Image Processing, 15*(10), 3089–3101. doi:10.1109/TIP.2006.877507 PMID:17022272

Dai, W., & Ji, W. (2014). A MapReduce implementation of C4.5 decision tree algorithm. *International Journal of Database Theory and Application, 7*(1), 49–60. doi:10.14257/ijdta.2014.7.1.05

Dalevi, D., Ivanova, N. N., Mavromatis, K., Hooper, S. D., Szeto, E., Hugenholtz, P., & Markowitz, V. M. et al. (2008). Annotation of metagenome short reads using proxygenes. *Bioinformatics (Oxford, England), 24*(16), i713. doi:10.1093/bioinformatics/btn276 PMID:18689842

Das, S., & Kundu, M. K. (2012). *Effective Management of Medical Information Through A Novel Blind Watermarking Technique*. Springer Science & Business Media, LLC.

Datta, R., Joshi, D., Li, J., & Wang, J. Z. (2008). Image Retrieval: Ideas, Influences, and Trends of the New Age. *ACM Computing Surveys, 40*(2), 1–60. doi:10.1145/1348246.1348248

Davis, W. B., Gfeller, K. E., & Thaut, M. H. (2008). *An introduction to music therapy: Theory and practice*. ERIC.

de Groot, N. M., Schalij, M. J., Zeppenfeld, K., Blom, N. A., Van der Velde, E. T., & Van der Wall, E. E. (2003). Voltage and activation mapping: How the recording technique affects the outcome of catheter ablation procedures in patients with congenital heart disease. *Circulation*, *108*(17), 2099–2106. doi:10.1161/01.CIR.0000092893.11893.38 PMID:14517169

De Luca, C. J. (1979). Physiology and mathematics of myoelectric signals. *Biomedical Engineering, IEEE Transactions on*, (6), 313-325.

De Oliveiraa, J., Machadob, A., & Chaveza, G. (2010). MammoSys: A content-based image retrieval system using breast density patterns. *Computer Methods and Programs in Biomedicine*.

Del Carpio Munoz, F., Buescher, T. L., & Asirvatham, S. J. (2010). Three-dimensional mapping of cardiac arrhythmias: What do the colors really mean? *Circulation: Arrhythmia and Electrophysiology*, *6*(6), 6–11. doi:10.1161/CIRCEP.110.960161 PMID:21156773

Demirhan, A., & Guler, I. (2011). Combining stationary wavelet transform and self-organizing maps for brain MR image segmentation. *Engineering Applications of Artificial Intelligence*, *24*(2), 358–367. doi:10.1016/j.engappai.2010.09.008

Depeursinge, A., Vargas, A., Gaillard, F., Platon, A., Geissbuhler, A., Poletti, P.A., et al (2012). Case-based lung image categorization and retrieval for interstitial lung diseases: Clinical workflows. *International Journal of Computer Assisted Radiology Surgery*, *7*(1), 97–110.

Derek Hill, L. G., & Philipp Batchelor, G. (2001). Medical image registration. *Physics in Medicine and Biology*, *46*(3), R1–R45. doi:10.1088/0031-9155/46/3/201 PMID:11277237

Desai, K., & Sankhe, M. S. (2012). *A real-time fetal ECG feature extraction using multiscale discrete wavelet transform.* Paper presented at the Biomedical Engineering and Informatics (BMEI), 2012 5th International Conference on. doi:10.1109/BMEI.2012.6512966

Detterbeck, F. C., Boffa, D. J., & Tanoue, L. T. (2009). The new lung cancer staging system. *Chest*, *136*(1), 260–271. doi:10.1378/chest.08-0978 PMID:19584208

Devaul, R. W., Sung, M., Gips, J., & Pentland, S. (2003). MIThril 2003: Applications and architecture. In *Proceedings of the International Semantic Web Conference (SWC)*.

Dey, N., Biswas, S., Das, P., Das, A., & Chaudhuri, S. S. (2012). *Feature analysis for the reversible watermarked electrooculography signal using low distortion prediction-error expansion.* Paper presented at the Communications, Devices and Intelligent Systems (CODIS), 2012 International Conference on. doi:10.1109/CODIS.2012.6422280

Dey, A., Banerjee, A., Bhattacharya, D., & Tibarewala, D. (2015). *Does Music Affect HRV Impulse? A Time Domain Study. In Computational Advancement in Communication Circuits and Systems* (pp. 453–461). Springer.

Dey, A., Palit, S. K., Bhattacharya, D., & Tibarewala, D. (2014). Significance Analysis of Different Time Domain Measures Of HRV to Differentiate Normal and On-Music States. *Significance*, *3*(3).

Dey, N., Ashour, A. S., Ashour, A. S., & Singh, A. (2015a). Digital Analysis of Microscopic Images in Medicine. *Journal of Advanced Microscopy Research*, *10*(1), 1–13. doi:10.1166/jamr.2015.1229

Dey, N., Ashour, A. S., & Hassanien, A. E. (2015b). *Generation of Feature Detectors and their Numerous Applications: A Recap. Image Feature Detectors Foundations, Innovations, and Applications. Springer.*

Dhasal, P., Shrivastava, S. S., Gupta, H., & Kumar, P. (2012). An Optimized Feature Selection for Image Classification Based on SVM-ACO. *International Journal of Advanced Computer Research*, *2*(3), 123–128.

Diagnostics and Interventional Radiology. (n.d.) *Computational Environment for Radiotherapy Research*. Retrieved from http://www.cerr.info

Dickhaus, H., & Heinrich, H. (1996). Classifying biosignals with wavelet networks[a method for noninvasive diagnosis]. *Engineering in Medicine and Biology Magazine, IEEE, 15*(5), 103–111. doi:10.1109/51.537066

Dilaveris, P. E., & Gialafos, J. E. (2001). P-wave dispersion: A novel predictor of paroxysmal atrial fibrillation. *Annals of Noninvasive Electrocardiology, 6*(2), 159–165. doi:10.1111/j.1542-474X.2001.tb00101.x PMID:11333174

Ding, D., & Cooper, R. (2005). Electric powered wheelchairs. *Control Systems, IEEE, 25*(2), 22–34. doi:10.1109/MCS.2005.1411382

Divi, K., & Liu, H. (2013, September). Modeling of wban and cloud integration for secure and reliable healthcare. In *Proceedings of the 8th International Conference on Body Area Networks* (pp. 128-131). ICST (Institute for Computer Sciences, Social-Informatics and Telecommunications Engineering). doi:10.4108/icst.bodynets.2013.253706

Dixit, S., & Callans, D. J. (2002). Role of contact and noncontact mapping in the curative ablation of tachyarrhythmias. *Current Opinion in Cardiology, 17*(1), 65–72. doi:10.1097/00001573-200201000-00010 PMID:11790936

Dixon, W. J., & Massey, F. J. (1969). *Introduction to statistical analysis* (Vol. 344). McGraw-Hill New York.

Doi, K. (2007). Computer-aided diagnosis in medical imaging: Historical review, current status and future potential. *Computerized Medical Imaging and Graphics, 31*(4–5), 198–211. doi:10.1016/j.compmedimag.2007.02.002 PMID:17349778

Do, M. N., & Vetterli, M. (2005). The Contourlet Transform: An Efficient Directional Multiresolution Image Representation. *IEEE Transactions on Image Processing, 14*(12), 2091–2106. doi:10.1109/TIP.2005.859376 PMID:16370462

Donoho, D. L., & Duncan, M. R. (2000). Digital curvelet transform: Strategy, implementation and experiments. Rpoc. *SPIE, 4056*, 12–29.

Donoho, L. (1998). *Orthonormal ridgelets and linear singularities. Tech. Report*. Department of Statistics, Stanford University.

Doukas, C., Pliakas, T., & Maglogiannis, I. (2010). Mobile Healthcare Information Management utilizing Cloud Computing and Android OS. In *Proc. IEEE Eng. Med. Bio. Soc.*

Dou, W. B., Ruan, S., Chen, Y. P., Bloyet, D., & Constans, J. M. (2007). A framework of fuzzy information fusion for the segmentation of brain tumor tissues on MR images. *Image and Vision Computing, 25*(2), 164–171. doi:10.1016/j.imavis.2006.01.025

Drakonaki, E. E., Allen, G. M., & Wilson, D. J. (2009). Real-time ultrasound elastography of the normal Achilles tendon: Reproducibility and pattern description. *Clinical Radiology, 64*(12), 1196–1202. doi:10.1016/j.crad.2009.08.006 PMID:19913130

Drost, G., Stegeman, D. F., van Engelen, B. G., & Zwarts, M. J. (2006). Clinical applications of high-density surface EMG: A systematic review. *Journal of Electromyography and Kinesiology, 16*(6), 586–602. doi:10.1016/j.jelekin.2006.09.005 PMID:17085302

Dudoit, S., & Fridyyand, J. (2002). A prediction-based resampling method for estimating the number of clusters in a dataset. *Genome Biology, 3*(7).

Dunlop, D. D., & Tamhane, A. C. (2000). *Statistics and data analysis: from elementary to intermediate*. Prentice Hall.

Dunn, J. (1974). Well Separated Clusters and Optimal Fuzzy Partitions. *Cybernetics, 4*(1), 95–104. doi:10.1080/01969727408546059

Dunn, J. C. (1973). A fuzzy relative of the ISODATA process and its use in detecting compact well-separated clusters. *Journal of Cybernetics*, *3*(3), 32–57. doi:10.1080/01969727308546046

Eakins, J. P., Boardman, J. M., & Graham, M. E. (1998). Similarity retrieval of trade mark images. *IEEE Multimedia*, *5*(2), 53-63.

Earley, M., Showkathali, R., Alzetani, M., Kistler, P. M., Gupta, D., Abrams, D. J., & Schilling, R. J. et al. (2006). Radiofrequency ablation of arrhythmias guided by non-fluoroscopic catheter location: A prospective randomized trial. *European Heart Journal*, *27*(10), 1223–1229. doi:10.1093/eurheartj/ehi834 PMID:16613932

Edge, S. B., Byrd, D. R., Compton, C. C., Frtiz, A. G., Greene, F. L., & Trotti Eds, A. (2010). *AJCC Cancer Staging Manual and Handbook*. New York: Springer.

Edwards (1992). *Discrete Wavelet Transforms: Theory and Implementation*. Academic Press.

Ehrenfeucht, A., Harju, T., Petre, I., Prescott, D. M., & Rozenberg, G. (2004). *Computation in Living Cells: Gene Assembly in Ciliates*. Springer. doi:10.1007/978-3-662-06371-2

El Khouli, R. H., Macura, K. J., Jacobs, M. A., Khalil, T. H., Kamel, I. R., Dwyer, A., & Bluemke, D. A. (2009). Dynamic contrast-enhanced MRI of the breast: Quantitative method for kinetic curve type assessment. *AJR. American Journal of Roentgenology*, *193*(4), W295-300. doi:10.2214/AJR.09.2483 PMID:19770298

El-Dansham, Hosny, & Salem. (2010). Hybrid intelligent techniques for MRI brain images classification. *Digital Signal Processing*, *20*, 433–441.

Ellis, R. J., & Thayer, J. F. (2010). Music and autonomic nervous system (dys) function. *Music Perception*, *27*(4), 317–326. doi:10.1525/mp.2010.27.4.317 PMID:21197136

El-Naqa, I., Yang, Y. Y., Wernick, M. N., Galatsanos, N. P., & Nishikawa, R. (2002). Support vector machine learning for detection of microcalcifications in mammograms. *IEEE Transactions on Medical Imaging*, *21*, 1552–1563. doi:10.1109/TMI.2002.806569 PMID:12588039

Eranki, A., Cortes, N., Feren, Z. G., & Sikdar, S. (2013). *A Novel Application of Musculoskeletal Ultrasound Imaging*. Academic Press.

Erdt, M., Steger, S., Sakas, G., & Fraunhofer, I. G. D. (2012). Regmentation: A New View Of Segmentation and Registration Germany, Technical University Darmstadt, Darmstadt, Germany. *Journal of Radiation Oncology Informatics*, *4*(1), 1-23.

Eschler, J., O'Leary, K., Kendall, L., Ralston, J. D., & Pratt, W. (2015). Systematic Inquiry for Design of Health Care Information Systems: An Example of Elicitation of the Patient Stakeholder Perspective. In *System Sciences (HICSS), 2015 48th Hawaii International Conference*. DOI: doi:10.1109/HICSS.2015.339

Estner, H. L., Deisenhofer, I., Luik, A., Ndrepepa, G., von Bary, C., Zrenner, B., & Schmitt, C. (2006). Electrical isolation of pulmonary veins in patients with atrial fibrillation: Reduction of fluoroscopy exposure and procedure duration by the use of a non-fluoroscopic navigation system (navx). *Europace*, *8*(8), 583–587. doi:10.1093/europace/eul079 PMID:16831837

Ewan, B., Michele, C., & Richard, D. (2004). *Gene wise and genome wise*. Genome Res.

Farina, D., Cescon, C., & Merletti, R. (2002). Influence of anatomical, physical, and detection-system parameters on surface EMG. *Biological Cybernetics*, *86*(6), 445–456. doi:10.1007/s00422-002-0309-2 PMID:12111273

Farshchi, S., Nuyujukian, P. H., Pesterev, A., Mody, I., & Judy, J. W. (2006). A TinyOS-Based Wireless Neural Interface. *Proceedings of the 26th Annual International Conference of the IEEE EMBS*, *53*(7), 1416-1424.

Fehr, L., Langbein, W. E., & Skaar, S. B. (2000). Adequacy of power wheelchair control i terfaces for persons with severe disabilities: A clinical survey. *Journal of Rehabilitation Research and Development*, *37*(3), 353–360. PMID:10917267

Feleppa, E. J., Mamou, J., Porter, C. R., & Machi, J. (2011). Quantitative ultrasound in cancer imaging. *Seminars in Oncology*, *38*(1), 136–150. doi:10.1053/j.seminoncol.2010.11.006 PMID:21362522

Felzer, T., & Freisleben, B. (2002). *HaWCoS: the hands-free wheelchair control system.* Paper presented at the fifth international ACM conference on Assistive technologies. doi:10.1145/638249.638273

Fergus, R., Fei-Fei, L., Perona, P., & Zisserman, A. (2005). *Learning object categories from Google's image search.* Academic Press.

Fernando, N., Seng, W. L., & Wenny, R. (2013). Mobile cloud computing: A survey. *Future Generation Computer Systems*, *29*(1), 84–106. doi:10.1016/j.future.2012.05.023

Ferreira, A., Silva, R., Celeste, W., Bastos Filho, T. F., & Sarcinelli Filho, M. (2007). *Human–machine interface based on muscular and brain signals applied to a robotic wheelchair.* Paper presented at the Journal of Physics: Conference Series.

Ferreira, A., Celeste, W. C., Cheein, F. A., Bastos-Filho, T. F., Sarcinelli-Filho, M., & Carelli, R. (2008). Journal of NeuroEngineering and Rehabilitation. *Journal of Neuroengineering and Rehabilitation*, *5*, 10. doi:10.1186/1743-0003-5-10 PMID:18366775

Fesmire, F. M., Percy, R. F., Bardoner, J. B., Wharton, D. R., & Calhoun, F. B. (1998). Usefulness of automated serial 12-lead ECG monitoring during the initial emergency department evaluation of patients with chest pain. *Annals of Emergency Medicine*, *31*(1), 3–11. doi:10.1016/S0196-0644(98)70274-4 PMID:9437335

Fezari, M., & Bousbia-Salah, M. (2007). Speech and sensor in guiding an electric wheelchair. *Automatic Control and Computer Sciences*, *41*(1), 39–43. doi:10.3103/S0146411607010063

Finan, R., Sapeluk, A., & Damper, R. (1996). *Comparison of multilayer and radial basis function neural networks for text-dependent speaker recognition.* Paper presented at the Neural Networks, 1996, IEEE International Conference on. doi:10.1109/ICNN.1996.549207

Fitzpatrick, J. M. (2010). The role of registration in accurate surgical guidance. Proceedings of the institution mechanical engineering Part H. *Journal of Engineering in Medicine*, *224*(5), 607–622. doi:10.1243/09544119JEIM589 PMID:20718266

Florea, F., Rogozan, A., Bensrhair, A., Dacher, J.-N., & Darmoni, S. (2005). *Recherche des images médicales par contenu et type de ressource dans un catalogue de santé en ligne. Laboratoire Perception, Systèmes et Information, CNRS FRE-2645*. France: INSA & Université de Rouen.

Forouzanfar, M., Forghani, N., & Teshnehlab, M. (2010). Parameter optimization of improved fuzzy c-means clustering algorithm for brain MR image segmentation. *Engineering Applications of Artificial Intelligence*, *23*(2), 160–168. doi:10.1016/j.engappai.2009.10.002

Fowlkes, C., Belongie, S., Fan, C., & Malik, J. (2004). Spectral grouping using the Nystrom method. *Pattern Analysis and Machine Intelligence. IEEE Transactions on*, *26*(2), 214–225.

Fowlkes, E. B., & Mallows, C. L. (1983). A method for comparing two hierarchical clusterings. *Journal of the American Statistical Association*, *78*(383), 553–584. doi: doi:10.1080/01621459.1983.10478008

Freund, Y., & Schapire, R. (1999). A Short Introduction to Boosting. *Journal of Japanese Society for Artificial Intelligence*, *14*(5), 771–780.

Friedman, P. A. (2002). Novel mapping techniques for cardiac electrophysiology. *Heart (British Cardiac Society)*, *87*(6), 575–582. doi:10.1136/heart.87.6.575 PMID:12010949

Friedman, P. A., Asirvatham, S. J., Grice, S., Glikson, M., Munger, T. M., Rea, R. F., & Hammill, S. C. et al. (2002). Noncontact mapping to guide ablation of right ventricular outflow tract tachycardia. *Journal of the American College of Cardiology*, *39*(11), 1808–1812. doi:10.1016/S0735-1097(02)01864-8 PMID:12039496

Fryer, R. M., Randall, J., Yoshida, T., Hsiao, L., Blumenstock, J., Jensen, K. E., & Gullansa, S. R. et al. (2002). Global Analysis of Gene Expression:Methods, Interpretation, and Pitfalls. *Experimental Nephrology*, *10*(2), 64–74. doi:10.1159/000049901 PMID:11937753

Fukuda, O., Tsuji, T., Ohtsuka, A., & Kaneko, M. (1998). *EMG-based human-robot interface for rehabilitation aid.* Paper presented at the Robotics and Automation, 1998. doi:10.1109/ROBOT.1998.680978

Fulford-Jones, T. R. F., Wei, & Welsh, M. (2004). A Portable, Low-Power & Wireless Two-Lead EKG System. *26th Annual International Conference of the IEEE EMBS.* doi:10.1109/IEMBS.2004.1403627

Gallegos-Funes, F. J., Gómez-Mayorga, M. E., Lopez-Bonilla, J. L., & Cruz-Santiago, R. (2009). Rank M-type radial basis function (RMRBF) neural network for Pap smear microscopic image classification. *Apeiron (Montreal, Quebec)*, *16*(4), 542–554.

Gan Lim, L. (2011). *Automatic Classification Of Colonic Histophathological Images Using Adaptive Neuro-Fuzzy Networks And Genetic Algorithms.* (PhD Thesis). Coventry University.

Gao, J., Zhou, M. C., & Zhang, C. (2001). 2D and 3D medical image database design.*Proceedings of the IEEE international conference on systems, man, and cybernetics* (vol. 3, pp. 2011-2015). IEEE.

Gargiulo, G., Bifulco, P., Cesarelli, M., Jin, C., McEwan, A., & van Schaik, A. (2010). Wearable dry sensors with Bluetooth connection for use in remote patient monitoring systems. *Studies in Health Technology and Informatics*, *161*, 57–65. PMID:21191158

Gens, P., Enrique, B., & Roderic, G. (2000). Geneid in drosophila. *Genome Research*, *10*(4), 511–515. doi:10.1101/gr.10.4.511 PMID:10779490

Gerdle, B., Karlsson, S., Day, S., & Djupsjöbacka, M. (1999). *Acquisition, processing and analysis of the surface electromyogram. In Modern techniques in neuroscience research* (pp. 705–755). Springer. doi:10.1007/978-3-642-58552-4_26

Geremia, E., Menze, B. H., & Ayache, N. (2012). Spatial decision forest for glioma segmentation in multi-channel MR images.*Proceedings MICCAI-BRATS.*

Ghofrani. (2015). Comparing Nonsubsampled Wavelet, Contourlet and Shearlet Transforms for Ultrasound Image Despkeckling. *International Journal of Image, Graphics and Signal Processing*, 15-22.

Ghose, S., Oliver, A., Marti, R., Llado, X., Vilanova, J. C., Freixenet, J., & Meriaudeau, F. et al. (2012). A survey of prostate segmentation methodologies in ultrasound, magnetic resonance and computed tomography images. *Computer Methods and Programs in Biomedicine*, *108*(1), 262–287. doi:10.1016/j.cmpb.2012.04.006 PMID:22739209

Giro-i-Nieto, X., Ventura, C., Jordi Pont-Tuset, C., & Marques, F. (2010). *Content-Based Image Retrieval as a Web Service. Technical University of Catalonia.* UPC.

Gletsos, M. (2003). A computer-aided diagnostic system to characterize CT focal liver lesions: design and optimization of a neural network classifier.*IEEE Transaction on Information Technology on Biomedicine*, *7*(3), 153–162.

Glotsos, D., Spyridonos, P., Petalas, P., Cavouras, D., Ravazoula, P., Dadioti, P., & Nikiforidis, G. et al. (2004). Computer-based malignancy grading of astrocytomas employing a support vector machine classifier, the who grading system and the regular hematoxylineosin diagnostic staining procedure. *Analytical and Quantitative Cytology and Histology*, *26*(2), 77–83. PMID:15131894

Gokgoz, E., & Subasi, A. (2015). Comparison of decision tree algorithms for EMG signal classification using DWT. *Biomedical Signal Processing and Control*, *18*, 138–144. doi:10.1016/j.bspc.2014.12.005

Gomes, L. (2014). *Machine-Learning Maestro Michael Jordan on the Delusions of Big Data and Other Huge Engineering Efforts, Big-data boondoggles and brain-inspired chips are just two of the things we're really getting wrong*. IEEE Spectrum.

Gomez-Gil, J., San-Jose-Gonzalez, I., Nicolas-Alonso, L. F., & Alonso-Garcia, S. (2011). Steering a tractor by means of an EMG-based human-machine interface. *Sensors (Basel, Switzerland)*, *11*(7), 7110–7126. doi:10.3390/s110707110 PMID:22164006

Gonzalez, R. C., & Richard, E. (2002). *Woods digital image processing* (2nd ed.). Upper Saddle River, New Jersey: Prentice Hall.

Gooch, C. L., Doherty, T. J., Chan, K. M., Bromberg, M. B., Lewis, R. A., & Stashuk, D. W. (2014). Motor unit number estimation: A technology and literature review. *Muscle & Nerve*, *50*(6), 884–893. PMID:25186553

Gordillo, N., Montseny, E., & Sobrevilla, P. (2013, October). State of the art survey on MRI brain tumor segmentation. *Magnetic Resonance Imaging*, *31*(8), 1426–1438. doi:10.1016/j.mri.2013.05.002 PMID:23790354

Gorgolewski, K. J., Storkey, A. J., Bastin, M. E., & Pernet, C. R. (2012). Adaptive thresholding for reliable topological inference in single subject fMRI analysis. *Frontiers in Human Neuroscience*, *6*(245), 1–14. PMID:22936908

Gornick, C., Adler, S., Pederson, B., Hauck, J., Budd, J., & Schweitzer, J. (1999). Validation of a new noncontact catheter system for electroanatomic mapping of left ventricular endocardium. *Circulation*, *99*(6), 829–835. doi:10.1161/01.CIR.99.6.829 PMID:9989971

Gou, H.U., Douze, M., & Schmid, C. (2010). Improving bag-of-features for large scale image search. *International Journal of Computer Vision*, *87*(3), 316–336.

Graps, A. (1995). An Introduction to Wavelets. *IEEE Computational Science & Engineering*, *2*(2), 50–61. doi:10.1109/99.388960

Gravel, P., Beaudoin, G., & DeGuise, J. A. (2004). A method for modeling noise in medical images. *IEEE Transactions on Medical Imaging*, *23*(10), 1221–1232. doi:10.1109/TMI.2004.832656 PMID:15493690

Greenblum, S., Turnbaugh, P. J., & Borenstein, E. (2011). Metagenomic systems biology of the human gut microbiome reveals topological shifts associated with obesity and inflammatory bowel disease. *Proceedings of the National Academy of Sciences of the United States of America*, *109*(2), 594–599. doi:10.1073/pnas.1116053109 PMID:22184244

Green, P., Lipman, D., Hillier, L., Waterston, R., States, D., & Claverie, J. M. (1993). Ancient conserved regions in new gene sequences and the protein databases. *Science*, *259*(5102), 1711–1716. doi:10.1126/science.8456298 PMID:8456298

Gurevitz, O. T., Glikson, M., Asirvatham, S., Kester, T. A., Grice, S. K., Munger, T. M., & Friedman, P. A. et al. (2005). Use of advanced mapping systems to guide ablation in complex cases: Experience with noncontact mapping and electroanatomic mapping systems. *Pacing and Clinical Electrophysiology*, *28*(4), 316–323. doi:10.1111/j.1540-8159.2005.09477.x PMID:15826266

Gyaw, T., & Ray, S. (1993). The wavelet transform as a tool for recognition of biosignals. *Biomedical Sciences Instrumentation, 30*, 63–68. PMID:7948651

Habermeyer, P., Krieter, C., Tang, K. L., Lichtenberg, S., & Magosch, P. (2008). A new arthroscopic classification of articular-sided supraspinatus footprint lesions: A prospective comparison with Snyder's and Ellman's classification. *Journal of Shoulder and Elbow Surgery, 17*(6), 909–913. doi:10.1016/j.jse.2008.06.007 PMID:18818103

Haissaguerre, M., Jais, P., Shah, D. C., Takahashi, A., Hocini, M., Quiniou, G., & Clémenty, J. et al. (1998). Spontaneous initiation of atrial fibrillation by ectopic beats originating in the pulmonary veins. *The New England Journal of Medicine, 339*(10), 659–666. doi:10.1056/NEJM199809033391003 PMID:9725923

Hamamci, A., & Unal, G. (2012). Multimodal brain tumor segmentation using the tumor-cut method on the BraTS dataset.*Proceeding MICCAI-BRATS.*

Han, J.-S., Bien, Z. Z., Kim, D.-J., Lee, H.-E., & Kim, J.-S. (2003). *Human-machine interface for wheelchair control with EMG and its evaluation.* Paper presented at the Engineering in Medicine and Biology Society.

Handelsman, J. (2007). *Committee on Metagenomics.* Challenges and Functional Applications The National Academies Press.

Haralick, R. M., Shanmugam, K., & Dinstein, I. (1973). Textural features for image classification. *IEEE Transactions on Systems, Man, and Cybernetics*, 3.

Harbaoui, A., Ghenima, M., & Sidhom, S. (2009). Enrichissement des contenus par la réindexation des usagers: un état de l'art sur la problématique. *SIIE'2009 International conference. HAL Id: inria-00426376.* Retrieved from https://hal.inria.fr/inria-00426376

Harold, L., & Kundel, M. P. (2003). Measurement of Observer Agreement. *Radiology, 228*(2), 303–308. doi:10.1148/radiol.2282011860 PMID:12819342

Harris-Love, M. O., Monfaredi, R., Ismail, C., Blackman, M. R., & Cleary, K. (2014). Quantitative ultrasound: Measurement considerations for the assessment of muscular dystrophy and sarcopenia. *Front Aging Neurosci, 6*, 172. doi:10.3389/fnagi.2014.00172 PMID:25071570

Hartigan, J. A. (1975). *Clustering Algorithms.* New York, NY: John Wiley & Sons.

Hassenpflug, P., Prager, R. W., Treece, G. M., & Gee, A. H. (2005). Speckle classification for sensorless freehand 3-D ultrasound. *Ultrasound in Medicine & Biology, 31*(11), 1499–1508. doi:10.1016/j.ultrasmedbio.2005.07.007 PMID:16286028

Hastie, T., Tibshirani, R., & Friedman, J. (2009). *The elements of statistical learning: Data mining, inference and prediction.* New York, NY: Springer-Verlag. doi:10.1007/978-0-387-84858-7

Haux, R. (2006). Health Information systems-Past, present, future. *International Journal of Medical Informatics, 75*(3–4), 268–281. doi:10.1016/j.ijmedinf.2005.08.002 PMID:16169771

He, C., Zhuo, T., Zhao, S., Yin, S., & Chen, D. (2015). Particle Filter Sample Texton Feature for SAR Image Classification. Geoscience and Remote Sensing Letters, 12(5). DOI: doi:10.1109/LGRS.2014.2386351

Heston, T. F. (2011). Standardizing predictive values in diagnostic imaging research. *Journal of Magnetic Resonance Imaging, 33*(2), 505. doi:10.1002/jmri.22466 PMID:21274995

Hildebrand, L., & Ploch, T. (2011). Image Based Analysis of Microstructures Using Texture Detection and Fuzzy Classifiers. In Integrated Systems, Design and Technology 2010, (pp. 313-319). doi:10.1007/978-3-642-17384-4_25

Hinton, G., Osindero, S., & Teh, Y. W. (2006). A fast learning algorithm for deep belief nets. *Neural Computation, 18*(7), 1527–1554. doi:10.1162/neco.2006.18.7.1527 PMID:16764513

Hiran & Doshi. (2013). An Artificial Neural Network Approach for Brain Tumor Detection Using Digital Image Segmentation. *IJETTCS, 2*(5).

Hiremath, P. S., & Iranna, Y. H. (2011). Fuzzy rule based classification of microscopic images of squamous cell carcinoma of esophagus. *International Journal of Computers and Applications, 25*(11), 30–33. doi:10.5120/3156-4366

Hodge, V. J., & Austin, J. (2004). A survey of outlier detection methodologies. *Artificial Intelligence Review, 22*(2), 85–126. doi:10.1023/B:AIRE.0000045502.10941.a9

Hoff, K. J., Lingner, T., Meinicke, P., & Tech, M. (2009). Orphelia:predicting genes in metagenomic sequencing reads. *Nucleic Acids Research, 37*(Web Server), 101–105. doi:10.1093/nar/gkp327 PMID:19429689

Hogrel, J.-Y. (2005). Clinical applications of surface electromyography in neuromuscular disorders. *Neurophysiologie Clinique. Clinical Neurophysiology, 35*(2), 59–71. doi:10.1016/j.neucli.2005.03.001 PMID:16087069

Holden, J. E., Finch, W. H., & Kelley, K. (2011). A comparison of two-group classification methods. *Educational and Psychological Measurement, 71*(5), 870–901. doi:10.1177/0013164411398357

Holland, J. H. (1975). *Adaptation in Natural and Artificial Systems*. University of Michigan Press.

Holt, A., Bichindaritz, I., Schmidt, R., & Perner, P. (2005). Medical applications in case-based reasoning. *The Knowledge Engineering Review, 20*(03), 289–292. doi:10.1017/S0269888906000622

Hooda, A., Sharma, S., & Sharma, A. (2013). Wireless body area network. *International Journal of Electronics, Communication & Instrumentation Engineering Research and Development, 3*(1), 203–210.

Hore, S., Chakroborty, S., Ashour, A. S., Dey, N., Ashour, A., Sifaki-Pistolla, D., & Chaudhuri, S. R. B. et al. (2015). Finding contours of Hippocampus Brain Cell using Microscopic Image Analysis. *Journal of Advanced Microscopy Research, 10*(2), 93–103. doi:10.1166/jamr.2015.1245

Horlings, R., Datcu, D., & Rothkrantz, L. J. (2008). *Emotion recognition using brain activity*. Paper presented at the 9th international conference on computer systems and technologies and workshop for PhD students in computing.

Horng, & Chen, S.-M. (2009). Multi-class Classification of Ultrasonic Supraspinatus Images based on Radial Basis Function Neural Network. *Journal of Medical and Biological Engineering, 29*(5), 242–250.

Horng, M.-H. (2013). The Glowworm Swarm Optimization for Training the Radial Basis Function Network in Ultrasonic Supraspinatus Image Classification. *Advanced Science Letters, 19*(9), 2724–2727. doi:10.1166/asl.2013.4977

Ho, S., Bullitt, E., & Gerig, G. (2002). *Level set evolution with region competition: automatic3-D segmentation of brain tumors*. Int Conf Pattern Rec.

Hota, H.S., Shukla S.P., & Kiran, G. K. (2013). Review of Intelligent Techniques Applied for classification and preprocessing of Medical Image Data. *International Journal of Computer Science Issues, 10*(3).

Hourigan, M. L., McKinnon, N. B., Johnson, M., Rice, C. L., Stashuk, D. W., & Doherty, T. J. (2015). Increased motor unit potential shape variability across consecutive motor unit discharges in the tibialis anterior and vastus medialis muscles of healthy older subjects. *Clinical Neurophysiology, 126*(12), 2381–2389. doi:10.1016/j.clinph.2015.02.002 PMID:25727901

Huang, H. K. (2004). PACS and Imaging Informatics: Basic Principles and Applications.New York: Wiley. doi:10.1002/0471654787

Hudgins, B., Parker, P., & Scott, R. N. (1993). A new strategy for multifunction myoelectric control. *Biomedical Engineering. IEEE Transactions on*, *40*(1), 82–94.

Hunter, J. (2008). Tracking the Progress of Multimedia Semantics – from MPEG-7 to Web 3.0. (Keynote Talk). In SAMT 2008 (LNCS), (vol. 5392). Springer-Verlag Berlin Heidelberg.

Hurst, J. W. (1998). Naming of the waves in the ECG, with a brief account of their genesis. *Circulation*, *98*(18), 1937–1942. doi:10.1161/01.CIR.98.18.1937 PMID:9799216

Huttenhower, C., Gevers, D., Knight, R., Abubucker, S., Badger, J. H., Chinwalla, A. T., & White, O. et al. (2012). Structure, function and diversity of the healthy human microbiome. *Nature*, *486*(7402), 207–214. doi:10.1038/nature11234 PMID:22699609

Iftekharuddin, K. M., Jia, W., & March, R. (2003). Fractal analysis of tumor in brain MR images. *Machine Vision and Applications*, *13*(5-6), 352–362. doi:10.1007/s00138-002-0087-9

Ikeda, N., Gupta, A., Dey, N., Bose, S., Shafique, S., Arak, T., & Suri, J. S. et al. (2015). Improved correlation between carotid and coronary atherosclerosis SYNTAX score using automated ultrasound carotid bulb plaque IMT measurement. *Ultrasound in Medicine & Biology*, *41*(5), 1247–1262. doi:10.1016/j.ultrasmedbio.2014.12.024 PMID:25638311

Ingole, P. V., & Kulat, K. D. (2012). A Chain Code Based Fuzzy Features for Brain MRI Retrieval. In *Emerging Trends in Engineering and Technology (ICETET),2012 Fifth International Conference*. DOI: doi:10.1109/ICETET.2012.50

Insana, M. F., & Hall, T. J. (1990). Characterising the microstructure of random media using ultrasound. *Physics in Medicine and Biology*, *35*(10), 1373–1386. doi:10.1088/0031-9155/35/10/003 PMID:2243842

International Agency for Research on Cancer (IARC). (2015). *OMS organization: statistics of dec. 2012*. Retrieved from http://www-dep.iarc.fr/

Ising, H., & Kruppa, B. (2004). Health effects caused by noise: Evidence in the literature from the past 25 years. *Noise & Health*, *6*(22), 5. PMID:15070524

Islam, M. J., Wu, Q. M. J., Ahmadi, M., & Sid-Ahmed, M. A. (2007). Investigating the Performance of Naive- Bayes Classifiers and K- Nearest Neighbor Classifiers.*International Conference on Convergence Information Technology*, 1541-1546. doi:10.1109/ICCIT.2007.148

Ivan Selesnick, W., Richard Baraniuk, G., & Nick Kingsbury, G. (2005). 2005. The Dual-Tree Complex Wavelet Transform. *IEEE Signal Processing Magazine*, *22*(nov), 123–150. doi:10.1109/MSP.2005.1550194

Iwanaga, M., & Tsukamoto, M. (1997). Effects of excitative and sedative music on subjective and physiological relaxation. *Perceptual and Motor Skills*, *85*(1), 287–296. doi:10.2466/pms.1997.85.1.287 PMID:9293589

Jafari-Khouzani, K., & Soltanian-Zadeh, H. (2003). Multiwavelet grading of pathological images of prostate. *IEEE Transactions on Bio-Medical Engineering*, *50*(6), 697–704. doi:10.1109/TBME.2003.812194 PMID:12814236

Jai-Andaloussi, S., Lamard, M., Cazuguel, G., Tairi, H., Meknassi, M., Cochener, B., & Roux, C. (2010). Content Based medical Image Retrieval based on BEMD: Optimization of a similarity metric. In *Engineering in Medicine and Biology Society (EMBC), 2010 Annual International Conference of the IEEE*. DOI: doi:10.1109/IEMBS.2010.5626134

Jain, S., & Mishra. (2012). Automated Brain Tumor Detection and Identification Using Image Processing and Probabilistic Neural Network Techniques. *International Journal of Image Processing and Visual Communication, 1*(2).

Jain, A. K., & Dubes, R. C. (1988). *Algorithms for Clustering Data*. Englewood Cliffs, NJ: Prentice-Hall.

Jais, P., Matsuo, S., Knecht, S., Weerasooriya, R., Hocini, M., Sacher, F., & Haïssaguerre, M. et al. (2009). A deductive mapping strategy for atrial tachycardia following atrial fibrillation ablation: Importance of localized reentry. *Journal of Cardiovascular Electrophysiology*, *20*(5), 480–491. doi:10.1111/j.1540-8167.2008.01373.x PMID:19207747

Jais, P., Shah, D. C., Haissaguerre, M., Hocini, M., Peng, J. T., Takahashi, A., & Clémenty, J. et al. (2000). Mapping and ablation of left atrial flutters. *Circulation*, *101*(25), 2928–2934. doi:10.1161/01.CIR.101.25.2928 PMID:10869265

Jayadevappa, D., Srinivas Kumar, S., & Murty, D. S. (2011). Medical Image Segmentation Algorithms using Deformable Models: A Review. *IETE Technical Review*, *28*(3), 248. doi:10.4103/0256-4602.81244

Ji, Sun, & Xia. (2011). A modified possibility fuzzy c-means clustering algorithm for bias field estimation and segmentation of brain MR image. *Computerized Medical Imaging and Graphics*, *35*, 383–397.

Jian, Sun, & Luo. (2012). Computer-aided diagnosis of breast microcalcifications based on dual-tree complex wavelet transform. *Biomedical Engineering Online*.

Jiang & Sha. (2013). Image De-Nosing Based on Non-Subsampled Contourlet Transform Domain in Multi-Bessel K Form Model. Research Journal of Applied Sciences. *Engineering and Technology*, *6*(18), 3400–3403.

Jiang, Y. G., Ngo, C. W., & Yang, J. (2007). Towards optimal bag-of-features for object categorization and semantic video retrieval. *6th ACM international conference on Image and video retrieval*, 494-501.

Jiang, J., Zhou, L., Rickson, D., & Jiang, C. (2013). The effects of sedative and stimulative music on stress reduction depend on music preference. *The Arts in Psychotherapy*, *40*(2), 201–205. doi:10.1016/j.aip.2013.02.002

Jiang, M., Wang, G., Skinner, M. W., Rubinstien, J. T., & Vannier, M. W. (2003). Blind deblurring of spiral CT images. *IEEE Transactions on Medical Imaging*, *22*(7), 837–845. doi:10.1109/TMI.2003.815075 PMID:12906237

Jia, W., Hu, R., Lei, X., Zhao, Y. K., & Gui, J. (2014). Histogram of oriented lines for palmprint recognition. *IEEE Transactions on Systems, Man, and Cybernetics. Systems*, *44*(3), 385–395.

Jovanov, E., Milenkovic, A., Otto, C., & Piet, C. G. (2005). A wireless body area network of intelligent motion sensors for computer assisted physical rehabilitation. *Journal of Neuroengineering and Rehabilitation*, 2–6. PMID:15740621

Jovanov, E., Raskovic, D., Price, J., Chapman, J., Moore, A., & Krishnamurthy, A. (2001). Patient Monitoring Using Personal Area Networks of Wireless Intelligent Sensors. *Biomedical Sciences Instrumentation*, 373–378. PMID:11347420

Jude Hemanth, D., Kezi Selva Vijila, C., & Anitha, J. (2010). Application of Neuro-Fuzzy Model for MR Brain Tumor Image Classification. *Biomedical Soft Computing and Human Sciences*, *16*(1), 95–102.

Jumb, V., Sohani, M., & Shrivas, A. (2014). Color image segmentation using k-means clustering and Otsu's adaptive thresholding. *International Journal of Innovative Technology and Exploring Engineering*, *3*(9), 72–76.

Junsheng, C., Dejie, Y., & Yu, Y. (2005). Time–energy density analysis based on wavelet transform. *NDT & E International*, *38*(7), 569–572. doi:10.1016/j.ndteint.2005.02.002

Jurrus, E., Paiva, A. R., Watanabe, S., Anderson, J. R., Jones, B. W., Whitaker, R. T., & Tasdizen, T. et al. (2010). Detection of neuron membranes in electron microscopy images using a serial neural network architecture. *Medical Image Analysis*, *14*(6), 770–783. doi:10.1016/j.media.2010.06.002 PMID:20598935

Kadah, Y. M., Farag, A. A., Zurada, J. M., Badawi, A. M., & Youssef, A. M. (1996). Classification algorithms for quantitative tissue characterization of diffuse liver disease from ultrasound images. *IEEE Transactions on Medical Imaging*, *15*(4), 466–478. doi:10.1109/42.511750 PMID:18215928

Kaili & Huang. (2003). A modified PCM clustering algorithm. In *Proceedings of the Second International Conference on Machine Learning and Cybernetics*.

Kanehisa, M., Goto, S., Sato, Y., Furumichi, M., & Tanabe, M. (2012). KEGG for integration and interpretation of large-scale molecular data sets. *Nucleic Acids Research*, *40*(D1), 109–114. doi:10.1093/nar/gkr988 PMID:22080510

Kang, K. T., Etheridge, S. P., Kantoch, M. J., Tisma-Dupanovic, S., Bradley, D. J., Balaji, S., & Sanatani, S. et al. (2014). Current management of focal atrial tachycardia in children: A multicenter experience. *Circulation: Arrhythmia and Electrophysiology*, *3*(4), 664–670. doi:10.1161/CIRCEP.113.001423 PMID:25015944

Kapa, S., & Asirvatham, S. J. (2014). You can't know where you're going until you know where you've been: The clinical relevance of differences in accurate assessment of catheter location with mapping technologies. *Journal of Cardiovascular Electrophysiology*, *25*(1), 84–86. doi:10.1111/jce.12287 PMID:24118496

Karaa, W. B. A., Ashour, A. S., Sassi, D. B., Roy, P., Kausar, N., & Dey, N. (2015). MEDLINE Text Mining: An Enhancement Genetic Algorithm based Approach for Document Clustering. In E. Hassanien, C. Grosan, & M. Fahmy Tolba (Eds.), *Applications of Intelligent Optimization in Biology and Medicine: Current Trends and Open Problems* (pp. 267–287). Springer International Publishing.

Karaa, W. B. A., & Dey, N. (Eds.). (2015). *Biomedical Image Analysis and Mining Techniques for Improved Health Outcomes*. Idea Group.

Karim, N., Hasan, J. A., & Ali, S. S. (2011). Heart rate variability–a review. *Journal of Basic and Applied Sciences*, *7*(1), 71–77.

Karim, R., Khaliluzzaman, M., & Mahmud, S. (2014). A Review of Image Analysis Techniques for Gene Spot Identification in cDNA Microarray Images. *International Journal of Artificial Intelligence & Application*, *5*, 1–7.

Kario, K., Yasui, N., & Yokoi, H. (2003). Ambulatory Blood Pressure Monitoring for Cardiovascular Medicine. *IEEE Engineering in Medicine and Biology Magazine*, *22*(3), 81–88. doi:10.1109/MEMB.2003.1213630 PMID:12845823

Karlof, C., Sastry, N., & Wagner, D. (2004). TinySec:A Link Layer Security Architecture for Wireless Sensor Networks. *Second ACM Conference on Embedded Networked Sensor Systems (SenSys '04)*. doi:10.1145/1031495.1031515

Karlsson, F. H., Tremaroli, V., Nookaew, I., Bergstrom, G., & Behre, C. J. (2013). Gut metagenome in European women with normal, impaired and diabetic glucose control. *Nature*, 4–10. PMID:23719380

Karlsson, S., & Gerdle, B. (2001). Mean frequency and signal amplitude of the surface EMG of the quadriceps muscles increase with increasing torque—a study using the continuous wavelet transform. *Journal of Electromyography and Kinesiology*, *11*(2), 131–140. doi:10.1016/S1050-6411(00)00046-8 PMID:11228426

Kass, M., Witkin, A., & Terzopoulos, D. (1987). Snakes: Active contour models. *Int Comput Vis*, *1*(4), 321–331. doi:10.1007/BF00133570

Katayose, M., & Magee, D. J. (2001). The cross-sectional area of supraspinatus as measured by diagnostic ultrasound. *The Journal of Bone and Joint Surgery. British Volume*, *83*(4), 565–568. doi:10.1302/0301-620X.83B4.11153 PMID:11380133

Kaufman, L., & Rousseeuw, P. J. (1990). *Finding Groups in Data: An Introduction to Cluster Analysis*. New York: Wiley. doi:10.1002/9780470316801

Kausar, N., Palaniappan, S., Al Ghamdi, B. S., Samir, B. B., Dey, N., & Abdullah, A. (2015). Systematic Analysis of Applied Data Mining Based Optimization Algorithms in Clinical Attribute Extraction and Classification for Diagnosis of Cardiac Patients. In A. Hassanien, C. Grosan, & M. F. Tolba (Eds.), *Applications of Intelligent Optimization in Biology and Medicine* (Vol. 96, pp. 217–231). Dordrecht: Springer. doi:10.1007/978-3-319-21212-8_9

Kautzner, J., & John Camm, A. (1997). Clinical relevance of heart rate variability. *Clinical Cardiology*, *20*(2), 162–168. doi:10.1002/clc.4960200214 PMID:9034646

Kay, G. N., Chong, F., Epstein, A. E., Dailey, S. M., & Plumb, V. J. (1993). Radiofrequency ablation for treatment of primary atrial tachycardias. *Journal of the American College of Cardiology*, *21*(4), 901–909. doi:10.1016/0735-1097(93)90345-2 PMID:8450158

Keijsers, N. L. W., Horstink, M. W. I. M., & Gielen, S. C. A. M. (2003). Online Monitoring of Dyskinesia in Patients with Parkinson's Disease. *IEEE Engineering in Medicine and Biology Magazine*, *22*(3), 96–103. doi:10.1109/MEMB.2003.1213632 PMID:12845825

Kekre, H. B., & Mishra, D. (2010). CBIR using Upper Six FFT Sectors of Color Images for Feature Vector Generation. *IACSIT International Journal of Engineering and Technology*.

Kemp, A. H., & Quintana, D. S. (2013). The relationship between mental and physical health: Insights from the study of heart rate variability. *International Journal of Psychophysiology*, *89*(3), 288–296. doi:10.1016/j.ijpsycho.2013.06.018 PMID:23797149

Kepa, K., & Abaid, N. (2015). *Development of a frequency-modulated ultrasonic sensor inspired by bat echolocation.* Paper presented at the SPIE Smart Structures and Materials+ Nondestructive Evaluation and Health Monitoring.

Khan, A., Deep, S., Li, J.-P., Kumar, K., Shaikh, R. A., & Hasan, F. (2014). Vision prehension with CBIR for cloud robo. In *Wavelet Active Media Technology and Information Processing (ICCWAMTIP), 2014 11th International Computer Conference*. doi:10.1109/ICCWAMTIP.2014.7073411

Khan, J. Y., Yuce, M. R., & Karami, F. (2008). Performance evaluation of a wireless body area sensor network for remote patient monitoring.*30th Annual International Conference of the IEEE Engineering in Medicine and Biology Society (EMBS)*. doi:10.1109/IEMBS.2008.4649394

Khare & Tiwary. (2006). A new method for deblurring and denoising of medical images using complex wavelet transform. Engineering in Medicine and Biology Society, IEEE.

Khare & Tiwary. (2006). Symmetric Daubechies Complex Wavelet Transform and its application to denoising and deblurring. *WSEAS Transactions on Signal Processing, 2*(5), 738 - 745.

Khare & Uma. (2006). A new method for deblurring and denoising of medical images using complex wavelet transform.*27th Annual International Conference of the Engineering in Medicine and Biology Society*, (pp. 1897 – 1900).

Khare, A., & Tiwary, U. S. (2005). Soft-thresholding for denoising of medical images – A multiresolution approach. *International Journal of Wavelets, Multresolution, and Information Processing*, *3*(4), 477–496. doi:10.1142/S021969130500097X

Khaykin, Y., Oosthuizen, R., Zarnett, L., Wulffhart, Z. A., Whaley, B., Hill, C., & Verma, A. et al. (2011). Carto-guided vs. Navx-guided pulmonary vein antrum isolation and pulmonary vein antrum isolation performed without 3-d mapping: Effect of the 3-d mapping system on procedure duration and fluoroscopy time. *Journal of Interventional Cardiac Electrophysiology*, *30*(3), 233–240. doi:10.1007/s10840-010-9538-9 PMID:21253840

Khotanlou, H., Colliot, O., Atif, J., & Bloch, I. (2009). 3D brain tumor segmentation in MRI using fuzzy classification, symmetry analysis and spatially constrained deformable models. *Fuzzy Sets and Systems*, *160*(6), 1457–1473. doi:10.1016/j.fss.2008.11.016

Khurshid, K., Siddiqi, I., Faure, C., & Vincent, N. (2009). Comparison of Niblack inspired binarization methods for ancient documents, *Proceedings SPIE 7247. Document Recognition and Retrieval, XVI*, 72470U, 72470U-9. doi:10.1117/12.805827

Kim & Park. (1999). Statistical textural features for detection of microcalcifications in digitized mammograms. IEEE Transactions Medical Imaging, 18(3), 231-238. DOI: doi:10.1109/42.764896

Kim, S., & Kim, D. (2009). Scene classification using PLSA with visterm spatial location.*Proceedings of the 1st ACM International Workshop on Interactive Multimedia for Consumer Electronics (IMCE '09)*, (pp. 57–66). doi:10.1145/1631040.1631050

Kingsbury, N.G. (1998). The dual-tree complex wavelet transform: a new technique for the shift invariance and directional filters. *IEEE Digital Signal Processing Workshop.*

Kirchhof, P., Loh, P., Eckardt, L., Ribbing, M., Rolf, S., Eick, O., & Haverkamp, W. et al. (2002). A novel nonfluoroscopic catheter visualization system (LocaLisa) to reduce radiation exposure during catheter ablation of supraventricular tachycardias. *The American Journal of Cardiology*, *90*(3), 340–343. doi:10.1016/S0002-9149(02)02481-5 PMID:12127630

Kistler, P. M., Rajappan, K., Jahngir, M., Earley, M. J., Harris, S., Abrams, D., & Schilling, R. J. et al. (2006). The impact of ct image integration into an electroanatomic mapping system on clinical outcomes of catheter ablation of atrial fibrillation. *Journal of Cardiovascular Electrophysiology*, *17*(10), 1093–1101. doi:10.1111/j.1540-8167.2006.00594.x PMID:16989651

Kitayoshi, H., Sawaya, K., & Kuwano, H. (2013). *Ultra low power wireless ECG sensor tag with wearable antenna.* Paper presented at the SENSORS, 2013 IEEE. doi:10.1109/ICSENS.2013.6688381

Kittler, J., & Illingworth, J. (1986). Minimum error thresholding. *Pattern Recognition*, *19*(1), 41–47. doi:10.1016/0031-3203(86)90030-0

Kleiger, R. E., Stein, P. K., & Bigger, J. T. (2005). Heart rate variability: Measurement and clinical utility. *Annals of Noninvasive Electrocardiology*, *10*(1), 88–101. doi:10.1111/j.1542-474X.2005.10101.x PMID:15649244

Kobayashi, H. (2011). *A ZigBee based wireless EMG/ECG streaming system for the universal interface.* Paper presented at the IECON 2011-37th Annual Conference on IEEE Industrial Electronics Society.

Kopelman, H., Prater, S., Tondato, F., Chronos, N. A., & Peters, N. S. (2003). Slow pathway catheter ablation of atrioventricular nodal re-entrant tachycardia guided by electroanatomical mapping: A randomized comparison to the conventional approach. *Europace*, *5*(2), 171–174. doi:10.1053/eupc.2002.0296 PMID:12633642

Kottkamp, H., Hugl, B., Krauss, B., Wetzel, U., Fleck, A., Schuler, G., & Hindricks, G. (2000). Electromagnetic versus fluoroscopic mapping of the inferior isthmus for ablation of typical atrial flutter. A prospective randomized study. *Circulation*, *102*(17), 2082–2086. doi:10.1161/01.CIR.102.17.2082 PMID:11044424

Kotyk, T., Ashour, A. S., Chakraborty, S., Dey, N., & Balas, V. E. (2015c). *Apoptosis Analysis in Classification Paradigm: A Neural Network based Approach.* Healthy World Conference 2015 - A Healthy World for a Happy Life, Kakinada, India.

Kotyk, T., Dey, N., Ashour, A. S., Balas-Timar, D., Chakraborty, S., Ashour, A. S., & Tavares, J. M. (2015a). Measurement of the Glomerulus Diameter and Bowman's Space Width of Renal Albino Rats.[In-press]. *Computer Methods and Programs in Biomedicine*. doi:10.1016/j.cmpb.2015.10.023 PMID:26796351

Kotyk, T., Dey, N., Ashour, A. S., Victoria, A. D. C., Hassanien, A. E., Gaber, T., & Snasel, V. (2015b) Detection of Dead stained microscopic cells based on Color Intensity and Contrast.*International Conference on Advanced Intelligent Systems and Informatics*. Beni Suef University.

Krinidis, S., & Chatzis, V. (2010). A Robust Fuzzy Local Information C-Means Clustering Algorithm. Image Processing. *IEEE Transactions on*, *19*(5), 1328–1337.

Krishnapuram, R., & Keller, J. (1996). The possibilistic c means algorithm: Insights and recommendations. *IEEE Transactions on Fuzzy Systems*, *4*(3), 385–393. doi:10.1109/91.531779

Krizhevsky, A., Sutskever, I., & Hinton, G. (2012). ImageNet Classification with Deep Convolutional Neural Networks. *Advances in Neural Information Processing Systems*, *25*, 1–14.

Kruk, M., Osowski, S., & Koktysz, R. (2007) Recognition of colon cells using ensemble of classifiers.*Proceedings of International Joint Conference on Neural Networks*, 288–293. doi:10.1109/IJCNN.2007.4370970

Kumar, Cai, & Feng. (2011). Multi modal Content Based Image Retrieval in Multi-modal Healthcare. Current Applications and Future Challenges.

Kumar, R., Srivastava, R., & Srivastava, S. (2015). Detection and Classification of Cancer from Microscopic Biopsy Images Using Clinically Significant and Biologically Interpretable Features. *Journal of Medical Engineering*, *2015*, 1–14. doi:10.1155/2015/457906

Kuribayashi, K., Shimizu, S., Okimura, K., & Taniguchi, T. (1993). A discrimination system using neural network for EMG-controlled prostheses-Integral type of EMG signal processing. Paper presented at the Intelligent Robots and Systems' 93, IROS'93.

Kurtzberg, J. M., & Lew, J. S. (2000). *Voice-controlled motorized wheelchair with sensors and displays*. Google Patents.

Kusserow, M., Amft, O., & Tröster, G. (2009). BodyANT: Miniature wireless sensors for naturalistic monitoring of daily activity.*4th Annual International ICST Conference on Body Area Networks*. doi:10.4108/ICST.BODYNETS2009.5899

Kwak, D. M. (2003). Content-based ultrasound image retrieval using a coarse to fine approach. *Annals of the New York Academy of Sciences*, 212–224. PMID:12594091

Kwon, S. H., Jeong, H. C., Seo, S. T., Lee, I. K., & Son, C. S. (2008). Histogram equalization-based thresholding. *Journal IEICE - Transactions on Information and Systems Archive, E91-D(11)*, 2751-2753.

Kwon, M., Han, Y., Shin, I., & Park, H. (2003). Segmentation of brain MR image using template matching and hierarchical fuzzy C-means. *Proc. of the Int. Society for Magnetic Resonance in Medicine*, *11*, 904.

Kwon, S. H. (1998). Cluster validity index for fuzzy clustering. *Electronics Letters*, *34*(22), 2176–2177. doi:10.1049/el:19981523

Kwon, S. H. (2004). Threshold selection based on cluster analysis. *Pattern Recognition Letters*, *25*(9), 1045–1050. doi:10.1016/j.patrec.2004.03.001

Labbé, E., Schmidt, N., Babin, J., & Pharr, M. (2007). Coping with stress: The effectiveness of different types of music. *Applied Psychophysiology and Biofeedback*, *32*(3-4), 163–168. doi:10.1007/s10484-007-9043-9 PMID:17965934

Ladak, H. M., Mao, F., Wang, Y., Downey, D. B., Steinman, D. A., & Fenster, A. (2000). Prostate boundary segmentation from 2D ultrasound images. *Medical Physics*, *27*(8), 1777–1788. doi:10.1118/1.1286722 PMID:10984224

Lahmiri & Boukadoum. (2013). Hybrid discrete wavelet transform and gabor filter banks processing for feature extraction from biomedical images, Hindawi Publishing Corporation. *Journal of Medical Engineering*.

Lanata, A., Valenza, G., Nardelli, M., Gentili, C., & Scilingo, E. P. (2015). Complexity Index From a Personalized Wearable Monitoring System for Assessing Remission in Mental Health. Biomedical and Health Informatics, 19(1). DOI: . Publication Year: 2015, pp: 132 - 139 doi:10.1109/JBHI.2014.2360711

Landis, K. G. Jr, & Koch, G. G. (1977). The measurement of observer agreement for categorical data. *Biometrics*, *33*(1), 159–174. doi:10.2307/2529310 PMID:843571

Latha, R., Srikanth, S., & Sairaman, H. (2014). Effect of music on heart rate variability and stress in medical students. *International Journal of Clinical and Experimental Physiology*, *1*(2), 131. doi:10.4103/2348-8093.137409

Latha, R., Tamilselvan, K., Susiganeshkumar, E., & Sairaman, H. (2015). Effect of Classical music on heart rate variability between genders. *International Journal of Biomedical Research*, *6*(3), 192–195. doi:10.7439/ijbr.v6i3.1841

Lauer, R. T., Peckham, P. H., & Kilgore, K. L. (1999). EEG-based control of a hand grasp neuroprosthesis. *Neuroreport*, *10*(8), 1767–1771. doi:10.1097/00001756-199906030-00026 PMID:10501572

Laufs, H., Krakow, K., Sterzer, P., Eger, E., Beyerle, A., Salek-Haddadi, A., & Kleinschmidt, A. (2003). Electroencephalographic signatures of attentional and cognitive default modes in spontaneous brain activity fluctuations at rest. *Proceedings of the National Academy of Sciences of the United States of America*, *100*(19), 11053–11058. doi:10.1073/pnas.1831638100 PMID:12958209

Laurikkala, J., Juhola, M., & Kentala, E. (2000). Informal identification of outliers in medical data. In *Fifth International Workshop on Intelligent Data Analysis in Medicine and Pharmacology* (vol.1, pp. 20-24). Berlin, Germany: IOS Press.

Law, A., Lam, F., & Chan, F. (2002). *A fast deformable region model for brain tumor boundary extraction.* Int Conf EMBS. doi:10.1109/IEMBS.2002.1106273

Lazebnik, S., Schmid, C., & Ponce, J. (2003). Affine-invariant local descriptors and neighborhood statistics for texture recognition. *Computer Vision*, 649–655.

Lazebnik, S., Schmid, C., & Ponce, J. (2006). Beyond bags of features: spatial pyramid matching for recognizing natural scene categories.*Proceedings of the IEEE Computer Society Conference on Computer Vision and Pattern Recognition (CVPR '06).* doi:10.1109/CVPR.2006.68

Ledesma-Carbayo, M. J., Kybic, J., Desco, M., Santos, A., Suhling, M., Hunziker, P., & Unser, M. (2005). Spatio-temporal nonrigid registration for ultrasound cardiac motion estimation. *IEEE Transactions on Medical Imaging*, *24*(9), 1113–1126. doi:10.1109/TMI.2005.852050 PMID:16156350

Lee, C. H., Schmidt, M., Murtha, A., Bistritz, A., Sander, J., & Greiner, R. (2005). Segmenting brain tumor with conditional random fields and support vector machines.*International Conference on Computer Vision.* doi:10.1007/11569541_47

Lee, K.-C., Chao, Y.-H., Yiin, J.-J., Hsieh, H.-Y., Dai, W.-J., & Chao, Y.-F. (2012). Evidence that music listening reduces preoperative patients' anxiety. *Biological Research for Nursing*, *14*(1), 78–84. doi:10.1177/1099800410396704 PMID:21278165

Lefohn, A., Cates, J., & Whitaker, R. (2003). Interactive GPU-based level sets for 3D brain tumor segmentation. Technical Report. University of Utah.

Leila, T., Oliver, R., Saurabh, G., Alexander, S., Michael, B., Serafim, B., & Burkhard, M. (2003). Agenda: Homology-based gene prediction. *Bioinformatics (Oxford, England)*, *19*(12), 1575–1577. doi:10.1093/bioinformatics/btg181 PMID:12912840

Lenza, M., Buchbinder, R., Takwoingi, Y., Johnston, R. V., Hanchard, N. C., & Faloppa, F. (2013). Magnetic resonance imaging, magnetic resonance arthrography and ultrasonography for assessing rotator cuff tears in people with shoulder pain for whom surgery is being considered. *Cochrane Database of Systematic Reviews*, *9*, CD009020. PMID:24065456

Leonardo, B. O., Diego, F. A., Eduardo, M., Felipe, D., Julio, L., & Ricardo, D. (2007). TinyTate:Identity-Based Encryption for Sensor Networks. *NCA*, *2007*(020), 318–323.

Lesh, M., Van Hare, G., Epstein, L., Fitzpatrick, A., Scheinman, M., Lee, R., & Griffin, J. C. et al. (1994). Radiofrequency catheter ablation of atrial arrhythmias. Results and mechanisms. *Circulation*, *89*(3), 1074–1089. doi:10.1161/01.CIR.89.3.1074 PMID:8124793

Leung, J. L., & Griffith, J. F. (2008). Sonography of chronic Achilles tendinopathy: A case-control study. *Journal of Clinical Ultrasound*, *36*(1), 27–32. doi:10.1002/jcu.20388 PMID:17721925

Leuthardt, E. C., Schalk, G., Moran, D. W., Wolpaw, J. R., & Ojemann, J. G. (2006). Brain computer interface: Google Patents.

Levenson, R. W. (2014). The autonomic nervous system and emotion. *Emotion Review*, *6*(2), 100–112. doi:10.1177/1754073913512003

Levine, S. P., Bell, D., Jaros, L., Simpson, R. C., Koren, Y., & Borenstein, J. (1999). The NavChair assistive wheelchair navigation system. *Rehabilitation Engineering. IEEE Transactions on*, *7*(4), 443–451.

Lewell, M., & Davis, M. (2011). *12 Lead ECG*. Academic Press.

Ley, R. E., Hamady, M., Lozupone, C., Turnbaugh, P. J., Ramey, R. R., Bircher, J. S., & Gordon, J. I. et al. (2008). Evolution of mammals and their gut microbes. *Science*, *320*(5883), 1647–1651. doi:10.1126/science.1155725 PMID:18497261

Li, C., Duan, G., & Zhong, F. (2015). Rotation Invariant Texture Retrieval Considering the Scale Dependence of Gabor Wavelet. IEEE Transactions on Image Processing, (99). DOI: doi:10.1109/TIP.2015.2422575

Li, C., Shirahama, K., Grzegorzek, M., Ma, F. J., & Zhou, B. (2013, September). Classification of environmental microorganisms in microscopic images using shape features and support vector machines. *2013 20th IEEE International Conference on Image Processing* (ICIP), (pp. 2435-2439).

Li, H. B., Takizawa, K. I., Zhen, B., & Kohno, R. (2007). Body area network and its standardization at IEEE 802.15. MBAN. 16th IST on mobile and wireless communications summit.

Liang, Y.-C., & Cuevas, J. R. (2013). An automatic multilevel image thresholding using relative entropy and meta-heuristic algorithms. *Entropy*, *15*(6), 2181–2209. doi:10.3390/e15062181

Liao, Y. Y., Li, C. H., Tsui, P. H., Chang, C. C., Kuo, W. H., Chang, K. J., & Yeh, C.-K. (2012). Strain-compounding technique with ultrasound Nakagami imaging for distinguishing between benign and malignant breast tumors. *Medical Physics*, *39*(5), 2325–2333. doi:10.1118/1.3700167 PMID:22559602

Liaw, A., & Wiener, M. (2002). Classification and regression by randomForest. *R News*, *2*(3), 18-22.

Li, C., Huang, R., Ding, Z., Gatenby, C., Metaxas, C., & Gore, J. (2011). A level set method for image segmentation in the presence of intensity in homogeneities with application to MRI. *IEEE Transactions on Image Processing*, *20*(7), 2007–2016. doi:10.1109/TIP.2011.2146190 PMID:21518662

Li, C., Kao, C., Gore, J., & Ding, Z. (2008). Minimization of region-scalable fitting energy for image segmentation. *IEEE Transactions on Image Processing*, *17*(10), 1940–1049. doi:10.1109/TIP.2008.2002304 PMID:18784040

Lijiya, A., Sreejithlal, G. S., & Govindan, V. K. (2013). M-FISH Image Segmentation and Classification using Fuzzy Logic. *International Journal of Computers and Applications*, *70*(25).

Lim, C. T., & Hong, J. G. C. (2009). *13th International Conference on Biomedical Engineering: ICBME 2008* (Vol. 23). Springer Science & Business Media.

Lin, J.-S., Chen, K.-C., & Yang, W.-C. (2010). *EEG and eye-blinking signals through a Brain-Computer Interface based control for electric wheelchairs with wireless scheme.* Paper presented at the New Trends in Information Science and Service Science (NISS), 2010 4th International Conference on.

Lin, Wu, & Chaovalitwongse. (2015). Integrating Human Behavior Modeling and Data Mining Techniques to Predict Human Errors in Numerical Typing. IEEE Transactions Human-Machine Systems, 45(1). DOI: doi:10.1109/THMS.2014.2357178

Lina, M. (1997). Image processing with complex Daubechies wavelets. *Journal of Mathematical Imaging and Vision*, *7*(3), 211–223. doi:10.1023/A:1008274210946

Lina, M., & Mayrand, M. (1995). Complex Daubechies Wavelets. *Journal of Applied and Computational Harmonic Analysis*, *2*(3), 219–229. doi:10.1006/acha.1995.1015

Liolios, C., Doukas, C., Fourlas, G., & Maglogiannis, I. (2010, June). An overview of body sensor networks in enabling pervasive healthcare and assistive environments. In *Proceedings of the 3rd International Conference on PErvasive Technologies Related to Assistive Environments* (p. 43). ACM. doi:10.1145/1839294.1839346

Liu, C.-L. (2010). *A tutorial of the wavelet transform.* Taiwan: NTUEE.

Liu, J., Udupa, J. K., Odhner, D., Hackney, D., & Moonis, G. (2005). A system for brain tumor volume estimation via MR imaging and fuzzy connectedness. *Computerized Medical Imaging and Graphics*, *29*(1), 21–34. doi:10.1016/j.compmedimag.2004.07.008 PMID:15710538

Li, w., Liu, J., Zhang, S., He, W., Chen, S., & Li, Z. (2015).Study on process technique of PCBs with ladder conductive lines. *Circuit World*, *41*(1). doi: doi:10.1109/IROS.1993.583873

Lizzi, F. L., Astor, M., Liu, T., Deng, C., Coleman, D. J., & Silverman, R. H. (1997). Ultrasonic spectrum analysis for tissue assays and therapy evaluation. *International Journal of Imaging Systems and Technology*, *8*(1), 3–10. doi:10.1002/(SICI)1098-1098(1997)8:1<3::AID-IMA2>3.0.CO;2-E

Lizzi, F. L., Greenebaum, M., Feleppa, E. J., Elbaum, M., & Coleman, D. J. (1983). Theoretical framework for spectrum analysis in ultrasonic tissue characterization. *The Journal of the Acoustical Society of America*, *73*(4), 1366–1373. doi:10.1121/1.389241 PMID:6853848

Loeckx, D., Slagmolen, P., Maes, F., Vandermeulen, D., & Suetens, P. (2006). *Automated non-rigid intra-patient image registration using B-Splines.* Paper presented at the Information Processing in Medical Imaging.

Lombaert, H., Criminisi, A., & Ayache, N. (2015). Spectral Forests: Learning of Surface Data, Application to Cortical Parcellation, In *Proceedings of 18th International Conference on Medical Image Computing and Computer-Assisted Intervention (MICCAI)* (LNCS), (vol. 9349, pp. 547-556). Springer. doi:10.1007/978-3-319-24553-9_67

Long, L. R., Antani, S., Deserno, T. M., & Thoma, G. R. (2009). Content-based image retrieval in medicine: Retrospective assessment, state of the art, and future directions. *International Journal of Healthcare Information Systems and Informatics*, *4*(1), 1–16. doi:10.4018/jhisi.2009010101 PMID:20523757

Lopes, A. C., Nunes, U., & Vaz, L. (2010). *Assisted navigation based on shared-control, using discrete and sparse human-machine interfaces.* Paper presented at the Engineering in Medicine and Biology Society (EMBC), 2010 Annual International Conference of the IEEE. doi:10.1109/IEMBS.2010.5626221

Lowe, D. (2004). Distinctive image features from scale-invariant keypoints. *International Journal of Scale Invariant Computer Vision*, *60*(2), 91–110.

Lu, H.-Y., Zhao, Q.-S., Xu, M.-Z., & Jin, T.-H. (2007). ECG monitoring module based on Bluetooth technology. *Chinese Medical Equipment Journal, 9*, 9.

Lu, K., He, N., & Li, L. (2012). Nonlocal Means-Based Denoising for Medical Images. Computational and Mathematical Methods in Medicine. doi:10.1155/2012/438617

Lu, F., & Ba, Q. (2010). A refined weighted K-Nearest Neighbors algorithm for text categorization. In *Proceedings of International Conference on Intelligent Systems and Knowledge Engineering* (pp. 326-330). Hangzhou, China: IEEE.

Luo, S., Li, R., & Ourselin, S. (2000). A new deformable model using dynamic gradient vector flow and adaptive balloon forces. In *APRSWorkshop on Dig Image Comp*.

Luo, S. (2006). Automated medical image segmentation using a deformable surface model. *Int J Comput Sci*, *6*(5), 109–115.

Luo, S., Li, X., & Li, J. (2014). Review on the Methods of Automatic Liver Segmentation from Abdominal Images. *Journal of Computer and Communications*, *2*(02), 1–7. doi:10.4236/jcc.2014.22001

Luo, T., Kramer, K., Goldgof, D. B., Hall, L. O., Samson, S., Remsen, A., & Hopkins, T. (2004). Recognizing plankton images from the shadow image particle profiling evaluation recorder. *IEEE Transactions on Systems, Man, and Cybernetics*, *34*(4), 1753–1762. doi:10.1109/TSMCB.2004.830340 PMID:15462442

Lu, Z., & Ip, H. S. S. (2009*).*Image categorization by learning with context and consistency. *Proceedings of the IEEE Computer Society Conference on Computer Vision and Pattern Recognition (CVPR '09).*

Macle, L., Jais, P., Scavee, C., Weerasooriya, R., Hocini, M., Shah, D. C., & Haïssaguerre, M. et al. (2003). Pulmonary vein disconnection using the LocaLisa three-dimensional nonfluoroscopic catheter imaging system. *Journal of Cardiovascular Electrophysiology*, *14*(7), 693–697. doi:10.1046/j.1540-8167.2003.03012.x PMID:12930247

MacQueen, J. B. (1967). Some methods for classification and analysis of multivariate observations. In *Proceedings of 5-th Berkeley Symposium on Mathematical Statistics and Probability* (vol. 1, pp. 281-297). Berkeley, CA: University of California Press.

Madabhushi, A., & Metaxas, D. N. (2003). Combining low-, high-level and empirical domain knowledge for automated segmentation of ultrasonic breast lesions. *IEEE Transactions on Medical Imaging*, *22*(2), 155–169. doi:10.1109/TMI.2002.808364 PMID:12715992

Mageswari, D. U., & Selvavinayagam, G. (2013). Wheelchair Motion Control Guide Using Eye Movement Based on EEG Signals. *International Journal of Engineering Sciences & Research Technology.*

Ma, J., & Plonka, G. (2010). The Curvelet Transform a Review of recent Applications. *IEEE Signal Processing Magazine*, *27*(2), 118–133. doi:10.1109/MSP.2009.935453

MajaTemerinac, O. (2010). *Tile-based Lucy-Richardson Deconvolution modeling a spatially-varying PSF for Fast Multiview Fusion of Microscopical images*. Teachnical Report 260.

Mamatha, M. (2015). *Development of Novel Architectures for Patient Care Monitoring System and Diagnosis. In Advancements of Medical Electronics* (pp. 333–342). Springer.

Mammographic Image Analysis Society (MIAS). (2015). Retrieved from http://skye.icr.ac.uk/miasdb/miasdb.html

Mamou, J., Coron, A., Oelze, M. L., Saegusa-Beecroft, E., Hata, M., Lee, P., & Feleppa, E. J. et al. (2011). Three-dimensional high-frequency backscatter and envelope quantification of cancerous human lymph nodes. *Ultrasound in Medicine & Biology*, *37*(3), 345–357. doi:10.1016/j.ultrasmedbio.2010.11.020 PMID:21316559

Maoguo, G., Yan, L., Jiao, S., Wenping, M., & Jingjing, M. (2013). Fuzzy C-Means Clustering With Local Information and Kernel Metric for Image Segmentation. Image Processing. *IEEE Transactions on*, *22*(2), 573–584.

Maoguo, G., Zhiqiang, Z., & Jingjing, M. (2012). Change Detection in Synthetic Aperture Radar Images based on Image Fusion and Fuzzy Clustering. Image Processing. *IEEE Transactions on*, *21*(4), 2141–2151.

Marcin, K., Materka, Strzelecki, & Szczypinski. (2001). Discrete Wavelet transform – derived features for digital image texture analysis. *Proc. Of International Conference on Signals and Electronic Systems*, (pp. 163 -168).

Marcus, C., Ladam-Marcus, V., Cucu, C., Bouché, O., Lucas, L., & Hoeffel, C. (2009). Imaging techniques to evaluate the response to treatment in oncology: Current standards and perspectives. *Critical Reviews in Oncology/Hematology*, *72*(3), 217–238. doi:10.1016/j.critrevonc.2008.07.012 PMID:18760935

Mardis, E. R. (2008). The impact of next-generation sequencing technology on genetics. *Trends in Genetics*, *24*(3), 133–141. doi:10.1016/j.tig.2007.12.007 PMID:18262675

Margulies, M., Eghol, M., Altman, W. E., Attiya, S., Bader, J. S., Bemben, L. A., & Rothberg, J. M. et al. (2005). Genome sequencing in microfabricated high-density picolitre reactors. *Nature*, *437*, 376–378. PMID:16056220

Marieb, E. N., & Hoehn, K. (2007). *Human anatomy & physiology*. Pearson Education.

Marinakis, Y., Marinaki, M., & Dounias, G. (2008). Particle swarm optimization for pap-smear diagnosis. *Expert Systems with Applications*, *35*(4), 1645–1656. doi:10.1016/j.eswa.2007.08.089

Marino, G., & Tarchi, D. (2014). MIMO radar imaging and geometrical target properties: A perspective from a classification point of view. In *EUSAR 2014; 10th European Conference on Synthetic Aperture Radar Proceedings*.

Mario, S., & Stephan, W. (2003). Gene prediction with a hidden markov model and a new intron submodel. Oxford University Press.

Marrouche, N. F., Martin, D. O., Wazni, O., Gillinov, A. M., Klein, A., Bhargava, M., & Natale, A. et al. (2003). Phased-array intracardiac echocardiography monitoring during pulmonary vein isolation in patients with atrial fibrillation: Impact on outcome and complications. *Circulation*, *107*(>21), 2710–2716. doi:10.1161/01.CIR.0000070541.83326.15 PMID:12756153

Marszałek, M., & Schmid, C. (2006). Spatial weighting for bag-of- features.*Proceedings of the IEEE Computer Society Conference on Computer Vision and Pattern Recognition (CVPR '06)*.

Martinek, M., Nesser, H. J., Aichinger, J., Boehm, G., & Purerfellner, H. (2007). Impact of integration of multislice computed tomography imaging into three-dimensional electroanatomic mapping on clinical outcomes, safety, and efficacy using radiofrequency ablation for atrial fibrillation. *Pacing and Clinical Electrophysiology*, *30*(10), 1215–1223. doi:10.1111/j.1540-8159.2007.00843.x PMID:17897124

Martin, G., David, K., Hari, T., & David, H. (2000). Genie–gene finding in drosophila melanogaster. *Genome Research*, 529–538.

Massich, J., Meriaudeau, F., Pérez, E., Martí, R., Oliver, A., & Martí, J. (2010). Lesion Segmentation in Breast Sonography. In J. Martí, A. Oliver, J. Freixenet, & R. Martí (Eds.), *Digital Mammography* (Vol. 6136, pp. 39–45). Springer Berlin Heidelberg. doi:10.1007/978-3-642-13666-5_6

Massich, J., Meriaudeau, F., Sentís, M., Ganau, S., Pérez, E., & Martí, R. et al.. (2012). Automatic Seed Placement for Breast Lesion Segmentation on US Images. In A. A. Maidment, P. Bakic, & S. Gavenonis (Eds.), *Breast Imaging* (Vol. 7361, pp. 308–315). Springer Berlin Heidelberg. doi:10.1007/978-3-642-31271-7_40

Matsumoto, O., Komoriya, K., Hatase, T., & Nishimura, H. (2006). *Autonomous Traveling Control of the "TAO Aicle" Intelligent Wheelchair.* Paper presented at the Intelligent Robots and Systems, 2006 IEEE/RSJ International Conference on.

Matsuo, S., Lim, K. T., & Haissaguerre, M. (2007). Ablation of chronic atrial fibrillation. *Heart Rhythm*, *4*(11), 1461–1463. doi:10.1016/j.hrthm.2007.07.016 PMID:17954407

Maybury, M. (2011). Information Graphics in Multimodal Documents. In Multimedia Information Extraction: Advances in Video, Audio, and Imagery Analysis for Search, Data Mining, Surveillance and Authoring. DOI: doi:10.1002/9781118219546.ch15

McCraty, R., Barrios-Choplin, B., Atkinson, M., & Tomasino, D. (1998). The effects of different types of music on mood, tension, and mental clarity. *Alternative Therapies in Health and Medicine*, *4*(1), 75–85. PMID:9439023

Mclnerney, T., & Terzopoulos, D. (2008). Deformable Models. In I. Bankman (Ed.), *Handbook of Medical Image Processing and Analysis* (2nd ed.; pp. 145–166). San Diego, CA: Academic Press.

Medi, C., Kalman, J. M., Haqqani, H., Vohra, J. K., Morton, J. B., Sparks, P. B., & Kistler, P. M. (2009). Tachycardia-mediated cardiomyopathy secondary to focal atrial tachycardia: Long-term outcome after catheter ablation. *Journal of the American College of Cardiology*, *53*(19), 1791–1797. doi:10.1016/j.jacc.2009.02.014 PMID:19422986

Meingast, M., Roosta, T., & Sastry, S. (2006). Security and Privacy Issues with Health Care Information Technology.*28th Annual International Conference of the IEEE Engineering in Medicine and Biology Society (EMBS 06)*. doi:10.1109/IEMBS.2006.260060

Mendez-Villanueva, A., Edge, J., Suriano, R., Hamer, P., & Bishop, D. (2012). The recovery of repeated-sprint exercise is associated with PCr resynthesis, while muscle pH and EMG amplitude remain depressed. *PLoS ONE*, *7*(12), e51977. doi:10.1371/journal.pone.0051977 PMID:23284836

Merletti, R., & Di Torino, P. (1999). Standards for reporting EMG data. *Journal of Electromyography and Kinesiology*, *9*(1), 3–4.

Merletti, R., & Parker, P. A. (2004). *Electromyography: physiology, engineering, and non-invasive applications* (Vol. 11). John Wiley & Sons. doi:10.1002/0471678384

Michailovich, O., & Adam, D. (2004). Phase unwrapping for 2-D blind deconvolution of ultrasound images. *IEEE Transactions on Medical Imaging*, *23*(1), 7–25. doi:10.1109/TMI.2003.819932 PMID:14719683

Miller, J. R., Koren, S., & Sutton, G. (2010). Assembly algorithms for nextgeneration sequencing data. *Genomics*, *95*(6), 315–327. doi:10.1016/j.ygeno.2010.03.001 PMID:20211242

Mitrea, D., Nedevschi, S., & Badea, R. (2014). The role of the Textural Microstructure Cooccurrence Matrices in the classification of the abdominal tumors, based on ultrasound images. In *Intelligent Computer Communication and Processing (ICCP),2014 IEEE International Conference*. doi:10.1109/ICCP.2014.6936972

Moghaddam, B., & Yang, M. H. (2002). Learning Gender with Support Faces. *IEEE Transactions on Pattern Analysis and Machine Intelligence*, *24*(5), 707–711. doi:10.1109/34.1000244

Mohamad, A., Jusoh Awang, N., Zaw, Z., & Shoon, L. W. (2014). Bayesian prokaryote classification from microscopic images. *Computer Applications: An International Journal*, *1*(1), 1–9.

Mohammad, I. K., Sarwar, K., & Linkon, C. (2015). MSuPDA: A Memory Efficient Algorithm for Sequence Alignment. *Interdisciplinary Sciences Computational Life Sciences*, *6*, 1.

Mohammed, N., & Squire, D. M. (2013). Efficient and accurate independent component filter-based features for texure similarity. In *Image Processing (ICIP), 2013 20th IEEE International Conference*. doi:10.1109/ICIP.2013.6738594

Mohana Shankar, P., Dumane, V. A., Reid, J. M., Genis, V., Forsberg, F., & Piccoli, C. W. (2001). Classification of ultrasonic B-mode images of breast masses using Nakagami distribution. *Ultrasonics, Ferroelectrics and Frequency Control. IEEE Transactions on*, *48*(2), 569–580.

Mohapatra, S., Patra, D., & Satpathi, S. (2010). Image analysis of blood microscopic images for acute leukemia detection.*2010 International Conference on Industrial Electronics, Control & Robotics (IECR)*, (pp. 215-219). doi:10.1109/IECR.2010.5720171

Moldovanu, S., Moraru, L., & Biswas, A. (2015). Robust skull stripping segmentation based on irrational mask for magnetic resonance brain images.Journal od Digital Imaging, 28(6) 738-747 PMID:25733013

Moldovanu, S., Obreja, C., & Moraru, L. (2014, November). *Threshold selection for classification of MR brain images by clustering method.* Paper presented at the meeting of the TIM 2014 Physics Conference, Timisoara, Romania.

Moldovanu, S., Moraru, L., & Nicolae, M. C. (2010). Comparative analysis of ultrasound image using gray level. *Annals of Dunarea de Jos University. Fascicle II*, *2*(33), 145–151.

Moldovanu, S., Punga Visan, M., & Moraru, L. (2015). Evaluation of outliers in acquired brain MR images. *Journal of Physics: Conference Series*, *574*, 012121. doi:10.1088/1742-6596/574/1/012121

Momen, K., Krishnan, S., & Chau, T. (2007). Real-time classification of forearm electromyographic signals corresponding to user-selected intentional movements for multifunction prosthesis control. *Neural Systems and Rehabilitation Engineering. IEEE Transactions on*, *15*(4), 535–542.

Moon, I., Lee, M., Chu, J., & Mun, M. (2005). *Wearable EMG-based HCI for electric-powered wheelchair users with motor disabilities.* Paper presented at the Robotics and Automation, 2005.

Moon, I., Lee, M., Chu, J., & Mun, M. (2005). *Wearable EMG-based HCI for electric-powered wheelchair users with motor disabilities.* Paper presented at the Robotics and Automation, 2005. ICRA 2005.

Moon, I., Lee, M., Chu, J., & Mun, M. (2005). *Wearable EMG-based HCI for electric-powered wheelchair users with motor disabilities.* Paper presented at the Robotics and Automation.

Morgan, X. C., Segata, N., & Huttenhower, C. (2012). Biodiversity and functional genomics in the human microbiome. *Trends in Genetics*, 1–8. PMID:23140990

Morissette, L., & Chartier, S. (2013). The k-means clustering technique: General considerations and implementation in mathematic. *Tutorials in Quantitative Methods for Psychology*, *9*(1), 15–24.

Mukherjee, A., Dey, G., Dey, M., & Dey, N. (2015). *Web-Based Intelligent EEG Signal Authentication and Tamper Detection System for Secure Telemonitoring. In Brain-Computer Interfaces* (pp. 295–312). Springer.

Mukherjee, S., Palit, S. K., Banerjee, S., & Bhattacharya, D. (2015). A Comparative Study on Three Different Types of Music Based on Same Indian Raga and Their Effects on Human Autonomic Nervous Systems *Chaos*[Springer.]. *Complexity and Leadership*, *2013*, 243–254.

Mukhopadhyaya, A., & Maulik, U. (2011). A multiobjective approach to MR brain image segmentation. *Applied Soft Computing*, *11*(1), 872–880. doi:10.1016/j.asoc.2010.01.007

Muller, U., Ligges, M., Georgiewa, P., Grnling, C., Kaiser, W. A., Witte, H., & Blanz, B. (2002). How to Avoid Spurious Cluster Validation? A Methodological Investigation on Simulated and fMRI Data. *NeuroImage*, *17*, 431–446.

Muller, H., Michoux, N., Bandon, D., & Geissbuhler, A. (2004). A review of content- based image retrieval systems in medical applications - Clinical benefits and future directions. *International Journal of Medical Informatics*, *73*(1), 1–23. doi:10.1016/j.ijmedinf.2003.11.024 PMID:15036075

Muller, H., Zhou, X., Depeursinge, A., Pitkanen, M., Iavindrasana, J., & Geissbuhler, A. (2007).Medical visual information retrieval: State of the art and challenges ahead.*Proceedings of the IEEE International Conference on Multimedia and Expo*. doi:10.1109/ICME.2007.4284742

Mulroy, S. J., Gronley, J. K., Newsam, C. J., & Perry, J. (1996). Electromyographic activity of shoulder muscles during wheelchair propulsion by paraplegic persons. *Archives of Physical Medicine and Rehabilitation*, *77*(2), 187–193. doi:10.1016/S0003-9993(96)90166-5 PMID:8607745

Mumford, D., & Shah, J. (1985). Boundary detection by minimizing functional. In *Proc.of IEEE Conference on Computer Vision and Pattern Recognition*. IEEE.

Mundy, J., Binford, T., Boult, T., Hanson, A., Beveridge, R., Haralick, R., . . . Strat, T. (1992). The image understanding environment program. *Computer Vision and Pattern Recognition, 1992. Proceedings CVPR '92.,1992 IEEE Computer Society Conference*. DOI: doi:10.1109/CVPR.1992.223157

Murtagh, F., & Legendre, P. (2014). Ward's hierarchical agglomerative clustering method: Which algorithms implement Ward's criterion? *Journal of Classification*, *31*(3), 274–295. doi:10.1007/s00357-014-9161-z

Murugavalli, S., & Rajamani, V. (2007). An improved implementation of brain tumor detection using segmentation based on neuro fuzzy technique. *Journal of Computer Science*, *3*(11), 41–846.

Nagashree, R. N., Aswini, N., Dyana, A., & Srinivas Rao, C. H. (2014). Detection and classification of ground penetrating radar image using textrual features. In *Advances in Electronics, Computers and Communications (ICAECC),2014 International Conference*. doi:10.1109/ICAECC.2014.7002403

Nakagawa, H., Shah, N., Matsudaira, K., Overholt, E., Chandrasekaran, K., Beckman, K. J., & Jackman, W. M. et al. (2001). Characterization of reentrant circuit in macroreentrant right atrial tachycardia after surgical repair of congenital heart disease: Isolated channels between scars allow "focal" ablation. *Circulation*, *103*(5), 699–709. doi:10.1161/01.CIR.103.5.699 PMID:11156882

Nakib, A., Oulhadj, H., & Siarry, P. (2007). Image histogram thresholding based on multiobjective optimization. *Signal Processing*, *87*(11), 2516–2534. doi:10.1016/j.sigpro.2007.04.001

Nandi, D., Ashour, A. S., Samanta, S., Chakraborty, S., Salem, M., & Dey, N. (2015). Principal Component Analysis in Medical Image Processing: A Study. *International Journal of Image Mining*, *1*(1), 65. doi:10.1504/IJIM.2015.070024

Naredo, E., Moller, I., Moragues, C., de Agustin, J. J., Scheel, A. K., & Grassi, W. (2006). Interobserver reliability in musculoskeletal ultrasonography: Results from a "Teach the Teachers" rheumatologist course. *Annals of the Rheumatic Diseases*, *65*(1), 14–19. doi:10.1136/ard.2005.037382 PMID:15941835

Natarajan, A., De Silva, B., Yap, K. K., & Motani, M. (2009). Link Layer Behavior of Body Area Networks at 2.4 GHz. In *15th Annual International Conference on Mobile Computing and Networking(MobiCom '09)*.

Nayak, S., Sahoo, S., Champaty, B., & Pal, K. (2014). *Effect of horror clips on the physiology of ANS & heart using ECG signal classification.* Paper presented at the Control, Instrumentation, Communication and Computational Technologies (ICCICCT), 2014 International Conference on. doi:10.1109/ICCICCT.2014.6993010

Nayak, S. K., Panda, I., Champaty, B., Bagh, N., Pal, K., & Tibarewala, D. (2015). *Automated Neural Network Based Classification of HRV and ECG Signals of Smokers: A Preliminary Study. In Advancements of Medical Electronics* (pp. 271–279). Springer.

Nazarpour, K., Al-Timemy, A. H., Bugmann, G., & Jackson, A. (2013). A note on the probability distribution function of the surface electromyogram signal. *Brain Research Bulletin*, *90*, 88–91. doi:10.1016/j.brainresbull.2012.09.012 PMID:23047056

Neto, A. F., Celeste, W. C., & Martins, V. R. (2006). *Human-machine interface based on electro-biological signals for mobile vehicles.* Paper presented at the Industrial Electronics, 2006 IEEE International Symposium on. doi:10.1109/ISIE.2006.296086

Ng, H. P., Ong, S. H., Foong, K. W. C., Goh, P. S., & Nowinski, W. L. (2006). Medical image segmentation using k-means clustering and improved watershed algorithm. In *Proceedings of the Symposium on Image Analysis and Interpretation* (pp. 61-65). Denver, CO: IEEE. doi:10.1109/SSIAI.2006.1633722

Niblack, W. (1986). *An introduction to digital image processing*. Denmark: Prentice Hall.

Nielsen, P. K., Jensen, B. R., Darvann, T., Jørgensen, K., & Bakke, M. (2000). Quantitative ultrasound image analysis of the supraspinatus muscle. Clinical Biomechanics, 15. *Supplement*, *1*(0), S13–S16.

Nielsen, P. K., Jensen, B. R., Darvann, T., Jorgensen, K., & Bakke, M. (2006). Quantitative ultrasound tissue characterization in shoulder and thigh muscles--a new approach. *BMC Musculoskeletal Disorders*, *7*(1), 2. doi:10.1186/1471-2474-7-2 PMID:16420695

Nimmy, S. F., & Kamal, M. S. (2015). Next generation sequencing under de novo genome assembly. *International Journal of Biomathematics*, *8*(05), 5. doi:10.1142/S1793524515300018

Nimmy, S. F., & Rahman, M. S. (2014). Algorithms for global protein–protein interaction network alignment. *Netw Model Anal Health Inform Bioinformatics*, *3*(1), 65. doi:10.1007/s13721-014-0065-y

Njeh, I., Ayed, I. B., & Hamida, A. B. (2012). A distribution-matching approach to MRI brain tumor segmentation.*9th IEEE International Symposium on Biomedical Imaging (ISBI)*. doi:10.1109/ISBI.2012.6235908

Noble, J. A., & Boukerroui, D. (2006). Ultrasound image segmentation: A survey. Medical Imaging. *IEEE Transactions on*, *25*(8), 987–1010.

Noble, J. A., & Wells, P. N. T. (2010). Ultrasound image segmentation and tissue characterization. *Proceedings of the Institution of Mechanical Engineers. Part H, Journal of Engineering in Medicine*, *224*(2), 307–316. doi:10.1243/09544119JEIM604 PMID:20349821

Noguchi, H., Park, J., & Takagi, T. (2006). MetaGene: Prokaryotic gene finding from environmental genome shotgun sequences. *Nucleic Acids Research*, *34*(19), 5623–5630. doi:10.1093/nar/gkl723 PMID:17028096

Noguchi, H., Taniguchi, T., & Itoh, T. (2008). Meta Gene Annotator: Detecting Species- Specific Patterns of Ribosomal Binding Site for Precise Gene Prediction in Anonymous Prokaryotic and Phage Genomes. *DNA Research*, *15*(6), 387–396. doi:10.1093/dnares/dsn027 PMID:18940874

Nowak, E., Jurie, F., & Triggs, B. (2006). *Sampling strategies for bag-of-features image classification* ECCV'06: 9th European Conference on Computer Vision: workshop on statistical Learning in Computer Vision.

Nowak, E., Jurie, F., & Triggs, B. (2006). Sampling strategies for bag-of-features image classification. In Computer Vision–ECCV 2006, (pp. 490-503). Springer Berlin Heidelberg. doi:10.1007/11744085_38

Nurhanim, K., Elamvazuthi, I., Vasant, P., Ganesan, T., Parasuraman, S., & Khan, M. A. (2014). Joint Torque Estimation Model of Surface Electromyography (sEMG) Based on Swarm Intelligence Algorithm for Robotic Assistive Device. *Procedia Computer Science*, *42*, 175–182. doi:10.1016/j.procs.2014.11.049

O'Donoghue, J., & Herbert, J. (2012). Data management within mHealth environments: Patient sensors, mobile devices, and databases. *Journal of Data and Information Quality*, *4*(1), 1–20. doi:10.1145/2378016.2378021

O'Donoghue, J., Herbert, J., & Fensli, R. (2006). Sensor Validation within a Pervasive Medical Environment. In *Proceedings of IEEE Sensors.*

Ohnishi, K., Weir, R. F., & Kuiken, T. A. (2007). Neural machine interfaces for controlling multifunctional powered upper-limb prostheses. *Expert Review of Medical Devices*, *4*(1), 43–53. doi:10.1586/17434440.4.1.43 PMID:17187470

Oktay, O., Schuh, A., Rajchl, M., Keraudren, K., Gomez, A., Heinrich, M. P., & Rueckert, D. et al. (2015). Structured Decision Forests for Multi-modal Ultrasound Image Registration. In *Proceedings of 18th International Conference on Medical Image Computing and Computer-Assisted Intervention (MICCAI)*, (LNCS), (vol. 9349, pp. 363–372). Springer. doi:10.1007/978-3-319-24571-3_44

Olshansky, B., Sabbah, H. N., Hauptman, P. J., & Colucci, W. S. (2008). Parasympathetic nervous system and heart failure pathophysiology and potential implications for therapy. *Circulation*, *118*(8), 863–871. doi:10.1161/CIRCULATIONAHA.107.760405 PMID:18711023

Opthof, T., Coronel, R., Wilms-Schopman, F. J., Plotnikov, A. N., Shlapakova, I. N., Danilo, P. Jr, & Janse, M. J. et al. (2007). Dispersion of repolarization in canine ventricle and the electrocardiographic T wave: T pe interval does not reflect transmural dispersion. *Heart Rhythm*, *4*(3), 341–348. doi:10.1016/j.hrthm.2006.11.022 PMID:17341400

Oral, H., Pappone, C., Chugh, A., Good, E., Bogun, F., Pelosi, F. Jr, & Morady, F. et al. (2006). Circumferential pulmonary vein ablation for chronic atrial fibrillation: A randomized, controlled study. *The New England Journal of Medicine*, *354*(9), 934–941. doi:10.1056/NEJMoa050955 PMID:16510747

Oral, H., Scharf, C., Chugh, A., Hall, B., Cheung, P., Good, E., & Morady, F. et al. (2003). Catheter ablation for paroxysmal atrial fibrillation: Segmental pulmonary vein ostial ablation versus left atrial ablation. *Circulation*, *108*(19), 2355–2360. doi:10.1161/01.CIR.0000095796.45180.88 PMID:14557355

Oren, B. (2008). *Defense of Nearest-Neighbor Based Image Classification.* Weizmann Institute of Science.

Osher, S., & Sethian, J. A. (1988). Fronts Propagating with Curvature-Dependent Speed: Algorithms Based on Hamilton-Jacobi Formulations. *Journal of Computational Physics*, *79*(1), 12–49. doi:10.1016/0021-9991(88)90002-2

Oskoei, M. A., & Hu, H. (2007). Myoelectric control systems—A survey. *Biomedical Signal Processing and Control*, *2*(4), 275–294. doi:10.1016/j.bspc.2007.07.009

Oskoei, M. A., & Hu, H. (2008). Support vector machine-based classification scheme for myoelectric control applied to upper limb. *Biomedical Engineering. IEEE Transactions on*, *55*(8), 1956–1965.

Otsu, N. (1979). A threshold selection method from gray-level histograms. *IEEE Transactions on Systems, Man, and Cybernetics*, *9*(1), 62–66. doi:10.1109/TSMC.1979.4310076

Ottenheijm, R. P., van't Klooster, I. G., Starmans, L. M., Vanderdood, K., de Bie, R. A., Dinant, G. J., & Cals, J. W. L. (2014). Ultrasound-diagnosed disorders in shoulder patients in daily general practice: A retrospective observational study. *BMC Family Practice*, *15*(1), 115. doi:10.1186/1471-2296-15-115 PMID:24916105

Oussalah, M. (2008). Content Based Image Retrieval: Review of State of Art and Future Directions. In Image Processing Theory, Tools and Applications, 2008. IPTA 2008. First Workshops. DOI: doi:10.1109/IPTA.2008.4743799

Packer, D. (2005). Three-dimensional mapping in interventional electrophysiology: Techniques and technology. *Journal of Cardiovascular Electrophysiology*, *16*(10), 1110–1116. doi:10.1111/j.1540-8167.2005.50161.x PMID:16191123

Pačnik, G., Benkič, K., & Brečko, B. (2005). *Voice operated intelligent wheelchair-VOIC.* Paper presented at the Industrial Electronics.

Pappone, C., Augello, G., Sala, S., Gugliotta, F., Vicedomini, G., Gulletta, S., & Santinelli, V. et al. (2006). A Randomized Trial of Circumferential Pulmonary Vein Ablation versus Antiarrhythmic Drug Therapy in Paroxysmal Atrial Fibrillation. The Ablation for Paroxysmal Atrial Fibrillation (APAF) Study. *Journal of the American College of Cardiology*, *48*(11), 2340–2347. doi:10.1016/j.jacc.2006.08.037 PMID:17161267

Pappone, C., Manguso, F., Vicedomini, G., Gugliotta, F., Santinelli, O., Ferro, A., & Santinelli, V. et al. (2004). Prevention of Iatrogenic Atrial Tachycardia following ablation of Atrial Fibrillation. A prospective randomized study comparing circumferential pulmonary vein ablation with a modified approach. *Circulation*, *110*(19), 3036–3042. doi:10.1161/01.CIR.0000147186.83715.95 PMID:15520310

Pappone, C., Rosanio, S., Augello, G., Gallus, G., Vicedomini, G., Mazzone, P., & Alfieri, O. et al. (2003). Mortality, Morbidity and Quality of Life after Circumferential Pulmonary Vein Ablation for Atrial Fibrillation. Outcomes from a Controlled not Randomized Long-Term Study. *Journal of the American College of Cardiology*, *42*(2), 185–197. doi:10.1016/S0735-1097(03)00577-1 PMID:12875749

Pappone, C., & Santinelli, V. (2006). How to perform encircling ablation of the left atrium. *Heart Rhythm*, *3*(9), 1105–1109. doi:10.1016/j.hrthm.2006.03.003 PMID:16945812

Pappone, C., Santinelli, V., Manguso, F., Vicedomini, G., Gugliotta, F., Augello, G., & Alfieri, O. et al. (2004). Pulmonary vein denervation enhances long-term benefit after circumferential ablation for paroxysmal atrial fibrillation. *Circulation*, *109*(3), 327–334. doi:10.1161/01.CIR.0000112641.16340.C7 PMID:14707026

Parati, G., Saul, J. P., Di Rienzo, M., & Mancia, G. (1995). Spectral analysis of blood pressure and heart rate variability in evaluating cardiovascular regulation a critical appraisal. *Hypertension*, *25*(6), 1276–1286. doi:10.1161/01.HYP.25.6.1276 PMID:7768574

Parikh, S. P., Grassi, V., Jr., Kumar, V., & Okamoto, J., Jr. (2005). *Usability study of a control framework for an intelligent wheelchair.* Paper presented at the Robotics and Automation. doi:10.1109/ROBOT.2005.1570853

Park, J. H., Zhou, S. K., Simopoulos, C., & Comaniciu, D. (2008). AutoGate: Fast and Automatic Doppler gate localization in B-mode echocardiogram, In *Proceedings of 11th International Conference on MICCAI* (LNCS), (vol. 5242, pp. 230-237). Springer Verlag Berlin Heidelberg. doi:10.1007/978-3-540-85990-1_28

Park, S.-H., & Lee, S.-P. (1998). EMG pattern recognition based on artificial intelligence techniques. *Rehabilitation Engineering. IEEE Transactions on*, *6*(4), 400–405.

Pascual-Montano, A., Donate, L. E., Valle, M., Barcena, M., Pascual-Marqui, R. D., & Carazo, J. M. (2001). A novel neural network technique for analysis and classification of EM single-particle images. *Journal of Structural Biology*, *133*(2), 233–245. doi:10.1006/jsbi.2001.4369 PMID:11472094

Patra, M. R., Das, R. K., & Padhy, R. P. (2012, October). CRHIS: cloud based rural healthcare information system. In *Proceedings of the 6th International Conference on Theory and Practice of Electronic Governance* (pp. 402-405). doi:10.1145/2463728.2463805

Peng, Y., Henry, C. M., Yiu, S. M., & Francis, Y. L. (2011). T-IDBA: A de novo iterative de Bruijn graph assembler for transcriptome. In Research in Computational Molecular Biology, Vancouver, Canada.

Pereira, F., Barros, C., Carvalho, V., Machado, J., Leão, C., & Soares, F. (2015). *Ambient Assisted Living Platform for Remote Monitoring of Bedridden People. In New Trends in Mechanism and Machine Science* (pp. 573–581). Springer.

Perez, J. E., Miller, J. G., Wickline, S. A., Holland, M. R., Waggoner, A. D., Barzilai, B., & Sobel, B. E. (1992). Quantitative ultrasonic imaging: Tissue characterization and instantaneous quantification of cardiac function. *The American Journal of Cardiology*, *69*(20), 104H–111H. doi:10.1016/0002-9149(92)90653-G PMID:1605115

Perrin, X. (2009). *Semi-autonomous navigation of an assistive robot using low throughput interfaces.* (Diss.). Eidgenössische Technische Hochschule ETH Zürich.

Pham, M., Mercier, G., & Michel, J. (2015). Pointwise Graph-Based Local Texture Characterization for Very High Resolution Multispectral Image Classification. Selected Topics in Applied Earth Observations and Remote Sensing, (99). DOI: doi:10.1109/JSTARS.2014.2386902

Phinyomark, A., Limsakul, C., & Phukpattaranont, P. (2011). Application of wavelet analysis in EMG feature extraction for pattern classification. *Measurement Science Review*, *11*(2), 45–52. doi:10.2478/v10048-011-0009-y

Phinyomark, A., Phukpattaranont, P., & Limsakul, C. (2012). Feature reduction and selection for EMG signal classification. *Expert Systems with Applications*, *39*(8), 7420–7431. doi:10.1016/j.eswa.2012.01.102

Phinyomark, A., Quaine, F., Charbonnier, S., Serviere, C., Tarpin-Bernard, F., & Laurillau, Y. (2013). EMG feature evaluation for improving myoelectric pattern recognition robustness. *Expert Systems with Applications*, *40*(12), 4832–4840. doi:10.1016/j.eswa.2013.02.023

Phukpattaranont, P., & Boonyaphiphat, P. (2006, October). Segmentation of cancer cells in microscopic images using neural network and mathematical morphology. *International Joint Conference SICE-ICASE*, (pp. 2312-2315). doi:10.1109/SICE.2006.315360

Phuong, L. T., & Binh, N. T. (2015). Human Object Classification Based on Nonsubsampled Contourlet Transform Combined with Zernike Moment. *4th EAI International Conference on Context-Aware Systems and Applications.* Springer.

Poon, Braun, Fahrig, Ginige, & Dorrell. (1994). Segmentation of Medical Images using an Active Contour Model Incorporating Region-based Images Features. In *Robb*, (pp. 90-97).

Pope, M., Aleksiev, A., Panagiotacopulos, N., Lee, J., Wilder, D., Friesen, K., & Goel, V. K. et al. (2000). Evaluation of low back muscle surface EMG signals using wavelets. *Clinical Biomechanics (Bristol, Avon)*, *15*(8), 567–573. doi:10.1016/S0268-0033(00)00024-3 PMID:10936428

Popuri, K., & Cobzas, D. (2009). *3D variational brain tumor segmentation on a clustered feature set.* SPIE Med Imaging.

Poty, H., Saoudi, N., Haïssaguerre, M., Daou, A., Clémenty, J., & Letac, B. (1996). Radiofrequency catheter ablation of atrial tachycardias. *American Heart Journal*, *131*(3), 481–489. doi:10.1016/S0002-8703(96)90526-8 PMID:8604627

Powell, S., Szklarczyk, D., Trachana, K., Roth, A., Kuhn, M., Muller, J., & Bork, P. et al. (2012). eggnog v3.0: Orthologous groups covering 1133 organisms at 41 different taxonomic ranges. *Nucleic Acids Research*, *40*(D1), 284–289. doi:10.1093/nar/gkr1060 PMID:22096231

Power, J. D., Cohen, A. L., Nelson, S. M., Wig, G. S., Barnes, K. A., Church, J. A., & Petersen, S. E. et al. (2011). Functional network organization of the human brain. *Neuron*, *72*(4), 665–678. doi:10.1016/j.neuron.2011.09.006 PMID:22099467

Prasad, A. M., Iverson, L. R., & Liaw, A. (2006). Newer classification and regression tree techniques: Bagging and random forests for ecological prediction. *Ecosystems (New York, N.Y.)*, *9*(2), 181–199. doi:10.1007/s10021-005-0054-1

Prasad, B. E., Gupta, A., Toong, H.-M., & Madnick, S. E. (1987). A microcomputer-based image database management system. *IEEE Transactions on Industrial Electronics*, *IE-34*(1), 83–88. doi:10.1109/TIE.1987.350929

Prastawa, M., Bullitt, E., Ho, S., & Gerig, G. (2004). A brain tumor segmentation framework based on outlier detection. *Medical Image Analysis*, *8*(3), 275–283. doi:10.1016/j.media.2004.06.007 PMID:15450222

Prastawa, M., Bullitt, E., Moon, N., Van Leemput, K., & Gerig, G. (2003). Automatic brain tumor segmentation by subject specific modification of atlas priors. *Academic Radiology*, *10*(12), 1341–1348. doi:10.1016/S1076-6332(03)00506-3 PMID:14697002

Pratik & Ladhake. (2013). Brain Tumor Detection Using Marker Based Watershed Segmentation from Digital MR Images. *International Journal of Innovative Technology and Exploring Engineering, 2*(5).

Prevost, R., Mory, B., Cuingnet, R., Correas, J.-M., Cohen, L., & Ardon, R. (2014). Kidney Detection and Segmentation in Contrast-Enhanced Ultrasound 3D Images. In A. S. El-Baz, L. Saba, & J. Suri (Eds.), *Abdomen and Thoracic Imaging* (pp. 37–67). Springer. doi:10.1007/978-1-4614-8498-1_2

Qian, G., Sural, S., & Pramanik, S. (2002). A comparative analysis of two distance measures in color image databases. In *Proceedings of the International Conference on Image Processing* (vol. 1, pp. I-401 - I-404). New York, NY: IEEE doi:10.1109/ICIP.2002.1038045

Qin, J., Li, R., Raes, J., Arumugam, M., Burgdorf, K. S., Manichanh, C., & Wang, J. et al. (2010). A human gut microbial gene catalogue established by metagenomic sequencing. *Nature*, *464*(7285), 59–65. doi:10.1038/nature08821 PMID:20203603

Qin, J., Li, Y., Cai, Z., Li, S., Zhu, J., Zhang, F., & Wang, J. et al. (2012). A metagenome-wide association study of gut microbiota in type 2 diabetes. *Nature*, *490*(7418), 55–60. doi:10.1038/nature11450 PMID:23023125

Quddus, A., & Basir, O. (2008). *Wavelet-based medical image registration for retrieval applications*. Paper presented at the International Conference on Biomedical Engineering and Informatics. doi:10.1109/BMEI.2008.257

Rahman, M. M., Desai, B.C., & Bhattacharya, P. (2006). Supervised machine learning based medical image annotation and retrieval. In Accessing Multilingual Information Repositories (LNCS) (pp. 692–701). Berlin: Springer.

Rahman, M., Wang, T., & Desai, B., C (2003). Medical image retrieval and registration: towards computer assisted diagnostics approach.*Proceedings of the fourth international workshop on design of reliable communication networks.*

Raina, N., Roshi, N., Chauhan, R., & Goudar, R. H. (2014). A fused features approach on Content-Based Image Retrieval based on Fuzzy rule-set. In *Advances in Computing, Communications and Informatics (ICACCI),2014 International Conference*. doi:10.1109/ICACCI.2014.6968407

Rajalakshmi, T., & Minu, R. I. (2014). Improving relevance feedback for content based medical image retrieval. In *Information Communication and Embedded Systems (ICICES),2014 International Conference Proceedings*. DOI: doi:10.1109/ICICES.2014.7033863

Ramos, J., Kockelkorn, T., Ramos, I., Ramos, R., Ginneken, B., Viergever, M., ... Grutters, J. (2015). Content Based Image Retrieval by Metric Learning from Radiology Reports: Application to Interstitial Lung Diseases. *IEEE Journal of Biomedical and Health Informatics*, (99). DOI: .10.1109/JBHI.2014.2375491

Rand, W. M. (1971). Objective criteria for the evaluation of clustering methods. *Journal of American Statisitics Association*, *66*(336), 846–850. doi:10.1080/01621459.1971.10482356

Rangayyan, R. M., Mudigonda, N. R., & Desautels, J. E. L. (2000). Boundary modelling and shape analysis methods for classification of mammographic masses.Revue: Medical and Biological Engineering and Computing, Collection: Engineering, 38(5), 487-496.

Rangayyan, R. M., Ayres, F. J., & Desautels, J. E. L. (2007). A Review of Computer-Aided Diagnosis of Breast Cancer: Toward the Detection of Subtle Signs. *Journal of the Franklin Institute*, *344*(3-4), 312–348. doi:10.1016/j.jfranklin.2006.09.003

Rao, P. S., & Raju, G. S. (2010). An approach for CBIR system through multilayer neural network. International Journal of Engineering Science and Technology, 2(4), 559-563.

Ravani, R., Mirali, M. R., & Baniasadi, M. (2010). *Parallel CBIR System Based on Color Coherence Vector*. In *17th International Conference on Systems, Signals and Image Processing*.

Raviv, T. R., Leemput, K. V., & Menze, B. H. (2012). Multi-modal brain tumor segmentation via latent atlases.*Proceeding MICCAIBRATS*.

Raya, R., Rocon, E., Urendes, E., Velasco, M. A., Clemotte, A., & Ceres, R. (2015). *Assistive Robots for Physical and Cognitive Rehabilitation in Cerebral Palsy. In Intelligent Assistive Robots* (pp. 133–156). Springer.

Reaz, M., Hussain, M., & Mohd-Yasin, F. (2006). Techniques of EMG signal analysis: Detection, processing, classification and applications. *Biological Procedures Online*, *8*(1), 11–35. doi:10.1251/bpo115 PMID:16799694

Rebsamen, B., Burdet, E., Guan, C., Zhang, H., Teo, C. L., & Zeng, Q. (2006). *A brain-controlled wheelchair based on P300 and path guidance*. Paper presented at the Biomedical Robotics and Biomechatronics, 2006. BioRob 2006. The First IEEE/RAS-EMBS International Conference on. doi:10.1109/BIOROB.2006.1639239

Rebsamen, B., Teo, C. L., Zeng, Q., Ang, M. H. Jr, Burdet, E., & Guan, C. (2007). Controlling a wheelchair indoors using thought. *IEEE Intelligent Systems*, *22*(2), 18–24. doi:10.1109/MIS.2007.26

Rechy-Ramirez, E. J., & Hu, H. (2014). A Flexible Bio-Signal Based HMI for Hands-Free Control of an Electric Powered Wheelchair. *International Journal of Artificial Life Research*, *4*(1), 59–76. doi:10.4018/ijalr.2014010105

Regniers, O., Bombrun, L., Guyon, D., Samalens, J.-C., & Germain, C. (2015). Wavelet-Based Texture Features for the Classification of Age Classes in a Maritime Pine Forest. Geoscience and Remote Sensing Letters, 12(3). DOI: doi:10.1109/LGRS.2014.2353656

Roberts-Thomson, K. C., Kistler, P. M., & Kalman, J. M. (2006). Focal atrial tachycardia II: Management. *Pacing and Clinical Electrophysiology*, *29*(7), 769–778. doi:10.1111/j.1540-8159.2006.00433.x PMID:16884515

Rockland, R. H., & Reisman, S. (1998). *Voice activated wheelchair controller.* Paper presented at the Bioengineering Conference.

Ronneberger, O., Heimann, U., Schultz, E., Dietze, V., Burkhardt, H., & Gehrig, R. (2000). Automated pollen recognition using gray scale invariants on 3D volume image data.*Second European Symposium on Aerobiology*.

Roth, H. R., Lu, L., Farag, A., Shin, H., Liu, J., Turkbey, E. B., & Summers, R. M. (2015). DeepOrgan: Multi-level Deep Convolutional Networks for Automated Pancreas Segmentation. In *Proceedings of 18th International Conference on Medical Image Computing and Computer-Assisted Intervention (MICCAI)*, (LNCS), (vol. 9349, pp. 556–564). Springer. doi:10.1007/978-3-319-24553-9_68

Rotter, M., Takahashi, Y., Sanders, P., Haissaguerre, M., Hsu, L. F., Sacher, F., & Hocini, M. et al. (2005). Reduction of fluoroscopy exposure and procedure duration during ablation of atrial fibrillation using a novel anatomical navigation system. *European Heart Journal*, *26*(14), 1415–1421. doi:10.1093/eurheartj/ehi172 PMID:15741228

Rubinov, M., & Sporns, O. (2011). Weight-conserving characterization of complex functional brain networks. *NeuroImage, 56*(4), 2068–2079. doi:10.1016/j.neuroimage.2011.03.069 PMID:21459148

Rueda, S., Fathima, S., Knight, C. L., Yaqub, M., Papageorghiou, A. T., Rahmatullah, B., & Noble, J. A. et al. (2014). Evaluation and comparison of current fetal ultrasound image segmentation methods for biometric measurements: A grand challenge. *IEEE Transactions on Medical Imaging, 33*(4), 797–813. doi:10.1109/TMI.2013.2276943 PMID:23934664

Rusch, D. B., Halpern, A. L., Sutton, G., Heidelberg, K. B., Williamson, S., Yooseph, S., & Venter, J. C. et al. (2007). The Sorcerer II Global Ocean Sampling expedition: Northwest Atlantic through eastern tropical Pacific. *PLoS Biology, 5*(3), e77. doi:10.1371/journal.pbio.0050077 PMID:17355176

Rutten, M. J., Jager, G. J., & Kiemeney, L. A. (2010). Ultrasound detection of rotator cuff tears: Observer agreement related to increasing experience. *AJR. American Journal of Roentgenology, 195*(6), W440-446. doi:10.2214/AJR.10.4526 PMID:21098177

Sahoo, P. K., Soltani, S., & Wong, A. K. C. (1988). A survey of thrsholding technique. *Computer Vision Graphics and Image Processing, 41*(2), 133–260. doi:10.1016/0734-189X(88)90022-9

Salton, G., Wong, A., & Yang, C. S. (1975). A Vector Space model for automatic indexing. *Model Communication of ACM., 18*(11), 613–620. doi:10.1145/361219.361220

Sampat, M. P., Markey, M. K., & Bovik, A. C. (2005). Computer-Aided Detection and Diagnosis in Mammography. In *Handbook of Image and Video Processing*. Amsterdam: Elsevier Academic Press. doi:10.1016/B978-012119792-6/50130-3

Sanei, S., & Chambers, J. A. (2013). *EEG signal processing*. John Wiley & Sons.

Santhosh Kumar, S., & Albert. (2014). Medical Image Segmentation using Kernel Weighted Fuzzy Clustering (KWFC) Algorithm. *International Journal of Inventions in Computer Science and Engineering, 1*(9).

Saoudi, N., Cosío, F., Waldo, A., Chen, S. A., Iesaka, Y., Lesh, M., & Schoels, W. et al. (2001). A classification of atrial flutter and regular atrial tachycardia according to electrophysiological mechanisms and anatomical bases; a Statement from a Joint Expert Group from The Working Group of Arrhythmias of the European Society of Cardiology and the North American Society of Pacing and Electrophysiology. *European Heart Journal, 22*(14), 1162–1182. doi:10.1053/euhj.2001.2658 PMID:11440490

Sapiro, G. (1997). Color snakes. *Computer Vision and Image Understanding, 2*(2), 247–253. doi:10.1006/cviu.1997.0562

Sauvola, J., & Pietikainen, M. (2000). Adaptive document image binarization. *Pattern Recognition, 33*(2), 225–236. doi:10.1016/S0031-3203(99)00055-2

Scheme, E., & Englehart, K. (2011). Electromyogram pattern recognition for control of powered upper-limb prostheses: State of the art and challenges for clinical use. *Journal of Rehabilitation Research and Development, 48*(6), 643. doi:10.1682/JRRD.2010.09.0177 PMID:21938652

Schenider, M., Ndrepepa, G., Dobran, I., Schreieck, J., Weber, S., Plewan, A., & Schmitt, C. et al. (2003). LocaLisa catheter navigation reduces fluoroscopy time and dosage in ablation of atrial flutter: A prospective randomized study. *Journal of Cardiovascular Electrophysiology, 14*(6), 587–590. doi:10.1046/j.1540-8167.2003.03017.x PMID:12875418

Scherr, D., Derval, N., Sohal, M., Pascale, P., Wright, M., Jadidi, A., & Knecht, S. et al. (2015). Length of the Mitral Isthmus But Not Anatomical Location of Ablation Line Predicts Bidirectional Mitral Isthmus Block in Patients Undergoing Catheter Ablation of Persistent Atrial Fibrillation: A Randomized Controlled Trial. *Journal of Cardiovascular Electrophysiology, 26*(6), 629–634. doi:10.1111/jce.12667 PMID:25786517

Schilling, R., Peters, N., & Davies, D. (1998). Simultaneous endocardial mapping in the human left ventricle using a noncontact catheter. Comparison of contact and reconstructed electrograms during sinus rhythm. *Circulation*, *98*(9), 887–898. doi:10.1161/01.CIR.98.9.887 PMID:9738644

Schmidt, B., Sinha, R., Beresford, B., & Puglisi, S. J. (2009). A fast hybrid short read fragment assembly algorithm. *Bioinformatics (Oxford, England)*, *25*(17), 2279–2280. doi:10.1093/bioinformatics/btp374 PMID:19535537

Schnorrenberg, F., Pattichis, C., Kyriacou, K., & Schizas, C. (1997). Computer-aided detection of breast cancer nuclei. *IEEE Transactions on Information Technology in Biomedicine*, *1*(2), 128–140. doi:10.1109/4233.640655 PMID:11020815

Scholten, R. R., Pillen, S., Verrips, A., & Zwarts, M. J. (2003). Quantitative ultrasonography of skeletal muscles in children: Normal values. *Muscle & Nerve*, *27*(6), 693–698. doi:10.1002/mus.10384 PMID:12766980

Schreier, G., Schwarz, M., Modre-Osprian, R., Kastner, P., Scherr, D., & Fruhwald, F. (2013). Design and evaluation of a multimodal mHealth based medication management system for patient self administration. In *Engineering in Medicine and Biology Society (EMBC), 2013 35th Annual International Conference of the IEEE*. doi:10.1109/EMBC.2013.6611236

Schwiebert, L., Gupta, S. S., & Weinmann, J. (2001). Research Challenges in Wireless Networks of Biomedical Sensors. *7th Annual International Conference on Mobile Computing and Networking*.

Sebestyenova, J., & Kurdel, P. (2014). Multimodal aspects of communication and data storage and managing systems. In *Intelligent Engineering Systems (INES), 2014 18th International Conference*. doi:10.1109/INES.2014.6909370

Sedghi, S., Sanderson, M., & Clough, P. (2012). How do health care professionals select medical images they need? *Aslib Proceedings*, *64*(4), 437–456. doi:10.1108/00012531211244815

Selesnick, I. W., & Sendur, L. (2000). Iterated oversampled filter banks and wavelet frames. Wavelet Applications VII. *Proceedings of the Society for Photo-Instrumentation Engineers*, 733–744. doi:10.1117/12.408663

Sellers, E. W., Ryan, D. B., & Hauser, C. K. (2014). Noninvasive brain-computer interface enables communication after brainstem stroke. *Science Translational Medicine*, *6*(257).

Semmlow, J. L., & Griffel, B. (2014). *Biosignal and medical image processing*. CRC Press.

Seo, S.-H., Jeon, I.-H., Cho, Y.-H., Lee, H.-G., Hwang, Y.-T., & Jang, J.-H. (2013). Surface EMG during the push-up plus exercise on a stable support or swiss ball: Scapular stabilizer muscle exercise. *Journal of Physical Therapy Science*, *25*(7), 833–837. doi:10.1589/jpts.25.833 PMID:24259864

Sergio, G. V., Xuedong, L., Cao, H., Min, C., & Leung, V. C. M. (2011). Body Area Networks: A Survey. *Springer Mobile Networks and Applications*, *16*(2), 171–193. doi:10.1007/s11036-010-0260-8

Sethian, J. A. (1999). *Level set methods and fast marching methods: evolving interface sin geometry, fluid mechanics, computer vision and materials science* (2nd ed.). Cambridge University Press.

Sevillano, J. L., Cascado, D., Cagigas, D., Vicente, S., Lujan, C., & Rio, F. (2009). *A real-time wireless sensor network for wheelchair navigation*. Paper presented at the Computer Systems and Applications, 2009. AICCSA 2009. IEEE/ACS International Conference on. doi:10.1109/AICCSA.2009.5069311

Sezgin, M., & Sankur, B. (2004). Survey over image thresholding techniques and quantitative performance evaluation. *Journal of Electronic Imaging*, *13*(1), 146–165. doi:10.1117/1.1631315

Shafait, F., Keysers, D., & Breuel, T. (2008). Efficient implementation of local adaptive thresholding techniques using integral image. In *Proceedings of the 15th Document Recognition and Retrieval Conference* (vol. 6815, pp. 651–660). San Jose, CA: SPIE.

Shaheen, S., & Umamakeswari, A. (2013). Intelligent Wheelchair For People With Disabilities. *IACSIT International Journal of Engineering and Technology*, *5*(1), 391–397.

Shanmugapriya, Poonguzhali, & Umamaheshwari. (2014). An intensity-based medical image registration using genetic algorithm, signal & Image Processing. *Signal & Image Processing: An International Journal*, *5*(3), 197–206.

Shekhar & Jawahar. (2012). *Word Image Retrieval using Bag of Visual Words* 10th IAPR Paper presented at the International Workshop on Document Analysis Systems IEEE Computer Society.

Shen, H., Hao, H., Wei, L., & Wang, Z. (2008, December). An image based classification method for cataract. *International Symposium on Computer Science and Computational Technology* (vol. 1, pp. 583-586). doi:10.1109/ISCSCT.2008.78

Shenoy, P., Miller, K. J., Crawford, B., & Rao, R. P. (2008). Online electromyographic control of a robotic prosthesis. *Biomedical Engineering. IEEE Transactions on*, *55*(3), 1128–1135.

Shyu, C. R., Brodley, C. E., Kak, A. C., Kosaka, A., Aisen, A. M., & Broderick, L. S. (1999). ASSERT: A physician-in-the-loop content-based image retrieval system for HRCT image databases. *Computer Vision and Image Understanding*, *75*(2), 111–132. doi:10.1006/cviu.1999.0768

Shyu, C. R., Kak, A., Brodley, C., & Broderick, L. S. (1999). Testing for human perceptual categories in a physician-in-the-loop CBIR system for medical imagery.*Proceedings of the IEEE Workshop on Content-based Access of Image and Video Libraries (CBAIVL)*. doi:10.1109/IVL.1999.781132

Sidhom, S., & David, A. (2007). Automatic indexing of multimedia documents as a starting point to annotation process. *ISKO: 9th International Conference*. Vienna, Austria: Ergon Verlag.

Siedliecki, S. L., & Good, M. (2006). Effect of music on power, pain, depression and disability. *Journal of Advanced Nursing*, *54*(5), 553–562. doi:10.1111/j.1365-2648.2006.03860.x PMID:16722953

Silka, M. J., Gillette, P. C., Garson, A. Jr, & Zinner, A. (1985). Transvenous catheter ablation of a right atrial automatic ectopic tachycardia. *Journal of the American College of Cardiology*, *5*(4), 999–1001. doi:10.1016/S0735-1097(85)80448-4 PMID:3973306

Silva, H., Lourenço, A., & Paz, N. (2011). *Real-time Biosignal Acquisition and Telemedicine Platform for AAL based on Android OS*. Paper presented at the AAL.

Simmons, Z. (2005). Management strategies for patients with amyotrophic lateral sclerosis from diagnosis through death. *The Neurologist*, *11*(5), 257–270. doi:10.1097/01.nrl.0000178758.30374.34 PMID:16148733

Simms, A. P. (2014). *Reading and Wirelessly Sending EEG Signals Using Arduinos and XBee Radios to Control a Robot*. Academic Press.

Simpson, J.T., Wong, K., Jackman, K., Schein, J.E., Jones, S.J., & Birol, I. (2009), A parallel assembler for short read sequence data, Res. ABySS.

Simpson, R. C. (2005). Smart wheelchairs: A literature review. *Journal of Rehabilitation Research and Development*, *42*(4), 423. doi:10.1682/JRRD.2004.08.0101 PMID:16320139

Simpson, R., LoPresti, E., Hayashi, S., Nourbakhsh, I., & Miller, D. (2004). The smart wheelchair component system. *Journal of Rehabilitation Research and Development*, *41*(3b3B), 429–442. doi:10.1682/JRRD.2003.03.0032 PMID:15543461

Singh, B. K., & Mazumdar, B. (2010). Content Retrieval From X-RAY Images Using Color & Texture Features. Department of Biomedical Engg. National Institute of Technology, Raipur (C.G).

Singh, J. P. (2012). Shoulder ultrasound: What you need to know. *Indian J Radiol Imaging*, *22*(4), 284–292. doi:10.4103/0971-3026.111481 PMID:23833420

Singh, S. (2013). Microscopic Image Analysis of Nanoparticles by Edge Detection Using Ant Colony Optimization. *IOSR Journal of Computer Engineering*, *11*(3), 84–89. doi:10.9790/0661-1138489

Sinha, D., Ahmed, M. T., & Greenspan, M. (2014). Image Retrieval Using Landmark Indexing for Indoor Navigation. *Computer and Robot Vision (CRV),2014 Canadian Conference*. doi:10.1109/CRV.2014.17

Sitara, K., & Remya, S. (2012). Image deblurring in bayesian framework using template based blur estimation. *The International Journal of Multimedia & Its Applications*, *4*(1), 137–153. doi:10.5121/ijma.2012.4112

Sivakamasundari, J., Kavitha, G., Natarajan, V., & Ramakrishnan, S. (2014). Proposal of a Content Based retinal Image Retrieval system using Kirsch template based edge detection. In *Informatics, Electronics & Vision (ICIEV),2014 International Conference*. DOI: doi:10.1109/ICIEV.2014.6850744

Sivicand, A., & Zisserman. (2003). *Video Google: A text retrieval approach to object matching in videos.* ICCV'05: 10th IEEE International Conference on Computer Vision.

Skånland, M. S. (2013). Music, health, and well-being. *International Journal of Qualitative Studies on Health and Well-being*, 8. PMID:23930993

Smitha, P., Shaji, L., & Mini, M. G. (2011). A review of medical image classification technique. In *International conference on VLSI, Communication & Intrumrnataiom*, (pp. 34-38).

Soares, A., Andrade, A., Lamounier, E., & Carrijo, R. (2003). The development of a virtual myoelectric prosthesis controlled by an EMG pattern recognition system based on neural networks. *Journal of Intelligent Information Systems*, *21*(2), 127–141. doi:10.1023/A:1024758415877

Soros, G., & Madrick, J. (1999). The international crisis: An interview. *The New York Review of Books*, *46*, 36–37.

Sporton, S., Earley, M., Nathan, A., & Schilling, R. J. (2004). Electroanatomic versus fluoroscopic mapping for catheter ablation procedures: A prospective randomized study. *Journal of Cardiovascular Electrophysiology*, *15*(3), 310–315. doi:10.1111/j.1540-8167.2004.03356.x PMID:15030422

Stanley, H. (2011). An Augmented Lagrangian Method for Total Variation Video Restoration. *IEEE Transactions on Image Processing*, *20*(11), 3097–3111. doi:10.1109/TIP.2011.2158229 PMID:21632302

Starck, L., Candès, E. J., & Donoho, D. L. (2002). The Curvelet Transform for Image Denoising. *IEEE Transactions on Image Processing*, *11*(6), 670–684. doi:10.1109/TIP.2002.1014998 PMID:18244665

Strang. (1989). Wavelets and dilation equations: A brief introduction. *SIAM Review, 31*(4).

Strobl, C., Malley, J., & Tutz, G. (2009). An introduction to recursive partitioning: Rationale, application, and characteristics of classification and regression trees, bagging, and random forests. *Psychological Methods*, *14*(4), 323–348. doi:10.1037/a0016973 PMID:19968396

Suapang, P., Puttanakit, V., & Yimman, S. (2013). Mammography Archiving and Web Viewer. In *SICE Annual Conference (SICE), 2013 Proceedings.*

Subasi, A., Yilmaz, M., & Ozcalik, H. R. (2006). Classification of EMG signals using wavelet neural network. *Journal of Neuroscience Methods*, *156*(1), 360–367. doi:10.1016/j.jneumeth.2006.03.004 PMID:16621003

Sum, K. W., & Cheung, Y. S. (2007). Boundary Vector Field for Parametric Active Contours. *Pattern Recognition*, *40*(6), 1635–1645. doi:10.1016/j.patcog.2006.11.006

Sun, A. Y., & Piccini, J. P. (2014). Validation of non-contact and point-to-point mapping in a single electroanatomic map. *Europace*, *16*, 371–375. PMID:24158252

Sung, W.-T., Chen, J.-H., & Chang, K.-Y. (2013). ZigBee based multi-purpose electronic score design and implementation using EOG. *Sensors and Actuators. A, Physical*, *190*, 141–152. doi:10.1016/j.sna.2012.11.028

Supardi, N. Z., Mashor, M. Y., Harun, N. H., Bakri, F. A., & Hassan, R. (2012). Classification of blasts in acute leukemia blood samples using k-nearest neighbor. *2012 IEEE 8th International Colloquium on Signal Processing and its Applications* (CSPA), (pp. 461-465). IEEE.

Suzuki, K. (2012b). Pixel-based Machine-Learning in Medical Imaging. *International Journal of Biomedical Imaging*. PMID:22481907

Suzuki, K. (Ed.). (2012a). *Machine Learning in Computer-Aided Diagnosis: Medical Imaging Intelligence and Analysis*. Hershey, PA: IGI Global.

Suzuki, K., Abe, H., MacMahon, H., & Doi, K. (2006). Image-processing technique for suppressing ribs in chest radiographs by means of massive training artificial neural network (MTANN). *IEEE Transactions on Medical Imaging*, *25*(4), 406–416. doi:10.1109/TMI.2006.871549 PMID:16608057

Suzuki, K., Li, F., Sone, S., & Doi, K. (2005). Computer-aided diagnostic scheme for distinction between benign and malignant nodules in thoracic low-dose CT by use of massive training artificial neural network. *IEEE Transactions on Medical Imaging*, *24*(9), 1138–1150. doi:10.1109/TMI.2005.852048 PMID:16156352

Sweidan, A. H., El-Bendary, N., Hassanien, A. E., Hegazy, O. M., & Mohamed, A. E.-K. (2015). Grey Wolf Optimizer and Case-Based Reasoning Model for Water Quality Assessment. *1st International Conference on Advanced Intelligent System and Informatics (AISI2015)*.

Tabesh, A., Teverovskiy, M., Pang, H. Y., Kumar, V. P., Verbel, D., Kotsianti, A., & Saidi, O. (2007). Multifeature prostate cancer diagnosis and Gleason grading of histological images. Medical Imaging. *IEEE Transactions on*, *26*(10), 1366–1378.

Tafa, Z., & Stojanovic, R. (2006). Bluetooth-based approach to monitoring biomedical signals. *WSEAS Transactions on Business and Economics*, *2*(3), 75–80.

Talab, A. M. A., Huang, Z., & Junfei, W. (2014). An enhanced Bernsen algorithm approaches for vehicle logo detection. *International Journal of Signal Processing. Image Processing and Pattern Recognition*, *7*(4), 203–210. doi:10.14257/ijsip.2014.7.4.20

Tanaka, K., Matsunaga, K., & Wang, H. O. (2005). Electroencephalogram-based control of an electric wheelchair. *Robotics. IEEE Transactions on*, *21*(4), 762–766.

Tan, C. C., & Wang, H. (2008). Body Sensor Network Security: An Identity-Based Cryptography Approach. In *Frist ACM Conference on Wireless Network Security (WiSec '08)*. doi:10.1145/1352533.1352557

Tang, J., Chen, Z., Wai-chee Fu, A., & Cheung, D. (2001). A robust outlier detection scheme for large data sets. In *The 6th Pacific-Asia Conference on Knowledge Discovery and Data Mining* (vol. 1, pp. 6-8). London, UK: Springer-Verlag.

Tatiraju, S., & Mehta, A. (2011). Image Segmentation using k-means clustering, EM and Normalized Cuts. In *ICIAP'11 Proceedings of the 16th International Conference on Image Analysis and Processing* (vol. 2, pp. 229-240). Genova, Italy: Springer-Verlag.

Tatusov, R. L., Fedorova, N. D., Jackson, J. D., Jacobs, A. R., Kiryutin, B., Koonin, E. V., & Natale, D. A. et al. (2003). The COG database: An updated version includes eukaryotes. *BMC Bioinformatics*, *4*(1), 41. doi:10.1186/1471-2105-4-41 PMID:12969510

Taxt, T. (1997). Comparison of cepstrum - based methods for radial blind deconvolution of ultrasound images. *IEEE Transactions on Ultrasonics, Ferroelectrics, and Frequency Control*, *44*(3), 666–674. doi:10.1109/58.658327

Teefey, S. A., Middleton, W. D., Bauer, G. S., Hildebolt, C. F., & Yamaguchi, K. (2000). Sonographic differences in the appearance of acute and chronic full-thickness rotator cuff tears. *Journal of Ultrasound in Medicine*, *19*(6), 377–378, quiz 383. PMID:10841058

Teefey, S. A., Rubin, D. A., Middleton, W. D., Hildebolt, C. F., Leibold, R. A., & Yamaguchi, K. (2004). Detection and quantification of rotator cuff tears. Comparison of ultrasonographic, magnetic resonance imaging, and arthroscopic findings in seventy-one consecutive cases. *The Journal of Bone and Joint Surgery. American Volume*, *86-A*(4), 708–716. PMID:15069134

Thatte, G., Li, M., Lee, S., Emken, A., Narayanan, S., Mitra, U., & Annavaram, M. et al. (2012). Knowme: An energy-efficient multimodal body area network for physical activity monitoring. *ACM Transactions on Embedded Computing Systems*, *11*(S2), 48. doi:10.1145/2331147.2331158

Thoma, M. V., La Marca, R., Brönnimann, R., Finkel, L., Ehlert, U., & Nater, U. M. (2013). The effect of music on the human stress response. *PLoS ONE*, *8*(8), e70156. PMID:23940541

Thomas, J., & Sael, L. (2015). Overview of integrative analysis methods for heterogeneous data. In *Big Data and Smart Computing (BigComp),2015 International Conference*. doi:10.1109/35021BIGCOMP.2015.7072811

Toews, M., & Arbel, T. (2007). A statistical parts-based model of anatomical variability. *IEEE Transactions on Medical Imaging*, *26*(4), 497–508. doi:10.1109/TMI.2007.892510 PMID:17427737

Tomari, M. R. M., Kobayashi, Y., & Kuno, Y. (2012). Development of smart wheelchair system for a user with severe motor impairment. *Procedia Engineering*, *41*, 538–546. doi:10.1016/j.proeng.2012.07.209

Tomonaga, T., Filipi, C. J., Lowham, A., & Martinez, T. (1999). Laparoscopic intracorporeal ultrasound cystic duct length measurement: A new technique to prevent common bile duct injuries. *Surgical Endoscopy*, *13*(2), 183–185. doi:10.1007/s004649900935 PMID:9918627

Tong, X., Xie, H., & Weng, Q. (2014). Urban Land Cover Classification With Airborne Hyperspectral Data: What Features to Use? Selected Topics in Applied Earth Observations and Remote Sensing, 7(10). DOI: doi:10.1109/JSTARS.2013.2272212

Tsui, C. S. L., Jia, P., Gan, J. Q., Hu, H., & Yuan, K. (2007). *EMG-based hands-free wheelchair control with EOG attention shift detection*. Paper presented at the Robotics and Biomimetics, 2007. ROBIO 2007. IEEE International Conference on.

Tuyet, V. T. H., & Binh, N. T. (2015). Reducing impurities in medical images based on curvelet domain. *Nature of Computation and Communication, Springer*, *144*, 306–319. doi:10.1007/978-3-319-15392-6_29

Tyson, G. W., Chapman, J., Hugenholtz, P., Allen, E. E., Ram, R. J., Richardson, P. M., & Banfield, J. F. et al. (2004). Community structure and metabolism through reconstruction of microbial genomes from the environment. *Nature*, *428*(6978), 37–43. doi:10.1038/nature02340 PMID:14961025

Ubeda, A., Ianez, E., & Azorín, J. M. (2011). Wireless and portable EOG-based interface for assisting disabled people. *Mechatronics, IEEE/ASME Transactions on*, *16*(5), 870-873.

Usakli, A. B., Gurkan, S., Aloise, F., Vecchiato, G., & Babiloni, F. (2010). On the use of electrooculogram for efficient human computer interfaces. *Computational Intelligence and Neuroscience*, *2010*, 1. doi:10.1155/2010/630649 PMID:19841687

Vallabhaneni, A., Wang, T., & He, B. (2005). *Brain—computer interface. In Neural engineering* (pp. 85–121). Springer. doi:10.1007/0-306-48610-5_3

Van Boxtel, A. (2001). Optimal signal bandwidth for the recording of surface EMG activity of facial, jaw, oral, and neck muscles. *Psychophysiology*, *38*(1), 22–34. doi:10.1111/1469-8986.3810022 PMID:11321618

Van De Sande, K. E. A., Gevers, T., & Snoek, C. G. M. (2011). Empowering visual categorization with the GPU. *IEEE Transactions on Multimedia*, *13*(1), 60–70. doi:10.1109/TMM.2010.2091400

Van Den Elsen, Pol, & Viergever. (1993). Medical image matching: a review with classification. *IEEE Engineering in Medicine and Biology, 12*(1), 26-39.

Van Hare, G. F., Velvis, H., & Langberg, J. J. (1990). Successful transcatheter ablation of congenital junctional ectopic tachycardia in a ten-month-old infant using radiofrequency energy. *Pacing and Clinical Electrophysiology*, *13*(6), 730–735. doi:10.1111/j.1540-8159.1990.tb02099.x PMID:1695353

van Ravenswaaij-Arts, C. M., Kollee, L. A., Hopman, J. C., Stoelinga, G. B., & van Geijn, H. P. (1993). Heart rate variability. *Annals of Internal Medicine*, *118*(6), 436–447. doi:10.7326/0003-4819-118-6-199303150-00008 PMID:8439119

Vapnik, V. N. (1995). *The Nature of Statistical Learning Theory*. Springer-Verlag. doi:10.1007/978-1-4757-2440-0

Varoquaux, G., Gramfort, A., Poline, J. B., & Thirion, B. (2012). *Markov models for fMRI correlation structure: is brain functional connectivity small world, or decomposable into networks? Journal of Physiology.*

Ventura, R., Rostock, T., Klemm, H., Lutomsky, B., Demir, C., Weiss, C., & Willems, S. et al. (2004). Catheter ablation of common-type atrial flutter guided by three-dimensional right atrial geometry reconstruction and catheter tracking using cutaneous patches: A randomized prospective study. *Journal of Cardiovascular Electrophysiology*, *15*(10), 1157–1161. doi:10.1046/j.1540-8167.2004.04064.x PMID:15485440

Voss, A., Kurths, J., Kleiner, H., Witt, A., & Wessel, N. (1995). Improved analysis of heart rate variability by methods of nonlinear dynamics. *Journal of Electrocardiology*, *28*, 81–88. doi:10.1016/S0022-0736(95)80021-2 PMID:8656135

W.Yinan, D. W. Renner, I. Albert, & M. L.SzparaL.(2015).VirAmp: a galaxy-based viral genome assembly pipeline GigaScience 4,19.

Wagner, F. C., Macovski, A., & Nishimura, D. G. (1988). A characterization of the scatter point-spread function in terms of air gaps. *IEEE Transactions on Medical Imaging*, *7*(4), 337–344. doi:10.1109/42.14517 PMID:18230487

Waluyo, A. B., Yeoh, W. S., Pek, I., Yong, Y., & Chen, X. (2010). Mobisense: Mobile body sensor network for ambulatory monitoring. *ACM Transactions on Embedded Computing Systems*, *10*(1), 13. doi:10.1145/1814539.1814552

Wang, D., Wang, Li, Liu, Li, & Zhang. (2007). Mapping Query to Semantic Concepts: Leveraging Semantic Indices for Automatic and Interactive Video Retrieval. In *Semantic Computing, 2007. ICSC 2007.International Conference*. DOI: doi:10.1109/ICSC.2007.105

Wang, Kong, Lu, Qi, & Zhang. (2008). A modified FCM algorithm for MRI brain image segmentation using both local and non-local spatial constraints. *Computerized Medical Imaging and Graphics, 32*, 685–698

Wang, Y., & Feng, D. (2009). Image Registration for Biomedical Information Integration. In Data Mining and Medical Knowledge Management: Cases and Applications (pp. 122-136). Hershey, PA: IGI Global. doi:10.4018/978-1-60566-218-3.ch006

Wang, G., Vannier, M. W., Skinner, M. W., Cavalcanti, M. G. P., & Harding, G. (1998). Spiral CT image deblurring for cochlear implantation. *IEEE Transactions on Medical Imaging*, *17*(2), 251–262. doi:10.1109/42.700737 PMID:9688157

Wang, H., Zheng, C., Li, Y., Zhu, H., & Yan, X. (2003). Application of support vector machines to classification of blood cells. *Sheng Wu Yi Xue Gong Cheng Xue Za Zhi, 20*(3), 484–487. PMID:14565019

Wang, J. Z. (2000). Pathfinder: Multiresolution region based searching of pathology images using IRM. *Proceedings of the AMIA Symposium, 2000*, 883–887. PMID:11080011

Wang, L., & Fu, X. (2006). *Data mining with computational intelligence*. Springer Science & Business Media.

Wang, M., Zhou, X., Li, F., Huckins, J., King, R. W., & Wong, S. T. C. (2008). Novel cell segmentation and online SVM for cell cycle phase identification in automated microscopy. *Bioinformatics (Oxford, England), 24*(1), 94–101. doi:10.1093/bioinformatics/btm530 PMID:17989093

Wang, S., Cho, H., Zhai, C. X., Berger, B., & Peng, J. (2015). Exploiting ontology graph for predicting sparsely annotated gene function. *Bioinformatics (Oxford, England), 31*(12), i357–i364. doi:10.1093/bioinformatics/btv260 PMID:26072504

Wang, T., Cheng, I., & Basu, A. (2009). Fluid vector flow and applications in brain tumor segmentation. *IEEE Transactions on Bio-Medical Engineering, 56*(3), 781–789. doi:10.1109/TBME.2009.2012423 PMID:19174335

Wang, X., Ritchie, C. J., & Kim, Y. (1996). Elevation direction deconvolution in three-dimensional ultrasound imaging. *IEEE Transactions on Medical Imaging, 15*(3), 389–394. doi:10.1109/42.500148 PMID:18215920

Wang, Z., Ouyang, J., Liang, Y., Jin, Z., Yang, G., Liang, M., & Han, Y. et al. (2015). Focal atrial tachycardia surrounding the anterior septum: Strategy for mapping and catheter ablation. *Circulation: Arrhythmia and Electrophysiology, 8*(3), 575–582. doi:10.1161/CIRCEP.114.002281 PMID:25908691

Wan, J., Zou, C., Ullah, S., Lai, C. F., Zhou, M., & Wang, X. (2013). Cloud-enabled wireless body area networks for pervasive healthcare. *IEEE Network, 27*(5), 56–61. doi:10.1109/MNET.2013.6616116

Warfield, S., Kaus, M., Jolesz, F., & Kikinis, R. (2000). Adaptive template moderated spatially varying statistical classification. *Medical Image Analysis, 4*(1), 43–55. doi:10.1016/S1361-8415(00)00003-7 PMID:10972320

Watanabe, K., Kouzaki, M., Merletti, R., Fujibayashi, M., & Moritani, T. (2012). Spatial EMG potential distribution pattern of vastus lateralis muscle during isometric knee extension in young and elderly men. *Journal of Electromyography and Kinesiology, 22*(1), 74–79. doi:10.1016/j.jelekin.2011.09.010 PMID:21996320

Wei, N., You, J., Friehs, K., Flaschel, E., & Nattkemper, T. W. (2007). An in situ probe for on-line monitoring of cell density and viability on the basis of dark field micfroscopy in conjunction with image processing and supervised machine learning. *Biotechnology and Bioengineering, 97*(6), 1489–1500. doi:10.1002/bit.21368 PMID:17274069

Wellens, H. J., Bär, F. W., & Lie, K. (2000). *The value of the electrocardiogram in the differential diagnosis of a tachycardia with a widened QRS complex*. Springer.

Wels, M., Carneiro, G., Aplas, A., Huber, M., Hornegger, J., & Comaniciu, D. (2008). A Discriminative model-constrained graph cuts approach to fully automated pediatric brain tumor segmentation in 3-D MRI. *Lecture Notes in Computer Science, 5241*, 67–75. doi:10.1007/978-3-540-85988-8_9 PMID:18979733

Wernick, M. N., Yang, Y., Brankov, J. G., Yourganov, G., & Strother, S. C. (2010). Machine learning in medical imaging: Drawing conclusions from medical images. *IEEE Signal Processing Magazine, 27*(July), 25–38. doi:10.1109/MSP.2010.936730 PMID:25382956

White, J. M. (1999). Effects of relaxing music on cardiac autonomic balance and anxiety after acute myocardial infarction. *American Journal of Critical Care, 8*(4), 220. PMID:10392221

Wijesoma, W. S., Wee, K. S., Wee, O. C., Balasuriya, A. P., San, K. T., & Soon, L. K. (2005). *EOG based control of mobile assistive platforms for the severely disabled.* Paper presented at the Robotics and Biomimetics (ROBIO). 2005 IEEE International Conference on. doi:10.1109/ROBIO.2005.246316

Wilber, D. J., Pappone, C., Neuzil, P., De Paola, A., Marchlinski, F., Natale, A., & Berry, D. A. et al. (2010). ThermoCool AF Trial Investigators. *Journal of the American Medical Association*, *303*, 333–340. doi:10.1001/jama.2009.2029 PMID:20103757

Wilke, A., Harrison, T., Wilkening, J., Field, D., Glass, E. M., Kyrpides, N., & Meyer, F. et al. (2012). The M5nr: A novel non-redundant database containing protein sequences and annotations from multiple sources and associated tools. *BMC Bioinformatics*, *13*(1), 141. doi:10.1186/1471-2105-13-141 PMID:22720753

Willems, S., Weiss, C., Ventura, R., Rüppel, R., Risius, T., Hoffmann, M., & Meinertz, T. (2000). Catheter ablation of atrial flutter guided by electroanatomic mapping (CARTO): A randomized comparison to the conventional approach. *Journal of Cardiovascular Electrophysiology*, *12*(11), 1223–1230. doi:10.1046/j.1540-8167.2000.01223.x PMID:11083243

Winterfield, J. R., Jensen, J., Gilbert, T., Marchlinski, F., Natale, A., Packer, D., & Wilber, D. J. et al. (2015). Lesion Size and Safety Comparison between the Novel Flex Tip on the FlexAbility Ablation Catheter and the Solid Tips on the ThermoCool and ThermoCool SF Ablation Catheters. *Journal of Cardiovascular Electrophysiology*, *11*(Sep). doi: doi:10.1111/jce.12835 PMID:26359632

Wolterink, J. M., Leiner, T., Takx, R. A., Viergever, M. A., & Isgum, I. (2015). Automatic Coronary Calcium Scoring in Non-Contrast-Enhanced ECG-Triggered Cardiac CT with Ambiguity Detection. *IEEE Transactions on Medical Imaging*, *34*(9), 1867–1878. doi:10.1109/TMI.2015.2412651 PMID:25794387

Won-Young, H. (2014). A Coherent View on Entropy. *Natural Science*, *6*(7), 540–544. doi:10.4236/ns.2014.67053

Wu, B.-F., Jen, C.-L., & Huang, T.-W. (2011). *Intelligent radio based positioning and fuzzy based navigation for robotic wheelchair with wireless local area networks.* Paper presented at the Robot, Vision and Signal Processing (RVSP), 2011 First International Conference on. doi:10.1109/RVSP.2011.61

Wu, C., Song, A., Ling, Y., Wang, N., & Tian, L. (2014). *A Control Strategy with Tactile perception Feedback for EMG Prosthetic Hand.* Academic Press.

Wu, L. M., Li, Z., Ma, W. Y., & Yu, N. (2007). Visual language modeling for image classification. *Proceedings of the 9th ACM SIG Multimedia International Workshop on Multimedia Information Retrieval (MIR '07).* doi:10.1145/1290082.1290101

Wu, D., Wu, M., Halpern, A., Rusch, D. B., Yooseph, S., Frazier, M., & Eisen, J. A. et al. (2011). Stalking the fourth domain in metagenomic data: Searching for, discovering, and interpreting novel, deep branches in marker gene phylogenetic trees. *PLoS ONE*, *6*(3), e18011. doi:10.1371/journal.pone.0018011 PMID:21437252

Xiangfei, K., Kuan, L., Qingxiong, Y., Liu, W., & Ming, H. Y. (2013). A New Image Quality Metric for Image Auto-Denoising.*IEEE International Conference on Computer Vision*, (pp. 2888-2895). IEEE.

Xie, T., Yu, H., & Wilamowski, B. (2011). *Comparison between traditional neural networks and radial basis function networks.* Paper presented at the IEEE International Symposium on Industrial Electronics. doi:10.1109/ISIE.2011.5984328

Xie, Yang, Zhan, & Zhu. (2005). Semi-automated brain tumor and edema segmentation using MRI. *Eur J Radiol*, *56.*

Xie, X., & Beni, G. (1991). A validity measure for fuzzy clustering. *IEEE Transactions on Pattern Analysis and Machine Intelligence*, *13*(8), 841–847. doi:10.1109/34.85677

Xie, Y., & Tao, X. (2011). White Matter Lesion Segmentation Using Machine Learning and Weakly Labeled MR Images, In *Proceedings of SPIE Medical Imaging 2011*, (vol. 7962) doi:10.1117/12.878237

Xin-bo, Z., & Jiang, L. (2009). An image segmentation algorithm based on fuzzy c-means clustering. *Digital Image Processing*, *1*, 22–26.

Xu, C., & Prince, J. L. (1998). Generalized Gradient Vector Flow External Force for Active Contours. *Signal Processing*, *71*(2), 71–79. doi:10.1016/S0165-1684(98)00140-6

Xu, J. W., & Suzuki, K. (2011). Massive-training support vector regression and Gaussian process for false-positive reduction in computer-aided detection of polyps in CT colonography. *Medical Physics*, *38*(4), 1888–1902. doi:10.1118/1.3562898 PMID:21626922

Xu, L., Chen, H., Hu, X., Zhang, R., Zhang, Z., & Luo, Z. W. (2006). Average Gene Length Is Highly Conserved in Prokaryotes and Eukaryotes and Diverges Only Between the Two Kingdoms. *Molecular Biology and Evolution*, *23*(6), 1107–1108. doi:10.1093/molbev/msk019 PMID:16611645

Yamashita, S., Iwai, K., Akimoto, T., Sugawara, J., & Kono, I. (2006). Effects of music during exercise on RPE, heart rate and the autonomic nervous system. *The Journal of Sports Medicine and Physical Fitness*, *46*(3), 425. PMID:16998447

Yang, J., Jiang, Y. G., Hauptmann, A., & Ngo, C. W. (2007). *Evaluating bag-of-visual-words representations in scene classification*, MIR'07. International workshop on Multimedia Information. doi:10.1145/1290082.1290111

Yang, S., & Naiman, D. Q. (2014). Multiclass cancer classification based on gene expression comparison. *Statistical Applications in Genetics and Molecular Biology*, *13*(4), 477–496. PMID:24918456

Yang, Y. (2007). Image Segmentation by fuzzy c-means clustering algorithm with a novel penalty term. *Computing and Informatics*, *26*, 17–31.

Yang, Z., Su, Z., Ji, F., Zhu, M., & Bai, B. (2014). Mechanisms of behavior modification in clinical behavioral medicine in China. *International Journal of Behavioral Medicine*, *21*(4), 580–583. doi:10.1007/s12529-014-9405-7 PMID:24842543

Yathunanthan, S., Chandrasena, L., Umakanthan, A., Vasuki, V., & Munasinghe, S. (2008). *Controlling a wheelchair by use of EOG signal.* Paper presented at the Information and Automation for Sustainability, 2008. ICIAFS 2008. 4th International Conference on. doi:10.1109/ICIAFS.2008.4783987

Yatsunenko, T., Rey, F. E., Manary, M. J., Trehan, I., & Dominguez, M. G. (2012). Human gut microbiome viewed across age and geography. *Nature*, 10. PMID:22699611

Ying, Q. M. L., Wei, Q., & Ren, X. (2014). A Registration Method for Multimodal Medical Images Using Contours Mutual Information. *International Journal of Advanced Research in Artificial Intelligence*, *3*(4), 2014.

Yin, Y. H., Fan, Y. J., & Xu, L. D. (2012). EMG and EPP-integrated human–machine interface between the paralyzed and rehabilitation exoskeleton. *Information Technology in Biomedicine. IEEE Transactions on*, *16*(4), 542–549.

Yuan, Y., Li, B., & Meng, M. Q.-H. (2015). Improved Bag of Feature for Automatic Polyp Detection in Wireless Capsule Endoscopy Images. IEEE Transactions Automation Science and Engineering, (99). DOI: doi:10.1109/TASE.2015.2395429

Yu, B. Y., Elbuken, C., Ren, C. L., & Huissoon, J. P. (2011). Image processing and classification algorithm for yeast cell morphology in a microfluidic chip. *Journal of Biomedical Optics*, *16*(6), 066008–066008. doi:10.1117/1.3589100 PMID:21721809

Yuzhen, Y., & Haixu, T. (2015). Utilizing de Bruijn graph of metagenome assembly for metatranscriptome analysis. *Bioinformatics (Oxford, England)*, 1–8.

Zaidi, H., Vees, H., & Wissmeyer, M. (2009). Molecular PET/CT imaging- guided radiation therapy treatment planning. *Academic Radiology*, *16*(9), 1108–1133. doi:10.1016/j.acra.2009.02.014 PMID:19427800

Zardoshti-Kermani, M., Wheeler, B. C., Badie, K., & Hashemi, R. M. (1995). EMG feature evaluation for movement control of upper extremity prostheses. *Rehabilitation Engineering. IEEE Transactions on*, *3*(4), 324–333.

Zarit, S. H., Reever, K. E., & Bach-Peterson, J. (1980). Relatives of the impaired elderly: Correlates of feelings of burden. *The Gerontologist*, *20*(6), 649–655. doi:10.1093/geront/20.6.649 PMID:7203086

Zennaro, D., Wellig, P., Koch, V. M., Moschytz, G. S., & Läubli, T. (2003). A software package for the decomposition of long-term multichannel EMG signals using wavelet coefficients. *Biomedical Engineering. IEEE Transactions on*, *50*(1), 58–69.

Zerbino, D. R., & Birney, E. (2008). Velvet: Algorithms for de novo short read assembly using de Bruijn graphs. *Genome Research*, *18*(5), 821–829. doi:10.1101/gr.074492.107 PMID:18349386

Zhang, H., Fritts, J., & Goldman, S. (2004). An entropy-based objective evaluation method for image segmentation. *Proc. SPIE- Storage and Retrieval Methods and Applications for Multimedia, 5307*, 38–49.

Zhang, J., Marszalek, M., Lazebnik, S., & Schmid, C. (2005). *Local features and kernels for classification of texture and object categories: A comprehensive study.* Technical Report RR-5737. Inria.

Zhang, Y., Zhang, J., & Luo, Y. (2011). *A novel intelligent wheelchair control system based on hand gesture recognition.* Paper presented at the Complex Medical Engineering (CME), 2011 IEEE/ICME International Conference on. doi:10.1109/ICCME.2011.5876761 doi:10.1109/ICCME.2011.5876761

Zhang, Z., Zhang, R., Yao, J., Pu, G., Knudson, P.E., Weinstock, R.S., & Krol, A. (2005). Medical data on demand with WebMIA. Engineering in Medicine and Biology Magazine, 24(3). DOI: doi:10.1109/MEMB.2005.1436469

Zhang, Z., Zhu, Q., & Xie, Y. (2012). MRI Segmentation of Brain Tissue Based on Spatial Prior and Neighboring Pixels Affinities. *21st International Conference on Pattern Recognition (ICPR 2012).* Retrieved from http://in.mathworks.com/help/images/gray-level-co-occurrence-matrix-glcm.html

Zhang, J. M. F., & Starck, J. L. (2008). Wavelets, ridgelets and curvelets for poisson noise removal. *IEEE Transactions on Image Processing*, *17*(7), 1093–1108. doi:10.1109/TIP.2008.924386 PMID:18586618

Zhang, W., Yu, F., & Hong-mi, G. (2009). Improved adaptive wavelet threshold for image denoising.*Control and Decision Conference, Chinese.* IEEE. doi:10.1109/CCDC.2009.5195268

Zhang, Y., Brady, M., & Smith, S. (2001). Segmentation of brain MR images through a hidden Markov random field model and the expectation-maximization algorithm. *IEEE Transactions on Medical Imaging*, *20*(1), 45–57. doi:10.1109/42.906424 PMID:11293691

Zhang, Z., Schwartz, S., Wagner, L., & Miller, W. (2000). A greedy algorithm for aligning DNA sequences. *Journal of Computational Biology*, *7*(1-2), 203–214. doi:10.1089/10665270050081478 PMID:10890397

Zhao, J., Xie, Z., Jiang, L., Cai, H., Liu, H., & Hirzinger, G. (2006). *EMG control for a five-fingered underactuated prosthetic hand based on wavelet transform and sample entropy.* Paper presented at the Intelligent Robots and Systems, 2006 IEEE/RSJ International Conference on. doi:10.1109/IROS.2006.282425

Zhao, M. Y. (2007, May). Lattice Boltzmann based PDE solver on the GPU. *The Visual Computer*, *24*(5), 323–333. doi:10.1007/s00371-007-0191-y

Zheng, J., Kuai, D., Liu, Z., Teng, Y., & Zhang, T. (2011). *Salient Feature Volume and Its Application in Brain MRI Image Registration.4th International Conference on Biomedical Engineering and Informatics (BMEI).*

Zheng, Y., Liu, D., Georgescu, B., Nguyen, H., & Comaniciu, D. (2015). 3D Deep Learning for Efficient and Robust Landmark Detection in Volumetric Data. In *Proceedings of 18th International Conference on Medical Image Computing and Computer-Assisted Intervention (MICCAI)* (LNCS), (vol. 9349, pp. 565–572). Springer. doi:10.1007/978-3-319-24553-9_69

Zhong, T., Tagare, H. D., & Beaty, J. D. (2006). Evaluation of Four Probability Distribution Models for Speckle in Clinical Cardiac Ultrasound Images. Medical Imaging. *IEEE Transactions on*, *25*(11), 1483–1491.

Zhou, W., & Bovik, A. C. (2002). A universal image quality index. *Signal Processing Letters, IEEE*, *9*(3), 81–84. doi:10.1109/97.995823

Zhuang, X., Yu, & Haralick. (1984). A new approach to the solution of the maximum entropy image reconstruction problem. In *Acoustics, Speech, and Signal Processing, IEEE International Conference on ICASSP '84*. DOI: doi:10.1109/ICASSP.1984.1172340

Zipes, D.P., Calkins, H., Williams, E.S., & Halperin, J.L. (2015, September 16). ACC/AHA/HRS Advanced Training Statement on Clinical Cardiac Electrophysiology (A Revision of the ACC/AHA 2006 Update of the Clinical Competence Statement on Invasive Electrophysiology Studies, Catheter Ablation, and Cardioversion). *Heart Rhythm*.

Zohreh, S., Saeid, A., Abdullah, G., & Rajkumar, B. (2013). Heterogeneity in Mobile Cloud Computing: Taxonomy and Open Challenges. *IEEE Communications Surveys and Tutorials*, (99): 1–24.

Zwarts, M. J., & Stegeman, D. F. (2003). Multichannel surface EMG: Basic aspects and clinical utility. *Muscle & Nerve*, *28*(1), 1–17. doi:10.1002/mus.10358 PMID:12811768

Zywietz, C. (2003). *A brief history of electrocardiography-progress through technology*. Hannover: Biosigna Institute for Biosignal Processing and Systems Research.

About the Contributors

Nilanjan Dey is an Assistant Professer in the Department of Information Technology in Techno India College of Technology, Rajarhat, Kolkata, INDIA. He holds an honorary position of Visiting Scientist at Global Biomedical Technologies Inc., CA, USA and Research Scientist of Laboratory of Applied Mathematical Modeling in Human Physiology, Territorial Organization-of-gientifig and Engineering Unions, BULGARIA. He is the Editor in Chief of Int. J. of Rough Sets and Data Analysis, IGI Global, US Managing Editor of International Journal of Image Mining (IJIM), Inderscience, Regional Editor-Asia of International Journal of Intelligent Engineering Informatics (IJIEI), Inderscience and Associated Editor of International Journal of Service Science, Management, Engineering, and Technology, IGI Global. His research interests include: Medical Imaging, Soft computing, Data mining, Machine learning, Rough set, Mathematical Modeling and Computer Simulation, Modeling of Biomedical Systems, Robotics and Systems, Information Hiding, Security, Computer Aided Diagnosis, Atherosclerosis. He has 8 books and 160 international conferences and journal papers. He chaired sessions in INDIACom, 2014 Delhi, IC3T 2015, Hyderabad. He is chairing sessions in IEEE World Congress on Computational Intelligence, 2016 in Canada. He is the Program chair of AISI'15, Egypt and Publication Co-chair of CREATE'15, India, General Chair of RICE 2016, and Session Chair of FuzzyIEEE- 2016, Canada. He is a life member of IE, UACEE, IS.

Amira S. Ashour is Assistant Professer and Vice Chair of Computers Engineering Department, Computers and Information Technology College, Taif University, KSA. She was the vice chair of Computer Science department, CIT college, Taif University, KSA for five years. She is in the Electronics and Electrical Communications Engineering, Faculty of Engineering, Tanta University, Egypt. She received her Ph.D in Smart Antenna (2005) in the Electronics and Electrical Communications Engineering, Tanta University, Egypt. She had her Masters in Enhancement of Electromagnetic Non-Destructive Evaluation Performance using Advanced Signal Processing Techniques in Faculty of Engineering, Egypt, 2000. Her research interests include: Image Processing, Medical Imaging, Computer Aided Diagnosis, Machine learning, Smart Antenna and Adaptive Antenna Arrays. She has several international conferences and journal papers. She is an Associated Editor of the International Journal of Rough Sets and Data Analysis, IGI Global, US.

* * *

Swarnambiga Ayyachamy earned her Ph.D from Anna University Chennai, she is currently working as Associate professor in the department of Electronics and Communication Engineering and research coordinator at SACS MAVMM Engineering College, Madurai. She is the serving as the editor for journal of health and medical informatics, United States of America. She is also serving as reviewer for several journals and in Conferences. She has presented seminars in various colleges. She also serves as recognized supervisor for Ph.D in Anna University Chennai. She has organized conferences and seminars. She is the member of ISTE. She has been invited as speaker for conferences from China and Japan and her publications has been quoted widely by other researchers. She has published 30 articles. Among that 6 International and 1 National journal and15 International and 8 National conferences Research Interest Dr Swarnambiga Ayyachamy research interest includes Machine vision, Image processing, Splines and Wavelet analysis in imaging, Biomedical Data Analysis and Bioinformatics, Computer intelligence, Signal Processing, Data Mining, Public Health systems research.

Samsad Beagum is working as a Lecturer in the Department of Computer Science, Taif University, Kingdom of Saudi Arabia. She is an external Research Scholar at Karpagam University, Coimbatore, India. She received her MPhil in Computer Science from Manonmanian Sundaranar University, Tirunelveli, India. She has previously worked as a Software Engineer in Singapore, developing middleware and application software for digital TVs and set-top boxes. Her research interests include image processing, algorithms and bioinformatics.

Nguyen Thanh Binh received the Bachelor of Engineering degree from Ho Chi Minh City University of Technology, VNU-HCM, Vietnam in 2000, the Master of Science degree and Doctor of Philosophy degree in computer science from University of Allahabad - India in 2005 and 2011. Now, he is a lecturer at Faculty of Computer Science and Engineering, Ho Chi Minh City University of Technology-Vietnam National University in Ho Chi Minh City. He has published more than 40 papers in international journals and conference proceedings. His research interests include recognition, image processing, multimedia information systems, decision support system, and time series data.

Anjan Biswas is an Associate Professor in the Department of Mathematical Sciences at Delaware State University in Dover, DE, USA. He earned his Ph.D. degree in Mathematics from the University of New Mexico, Albuquerque, NM. His main research interests are in Theory of Solitons and Nonlinear Optics. To date, he has published more than 500 papers in several peer-reviewed journals, and two books on Optical Solitons. He is also serving as the editorial board member of more than 10 journals.

Noureddine Bourkache is an academic assistant at the M'hamed bouguerra University (Boumerdes) Algeria, while preparing his doctoral thesis at the Mouloud Mammeri University (Tizi-Ouzou Algeria). He is engineerin electronic -informatics and holds a Magister Diploma in the discipline.

Sayan Chakraborty has completed M.Tech from Computer Science & Engineering, JIS College of Engineering. He also completed his B. Tech. from the same college. His research area is digital image processing, nature inspired algorithms and mobile communication. He has about 30 research papers published in international conferences on optimization and digital image processing. He has 12 research paper published in International conference and 7 research paper in International Journal.

Biswajeet Champaty received his B.Tech degree in Biomedical Engineering from Trident Academy of Technology, Bhubaneswar, Odisha, India in 2010, M.Tech degree in Biomedical Engineering from SRM University, Chennai, India in 2012. Currently, he is pursuing his PhD degree in Biomedical Engineering from the National Institute of Technology Rourkela, India. His area of research includes biomedical instrumentation and signal processing for designing human-computer interface devices mainly for rehabilitation and assistive purposes.

Linkon Chodhury received the B.Sc (Hons) in computer science and engineering from University of Chittagong Bangladesh in 2011. Since 2011, he has been serving as a faculty member in the Department of Computer Science and Engineering at BGC Trust University Bangladesh Chittagong. Now he is M.Sc (Engineering) student in the Department of Computer Science and Engineering at Chittagong University of Engineering & Technology (CUET), Chittagong, Bangladesh. His research interest includes Bioinformatics, Data mining and Artificial Intelligence.

Simonetta Crisa, Clinical Engineer, Robotic remote approach for ablation of supraventricular tachyarrhythmias, including WPW syndrome, Robotic remote approach for the identification of the best site and lead positioning within coronary sinus during Biventricular implantation in patients with Heart Failure, Diagnostic and Therapeutic Telemedicine (home ECG and remote device monitoring and interrogation).

Kaushik Dev: B.Tech. in CSE (Russia), M.Tech. in CSE(Russia), PhD (South Korea); Field of Interests: Computer Vision, Digital Image Processing, Pattern Recognition, Human Computer Interaction, License plate recognition and Intelligent transportation system.

Irraivan Elamvazuthi obtained his PhD from Department of Automatic Control & Systems Engineering, University of Sheffield, UK in 2002. He is currently an Associate Professor at the Department of Electrical and Electronic Engineering, Universiti Teknologi PETRONAS (UTP), Malaysia. His research interests include Control, Robotics, Mechatronics, Power Systems and Bio-medical Applications.

Carmine Garzillo -- Fellow Researcher at University of Naples Federico II in Medical Statistics and Informatics Education: Fellowship in "Multi-scale Methods for applications in Life Sciences", 2006-8 Specialization courses in Statistics and Informatics in Health Sciences, 2004-6 Biochemical fellow at Regina Elena Cancer Research Institute in Rome, 2000-2003 Post doctoral fellow (VII cicle), 1997-99 Ph.D., Chemical Sciences, University of Naples Federico II, 1996 Concentrations: Theoretical Chemistry, Quantum Chemistry Dissertation: Theoretical Methods in the determination of the structure and the function of biomolecules. Practitioner in a Clinical Chemistry laboratory Degree: Chemistry, University of Naples Federico II, 1987 Concentrations: Bio-crystallography, Quantum Biochemistry Thesis: Refinement of the crystal structure of BS Rnase: interactions with water, ions, and substrate analogous Teaching: Instructor, 2009-2010, 2010 – 2011, 2012-2013, 2013-2014 University of Naples Federico II Courses: Medical Statistics, Informatics Research Skills: Extensive knowledge of molecular modeling software, statistical programs.

John George is Head of Musculoskeletal Radiology at the Department of Biomedical Imaging, University of Malaya Medical Centre in Kuala Lumpur, Malaysia. He has spoken at several International Conferences and runs annual Musculoskeletal MRI and ultrasound workshops in Penang Island. He has authored about 35 ISI cited publications and his research interests are in menisco-capsular tears of the knee, knee cartilage imaging and classification, MRI for age estimation used by FIFA and use of High Resolution of Ultrasound for arthritis screening.

Srijan Goswami has received M.Sc degree (2012) in Medical Biotechnology from The West Bengal University of Health Sciences, Kolkata, India. He also completed Post Graduate Diploma in Software Engineering from West Bengal Electronics Industry Development Corporation Limited, West Bengal, India and A-Level in Information Technology from National Institute of Electronics and Information Technology, Govt. of India. He is currently appointed as a Faculty in the Dept. of Information Technology at Webel Informatics Limited, Basirhat College. His research area is Bioinformatics, Medical Information Technology and Medical Genetics. He has around 4 research publications.

Rishu Gupta was born in Gonda, UP, India, in 1984. He received his B. Tech degree in Electronics and Communications Engineering fromBundelkhand Institute of Engineering and Technology in 2009 and M.S degree in Visual Contents from Dongseo University, South Korea. Currently, he is working toward the PhD Degree from UniversitiTeknologi Petronas, Malaysia. He is active IEEE student member since 2012. His research interests include medical ultrasound image processing and Visual Contents.

Uvanesh K. received the B.E degree in Biomedical Engineering from Rajalakshmi Engineering College, Anna University, Tamil Nadu, India, in 2013 and the M.Tech degree in Biomedical Engineering from National Institute of Technology-Rourkela, Odisha, India, in 2015. Now, he joined as a research scholar in School of Biomedical Engineering, Indian Institute of Technology (BHU), Uttar Pradesh, India. His research interests include Biomedical signal acquisition, processing & analysis, Bioinstrumentation and Circuit design.

Md. Sarwar Kamal working as a Senior Lecturer at Computer Science and Engineering department in East West University Bangladesh. He has completed his M.Sc (Eng) in Computer Science and Engineering from Chittagong University of Engineering and Technology. His research interest is Bioinformatics and Data Mining.

Mohammad Ibrahim Khan is the professor at Computer Science and Engineering department in Chittagong University of Engineering and Technology, Bangladesh.

P. Mohan Kumar has completed his undergraduate in Computer Science and Engineering in MS University, post graduate in Computer Science and Engineering in Anna University and PhD in Computer Science and Engineering at Sathyabama University. He is in the teaching field for the past 14 years. Currently he is working as Professor in the Department of Information Technology, Jeppiaar Engineering College.

Mourad Laghrouche is professor at the university Mouloud Mammeri (Tizi-Ouzou) in Algeria. He is the head of department in electronics-informatics (Lampa Lab.). His main research is in the domain of image processing and analysis. Currently, he is the Vice-President of the University Mouloud Mammeri in Algeria.

Biswajit Mohapatra is practising surgeon at Vesaj Patel Hospital, Rorurkela, India. Present designation consultant laparoscopic surgeon and endoscopist. Eductional qualification: MBBS Utkal University 1990, MS University, Boroda, Gujurat 1995, DIP. in Lap Surgery Indian Laparoscopic Institute, Coimbatore 2004, Endoscopy Fellowship K E M Hospital Mumbai and SMS Endoscopy Center - Mumbai 1997, FMAS Amasi 2010. Working experience - 15 years hospital place designation 1996-1997 Trust Hospital Bharuch (GUJURAT) consultant 1997-1997(DEC) Maniben Nagarji Hospital VAPI(Gujurat) Consultant 1998(JANUARY) – till date Vesaj Patel Hospital Rourkela consultant (private practice).

Simona Moldovanu got her MSc degrees in IT in 2006 and PhD in 2012 from University Dunarea de Jos of Galati. Currently, she is occupying a Post Doctoral position at University Dunarea de Jos of Galati. She has published 22 scientific papers as first author and co-author in national and international journals. Her current research interests are 2D/3D image segmentation, features extraction and, images characterization and classification by using CAD software. Her computer skills and competence filed includes experienced programmer in Matlab, Java, C++, databases MySQL, SPSS Statistics and Macromedia.

Luminita Moraru is Ph.D Professor in the Department of Chemistry, Physics and Environment at Dunarea de Jos University of Galati. She obtained her BSc degree in 1986 from University of Bucharest and Ph.D in 1997 from Dunarea de Jos University of Galati. Her areas of interest are image processing, features extraction, segmentation and medical imaging processing. She is the author and the co-author of more than 160 research journals in national and international conferences and journals. She is a member of the Board of External Examiners for international Ph.D thesis—Annamalai University, India.

Anand Narasimhamurthy completed his B.E. from University Visvesvaraya College of Engineering (UVCE) in Bangalore University in 1998. He obtained the M.Eng. and Ph.D. degrees from the Department of Computer Science, Penn State University, Pennsylvania,USA. His Ph.D. work was mostly in areas of applied machine learning, more specifically on classifier ensembles. He worked as a post doctoral researcher for a year each at two institutions, namely Bangor University, Wales, UK and University College Dublin (UCD) in Dublin, Ireland. He worked as a research scientist at GE Global Research, Bangalore in a Medical Image Analysis group for about five years since late 2008 and subsequently as a faculty in the Department of Computer Science and Engineering at PESIT Bangalore South Campus. He has recently joined the Computer Science and Information Systems department at BITS Pilani, Hyderabad campus. His research interests include Machine Learning, graph based algorithms and image analysis.

Suraj Kumar Nayak is a Ph.D scholar in Biomedical Engineering at NIT, Rourkela. He received his B.Tech in Electrical Engineering from Government college of Engineering Keonjhar, Odisha, India and M.Tech in Biomedical Engineering from NIT Rourkela, Odisha, India. His research interests include Bimedical Instrumentation, Biomedical Signal & Image Processing, Artificial Neural Network and Trans-dermal Drug Delivery.

Kunal Pal is an Assistant Professor in Biomedical Engineering at NIT Rourkela.

Ipsita Panda is a B.Tech in Biomedical Engineering from NIT Rourkela.

Carlo Pappone - Current Position Director, Department of Arrhythmology, Fields of Expertise Electrophysiology; Catheter ablation of cardiac arrhythmias; Ablation of atrial fibrillation; Nonfluoroscopic mapping; Cardiac pacing; Biventricular pacing; Nonexcitatory cardiac contractility modulation. Cardiology Specialty Degree 1986-1990. University of Naples Federico II. Thesis: "Transcatheter radiofrequency ablation of post-infarction ventricular tachycardias." Score: 70/70 with honors. Electrophysiology Training 1988-89. Interventional Electrophysiology, Hospital Policlinico San Matteo, Pavia. July – September 1991. Division of Cardiology, Univ. of Michigan Medical Center, Ann Arbor, Michigan (Chief: F. Morady, MD) July – August 1992. Division of Cardiology, University of Oklahoma Health Sciences Center, Oklahoma City, OK (Chief: W.M. Jackman, MD) PhD doctoral studies 1991-1995. Doctorate in Cardiovascular Pathophysiology, University "Tor Vergata", Rome PhD degree Oct. 1995, with honors Thesis: "Transcatheter radiofrequency ablation of atrial tachycardia: mapping techniques."

Manjula Pushparaj received M.E. degree in computer science and engineering from Anna University, Chennai in 2015 and the B. Tech. degree in information technology from Anna University, Chennai in 2013. Research interest in image processing, pattern recognition, neural network and data mining.

Sweta Rani obtained her Bachelor of Medicine and Bachelor of Surgery from Nobel Medical College and Teaching Hospital, Biratnagar (Nepal) in 2014. Her area of research ultrasonography, abdominal CT scans, Magnetic Resonance Imaging scans and activity surveys.

J. Arokia Renjit, B.E., M.E., Ph.D., works as Professor and Head(PG Studies- CSE), Jeppiaar Engineering College, Tamilnadu, India. He has more than 14 years of teaching experience. His areas of Specialization includes Image Processing, Network Security, Data Mining, Cloud Computing.

Payel Roy has completed MCA from Computer Application, JIS College of Engineering, India. She has also completed her B.sc from West Bengal State University, India. Professionally, she was employed as a Guest Faculty in JIS College of Engineering, Kalyani, West Bengal in the Department of Computer Application. Her research area is digital image processing and Networking. She has 10 research paper publications in international conference and journals.

Vincenzo Santinelli - MD Degree 29 July 1971 School of Medicine, Score: 110/110 with honors University of Naples. Cardiology Specialty Degree 1971-1974. School of Medicine Score: 110/110 with honors, University of Naples. Internal Medicine Specialty Degree 1974-1979. School of Medicine, Score: 110/110. University of Naples. Electrophysiology training 1980 Policlinico S. Matteo Pavia 1992 Division of Cardiology University of Michigan Medical Center Ann Arbor Michigan (Chief Fred Morady, MD) as Visiting Professor Fields of Expertise Primary research interests include catheterbased treatment of cardiac arrhythmias, electrical therapies in patients with heart failure, and electrophysiologic effects of antiarrhythmic drugs. Clinical experience Total number of procedures performed as first operator Total EP studies: ~ 7.000 Ablation procedures: ~ 1.000 PM implantation: ~ 2.000 ICD implantation: ~ 250 Biventricular PM: ~ 100 Employment history 1971-1975 Voluntary Physician University of Naples

1975-1994 Assistant Professor of Cardiology and Internal Medicine University Federico II Naples 1982-2003 Professor of Cardiology Medical School University Federico II Naples Professor of Cardiology at Cardiology Specialty Professor of Cardiology at Cardiac Surgery Specialty Professor of Cardiology at Thoracico-pulmonary Surgery Professor of Cardiology for Nursing Sciences trainings 1980-1990 Director of EP Lab – Clinical Researcher Naples Professor of Cardiology 1990-2003 Director of the Center of Arrhythmology University Federico II Naples 2003-Dec 2009 Scientific Director of Arrhythmology at the San Raffaele University-Hospital, Milan, Italy Professor of Cardiology at Cardiology Specialty at San Raffaele University-Hospital, Milan, Italy.

Abahan Sarkar is a Research Scholar in the department of Electrical Engineering in National Institute of Technology Silchar, Assam, India. Mr. Sarkar worked as Faculty member in Faculty of Science and Technology, The ICFAI University Tripura from 2007 to 2012. He has obtained his B.Tech degree in Electronics and Communication Engineering from North Eastern Regional Institute of Science and Technology, Nirjuli, Arunachal Pradesh, India in 2003. He has completed his Master of Technology in Computer Science and Technology from Tripura University, Suryamaninagar, Tripura, India in 2008. Mr. Sarkar's research interest includes Industrial automation, and Image processing and Machine vision.

Sahbi Sidhom is Associate Professor in Computer Science and in Information and Communication Sciences at Lorraine University (Nancy) in France and he is a Senior Researcher at LORIA laboratory in Computer Science and its applications (research team KIWI: Knowledge, Information and Web Intelligence). His main research fields are in natural language processing (NLP), Knowledge representation (content indexing, information retrieval systems, re-indexing in the social web), information and knowledge management (KM) and skills in economic intelligence (EI) or competitive intelligence (CI). He is the founder and president of two international projects: SIIE, the international conference in information systems and economic intelligence (www.siie.fr) and ISKO-Maghreb, is the chapter of Maghreb in ISKO Society for Knowledge Organization (www.isko-maghreb.org).

Fazal A. Talukdar obtained his B. E (Hons) from REC Silchar (Now National Institute of Technology, Silchar (India)) in 1987. He obtained his M. Tech in 1993 and Ph.D. in 2002-2003 from Indian Institute of Technology Delhi and Jadavpur University respectively. Currently, he is working as Professor in Electronics and Communication Engineering, National Institute of Technology, Silchar (India). His area of interest is power electronics, image processing and analog VLSI circuits.

Goutam Thakur is an Associate Professor in Biomedical Engineering at Manipal Institute of Technology (Manipal), India.

D. N. Tibarewala is a Professor of Biomedical Engineering at Jadavpur University. Presently a Professor of Biomedical Engineering at Jadavpur University, Kolkata, India since August 1996, Dr. D. N. Tibarewala has earlier served as Director in the School of Bioscience & Engineering of the same University during the period May 2004-November 2011. He did his BSc (Honours) in 1971 and B. Tech (Applied Physics) in 1974 from the Calcutta University, India. He was admitted to the Ph.D. (Tech) degree of the same University in 1980. Having professional, academic and research experience of more than 35 years, Dr. Tibarewala has contributed about 250 research papers in the areas of Rehabilitation Technology, Biomedical Instrumentation and, related branches of Biomedical Engineering.

Vo Thi Hong Tuyet received the Bachelor from Ho Chi Minh City University of Pedagogical - Vietnam in 2011, the Master's degree Ho Chi Minh city University of Technology - Vietnam National University in Ho Chi Minh City in 2015. Now, she is a lecturer at Faculty of Information Technology, Ho Chi Minh City Open University, VietNam. She research interests include recognition, image processing.

Index

G

H

I

K

L

M

N

P

Q

R

S

T

U

V

W

www.ingramcontent.com/pod-product-compliance
Lightning Source LLC
LaVergne TN
LVHW080531300926
849162LV00007B/1586